Understanding Epilepsy

Understanding Epilepsy

A Study Guide for the Boards

Edited by

Vibhangini S. Wasade, MD
Senior Staff Neurologist Henry Ford Medical Group – HFHS
Detroit, MI, USA
Clinical Associate Professor,
Wayne State University
MI, USA

Marianna V. Spanaki, MD, PhD, MBA
Senior Staff Neurologist Henry Ford Medical Group – HFHS
Detroit, MI, USA
Clinical Associate Professor,
Wayne State University
MI, USA

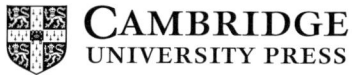
CAMBRIDGE
UNIVERSITY PRESS

CAMBRIDGE
UNIVERSITY PRESS

University Printing House, Cambridge CB2 8BS, United Kingdom

One Liberty Plaza, 20th Floor, New York, NY 10006, USA

477 Williamstown Road, Port Melbourne, VIC 3207, Australia

314–321, 3rd Floor, Plot 3, Splendor Forum, Jasola District Centre,
New Delhi – 110025, India

79 Anson Road, #06–04/06, Singapore 079906

Cambridge University Press is part of the University of Cambridge.

It furthers the University's mission by disseminating knowledge in the
pursuit of education, learning, and research at the highest international
levels of excellence.

www.cambridge.org
Information on this title: www.cambridge.org/9781108718905
DOI: 10.1017/9781108754200

First published 2020

Printed in Singapore by Markono Print Media Pte Ltd

A catalogue record for this publication is available from the British
Library.

ISBN 978-1-108-71890-5 Paperback

Contents

Contents

Contributors

Elie Abdelnour, MD
Division of Pediatric Neurology
Duke Children's Hospital and
Health Center
Durham, NC, USA

Ellen L. Air, MD, PhD, FAANS
Co-Director Functional Neurosurgery
Department of Neurosurgery
Henry Ford Hospital, Detroit,
MI, USA

Rushna Ali, MD
Department of Neurosurgery
Spectrum Health Medical Group
Grand Rapids, MI, USA

Ramon Edmundo D. Bautista, MD, MBA
Professor and Associate Chairman of
Neurology
Director, Comprehensive
Epilepsy Program
University of Florida Health Sciences
Center Jacksonville
Jacksonville, Florida, USA

Selim Benbadis, MD
Professor of Neurology and Director
Comprehensive Epilepsy Program
University of South Florida and Tampa
General Hospital
Tampa, FL, USA

Paul Brady, MD
Fellow
Neuro-Intensive Care Unit
Henry Ford Hospital
Detroit, MI, USA

Dana R. Connor, PhD
Neuropsychologist
Henry Ford Health System
Detroit, MI, USA

Jules E. C. Constantinou, MB ChB, FRACP
Division Head, Pediatric Neurology
Henry Ford Health System
Detroit, MI, USA
    and
Clinical Associate Professor
Wayne State University
Detroit, MI, USA

Russell A. Derry, MPH
Director of Education
Epilepsy Foundation of Michigan
Southfield, MI, USA

Michael DiSano, MD
Fellow Pediatric Epilepsy
Cleveland Clinic
Cleveland, OH, USA

Dawn Eliashiv, MD
Professor, Department of Neurology
David Geffen School of Medicine at UCLA
Co-director, UCLA Seizure Disorder
Center
UCLA Department of Neurology
Los Angeles, CA, USA

Kost Elisevich, MD, PhD
Chair
Department of Clinical Neurosciences
Spectrum Health, Grand Rapids, MI, USA
Michigan State University, MI, USA

Imran Farooqui, MD
University of Florida Health Sciences
Center Jacksonville
Jacksonville, Florida, USA

Anthony L. Fine, MD
Instructor
Division of Child and Adolescent Neurology
Department of Neurology
Mayo Clinic, Rochester, MN, USA

Stephen Fulton, MD
Associate Professor of Neurology and
Pediatrics
University of Tennessee Health Science
Center
Le Bonheur Comprehensive Epilepsy
Program
Le Bonheur Children's Hospital
Memphis, TN, USA

Brent A. Funk, PhD
Neuropsychologist
Henry Ford Health System
Detroit, MI, USA

Shailaja Gaddam, MD
Senior Staff Neurologist
Henry Ford Hospital
Detroit, MI, USA

Samuel S. Giles, MD
University of Florida Health Sciences
Center Jacksonville
Jacksonville, Florida, USA

L. John Greenfield Jr., MD, PhD
Professor and Chair of Neurology
UConn Health
Farmington, CT, USA
           and
Department of Neurology
University of Arkansas for
Medical Science
Little Rock, AR, USA

Ajay Gupta, MD
Associate Professor
The Cleveland Clinic Lerner College of
Medicine
Case Western Reserve University
           and
Section Head of Pediatric Epilepsy
Epilepsy Center/Neurological Institute
Cleveland, OH, USA

Naoum P. Issa, MD, PhD
Department of Neurology and Adult
Epilepsy Center

University of Chicago
Chicago, IL, USA

Kenneth Jenrow, PhD
Associate Professor of Neuroscience
Department of Psychology
Central Michigan University
Mt. Pleasant, MI, USA

Tasleema Khan, MD
Fellow
Yale University
New Haven, CT, USA

David King-Stephens, MD
Medical Director
Sutter Pacific Epilepsy Program at
California Pacific Medical Center in San
Francisco, CA, USA

William J. Kupsky, MD
Professor of Pathology
Wayne State University School of Medicine
Detroit, MI, USA

David M. Labiner
Professor and Head of Neurology
Department of Neurology
University of Arizona, Tuscon, AZ, USA

Shannon M. LaBoy, MD, MSMS
University of Florida Health Sciences
Center Jacksonville
Jacksonville, Florida, USA

Sang-Hun Lee, PhD
Department of Neurology
University of Arkansas for Medical Science
Little Rock, AR, USA

Sidrah Mahmud, MD
Epilepsy and Clinical Neurophysiology
Fellow
Yale University School of Medicine
New Haven, CT, USA

Richard H. Mattson, MD
Professor Emeritus of Neurology
Yale University School of Medicine
New Haven, CT, USA

Chandan B. Mehta, MD
Staff Neuro-Intensivist
Henry Ford Hospital
Detroit, MI, USA

Mohamad Mikati, MD
Wilburt C. Davison Professor of Pediatrics
Professor of Neurobiology
Chief, Division of Pediatric Neurology and
Developmental Medicine
Director of Pediatric Epilepsy Program
Duke University Medical Center
Durham, NC, USA

Georgia Montouris, MD
Clinical Associate Professor of
Neurology
Boston University School of Medicine
Director of Epilepsy Services
Boston Medical Center
Boston, MA, USA

Basanagoud Mudigoudar, MD
Assistant Professor of Pediatric Neurology
University of Tennessee Health Science
Center
Le Bonheur Comprehensive Epilepsy
Program
Le Bonheur Children's Hospital
Memphis, TN, USA

Wolfgang G. Muhlhofer, MD
Assistant Professor
UAB Epilepsy Center
Birmingham, AL, USA

Katherine C. Nickels, MD
Associate Professor
Divisions of Child and Adolescent
Neurology and Epilepsy
Department of Neurology
Mayo Clinic, Rochester,
MN, USA

Marc R. Nuwer, MD, PhD
Professor and Vice Chair, Department of
Neurology

Department Head, Department of Clinical
Neurophysiology
Ronald Reagan UCLA
Medical Center
Los Angeles, CA, USA

Patricia E. Penovich, MD
Minnesota Epilepsy Group PA
Adjunct Professor
Department of Neurology
University of Minnesota
St Paul, MN, USA

Elia Pestana-Knight, MD
Staff Pediatric Epilepsy
Cleveland Clinic
Cleveland, OH, USA

Amit Ray, MD
Director Neurology and
Epilepsy Program
Aurora Healthcare
Kenosha WI, USA

Monisha Sachdev, MD
Yale University
New Haven, CT, USA

Kamal Shouman, MD
Fellow, Division of Autonomic
Disorders
Department of Neurology
Mayo Clinic, Rochester
MN, USA

Vladimir Shvarts, MD
Director of Epilepsy and Clinical
Neurophysiology Fellowship
Director of Intraoperative Monitoring
Program
Assistant Professor of Clinical Neurology
Barrow Neurological Institute
Associate Professor of Neurology
Creighton Medical School
            and
Associate Professor of Neurology
University of Arizona, Pheonix,
AZ, USA

Yeeck Sim, MD
Department of Neurology
University of Arizona, Tuscon,
AZ, USA

Maria Stefanidou, MD, MSc
Assistant Professor of Neurology
Boston University School of Medicine
Boston, MA, USA

John Stern, MD
Professor, Department of Neurology
David Geffen School of Medicine
at UCLA
Co-director, UCLA Seizure Disorder Center
UCLA Department of Neurology
Los Angeles, CA, USA

Jerzy P. Szaflarski, MD
Professor of Neurology and Neurobiology
and Director
UAB Epilepsy Center
Birmingham, AL, USA

Ashley E. Thomas, MD
Assistant Professor
UAB Epilepsy Center
Birmingham, AL, USA

Vibhangini S. Wasade, MD
Senior Staff Neurologist,
Henry Ford Hospital
Detroit, MI, USA
Clinical Associate Professor
Wayne State University
Detroit, MI, USA

Sarah Weatherspoon, MD
Assistant Professor of Neurology and
Pediatrics
University of Tennessee Health Science
Center
Le Bonheur Comprehensive Epilepsy
Program

Le Bonheur Children's Hospital
Memphis, TN, USA

Peter Weber, MD
Surgical Director
Sutter Pacific Epilepsy Program at
California Pacific Medical Center in San
Francisco, CA, USA

James W. Wheless, MD
Professor and Chief of Pediatric
Neurology
Le Bonheur Chair in Pediatric Neurology
University of Tennessee Health Science
Center
Director, Le Bonheur Comprehensive
Epilepsy Program and Neuroscience
Institute
Le Bonheur Children's Hospital
Memphis, TN, USA

Elaine C. Wirrell, MD
Professor
Divisions of Child and Adolescent
Neurology and Epilepsy
Department of Neurology,
Mayo Clinic, Rochester, MN, USA

Alma Yum, MD
Assistant Professor
Department of Neurology
Denver Health Medical Center and The
University of Colorado Denver,
CO, USA

Andrew Zillgitt, DO
Director
Adult Epilepsy Program
Associate Professor
Oakland University
Beaumont School of Medicine,
Royal Oak, MI, USA

Preface

Epilepsy is one of the oldest recognized neurological conditions dating back to 2000 BC. Historical reports have documented famous people suspected to suffer from the disease. They come from all realms of vocation, from leaders (Julius Caesar, President Roosevelt), philosophers (Socrates), authors (Fyodor Dostoevsky, Charles Dickens), poets (Lord Byron), athletes (Glover Cleveland Alexander, Florence Griffith Joyner), artists (Vincent van Gogh), actors (Richard Burton, Hugo Weaving) and singers (Susan Boyle, Lil Wayne) to name a few. Epilepsy remains one of the most common neurological conditions affecting nearly 50 million people worldwide. Development in epilepsy management started occurring 100 years ago in the diagnostic field after Hans Berger invented electroencephalography (EEG), and most remarkably after the advent of magnetic resonance imaging (MRI) and other diagnostic tests in the past few decades. Since then, plentiful medications with novel mechanisms of action and minimal side effects have been available.

The information about epilepsy is vast and easily accessible via digital media on the internet. Numerous books have been published for those interested in epilepsy, varying from reference textbooks delving deeper in the field to those with practical approaches and primers. There are books that focus on EEG and are popular EEG atlases, and other books that review technical aspects of EEG or clinical aspects of epilepsy. Being involved in the fellowship program at Henry Ford Hospital, we realized the need for a book to aid our trainees during their rotation. This book will help bridge this gap for those preparing for board certification as well as those fellows, residents, physicians, or nurse practitioners who want to learn more about epilepsy and EEG in a more methodical fashion. The topics aim to comprehensively cover the field of epilepsy so as to eliminate the necessity of surfing multiple books to grasp the subject. This book will provide a more updated, systematic, and comprehensive approach to understanding epilepsy.

This book represents the work of our authors in their field of expertise. We are deeply grateful to each one of them for their time, hard work, and commitment to our effort.

We are very thankful to Stephanie Stebens from Henry Ford library services for her invaluable viewpoints and support. We would like to acknowledge the encouragement and input we received from Anna Whiting from Cambridge University Press during critical steps in the process of this project, and the ongoing help from Emily Jones, Nigel Graves, and the entire team at Cambridge University Press. Without their support, this book would not have been brought into existence. Lastly, our husbands – Sanjay and Panayiotis – who have been forever inspiring with no limits, stepping up to support us; our children – Vedant and Eleni – with whom we couldn't spent much time, but did marvelously in our absence and have matured beyond their years; encouraging siblings and doting parents, all comforting and positive throughout – we thank and love you all!

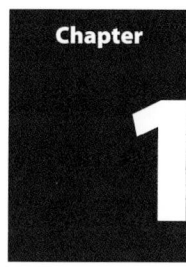

Chapter 1

Pathophysiology of Epilepsy

Kenneth Jenrow and Kost Elisevich

1.1 Introduction and Definitions

A *seizure* is a situational clinical event that may be instigated by any number of extrinsic or intrinsic precipitating factors and that results in an excessive, hypersynchronous discharge of a cortical neuronoglial population and manifests in the brain in either a localized or widespread manner. This abnormal activity takes over the normal functioning of one or more brain networks to result in seizures that characterize over 40 recognized epileptic syndromes.[1]

Epilepsy, is a central nervous system disorder characterized by recurrent seizures that manifest over a duration of time, even perpetually, and may occur spontaneously.

Epileptogenicity refers to the expression of the epilepsy as it may appear in electrographic recordings while *epileptogenesis* identifies the mechanism by which it comes about and is then perpetuated as a result of changes in cellular properties, gene expression, neuronoglial interactions and network reorganization.[2,3]

Brain function involves several incongruent parallel networks, cortical and subcortical, that align in a variety of ways to achieve different ends (e.g., cognition, language, sensory integration, locomotor execution). Epilepsy, once established, occasionally subsumes and, at times, overtakes some or most of these in often reproducible patterns in the form of seizures.

1.2 Cerebrocortical Anatomy

1.2.1 Cerebral Microstructure

The human cerebral cortex comprises 82% of total brain mass, while containing only 19% of the neurons in the brain. The greater relative cortical size, therefore, does not reflect an increased relative number of cortical neurons compared with other primates. The ratio of cerebrocortical glial cells to neurons (3.76:1) remains similar to that in other primates, despite astrocytes increasing progressively in size and number throughout evolution. Since Cajal, the brain has been primarily considered in a neuronal context, but it has become increasingly evident that glial cells, particularly astrocytes, serve a much greater role than once thought, so that it is important for us to consider the brain more as a neuronoglial entity in the context of functional expression, as well as in its disorders.

The neuronal cytoarchitecture of the human cerebral cortex varies by region and was originally mapped in detail and reported by Brodmann in 1908–9. Its width is upwards of 5 mm and it contains 16.34 billion neurons and 60.84 billion astrocytes spread throughout its considerable, highly-convoluted mantle.[4] A distinct stratification is noted with three to six layers that are differently constituted by region. The neopallium or neocortex, with its six cellular layers, occupies the majority of the surface area, while the archipallium or archicortex, represented by the hippocampus and dentate gyrus situated in the mesial temporal lobe, with their three layers, is the phylogenetically oldest part of the cerebral cortex. A transitional cortex or paleocortex, represented by the piriform area and entorhinal cortex, with its five layers, bridges the neocortex and archicortex.

The mesial temporal lobe, well known for its propensity toward epileptogenicity, is composed of the uncus, including the amygdala, the piriform area, the parahippocampal gyrus with its subicular complex and entorhinal cortex, the hippocampus, and the dentate gyrus. The hippocampus is composed of four subregions, CA1–4, with a layered structure that varies, to a degree, by subregion (Figure 1.1). CA3 has the following strata – lacunosum-moleculare,

(A)

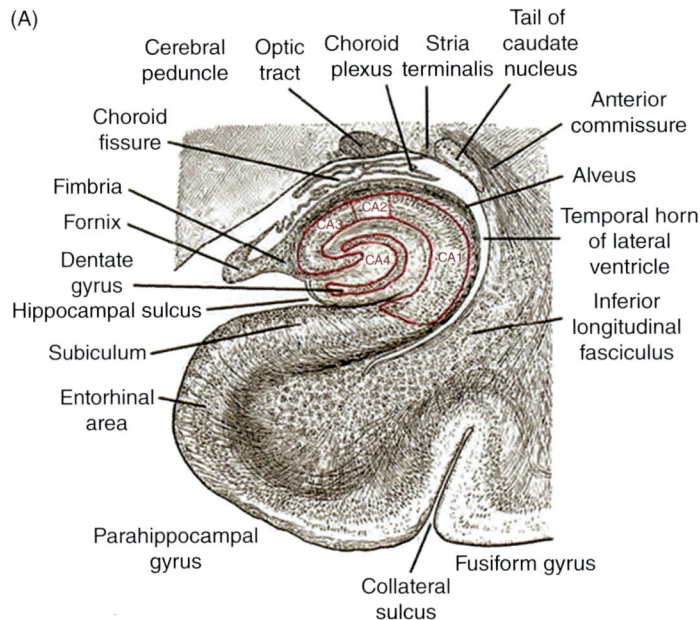

(B)

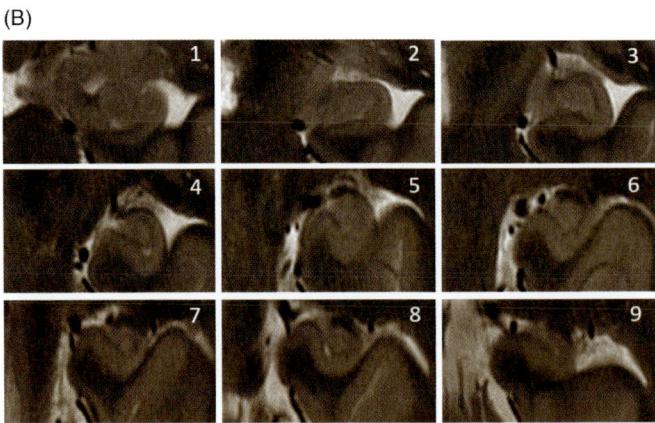

Figure 1.1 (A) Schematic representation of the right hippocampus and parahippocampal gyrus. (B) T2-weighted magnetic resonance images of the left hippocampus shown sequentially from anterior (1) to posterior (9). The most posterior image is immediately beyond the level of the midbrain tectum.

radiatum, lucidum, pyramidal, and oriens – while CA1 and CA2 lack the lucidum stratum. CA4 extends into the hilum of the dentate gyrus, which itself is composed of layers – the molecular, inner molecular, and granular – arranged in two blades joined in a V-shape containing the hilum. The primary input is from the entorhinal cortex (EC) via the perforant pathway, which also provides some reciprocal connections. The EC is widely and reciprocally connected to cortical and subcortical areas and therefore provides a conduit for input from a diversity of sources, initially to the dentate gyrus, which serves as a gatekeeper for the remainder of the hippocampus. The perforant pathway originates in layer II of the EC and extends to the dentate granular layer with some axons also extending to CA3 and fewer to CA1. Axons of dentate granule cells (e.g., mossy fibers) synapse with hilar and CA3 pyramidal cell dendrites, and the corresponding pyramidal axons extend to other CA3 neurons via immediate collaterals, to the contralateral hippocampus and to CA1 neurons (e.g., Schaffer collaterals) which, in turn, will synapse upon neurons of the subicular complex that will project back to the entorhinal cortex. Other projections to the prefrontal cortex, lateral septal area, and mammillary body extend the influence of the hippocampus upon functionally distinct areas.

In hippocampal sclerosis, neuronal loss and gliosis occur primarily in the dentate hilus (i.e., CA4 subregion) and CA1 subregion with less change in the CA3 subregion. The resulting loss of hilar interneurons and CA1 pyramidal neurons induces a synaptic reorganization (e.g., mossy fiber sprouting) with aberrant innervation of the dentate gyrus itself. Ostensibly, this results in a recurrent hyperexcitable situation that may be triggered by a yet undefined mechanism. Several initial events may bring about a relatively selective injury to this vulnerable area of the brain, including such events as trauma,[5,6] early protracted fever,[7] and hypoxia.[8]

The neocortex has primary areas that subserve the various sensory modalities and both locomotor and oculomotor action, and these lie adjacent to association areas that undertake more complex functions such as abstraction, creativity, and integrative aspects of locomotor function. The six layers are characterized by the different neuronal shapes, sizes, density, and distribution of nerve fibers. They constitute the following, from outer to inner layer:

I   molecular layer
II   external granular layer
III   external pyramidal layer
IV   internal granular layer
V   internal pyramidal layer
VI   multiform layer.

These may be organized functionally into three areas according to their projections:

1. *Supragranular (layers I–III):* origins and terminations of intracortical connections identified as associational (i.e., within the same hemisphere) or commissural (i.e., interhemispheric); most highly developed in humans
2. *Internal granular (layer IV):* termination of thalamocortical fibers, particularly evident in the sensory cortex
3. *Infragranular (layers V, VI):* primarily origin of subcortical projections with layer V comprising principal efferent projections to basal ganglia, brainstem, and spinal cord, and layer VI projecting to thalamus; motor areas bear very small to absent granular layers.

The interneuronal population of the cerebral cortex is characterized by morphology and includes, but is not limited to, basket cells, Martinotti cells, chandelier cells, bouquet cells, bipolar cells, and neurogliaform cells.[9] The molecular layer (layer I) is an important synaptic field of the cortex, with most dendrites originating in pyramidal cells and axons from elsewhere in the ipsi- and contralateral hemispheres and thalamus.[10] Martinotti cells in the deeper cortical layers also contribute axons to the molecular layer, where horizontal Retzius–Cajal cells and stellate cells may be found. Basket cells constitute 5–10% of cells in the cerebral cortex and are found in layers II–VI.[11] They form extensive axosomatic connections with pyramidal neurons. The external granular layer contains both small pyramidal and stellate cells from which dendrites extend into the molecular layer and axons into the deeper layers for intracortical distribution. The external pyramidal layer contains progressively larger pyramidal cells whose apical dendrites extend into the molecular layer and axons project to other cortical destinations. Stellate (i.e., granule) cells are most prominent in layer IV (internal granular layer). Their axons remain within the cortex and synapse with en passage dendrites from layers V and VI, other stellate and Martinotti cells. Layers V and VI are considered phylogenetically older than the more superficial layers. The internal pyramidal layer contains pyramidal cells that intermingle with stellate and Martinotti cells. The giant Betz cells reside here in the primary motor area. The multiform layer contains predominantly fusiform cells.

Approximately 80–90% of cerebrocortical neurons are glutamatergic while 10-20% are GABA-ergic interneurons, which exert inhibitory control and influence rhythmic network oscillations.[12] About 40% of interneurons, largely basket cells, express parvalbumin (PV), while 30%, largely Martinotti cells, express somatostatin, and the remaining 30%, largely bouquet and neurogliaform cells, express the serotonergic receptor, 5HT3A.[13,14] PV-expressing basket cells are fast-spiking, showing high-frequency spike trains exceeding 200 Hz, and have been implicated in the development of epilepsy in both genetic and lesional models.[15] Martinotti cells participate in a disynaptic surround inhibition of pyramidal cells.[16] The nicotinic acetylcholine receptor α2 subunit specifically marks layer V Martinotti cells projecting to layer I, where they target certain pyramidal cells, synchronizing them in a frequency-dependent manner.[17] Loss of this important central mechanism may bias the local circuitry toward excitability, as was seen in a mouse model of Dravet syndrome wherein excitability in both fast-spiking, PV-expressing basket cells and somatostatin-expressing Martinotti cells resulted in a disinhibition of cortical output.[18]

1.2.2 Cerebral Connectivity

For over a century, the neuron and its connectivity has been regarded, quite rightly, as the primary structural entity underlying function. The study of local non-neuronal cellular and extracellular compartmental influences upon its behavior has introduced a greater complexity to our still incomplete understanding of both normal and abnormal expression. This section will therefore review both the traditional synapse-mediated connectivity that has been identified and the nonsynaptic influences that have been more recently investigated.

1.2.2.1 Large-Scale Connectivity

The cerebral white matter contains three types of axons that constitute association, commissural, and projection fibers. Association fibers connect parts of one hemisphere over short intergyral distances via subcortical arcuate fibers and more longitudinally oriented interlobar bundles. The cingulum services the limbic lobe and interconnects the cingulate and parahippocampal gyri and the septal area. The superior longitudinal fasciculus, situated above the insula, interconnects all the lobes and includes the arcuate fasciculus that descends into the temporal lobe. Processed visual and proprioceptive signals pass anteriorly to the frontal cortex to execute appropriate locomotor responses when needed. Similarly, receptive and expressive language areas of the temporal and frontal cortices are interconnected by arcuate fibers. The much smaller inferior longitudinal fasciculus lies beneath the insula interconnecting the occipital and temporal cortices. The inferior occipitofrontal and uncinate fasciculi are part of the same association bundle lying beneath the insula and striatum with the shorter uncinate fasciculus passing along the stem of the Sylvian fissure interconnecting the temporal pole and the orbitofrontal cortex. The superior occipitofrontal fasciculus interconnects the frontal with the parieto-occipital cortices dorsally and mesially.

Commissural fibers largely traverse the corpus callosum with the forceps frontalis drawing fibers from the frontal lobes into the genu of the callosum anteriorly, which tapers inferiorly into the rostrum, and the forceps occipitalis connecting the occipital lobes through the splenium posteriorly. Direct connections are made between topographically and functionally similar regions of both hemispheres. Indirect connections exist for the hand area of the primary sensory cortex and parts of the primary visual cortex via callosal fibers passing from their respective association cortices to which they are primarily connected. The anterior commissure interconnects the middle and inferior gyri and the uncus of both temporal lobes. The fornices are symmetric bundles that originate along each hippocampus, leaving its posterior end to connect the hippocampal formation from each side with the hypothalamus and septal area. The forniceal or hippocampal commissure connects the two hippocampi across the midline.

Projection fibers connect the cerebral cortex with subcortical structures, appearing as the corona radiata in both hemispheres, and are afferent or efferent in relation to the cortex. Most afferent or corticofugal connections arise in the thalamus, with a few originating in the hypothalamus and brainstem. The thalamic radiations – anterior, middle, posterior, and inferior – are reciprocal and distribute between prefrontal, parietal, occipital, and temporal cortices, respectively. The corticofugal motor projection fibers do not constitute an integral aspect of the epileptogenic network, although they constitute the means by which some semiological features manifest.

1.2.2.2 Nonsynaptic Features

The Extracellular Space

The promotion of excitability and neuronoglial synchrony may be initiated and perpetuated by alterations in the extracellular space. Interference with Na^+-K^+ pump function by hypoxia or ischemia in hippocampal CA1 pyramidal neurons, known to be sensitive to changes in membrane K^+ currents,[19] can induce a transition to a state of excitability. Likewise, the transmembrane Cl^- gradient may be compromised by alteration of the Cl^--K^+ cotransport mechanism resulting in a compromise of GABA-activated inhibitory Cl^- currents.[20] Shrinkage of the extracellular space alone through changes in osmolality have also been shown to induce epileptiform bursting among hippocampal CA1 neurons.[21] Ephaptic transmission is enhanced by such circumstances, promoting wider field activation.[22] Spontaneous synchronous field bursts among these same neurons have been reported in hippocampal slice models exposed to a low Ca^{2+} environment designed to block chemical synaptic activity.[23] The extrasynaptic space can also be considered a medium for diffusion of neurotransmitters that affect extrasynaptic receptors and transporters to influence cells without mediation by frequency-coded neurotransmission.[24] Extrasynaptic nicotinic acetylcholine receptors, in particular, provide a fast form of transmission through ligand-gated ion channels and can interfere with dendritic signal integration after synaptic activation has occurred.[25]

Gap Junctions

These membrane channels, composed of connexin proteins, vary widely in distribution throughout the cerebral cortex and ostensibly underlie the functional organization of the neuronoglial environment in different areas.[26] There is some indication that gap junctions are up-regulated in epilepsy and that seizure duration may be influenced by gap-junction blockade,[27] although mRNA and protein expression of constituent glial connexins appears not to be altered.[28] Faster propagation may promote the hypersynchronous activity that characterizes ictal expression. Although different connexin protein subunits of gap-junction hemichannels predominate in neurons and glia, heterologous junctions have been identified and, indeed, glutamate release from neurons has been shown to evoke calcium waves in astrocytes, spreading via gap junctions, that may, in turn, activate neurons at a distance.[29] Moreover, the same syncytial junctional arrangement of astrocytes may serve to buffer excess extracellular K^+ to reduce excitability in a limited area of the cerebral cortex by creating a more efficient voluminous sink.[30] Hence, disturbance of such an arrangement by trauma or ischemia may alter its capacity and render a particular site more susceptible to the induction and maintenance of epileptogenicity.

Neuronal gap junctions appear predominantly in inhibitory interneurons. The two patterns of expression are identified between parvalbumin-positive multipolar bursting (Pb^+MB) cells,[31,32] and calretinin-positive multipolar ($Calr^+M$) cells and Pb^+MB cells. The Pb^+MB cells synapse upon the soma and proximal dendrites of cortical pyramidal cells.[31] Gap junctional blockade of these inhibitory interneurons may lead to pyramidal cell excitation, either by interfering with the timing of inhibition of pyramidal cells,[33] or releasing inhibition of pyramidal cells through blockade between Pb^+MB and $Calr^+M$ cells.[34] Fast ripples, field potentials of hypersynchronous pyramidal cell activity with frequencies of 250–600 Hz, are implicated in ictogenesis,[35] and are thought to be partly a product of inhibitory interneuronal behavior adversely influenced by altered gap junctional communication.[36] Likewise, hippocampal pyramidal axoaxonal gap junctional connections have been identified and modeling studies have implicated these in generating fast ripples as well.[37]

1.3 Cerebrocortical Biochemistry and Electrophysiology

Our understanding regarding the biochemical basis of epileptic seizures remains rooted in the early idea that they reflect an imbalance of inhibitory and excitatory influences in the brain, resulting in an increase in excitation and/or a decrease in inhibition. Consistent with this view are now well-established seizure-associated changes in synaptic communication mediated by glutamate and gamma-aminobutyric acid (GABA), the main excitatory and inhibitory neurotransmitters in the mammalian brain, respectively.[38]

Intracellular glutamate is synthesized primarily from glucose through glycolysis and the Kreb's cycle. Upon depolarization of the presynaptic terminal, opening of voltage-gated calcium channels and the resultant influx of calcium ions facilitates vesicular release of glutamate into the synaptic cleft. Glutamate can bind to multiple receptors, including both ionotropic and metabotropic varieties. Ligand-gated ion channels activated by glutamate include alpha-amino-3-hydroxyl-5-methyl-4-isoxazole-propionate (AMPA), *N*-methyl-D-aspartate (NMDA), and kainate receptors. AMPA activation mediates fast synaptic transmission and causes a rapid and transient depolarization of the postsynaptic cell. If sustained, depolarization of the postsynaptic cell by AMPA activation causes the expulsion of magnesium ions from coactivated NMDA receptors, permitting the movement of sodium, potassium, and calcium ions down their concentration gradients and depolarizing the cell. NMDA receptors are the primary means by which calcium ions enter the postsynaptic cell, a critical step in the initiation of secondary messenger systems involved in synaptic plasticity.[39]

Metabotropic glutamate receptors are divided into three groups: Group I (mGLuR1, 5), Group II (mGluR2, 3), and Group III (mGluR4, 6, 8). Group I receptors are primarily postsynaptic and their activation is both excitatory and inhibitory, modulating the conductance of sodium, potassium, and voltage-gated calcium channels. Group II and III are primarily presynaptic and their activation inhibits adenylate cyclase and decreases cyclic adenosine monophosphate (cAMP) concentrations, limiting the presynaptic release of glutamate. AMPA-mediated neurotransmission at certain synapses on principal cells in the neocortex, hippocampus, and striatum can also induce mGLuR-dependent long-term potentiation (LTP), particularly following strong repeated stimulation protocols.[40]

Removal of glutamate from the extracellular space is an active process involving glia and postsynaptic neuronal uptake via excitatory amino acid transporters (EAATs), of which there are five subtypes. Replenishing glutamate in the presynaptic terminal is achieved by shuttling glutamate back to the original cell via the glutamate–glutamine cycle. Within glia, glutamine synthetase converts intracellular glutamate to glutamine, which is then released into the intracellular space. Glutamine is then transported into the presynaptic cell, where it is converted back to glutamate by glutaminase and transported into vesicles by vesicular glutamate transporters (VGLUTs).[41]

GABA is synthesized within presynaptic terminals by the enzyme glutamic acid decarboxylase (GAD), which removes a carboxyl group from the α carbon of L-glutamate. Upon depolarization of the presynaptic terminal, opening of voltage-gated calcium channels and the resultant influx of calcium ions facilitates vesicular release of GABA into the synaptic cleft. Binding of GABA to GABA$_A$ receptors on the post-synaptic membrane facilitates the influx of chloride ions into the postsynaptic cell resulting in hyperpolarization, whereas binding to metabotropic GABA$_B$ receptors facilitates a G-protein-mediated activation of adenylate cyclase. This results in a cAMP-mediated increase in potassium channel conductance and the release of potassium ions from the cell, again resulting in hyperpolarization. GABA is removed from the extracellular space by GABA transporters (GATs) located on perisynaptic glia and the presynaptic neuron. GABA transport is accompanied by the influx of two sodium ions and one chloride ion. Reversal of GATs has also been implicated as a nonsynaptic mechanism of GABA receptor activation.[42,43]

Prolonged depolarization of neurons within epileptic foci can result in a paroxysmal depolarization shift (PDS), characterized by the repetitive firing of sodium-dependent action potentials. These represent the intracellular correlate of epileptiform discharges measured extracellularly via the EEG. Burst activity associated with PDS is commonly followed by GABA-mediated hyperpolarization, which suppresses seizure activity. However, if this inhibition fails, PDS can propagate to affect multiple brain regions and may generalize to the entire brain. The most common form of epilepsy associated with focal seizures is mesial temporal lobe epilepsy (mTLE). mTLE is frequently linked to mesial temporal sclerosis (MTS), characterized by neuronal loss and astrogliosis within the hippocampus and other neighboring structures, including the entorhinal cortex and amygdala.

Other hippocampal pathologies associated with mTLE include loss of hilar mossy cells and somatostatin-expressing GABAergic interneurons in the hilus, dispersion of the granule cells layer, and aberrant sprouting of granule cell axons. These pathologies are known to disrupt glutamate and GABA transmission within these networks and are widely believed to be pathophysiological.[44]

In contrast to the localized imbalance of GABAergic and glutamergic neurotransmission and seizure propagation characteristic of focal epilepsies, seizures associated with generalized epilepsies typically arise in multiple brain areas simultaneously and are caused by an abnormal activation of thalamocortical circuits. This reflects a dysregulation of GABAergic thalamic relay neurons, which project broadly throughout neocortex to influence the activity of glutamergic pyramidal neurons. Such seizures are characterized by a "spike and wave" pattern of ictal activity, which is also seen during absence epilepsy.[45]

In addition to the prominent roles of glutamate and GABA neural transmission in epileptogenesis, catecholamine neurotransmitters have also been implicated as modulators of epileptogenic pathophysiology within the brain. Abnormalities of dopaminergic neural transmission have been implicated in temporal lobe epilepsy, juvenile myoclonic epilepsy, and autosomal dominant nocturnal frontal lobe epilepsy. The nigrostriatal dopamine pathway has been implicated in modulating thalamocortical loops involved in generalized epilepsies. The mesocorticolimbic dopamine projection from the ventral tegmental area to the frontal cortex has been implicated in motor and behavioral symptoms associated with epilepsy.[46,47] Among the various noradrenergic brainstem nuclei, ascending pathways from the locus coeruleus (LC) have been implicated as having antiepileptic modulatory effects. These pathways branch extensively to innervate the entire cerebrum, where they exert an inhibitory influence on seizure activity. Common antiepileptic drugs, including phenobarbital, carbamazepine, valproic acid, and phenytoin, produce an increase in noradrenaline in some brain regions. Similarly, increased noradrenaline has been implicated in the antiepileptic effects of vagal nerve stimulation, perhaps in combination with galanin, neuropeptide Y, and adenosine, which are coreleased with noradrenaline.[48]

As illustrated by the kindling model of epilepsy, pathophysiological behavior in otherwise normal brain networks can result from aberrant induction of synaptic plasticity within these networks via a LTP-like phenomenon. Kindling results from repetitive seizure activity induced by either chemical or electrical stimulation of a discrete locus within the brain, which spreads with increasing efficiency to associated brain structures via established synaptic pathways. As the propagation of seizure activity via these networks expands, the electrographic activity and accompanying behavioral manifestations become increasingly complex. Once established, the kindled state persists for many months and pathophysiological behavior re-emerges rapidly if additional stimulation is applied to the kindled focus. The progression of seizure propagation associated with the kindling model has given rise to the assertion that seizure activity alone may be sufficient to promote epileptogenesis, that seizures beget seizures. While this is certainly true in the case of status epilepticus resulting in diffuse brain injury, it remains controversial whether brief clinical seizures analogous to those produced during the kindling process are sufficient to promote epileptogenesis.[49,50]

1.4 Genomics

The past two decades have witnessed an acceleration in our understanding of the role of genetics in rendering vulnerability toward various categories of epileptogenicity. Several linkage analyses and association studies have contributed to the wealth of information, now supplemented by chromosome microarrays and next-generation sequencing. Upwards of 80% of epilepsy cases are thought to be related to genetic factors.[51] Epilepsy has been grouped into three broad classes defined as genetic generalized epilepsy (GGE), focal epilepsy (FE), and epileptic encephalopathy (EE), with specific syndromes assigned to each group according to specific manifestations, EEG features, age of onset, and manner of progression.[52] A 22q11.2 deletion appears to lower seizure threshold in nonepileptic patients but has also been shown to manifest in patients with GGE and with FE.[53] Many of the current discoveries of genes involved in epileptogenesis support a channelopathy hypothesis, although a host of others are involved in transcriptional regulation, trafficking of synaptic vesicles, and mammalian target of rapamycin (mTOR) signaling suggesting a considerable genetic heterogeneity.

1.4.1 Genetic Generalized Epilepsies

Juvenile myoclonic epilepsy and childhood absence epilepsy exemplify this category and are early-life onset conditions with bihemispheric expression. Large recurrent deletions at chromosomes 15q13.3, 16p13.11, and 15q11.2 have been identified in GGE patients,[54,55] but with variable inheritance patterns and incomplete penetrance.[56] An association with autism and schizophrenia has also been found with these same three deletions. A severe early myoclonic epilepsy with hypotonia and developmental delay has been shown to bear a de novo mutation in *EEF1A2*,[57] which encodes the α2 subunit of eukaryotic elongation factor 1 and is also involved in actin cytoskeletal remodeling via protein kinase B.[58] Exome-sequencing has failed to provide statistically relevant genetic risk factors, despite several candidate sequence variants in affected patients.[59]

1.4.2 Focal Epilepsies

Heritable conditions such as familial mesial temporal lobe epilepsy (FMTLE), autosomal dominant lateral temporal epilepsy (ADLTE), autosomal dominant nocturnal frontal lobe epilepsy (ADNFLE), genetic epilepsy with febrile seizure plus (GEFS+), and autosomal dominant partial epilepsy with auditory features (ADPEAF) represent linkages in a number of chromosomes. FMTLE is not associated with hippocampal sclerosis or with febrile seizures and shows an autosomal dominant inheritance with incomplete penetrance.[60] Only one linkage has been identified on 4q13.2-21.3 in a four-generation family with 12 patients.[61] Linkage analysis in a three-generation family with 11 patients with ADLTE or ADPEAF provided a localization onto 10q.[62] Mutations of the *leucine-rich glioma-inactivated 1* (*LGI1*) gene at the 10q24 locus were subsequently identified.[63] Likewise, mutations in *CHRNA4*, encoding the α4 subunit of the pentameric nicotinic acetylcholine receptor, have been shown to cause ADNFLE. The gene is mapped to 20q13 and found in all layers of the frontal cortex.[64] Both 15q11.2 and 16p13.11 deletions have been found in patients with focal and other epilepsies.[59] The *NDE1* gene inhabits the latter deletion site and encodes a protein important for cell-positioning during cortical development. Neuro-pathological review of two cases of mesial temporal epilepsy with the same heterozygous *NDE1*-containing 16p13.11 deletion were found not to have evidence of cortical dyslamination or abnormality in cytoarchitectonics, although a cortical hamartia was present in one and hippocampal sclerosis in the other.[65] Mutations in *DEPDC5* on 22q12.2 have been implicated in familial FE with variable foci (FFEVF),[66,67] childhood FE,[68] and ADNFLE.[69]

Unlike the situation with *NDE1* deletion, brain malformations have been identified with *DEPDC5* mutations in the form of bottom of sulcus and focal cortical dysplasias, heterotopias, and hemimegelencephaly.[70] The *DEPDC5* gene is responsible for a protein belonging to the GATOR1 complex which regulates the mTOR pathway through its inhibition of mTOR complex 1 and, through this, cell growth, division, and plasticity. Dysregulation gives rise to several disorders, including tuberous sclerosis, focal cortical dysplasia, and hemimegelencephaly[71] and an accompanying intractable epilepsy.

1.4.3 Epileptic Encephalopathies

Early notions of ion-channelopathies resulting from gene mutations and giving rise to epilepsy came from studies that identified *KCNQ2* in benign familial neonatal epilepsy,[72] *SCN2A* in benign familial infantile epilepsy,[73] and *SCN1A* in Dravet syndrome.[74] Different mutational sites are found for these conditions from either GGE or FE.[75] Other genes clearly implicated in EE include *STXBP1* and *CDKL5*. These more severe disorders are attributable to highly penetrant single gene or copy number variant mutations.[52] Exome sequencing has proven to be of great value in confirming the presence of de novo mutations and drawing attention to the genetic heterogeneity of conditions such as Dravet syndrome or severe myoclonic epilepsy of infancy. Such studies have identified *HCN1* involved with hyperpolarization-activated, cyclic-nucleotide-gated channels,[76] *GABRA1* encoding the α1 subunit[77] and *GABRB3* encoding the β3 subunit[78] of the $GABA_A$ receptor, *STXBP1* encoding the syntaxin-binding protein required for presynaptic vesicle fusion,[77] and *KCNB1* encoding a voltage-gated potassium channel,[79] all of which are critical for neuronal transmission and regulating excitability.

Encoding of proteins involved in chromatin remodeling and transcriptional regulation has been perturbed by deletions and duplications of variable lengths of DNA (i.e., copy number variants), as with de novo mutation in *CHD2* that encodes a chromatin remodeling factor[80] in both EE[81] and GGE.[82]

1.5 Neuronoglial Migrational Disorders

Both genetic and developmental aspects of cellular organization of the cerebral cortex constitute an important consideration regarding epileptogenesis, as disorganization, whether micro- or macroscopic, is a familiar substrate for epileptogenic expression. A number of genes regulating microtubular function (i.e., *LIS1*, *TUBA1A*, *TUBB3*, *DCX*) and actin (i.e., *FilaminA*) have been implicated in cerebrocortical disorganization and a resultant intractable epilepsy.[83] Periventricular heterotopia (PVH) itself has been shown to result from mutations in the filamin 1 gene which prevent cellular migration.[84,85] Doublecortin (DCX), a microtubule-associated protein that regulates radial and tangential migration of neurons in cortical development, shows a characteristic expression pattern in focal cortical dysplasia Ia suggesting abnormal cortical maturation.[86] Neuroimaging often readily identifies lissencephaly, pachygyria, subcortical band heterotopia, and periventricular nodular heterotopias, and may overlook minor focal failures of cellular migration (e.g., microdysgenesis) because of limits of resolution. Associated cortical network hyperexcitability may arise from singular or multiple anomalous sites,[87] with both increased postsynaptic glutamate and decreased $GABA_A$ receptors.[88]

Tuberous sclerosis complex (TSC) is a genetic disorder caused by mutations in one of two tumor suppressor genes, *TSC1* and *TSC2*, resulting in disordered neuronal migration.

Protein products of *TSC1* and *TSC2*, hamartin and tuberin, respectively, form a functional complex in the mTOR pathway that controls cell growth and proliferation. Approximately 90% of patients with TSC typically develop an early-onset epilepsy, often as infantile spasms. These may reflect a variety of brain pathologies, including cortical tubers, subependymal nodules, and giant cell astrocytomas. TSC is also associated with autism and other developmental delays.

1.5.1 Childhood Epilepsies

The highest incidence of childhood epilepsy occurs during the first few years of life. This increased excitability within the developing brain often reflects an imbalance between the maturation of excitatory and inhibitory circuits.[89] In particular, participation of the main ionotropic receptors, AMPA, NMDA, and $GABA_A$, in neuronal excitation within the neonatal hippocampus exhibits a distinct developmental pattern.[90] During the early stages of postnatal development, GABA, acting on postsynaptic $GABA_A$ receptors, provides the main excitatory input to the hippocampus, reflecting a chloride gradient that depolarizes immature neurons. Inhibitory responses associated with postsynaptic $GABA_B$ receptors, adenosine and 5-hydroxytryptamine–G-protein-coupled potassium channels, are delayed in their maturation such that neurotransmitter-mediated inhibition is significantly compromised in the neonatal hippocampus. Presynaptic GABA- and adenosine-mediated inhibitory responses, on the other hand, are fully established at birth, suggesting that inhibition in the neonatal hippocampus is mediated primarily by control of neurotransmitter release.[91]

The incidence of epilepsy is even higher in children with developmental disabilities and, in most cases, the pathogenesis responsible for the disability also facilitates the development of epilepsy. In general, the risk for developing epilepsy increases proportional to the severity of the developmental pathology. Conversely, in some cases, the epileptic condition precipitates the developmental disorder, particularly those involving impaired cognitive development and/or cognitive decline.[92] These are generally described as epileptic encephalopathies and include such disorders as infantile spasms, Lennox–Gastaut syndrome, and Landau–Kleffner syndrome. Both clinical data and data derived from animal models suggests that these disorders should be treated aggressively to prevent the development of more severe and long-term cognitive impairment.

1.5.2 Mental Retardation and Cerebral Palsy

Between 15 and 30% of childhood epilepsy cases are associated with mental retardation and cerebral palsy. The incidence of epilepsy in children with mental retardation and cerebral palsy is substantially higher than for the general population and the risk for developing epilepsy in this population remains elevated for the first 20 years of life. Epilepsy in this patient population is characterized by early-onset seizures of varying expression and severity, and with a high seizure frequency in the early stages. These seizures also tend to be resistant to drug therapy and have a higher rate of recurrence when therapy is terminated.[93]

1.6 Metabolic Disorders

In addition to the genetic disorders described previously, which promote epileptogenesis by directly affecting synaptic transmission, several metabolic disorders result from genetic abnormalities that promote epileptogenesis indirectly by negatively impacting cellular function. These disorders are often difficult to diagnose, but should be considered whenever developmental disabilities, cognitive impairment, and epilepsy are present in children. Inborn metabolic defects, in aggregate, amount to a considerable list of conditions promoting epileptogenicity.[94] The resulting persistent brain disturbance can be categorized into two groups. Small-molecule disorders involve amino, organic, and fatty acids, neurotransmitters, urea cycle constituents, vitamers, and cofactors and are represented by a variety of amino acidopathies, organic acidemias (e.g., methylmalonic acidemia), demyelinative conditions (e.g., Canavan disease), defective GABA metabolism (e.g., succinic semialdehyde dehydrogenase deficiency), mitochondrial disorders (e.g., myoclonic epilepsy with ragged red fibers), cerebral folate deficiency, glucose transporter 1 deficiency, glycine encephalopathy, and homocyteinemias to name a few. The large-molecule disorders involve lysosomal storage, peroxisomal and glycosylation disorders, as well as the leukodystrophies. These will involve also a wide variety of metabolopathies, including glycoprotein and membrane transporter deficiencies, ganglioside degradation, and aberrations of lipid metabolism. The effects range from cellular degeneration and dysmyelination to disorders of neuronal migration.

1.7 Inflammatory Mediators

Recent interest has centered upon neuroinflammation as both a precipitant of epileptogenesis and a means of perpetuating epileptogenicity.[95–97] A variety of mediators (i.e., cytokines, chemokines, eicosanoids) may act as activators of microglia and astrocytes, chemoattractants, promoters of cellular proliferation and death, as well as agents affecting microcirculatory function, ionic flux, and intercellular communication. Brain injury promotes an infiltration of blood cells,[98–100] and sites of epileptogenicity marked by neuronal death or dysfunction have shown increased leukocyte numbers[101] and altered central[102] and peripheral blood inflammatory mediators.[97,101,103–105]. Moreover, resection of epileptogenic sites has resulted in reduction of peripheral proinflammatory mediators.[105]

In a large series of mesial temporal lobe epilepsy cases, the hippocampus was found to have the majority of inflammatory mediator increases compared to the entorhinal and convexity neocortical regions and had the majority (70%) of inter-regional associations identifying a possible focus of inflammatory control between regions.[106] Hippocampal eotaxin, IL-2, IL-4, IL-12p70, IL-17A, TNFα, IFNγ, and ICAM1 were found to be higher. Blood levels of most of these proinflammatory mediators had been found to be more detectable in epilepsy patients than in age-matched controls.[107] Eotaxin is a potent chemoattractant of eosinophils and capable of rapid transport across the blood–brain barrier.[108] IFNγ, a macrophage activator and inducer of major histocompatibility II inflammatory activity, is involved in autoimmune mechanisms. IL-17A, also a proinflammatory mediator, has synergistic effects with IFNγ, IL-1, and TNFα[109]. The vasoactive cell adhesion molecules, ICAM1 and ICAM5, which are endothelial-, leukocyte- and tissue-associated proteins, have been found to be low in certain locations, such as the entorhinal cortex in epilepsy patients and in the peripheral blood, compared to age-matched controls.[106,110,111]

1.8 Conclusions

The pathophysiology of epilepsy must be understood as a process that leads to and sustains a condition in which recurrent seizures are perpetuated and that, although these may be triggered by local events through vulnerabilities that exist in cerebrocortical microcircuitry, their clinical manifestation will reflect whether the abnormally excessive, hypersynchronous activity remains local or propagates to distant nodal sites to engage other circuits in a widening network. An understanding of the nature of both the local and wider situations is driving current therapeutic intervention.

References

1. Berg AT, Berkovic SF, Brodie MJ, et al. Revised terminology and concepts for organization of seizures and epilepsies: report of the ILAE Commission on Classification and Terminology, 2005–2009. *Epilepsia.* 2010;51(4):676–685.

2. McNamara JO. Cellular and molecular basis of epilepsy. *J Neurosci.* 1994;14(6):3413–3425.

3. Tasker JG, Hoffman NW, Kim YI, et al. Electrical properties of neocortical neurons in slices from children with intractable epilepsy. *J Neurophysiol.* 1996;75(2):931–939.

4. Azevedo FA, Carvalho LR, Grinberg LT, et al. Equal numbers of neuronal and nonneuronal cells make the human brain an isometrically scaled-up primate brain. *J Comp Neurol.* 2009;513(5):532–541.

5. Hartzfeld P, Elisevich K, Pace M, Smith B, Gutierrez JA. Characteristics and surgical outcomes for medial temporal post-traumatic epilepsy. *Br J Neurosurg.* 2008;22(2):224–230.

6. Kotapka MJ, Gennarelli TA, Graham DI, et al. Selective vulnerability of hippocampal neurons in acceleration-induced experimental head injury. *J Neurotrauma.* 1991;8(4):247–258.

7. Nelson KB, Ellenberg JH. Prognosis in children with febrile seizures. *Pediatrics.* 1978;61(5):720–727.

8. Lynch NE, Stevenson NJ, Livingstone V, et al. The temporal evolution of electrographic seizure burden in neonatal hypoxic ischemic encephalopathy. *Epilepsia.* 2012;53(3):549–557.

9. Markram H, Toledo-Rodriguez M, Wang Y, et al. Interneurons of the neocortical inhibitory system. *Nat Rev Neurosci.* 2004;5(10):793–807.

10. Kiernan JA. *Barr's The Human Nervous System: An Anatomical Viewpoint.* 9th edn. Baltimore: Lippincott Williams & Wilkins; 2009.

11. Wang Y, Gupta A, Toledo-Rodriguez M, Wu CZ, Markram H. Anatomical, physiological, molecular and circuit properties of nest basket cells in the developing somatosensory cortex. *Cereb Cortex.* 2002;12(4):395–410.

12. Chu J, Anderson SA. Development of cortical interneurons. *Neuropsychopharmacology.* 2015;40(1):16–23.

13. Benarroch EE. Neocortical interneurons: functional diversity and clinical correlations. *Neurology.* 2013;81(3):273–280.

14. Rudy B, Fishell G, Lee S, Hjerling-Leffler J. Three groups of interneurons account for nearly 100% of neocortical GABAergic neurons. *Dev Neurobiol.* 2011;71(1):45–61.

15. Jiang X, Lachance M, Rossignol E. Involvement of cortical fast-spiking parvalbumin-positive basket cells in epilepsy. *Prog Brain Res.* 2016;226:81–126.

16. Silberberg G, Markram H. Disynaptic inhibition between neocortical pyramidal cells mediated by Martinotti cells. *Neuron.* 2007;53(5):735–746.

17. Hilscher MM, Leao RN, Edwards SJ, Leao KE, Kullander K. Chrna2-Martinotti cells synchronize layer 5 type a pyramidal cells via rebound excitation. *PLoS Biol.* 2017;15(2):e2001392.

18. Tai C, Abe Y, Westenbroek RE, Scheuer T, Catterall WA. Impaired excitability of somatostatin- and parvalbumin-expressing cortical interneurons in a mouse model of Dravet syndrome. *Proc Natl Acad Sci USA.* 2014;111(30):E3139–E3148.

19. Rutecki PA, Lebeda FJ, Johnston D. Epileptiform activity induced by changes in extracellular potassium in hippocampus. *J Neurophysiol*. 1985;54(5):1363–1374.

20. Prince DA, Connors BW, Benardo LS. Mechanisms underlying interictal-ictal transitions. *Adv Neurol*. 1983;34:177–187.

21. Dudek FE, Obenaus A, Tasker JG. Osmolality-induced changes in extracellular volume alter epileptiform bursts independent of chemical synapses in the rat: importance of non-synaptic mechanisms in hippocampal epileptogenesis. *Neurosci Lett*. 1990;120(2):267–270.

22. Traub RD, Dudek FE, Taylor CP, Knowles WD. Simulation of hippocampal afterdischarges synchronized by electrical interactions. *Neuroscience*. 1985;14(4):1033–1038.

23. Jefferys JG, Haas HL. Synchronized bursting of CA1 hippocampal pyramidal cells in the absence of synaptic transmission. *Nature*. 1982;300 (5891):448–450.

24. Vizi ES, Fekete A, Karoly R, Mike A. Non-synaptic receptors and transporters involved in brain functions and targets of drug treatment. *Br J Pharmacol*. 2010;160(4):785–809.

25. Lendvai B, Vizi ES. Nonsynaptic chemical transmission through nicotinic acetylcholine receptors. *Physiol Rev*. 2008;88(2):333–349.

26. Jin MM, Chen Z. Role of gap junctions in epilepsy. *Neurosci Bull*. 2011;27(6):389–406.

27. Elisevich K, Rempel SA, Smith BJ, Edvardsen K. Hippocampal connexin 43 expression in human complex partial seizure disorder. *Exp Neurol*. 1997;145(1):154–164.

28. Nadarajah B, Thomaidou D, Evans WH, Parnavelas JG. Gap junctions in the adult cerebral cortex: regional differences in their distribution and cellular expression of connexins. *J Comp Neurol*. 1996;376(2):326–342.

29. Venance L, Piomelli D, Glowinski J, Giaume C. Inhibition by anandamide of gap junctions and intercellular calcium signalling in striatal astrocytes. *Nature*. 1995;376(6541):590–594.

30. Trachtenberg MC, Pollen DA. Neuroglia: biophysical properties and physiologic function. *Science*. 1970;167 (3922):1248–1252.

31. Deans MR, Gibson JR, Sellitto C, Connors BW, Paul DL. Synchronous activity of inhibitory networks in neocortex requires electrical synapses containing connexin36. *Neuron*. 2001;31(3):477–485.

32. Baude A, Bleasdale C, Dalezios Y, Somogyi P, Klausberger T. Immunoreactivity for the GABAA receptor alpha1 subunit, somatostatin and Connexin36 distinguishes axoaxonic, basket, and bistratified interneurons of the rat hippocampus. *Cereb Cortex*. 2007;17(9):2094–2107.

33. Steyn-Ross ML, Steyn-Ross DA, Sleigh JW. Modelling general anaesthesia as a first-order phase transition in the cortex. *Prog Biophys Mol Biol*. 2004;85(2–3):369–385.

34. Voss LJ, Sleigh JW. Gap junctions regulate seizure activity – but in unexpected ways. In: Dere E, ed. *Gap Junctions in the Brain: Physiological and Pathological Roles*. Waltham, MA: Academic Press; 2013:217–229.

35. Grenier F, Timofeev I, Steriade M. Focal synchronization of ripples (80-200 Hz) in neocortex and their neuronal correlates. *J Neurophysiol*. 2001;86(4):1884–1898.

36. Schmitz D, Schuchmann S, Fisahn A, et al. Axo-axonal coupling. a novel mechanism for ultrafast neuronal communication. *Neuron*. 2001;31(5):831–840.

37. Traub RD, Whittington MA, Buhl EH, et al. A possible role for gap junctions in generation of very fast EEG oscillations preceding the onset of, and perhaps initiating, seizures. *Epilepsia*. 2001;42(2):153–170.

38. Van Rijn C, Meinardi H. Neurochemistry and epileptology. *Epilepsia*. 2009;50(Suppl 3):17–29.

39. Meldrum BS. Glutamate as a neurotransmitter in the brain: review of

physiology and pathology. *J Nutr.* 2000;130 (4S Suppl):1007s–1015s.

40. Anwyl R. Metabotropic glutamate receptor-dependent long-term potentiation. *Neuropharmacology.* 2009;56(4):735–740.

41. Danbolt NC. Glutamate uptake. *Prog Neurobiol.* 2001;65(1):1–105.

42. Jones EA, Yurdaydin C, Basile AS. The GABA hypothesis: state of the art. *Adv Exp Med Biol.* 1994;368:89–101.

43. Mathern GW, Mendoza D, Lozada A, et al. Hippocampal GABA and glutamate transporter immunoreactivity in patients with temporal lobe epilepsy. *Neurology.* 1999;52(3):453–472.

44. Bradford HF. Glutamate, GABA and epilepsy. *Prog Neurobiol.* 1995;47(6):477–511.

45. Blumenfeld H. Cellular and network mechanisms of spike-wave seizures. *Epilepsia.* 2005;46(Suppl 9):21–33.

46. Haut SR, Albin RL. Dopamine and epilepsy: hints of complex subcortical roles. *Neurology.* 2008;71(11):784–785.

47. Starr MS. The role of dopamine in epilepsy. *Synapse.* 1996;22(2):159–194.

48. Giorgi FS, Pizzanelli C, Biagioni F, Murri L, Fornai F. The role of norepinephrine in epilepsy: from the bench to the bedside. *Neurosci Biobehav Rev.* 2004;28 (5):507–524.

49. McNamara JO, Byrne MC, Dasheiff RM, Fitz JG. The kindling model of epilepsy: a review. *Prog Neurobiol.* 1980;15 (2):139–159.

50. Avanzini G. Do seizures promote epileptogenesis and cause cognitive decline? *Eur Neurol Rev.* 2015;9(2).

51. Hildebrand MS, Dahl HH, Damiano JA, et al. Recent advances in the molecular genetics of epilepsy. *J Med Genet.* 2013;50(5):271–279.

52. Myers CT, Mefford HC. Advancing epilepsy genetics in the genomic era. *Genome Med.* 2015;7(1):91.

53. Wither RG, Borlot F, MacDonald A, et al. 22q11.2 deletion syndrome lowers seizure threshold in adult patients without epilepsy. *Epilepsia.* 2017;58(6):1095–1101.

54. de Kovel CG, Trucks H, Helbig I, et al. Recurrent microdeletions at 15q11.2 and 16p13.11 predispose to idiopathic generalized epilepsies. *Brain.* 2010;133(Pt 1):23–32.

55. Helbig I, Mefford HC, Sharp AJ, et al. 15q13.3 microdeletions increase risk of idiopathic generalized epilepsy. *Nat Genet.* 2009;41(2):160–162.

56. Helbig I, Hodge SE, Ottman R. Familial cosegregation of rare genetic variants with disease in complex disorders. *Eur J Hum Genet.* 2013;21(4):444–450.

57. de Ligt J, Willemsen MH, van Bon BW, et al. Diagnostic exome sequencing in persons with severe intellectual disability. *N Engl J Med.* 2012;367(20):1921–1929.

58. Abbas W, Kumar A, Herbein G. The eEF1A proteins: at the crossroads of oncogenesis, apoptosis, and viral infections. *Front Oncol.* 2015;5:75.

59. Heinzen EL, Radtke RA, Urban TJ, et al. Rare deletions at 16p13.11 predispose to a diverse spectrum of sporadic epilepsy syndromes. *Am J Hum Genet.* 2010;86(5):707–718.

60. Crompton DE, Scheffer IE, Taylor I, et al. Familial mesial temporal lobe epilepsy: a benign epilepsy syndrome showing complex inheritance. *Brain.* 2010;133 (11):3221–3231.

61. Hedera P, Blair MA, Andermann E, et al. Familial mesial temporal lobe epilepsy maps to chromosome 4q13.2-q21.3. *Neurology.* 2007;68(24):2107–2112.

62. Ottman R, Risch N, Hauser WA, et al. Localization of a gene for partial epilepsy to chromosome 10q. *Nat Genet.* 1995;10 (1):56–60.

63. Kalachikov S, Evgrafov O, Ross B, et al. Mutations in LGI1 cause autosomal-dominant partial epilepsy with auditory features. *Nat Genet.* 2002;30(3):335–341.

64. Steinlein OK, Mulley JC, Propping P, et al. A missense mutation in the neuronal nicotinic acetylcholine receptor alpha 4 subunit is associated with autosomal

dominant nocturnal frontal lobe epilepsy. *Nat Genet.* 1995;11(2):201–203.

65. Liu JY, Kasperaviciute D, Martinian L, Thom M, Sisodiya SM. Neuropathology of 16p13.11 deletion in epilepsy. *PLoS One.* 2012;7(4):e34813.

66. Ishida S, Picard F, Rudolf G, et al. Mutations of DEPDC5 cause autosomal dominant focal epilepsies. *Nat Genet.* 2013;45(5):552–555.

67. Dibbens LM, de Vries B, Donatello S, et al. Mutations in DEPDC5 cause familial focal epilepsy with variable foci. *Nat Genet.* 2013;45(5):546–551.

68. Lal D, Reinthaler EM, Schubert J, et al. DEPDC5 mutations in genetic focal epilepsies of childhood. *Ann Neurol.* 2014;75(5):788–792.

69. Picard F, Makrythanasis P, Navarro V, et al. DEPDC5 mutations in families presenting as autosomal dominant nocturnal frontal lobe epilepsy. *Neurology.* 2014;82(23):2101–2106.

70. D'Gama AM, Geng Y, Couto JA, et al. Mammalian target of rapamycin pathway mutations cause hemimegalencephaly and focal cortical dysplasia. *Ann Neurol.* 2015;77(4):720–725.

71. Lim JS, Kim WI, Kang HC, et al. Brain somatic mutations in MTOR cause focal cortical dysplasia type II leading to intractable epilepsy. *Nat Med.* 2015;21 (4):395–400.

72. Singh NA, Charlier C, Stauffer D, et al. A novel potassium channel gene, KCNQ2, is mutated in an inherited epilepsy of newborns. *Nat Genet.* 1998;18(1):25-29.

73. Heron SE, Crossland KM, Andermann E, et al. Sodium-channel defects in benign familial neonatal-infantile seizures. *Lancet.* 2002;360(9336):851–852.

74. Claes L, Del-Favero J, Ceulemans B, et al. De novo mutations in the sodium-channel gene SCN1A cause severe myoclonic epilepsy of infancy. *Am J Hum Genet.* 2001;68(6):1327–1332.

75. Mefford HC. CNVs in epilepsy. *Curr Genet Med Rep.* 2014;2(3):162–167.

76. Nava C, Dalle C, Rastetter A, et al. De novo mutations in HCN1 cause early infantile epileptic encephalopathy. *Nat Genet.* 2014;46(6):640–645.

77. Carvill GL, Weckhuysen S, McMahon JM, et al. GABRA1 and STXBP1: novel genetic causes of Dravet syndrome. *Neurology.* 2014;82(14):1245–1253.

78. Moller RS, Wuttke TV, Helbig I, et al. Mutations in GABRB3: from febrile seizures to epileptic encephalopathies. *Neurology.* 2017;88(5):483–492.

79. Torkamani A, Bersell K, Jorge BS, et al. De novo KCNB1 mutations in epileptic encephalopathy. *Ann Neurol.* 2014;76(4):529–540.

80. Carvill GL, Heavin SB, Yendle SC, et al. Targeted resequencing in epileptic encephalopathies identifies de novo mutations in CHD2 and SYNGAP1. *Nat Genet.* 2013;45(7):825–830.

81. Suls A, Jaehn JA, Kecskes A, et al. De novo loss-of-function mutations in CHD2 cause a fever-sensitive myoclonic epileptic encephalopathy sharing features with Dravet syndrome. *Am J Hum Genet.* 2013;93(5):967–975.

82. Galizia EC, Myers CT, Leu C, et al. CHD2 variants are a risk factor for photosensitivity in epilepsy. *Brain.* 2015;138(Pt 5):1198–1207.

83. Liu JS. Molecular genetics of neuronal migration disorders. *Curr Neurol Neurosci Rep.* 2011;11(2):171–178.

84. Fox JW, Lamperti ED, Eksioglu YZ, et al. Mutations in filamin 1 prevent migration of cerebral cortical neurons in human periventricular heterotopia. *Neuron.* 1998;21(6):1315–1325.

85. Sheen VL, Dixon PH, Fox JW, et al. Mutations in the X-linked filamin 1 gene cause periventricular nodular heterotopia in males as well as in females. *Hum Mol Genet.* 2001;10 (17):1775–1783.

86. Srikandarajah N, Martinian L, Sisodiya SM, et al. Doublecortin expression in focal cortical dysplasia in epilepsy. *Epilepsia.* 2009;50(12):2619–2628.

87. Chevassus-au-Louis N, Baraban SC, Gaiarsa JL, Ben-Ari Y. Cortical malformations and epilepsy: new insights from animal models. *Epilepsia.* 1999;40(7):811–821.

88. Jacobs KM, Kharazia VN, Prince DA. Mechanisms underlying epileptogenesis in cortical malformations. *Epilepsy Res.* 1999;36(2–3):165–188.

89. Hauser WA. Seizure disorders: the changes with age. *Epilepsia.* 1992;33(Suppl 4): S6–S14.

90. Gaiarsa JL, Tseeb V, Ben-Ari Y. Postnatal development of pre- and postsynaptic GABAB-mediated inhibitions in the CA3 hippocampal region of the rat. *J Neurophysiol.* 1995;73(1):246–255.

91. Leinekugel X, Medina I, Khalilov I, Ben-Ari Y, Khazipov R. Ca^{2+} oscillations mediated by the synergistic excitatory actions of GABA(A) and NMDA receptors in the neonatal hippocampus. *Neuron.* 1997;18(2):243–255.

92. Holmes GL, Ben-Ari Y. Seizures in the developing brain: perhaps not so benign after all. *Neuron.* 1998;21(6):1231–1234.

93. Edebol-Tysk K. Epidemiology of spastic tetraplegic cerebral palsy in Sweden. I. Impairments and disabilities. *Neuropediatrics.* 1989;20(1):41–45.

94. Yu JY, Pearl PL. Metabolic causes of epileptic encephalopathy. *Epilepsy Res Treat.* 2013;2013:124934.

95. Vezzani A, Granata T. Brain inflammation in epilepsy: experimental and clinical evidence. *Epilepsia.* 2005;46(11):1724–1743.

96. Li G, Bauer S, Nowak M, et al. Cytokines and epilepsy. *Seizure.* 2011;20(3):249–256.

97. Nowak M, Bauer S, Haag A, et al. Interictal alterations of cytokines and leukocytes in patients with active epilepsy. *Brain Behav Immun.* 2011;25(3):423–428.

98. Hirschberg DL, Moalem G, He J, et al. Accumulation of passively transferred primed T cells independently of their antigen specificity following central nervous system trauma. *J Neuroimmunol.* 1998;89(1–2):88–96.

99. Holmin S, Soderlund J, Biberfeld P, Mathiesen T. Intracerebral inflammation after human brain contusion. *Neurosurgery.* 1998;42(2):291–298; discussion 298–299.

100. Lenzlinger PM, Hans VH, Joller-Jemelka HI, et al. Markers for cell-mediated immune response are elevated in cerebrospinal fluid and serum after severe traumatic brain injury in humans. *J Neurotrauma.* 2001;18(5):479–489.

101. Ravizza T, Gagliardi B, Noe F, et al. Innate and adaptive immunity during epileptogenesis and spontaneous seizures: evidence from experimental models and human temporal lobe epilepsy. *Neurobiol Dis.* 2008;29(1):142–160.

102. Mukherjee S, Bricker PC, Shapiro LA. Alteration of hippocampal cytokines and astrocyte morphology observed in rats 24 hour after fluid percussion injury. *J Neurol Disord Stroke.* 2014;2(4):1078.

103. Vezzani A, Ravizza T, Balosso S, Aronica E. Glia as a source of cytokines: implications for neuronal excitability and survival. *Epilepsia.* 2008;49(Suppl 2):24–32.

104. Alapirtti T, Rinta S, Hulkkonen J, et al. Interleukin-6, interleukin-1 receptor antagonist and interleukin-1beta production in patients with focal epilepsy: a video-EEG study. *J Neurol Sci.* 2009;280(1–2):94–97.

105. Quirico-Santos T, Meira ID, Gomes AC, et al. Resection of the epileptogenic lesion abolishes seizures and reduces inflammatory cytokines of patients with temporal lobe epilepsy. *J Neuroimmunol.* 2013;254(1–2):125–130.

106. Strauss KI, Elisevich KV. Brain region and epilepsy-associated differences in inflammatory mediator levels in medically refractory mesial temporal lobe epilepsy. *J Neuroinflammation.* 2016;13(1):270.

107. Sinha S, Patil SA, Jayalekshmy V, Satishchandra P. Do cytokines have any role in epilepsy? *Epilepsy Res.* 2008;82(2–3):171–176.

108. Erickson MA, Morofuji Y, Owen JB, Banks WA. Rapid transport of CCL11 across the blood-brain barrier: regional variation and

importance of blood cells. *J Pharmacol Exp Ther.* 2014;349(3):497–507.

109. Sutton C, Brereton C, Keogh B, Mills KH, Lavelle EC. A crucial role for interleukin (IL)-1 in the induction of IL-17-producing T cells that mediate autoimmune encephalomyelitis. *J Exp Med.* 2006;203(7):1685–1691.

110. Pollard JR, Eidelman O, Mueller GP, et al. The TARC/sICAM5 ratio in patient plasma is a candidate biomarker for drug resistant epilepsy. *Front Neurol.* 2012;3:181.

111. Lyck R, Enzmann G. The physiological roles of ICAM-1 and ICAM-2 in neutrophil migration into tissues. *Curr Opin Hematol.* 2015;22(1):53–59.

Physiologic Basis of Epileptic EEG Patterns

L. John Greenfield Jr. and Sang-Hun Lee

2.1 Introduction

Much of our attention as electroencephalographers is devoted to the identification and localization of spikes and seizures. Atlases, primers, and texts of electroencephalogram (EEG) interpretation provide a wealth of information to guide seizure identification, but often the diagnosis is based on the same principle as Justice Potter Stewart's maxim for identifying obscenity in *Jacobellis v. Ohio*: "I know it when I see it."[1] Virtually all of the mathematical seizure detection algorithms currently in use are based on empiric observations of EEG activity that occurs contemporaneously with behavioral seizures, or resembles the electrical activity we see during such behaviors. Ideally, we should be able to derive the parameters for identifying electrographic seizures from a detailed understanding of the underlying neuronal pathophysiology that generates abnormal rhythmic activity, disrupting normal brain circuit functions and behaviors. Unfortunately, we are not there yet. In many cases, however, we have at least a rudimentary knowledge of the neurons and brain structures involved in seizure generation. This chapter will review what we know about how seizures are generated and how that translates into the patterns we observe in EEG recordings.

2.2 Sources of EEG Potentials and Brain Rhythms

Brain rhythms are more than the epiphenomena of neuronal activity; they are the physiologic structure from which all thought and behavior derives.[2] The brain rhythms we are able to record using scalp and intracranial electrodes are measurable due to temporal and spatial summation of coactivated synapses on the tightly packed forest of "vertically" oriented principal neurons (orthogonal to the cortical surface) in the superficial cortical layers. The currents generated by individual neurons are very tiny, on the order of picoamps (10^{-12} A) for single channels to nanoamps (10^{-9} A) for polysynaptic potentials, and it takes many thousands of coactivated synapses to generate currents and potential differences that are large enough (microvolts) to measure with macroscopic electrodes. Despite the higher voltage (100 mV or more) generated by action potentials (APs), their brief time course (0.5 to 3 ms) makes temporal summation less likely, and the quantity of current passed is small. Synaptic currents last significantly longer, facilitating temporal summation that is necessary to generate macroscopic field potential signals.

2.2.1 Neurotransmitter Receptor Mechanisms

Excitatory postsynaptic potentials (EPSPs) have a rise time and decay that depends on which type of postsynaptic glutamate receptors are activated. Depolarizing currents mediated by postsynaptic AMPA (α-amino-3-hydroxyl-5-methyl-4-isoxazole-propionate) and kainic acid receptors have very rapid rise and then decay over 10 to 25 ms, while those mediated by NMDA (*N*-methyl-D-aspartate) receptors have slower rise time (15–25 ms) and longer decay over 75–100 ms. NMDA receptors, which conduct both Na^+ and Ca^{2+} ions, are blocked by Mg^{2+} ions unless the postsynaptic cell is depolarized, usually by prior or simultaneous activation of AMPA receptors. NMDA receptors are critical for strengthening coactivated synapses by Ca^{2+}-dependent mobilization of intracellular AMPA receptors to the cell surface, in a form of synaptic plasticity known as long-term potentiation (LTP). LTP is an important mechanism for stabilizing and strengthening synaptic pathways involved in learning and memory, and likely also participates in strengthening abnormal synaptic activity involved in epileptogenesis. Additionally, three types of metabotropic (G-protein-mediated) glutamate receptors have modulatory effects that can increase or decrease neuronal excitability. Inhibitory postsynaptic potentials (IPSPs) have very rapid rise time (under 1 ms) and decay (tens of ms) when mediated by ionotropic $GABA_A$ receptors, but are slower in onset and last up to 150 ms when mediated by metabotropic $GABA_B$ receptors. Inhibition can also be mediated by activation of voltage- or second-messenger-gated potassium channels.

The temporal and spatial summation of these tiny excitatory and inhibitory potentials generate electrical fields detectable by intracranial or scalp EEG electrodes. Microelectrode recordings of single neurons performed simultaneously with macroelectrode EEG activity demonstrate strong correlations between synaptic events and specific types of EEG waves.[3,4] EPSPs correlate with surface-negative EEG waves, while IPSPs correlate with surface-positive EEG waves. Single APs or bursts of APs recorded in cortical neurons do not tightly correlate with waveforms detected by scalp electrodes. However, more recent microelectrode array studies in both humans and animals have begun to elucidate how neuronal firing participates in generation of normal EEG activity and seizures, as we will discuss below.

2.2.2 Brain Rhythms and Cortical Structure

The generation of detectable rhythms depends on the phasic activation of thousands to millions of neurons at (mostly) the same time, otherwise the cacophony of unsynchronized neuronal activity would create only noise, not an identifiable rhythmic signal. Studies in both animal models and humans demonstrate that the 8–13 Hz alpha-frequency rhythm recorded during quiet wakefulness is driven by interactions between thalamic nuclei (particularly lateral geniculate) and associated cortex.[5] The cortex is organized physiologically into vertically oriented functional columns, determined primarily by thalamocortical inputs representing specific sensory fields, which are usually about 0.5 mm in diameter and contain about 10 000 neurons and perhaps 100 000 synapses each. Since columns are defined by their thalamocortical inputs, they behave as physiological units. EEG signals represent the summated electrical field potentials generated by these columns.

Brain rhythms are generated by recurrent synaptic loops that involve both excitatory and inhibitory elements. The simplest oscillatory circuit requires two components: an excitatory neuron that depolarizes and activates the cells it contacts, and an inhibitory neuron that is excited by the first cell and synapses back onto it to provide negative feedback. When the excitatory neuron activates the inhibitory one, it stimulates the second cell to inhibit the first and turn off the excitatory stimulation. As the inhibitory signal dissipates, the excitatory neuron then resumes activity, and the circuit begins to cycle. Since most neurons in the neocortex are either excitatory or inhibitory but not both, oscillatory circuits are built into the neuronal architecture of cortical structures. The circuit described above involves feedback inhibition; there can also be "feedforward" inhibition that reduces activity in downstream structures or circuits. Some neurons are also intrinsic oscillators or "pacemaker cells" based on their internal tendency to oscillate, which can be due to the biophysics of their voltage-gated ion channels (with spontaneous excitation resulting from time-dependent release from inactivation), internal biochemical feedback systems, or auto-stimulation by recurrent synapses. Whatever the mechanism, rhythm generators require combinations of excitatory and inhibitory components.

2.3 Anatomical Substrates of Focal Epileptiform Activity and Seizures

The cytoarchitecture and connectivity of cerebral cortex and hippocampus function to generate rhythmic brain activity. Defects in the rhythm-generating circuits are responsible for epilepsy and possibly other neurological and psychiatric disorders.

The hippocampus has served as a robust model system for studying epileptiform activity due to its simplified architecture and its proclivity to generate seizures. The basic structure of the hippocampus, when laid lengthwise and sliced like a loaf of bread, reveals interlocking horseshoes consisting of the cell body and dendritic "molecular" layers of the dentate gyrus (DG) and the cornu ammonis (CA) layers of the hippocampus proper. A trisynaptic excitatory pathway passes through the hippocampus within the plane of the slice, allowing unidirectional information throughput.[6] Excitatory input from the entorhinal cortex (EC) passes into the DG via the perforant pathway and synapses onto DG granule cell neurons. The axons of DG granule cells, called mossy fibers, project through the dentate hilus (the space enclosed by the horseshoe of granule cells) to the pyramidal cells of the CA3 region. The axons of the CA3 cells, called Schaffer collateral fibers, in turn pass around the hippocampal horseshoe to the pyramidal cells of the CA1 region. The axons of CA1 pyramidal cells in turn pass information either directly back to the EC or via the subiculum, a transitional cortical layer. Recurrent excitatory connections within the CA3 cell layer reinforce the excitatory throughput, and lead to discrete bursting of APs, a behavior that can produce lasting synaptic strengthening at downstream synapses by the mechanism known as LTP.

The positive feedback loop (from EC to DG to CA3 to CA1 (to subiculum) to EC) would produce runaway excitation in the absence of inhibitory feedback. To prevent this, feedback and feedforward inhibitory loops exist at multiple points in the circuit. In the DG, the mossy fibers from dentate granule neurons excite "mossy cells" in the dentate hilus, which in turn excite inhibitory basket cells that strongly inhibit dentate granule cells in a "surround" fashion. This inhibitory system has been called the "dentate gate"[7–9] as it limits and focuses excitatory input into the hippocampus. Elsewhere in the hippocampus, and throughout the cerebral cortex, GABAergic interneurons with varied morphological, neurochemical, and electrophysiological properties are critical for maintaining the balance of excitation and inhibition required to generate normal brain rhythms, and their dysfunction is implicated in disorders including epilepsy, autism, and schizophrenia.[10]

2.3.1 Epileptic EEG patterns in Temporal Lobe Epilepsy

The epilepsy-associated structural changes contribute to electrophysiological changes at the single cell, local field, and EEG levels. The normal hippocampus typically generates theta-frequency activity in concert with the overlying EC and parahippocampal gyrus. In the rat, hippocampal theta-activity occurs during exploratory behaviors such as sniffing, rearing, walking, and during REM sleep. Intracellular recordings performed during simultaneous field potential measurements demonstrate that interneuron firing is phase linked to theta oscillations.[11,12] In contrast, hippocampal pyramidal cells are typically silent or fire at specific spatial locations associated with a neuronal map of the spatial environment, which is critical for episodic memory processing.[13–15] In the absence of theta activity, intermittent sharp waves of 40–120 ms duration are observed, which typically occur during feeding, behavioral immobility, and slow wave sleep, and are recorded in the CA1 stratum radiatum.[16,17] Hippocampal sharp waves occur with a frequency of one per minute to about three per second, and reflect the synchronous discharge of a large number of CA3 pyramidal neurons and consequent depolarization of CA1 pyramidal cells. Hippocampal sharp waves frequently have superimposed gamma-frequency "ripple" oscillations (known as spike wave-ripple complexes) and intracellular recordings in CA1 hippocampal pyramidal cells display bursts of 200 Hz oscillations.[18] The sharp wave appears to be generated in the CA3 region by a highly synchronized discharge of CA3 pyramidal neurons, which then projects via Schaffer collaterals into the CA1 region and activates rhythmic 200 Hz ("ripple") IPSPs in CA1 pyramidal neurons via feedforward inhibition.[19] These high frequency IPSPs are likely mediated by fast-spiking, parvalbumin-expressing (PV+) basket cells (PVBCs).[20] Functionally, the sharp wave ripple discharges appear to be critical for spatial learning and memory, possibly by replaying sequenced neuronal activity in a compressed manner.[21] In the setting of decreased inhibition or excessive synchronization, they may also be related to the physiological mechanisms that are augmented to generate interictal EEG spikes in the temporal lobe, though the physiological sharp wave discharges are clearly distinct from epileptiform activity. They may also contribute to high frequency oscillations (HFOs), which we will discuss in greater detail below.

2.3.2 Basis of Focal Interictal Spike-and-Wave Discharges

The EEG hallmark of focal epilepsies is the interictal spike. Spikes are typically brief (70–200 ms), focal, often high amplitude waveforms that are most often arrhythmic, occurring independently of other brain rhythms and tending to locally disrupt them. They can occur on a normal background or in the context of focal delta slowing in the same region. The intracellular correlate of the interictal spike is a high-amplitude depolarizing potential associated with a burst of APs, known as the paroxysmal depolarizing shift (PDS).[22,23] Early animal studies of spike discharges found that penicillin, bicuculline, or other agents that blocked GABA$_A$ receptors, when applied to the cortical surface or the *in vitro* hippocampal slice,[24] resulted in spike-and-wave discharges on EEG that corresponded to PDS events recorded intracellularly. The PDS is essentially a high amplitude EPSP, generated by synaptically driven[24] synchronous depolarization and bursting of CA3 pyramidal neurons, and mediated by recurrent activation of non-NMDA (AMPA, kainate) and NMDA glutamatergic ionotropic receptors. The bursting activity resulting from the high amplitude synaptic depolarization is due to influx of extracellular Ca^{2+} through NMDA receptors and voltage-gated calcium channels, with subsequent opening of voltage-gated Na$^+$ channels and generation of repetitive or bursting Na$^+$ channel-dependent APs. The burst of APs results in rapid spread of depolarization and activation of other excitatory cells through the hippocampus and parahippocampal gyrus, generating the local field potential that underlies the spike component of the spike-and-wave discharge seen on EEG.[25]

After the high-amplitude depolarization of the PDS, the subsequent prolonged hyper-polarizing afterpotential is mediated by fast $GABA_A$ receptor/chloride channels, slower metabotropic $GABA_B$ receptors, and Ca^{2+}-dependent K^+ channels activated by the influx of Ca^{2+} during the PDS. The activation of Ca^{2+}-dependent K^+ channels can prolong the hyperpolarization to 1 s or more.[26] The large spatial extent of the hyperpolarizing after-potential is driven by PDS-induced activation of GABAergic interneurons, predominantly basket cells that produce strong perisomatic inhibition on a large number of neighboring principal neurons, creating an "inhibitory surround" that broadly silences excitatory activity for up to hundreds of milliseconds. At the macroscopic EEG level, the afterhyperpolar-ization is the slow "wave" of the spike-and-wave complex, and the silencing of excitatory activity by this wave of inhibition explains why spike-and-wave complexes disrupt the local background EEG rhythm.

In order to generate a signal large enough to be detected by surface EEG, a relatively large area of cortex must be activated. Modeling the transmission of electrical signals across the skull and scalp, Cooper et al.[27] proposed that "at least 6 cm^2 must be involved in synchronous or near synchronous activity before the scalp EEG is observed." More direct results of combined subdural (cortical surface) and scalp EEG recordings by Tao et al.[28] found that cortical spike sources of 10 cm^2 or more commonly resulted in scalp-recordable interictal spikes. This corresponds to a circle with radius of 1.8 cm, or the simultaneous activation of more than 5000 cortical columns, each composed of thousands of neurons. Prominent scalp spikes on surface EEG were associated with the activation of 20 to 30 cm^2 of cortex, an area covering as much as 70% of the temporal lobe gyral cortex. Clearly, massive synchronization of cortical activity is involved.

2.3.3 Relationship of Spikes and Rhythmic Slowing

Focal intermittent slowing in a region that generates spike discharges may represent interictal epileptiform activity with insufficient cortical synchrony, spatial extent or scalp proximity (e.g., due to arising in the mesial temporal lobe) to produce an observable spike at scalp electrodes, with the slow waves arising from the potent, more spatially extended and much longer lasting inhibitory surround. Rhythmic focal slowing, particularly involving the temporal lobe (temporal intermittent rhythmic delta activity, TIRDA), is so commonly associated with epileptiform activity, focal pathology, and seizures that it is felt to be a *forme fruste* of epileptiform activity with lateralizing if not localizing value.[29–31] As noted above, such activity appears to be generated by rhythmic spike-and-wave discharges in which the spike component is not observable. The specificity for seizures is also reasonably strong for intermittent rhythmic delta activity involving the occipital lobe (OIRDA) which occurs almost exclusively in children with epilepsy,[32,33] but not in the frontal lobe (FIRDA) where it is nonspecific and usually associated with encephalopathy.[34,35]

2.3.4 Rhythmic or Periodic Spike-and-Wave Discharges

Focal interictal spike-and-wave discharges are usually sporadic, but may also occur period-ically or rhythmically, as seen with pseudoperiodic lateralized epileptiform discharges (PLEDs). The generation of such rhythms likely arises from the structure and physiology of the irritable focus itself. Using the cortical surface penicillin model, Witte[26] noted that cortical neurons in the focus region have a high negative resting potential and are often silent until they are driven to paroxysmal bursting by synaptic input from neurons in the "inhibitory surround" region. Indeed, the firing pattern of neurons in the surround show markedly increased activity during the 100 ms just *before* the spike discharge, and are silent immediately afterwards for up to 1 s before resuming stochastic firing patterns. It is easy to see how this relationship between a central paroxysmal focus and an inhibited surround could generate rhythmic spike patterns. Neurons in the surround recovering from strong inhibition synaptically activate hyperexcitable neurons in the central epileptic focus and trigger a PDS, resulting in a focal paroxysmal discharge and strong inhibition in the surround neurons. When the recurrent inhibition dissipates, recovery from hyperpolarization triggers a new PDS in the focus. The period of the discharge cycle results from the refractory period of the neurons in the focus, which can last for up to several seconds due to the accumulation of calcium during the PDS and associated calcium-dependent K^+ currents. The timing of such periodicity nicely correlates with the 0.5–2 s period usually associated with PLEDs, and suggests that this rhythm is intrinsic to the epileptic focus, though the mechanism producing it is obviously different from the artificial scenario produced by focal application of penicillin. PLEDs are often associated with focal irritative or structural lesions such as acute stroke, encephalitis, or brain tumors, consistent with the concept that the PLED epileptic focus is the result of acute or chronic cortical injury.[36] Whether these discharges represent seizures in themselves has been long debated,[37] and veers from the purely scientific into philosophical territory. PLEDs are often associated with electrographic and clinical seizures,[38] and can occur as a pattern associated with status epilepticus.[39] More recently, the concept that PLED discharges are epileptiform has been questioned, and the currently accepted term endorsed by the American Clinical Neurophysiology Society is lateralized periodic discharges (LPD), discarding the "epileptiform" designation.[40] Despite the official change in terminology, the association of this EEG pattern with seizures is strong. The connection becomes murkier with generalized periodic discharges and periodic triphasic waves, which are far less associated with seizures,[41] even though they often have an initial sharp component. These patterns are more often associated with metabolic disturbances or diffuse brain injury,[42] particularly resulting from hypoxia-ischemia,[43] where they confer a poor prognosis for survival and cortical recovery.[44]

2.3.5 Repetitive Focal Spikes and Seizures

Using the focal cortical penicillin model, Witte and colleagues observed distinct patterns of epileptiform discharges: irregular, occurring from 1.7 to 4.8 s apart, "composed," with several discharges occurring at intervals of about 300 ms separated by longer irregular intervals, regular 1 Hz spike discharges, and ictal evolving seizure discharges. These patterns occurred in an ordered sequence indicating that the different rhythms are activated by a progressive enlargement of the focus and duration of focal activity, and suggest that different interictal discharge patterns can occur within the same brain regions and may represent characteristic "resonance" frequencies for specific brain regions susceptible to seizure generation. Changes in the pattern of spike discharges occur over the course of minutes to hours in the penicillin model, and are specific to this model. However, such changes might be analogous to the gradual recruitment of surrounding tissues into epileptic circuits due to progressive loss of inhibition or synaptic learning mechanisms such as long-term potentiation. Such recruitment has been demonstrated in animals using the process known as "kindling," in which subthreshold excitatory stimulation with electrical pulse trains (usually in the hippocampus or amygdala) sufficient to produce a brief rhythmic afterdischarge (a train of spikes that continues after the end of the stimulus), but no behavioral change or sustained electrographic seizure is used. When repeated daily, each stimulation gradually produces longer and longer afterdischarges. Eventually these produce increasingly severe behavioral seizures, beginning with freezing and staring, progressing through facial twitching automatisms and forepaw clonic jerking, to rearing and falling, the rodent equivalent of a generalized tonic–clonic seizure.[45] The evolution of seizure semiology and severity seen in kindling has never been directly demonstrated in humans. However, many epilepsies gradually worsen in seizure frequency and severity over time, and the latent period between brain injury and the onset of post-traumatic epilepsy may be 10 years or longer. These observations provide indirect evidence that a similar phenomenon may occur in people with epilepsy.

2.3.6 Interictal to Ictal Transition

What is the relationship between spike-and-wave discharges and the sustained, evolving rhythmic activity that constitutes a seizure? The mechanisms underlying the transition from interictal to ictal state at the onset of a focal seizure are poorly understood. On scalp EEG, the onset of focal seizures is frequently associated with a reduction in the amplitude of background alpha or theta frequencies and a "flattening" of the EEG amplitude. As recorded with stereotactic EEG depth electrodes or grid/strip subdural electrodes in patients with either TLE or extratemporal neocortical epilepsies, this loss of amplitude corresponds to the appearance of low amplitude fast activity in the beta- to low gamma-frequency range (15–40 Hz).[46] This change in background may be preceded by either a reduction in interictal spike frequency or increased spike frequency, with discharges of higher than usual amplitude, often occurring in brief clusters. Low-voltage fast activity may be mediated by spatial desynchronization of cortical networks due to excessive inhibition, as seen after a high-amplitude spike discharge encompassing a broad area of cortex.[47]

That initial hyperpolarizing stimulus may be produced by a strong and prolonged PDS. Early experiments by Ayala and colleagues[22,25] using the topical penicillin model found that the seizure focus transitioned from sporadic interictal spike/PDS complexes to PDS discharges of increasing frequency and longer depolarizations, with reduction or loss of afterhyperpolarization, suggesting a change in the balance of excitatory and inhibitory synaptic drive. The hypothesis that seizures are generated from a prolongation of the PDS[36] set the stage for many subsequent investigations into ictal mechanisms. However, some neurons were strongly hyperpolarized even during clonic seizures, with reversal potential suggesting increased K^+ conductance. Ayala et al. postulated that the hyperpolarization during the clonic seizure phase was related to the termination of the seizure, though it is also possible that hyperpolarization contributes to the spatial desynchronization of cortical rhythms that sets the stage for ictal onset.

The concept that seizures are the product of excess synchrony and a loss of the "balance of excitation and inhibition" is an oversimplification. The loss of normal cortical rhythms may allow pathological rhythmic activity in the seizure focus to recruit neighboring and connected cortical regions into the pathological evolving rhythm that constitutes a seizure. Recruitment of additional brain areas into the seizure increases synchrony over the course of the seizure, which is maximal near the time of seizure termination.

The mechanisms underlying seizure termination are also uncertain. As seizures progress, rhythms typically slow into the delta-frequency range, consistent with greater spatial extent and longer reactivation pathways for spiraling cycles of recurrent excitation and inhibition. In the cat model of spontaneous spike-and-wave seizures, as in many focal-onset seizures in humans and other animal models, synchronous activity towards the end of the seizures slows to ~1 Hz high-amplitude oscillations. Timofeev and Steriade found that these discharges were synchronized by EPSPs, but paced by intrinsic neuronal oscillations. Each cycle was initiated by hyperpolarization-activated depolarizing current (I_h) and then enhanced by voltage-gated Na^+ and Ca^{2+} currents, which then activate hyperpolarizing potassium currents (I_K). Eventually, Ca^{2+}-dependent hyperpolarizing currents overwhelm the depolarizing effect of the I_h component of the oscillation, resulting in seizure termination.[48,49] An alternative hypothesis is that pH changes induced by synchronous discharging of neurons during the periodic bursting typical of the late clonic seizure phase may promote synchronous postictal depression of principal cell activity via decoupling of gap junctions, leading to synchronization of inhibition and contributing to seizure termination.[49] In support of this mechanism, an extracellular alkaline shift has been observed in the piriform cortex of the isolated guinea pig brain associated with rhythmic interictal spikes, which correlated with interspike periodicity. It is likely that multiple electrophysiological and metabolic mechanisms contribute to both seizure onset and termination.

2.3.7 Single-Unit Recordings

The first single-unit recordings in human neocortex were obtained using glass micropipettes inserted into the posterior temporal lobe during an operation to locate the epileptogenic area.[50,51] The hallmark of epileptiform activity in focal epilepsies was bursts of APs in the recorded neurons. Bursting units were also found in the contralateral cortex homotopic to the seizure focus and in adjacent ipsilateral cortex, presumably areas driven by axonal projections from the focus, which suggested the misleading concept of a "mirror focus." Subsequent recordings with multiple electrodes (and later confirmed with microelectrode arrays) demonstrated that spread of seizure activity on the EEG was associated with involvement of more and more neurons, in agreement with increased synchrony between neurons in the participating cortical regions. As a seizure approaches, the clustering of APs becomes more prominent, more regularly periodic, and more consistently associated with the ictal EEG waves as they increase in amplitude and duration.[52] Many neurons in the focus, as well as some in the surrounding area, fire synchronously with the surface sharp waves.[53]

2.3.8 Microelectrode Array Recordings: Microdischarges and Microseizures

Simultaneous recordings using both multichannel microelectrodes (to record APs of single neurons) and macroelectrode contacts (to record cortical local field potentials or intracranial EEG) have improved our understanding of how neuronal firing patterns participate in the generation of seizure activity. These recordings are typically performed in patients undergoing invasive video-EEG monitoring for possible resective surgery, using microwire arrays such as the 16 mm² Behnke–Fried microelectrode array (Adtech) that includes 96 microcontacts that are 400 μm apart at the distal end of a conventional depth electrode,[54] or the "Utah" array (Blackrock) with 10×10 1.2 mm long needle electrodes projecting from a 4.2 mm square silicon frame, minus electrodes at the corners.[54] These microelectrode arrays, with the ability to resolve single neuron firing patterns and local field potentials, are implanted along with more standard strip, grid, or depth electrodes with contacts spaced about 1 cm apart. "MicroEEG" signals recorded from within the putative epileptogenic zone typically demonstrate discharges resembling both interictal epileptiform activity ("micro-discharges") and electrographic seizures ("microseizures") that are confined to cortical regions as small as 200 μm^2.[55] Microdischarges consisted of focal sharp activity involving 1–18 microcontacts, which were not usually detected by intracranial EEG electrodes, though discharges seen across all microelectrode contacts simultaneously were highly correlated with interictal discharges recorded with the conventional intracranial EEG.[55] Microseizures consisted of runs of repetitive sharp waveforms or continuous rhythmic activity, evolving in frequency, amplitude, and morphology, the same properties that characterize electrographic seizures in conventional macroelectrode EEG recordings. Most microseizures did not have intracranial EEG or behavioral correlate and remained highly localized to specific contacts/regions of the microarray, and when seen at the same time as a macroscopic seizure event, were often asynchronous with macroscopic ictal discharges until near the end of the seizure.[55] These findings suggest that seizure onset may occur at an extremely fine circuit level, as small as individual cortical columns, with clinical seizures occurring when microseizures spread to involve nearby hyperexcitable or normal (non-epileptic) brain regions.

Microarray recordings of individual neuron activities are more difficult to interpret. Neuronal firing during seizure initiation and spread as well as during interictal discharges is highly heterogeneous; most recorded neurons do not change their firing rates throughout the entire seizure, including neurons located within the seizure-onset zone.[56] Increased neuronal synchrony does occur, primarily following seizure onset, with some neurons increasing their firing rates near seizure onset or interictal discharge, while others decrease firing. At the end of a seizure, most cells stop firing for 5 to 30 s, with a gradual return to normal firing rates.[51] For interictal discharges, changes in firing rate sometimes occur up to 300 ms prior to spike onset in the seizure focus. Some neurons increased firing rate during the spike and some decreased during the aftergoing slow wave, but most did not change firing rate. The heterogeneous behavior of individual neurons reinforces early findings that neuronal synchrony during seizures likely involves only a subset of "active" neurons (about 30%) with the rest being "inactive" or silent during seizure activity.[57] Thus, it appears unlikely that individual neuronal activities will be of high predictive value for spike and seizure detection unless they can be more explicitly identified.

2.3.9 High-Frequency Oscillations (HFOs)

As mentioned in our discussion above regarding spike-and-wave discharges, bursts of high to very high frequency EEG activity, well above the usual "Berger band" frequencies (delta, theta, alpha, beta, or about 0.5–25 Hz) can be recorded under appropriate conditions. Faster frequencies were first appreciated in intracranial recordings not limited by skull and scalp filtering.[58]* There is no clear consensus on the terminology for these frequencies, and

---

* High frequencies above 30 Hz were not observed in early recordings largely due to the limitations of the pen-and-ink recorders, which could not respond quickly enough to track high-frequency oscillations above 30 Hz or so (and at 30 Hz would appear as a solid smear of ink). When EEG recordings became digital in the 1990s, recording systems were designed to measure the frequencies that were routinely used to interpret clinical EEG; the presence of higher-frequency activity was felt to be primarily "noise" due to muscle activity or from other sources (e.g. 50–60 Hz power-line

investigators use different cut-off frequencies to define frequency bands with similar names. Frequencies above 30 and below 100–150 Hz (sometimes up to 400 Hz) are called gamma. There are "lumpers" and "splitters," with some papers dividing gamma into low-gamma (30–50 Hz), mid-gamma (50–90 Hz), and high-gamma (90–150 Hz),[60] while other authors do not use a mid-range (e.g. 50–150 Hz is high-gamma) or limit gamma to <80 Hz. Due to the low amplitude of these fast oscillations, they have also been labeled "ripples" (typically 80–200 Hz,[18] sometimes 150–250 Hz) and "fast ripples" (200–400 Hz, 250–600 Hz, or higher).[61] Others divide these spectra into gamma (30–100 Hz), "fast" (100–400 Hz), and "ultrafast" (400–800 Hz).[62] The lack of consensus can make comparisons between studies difficult. There is some agreement that the low end of these fast activities (below 200 Hz) are mostly normal physiological phenomena that are critically important for "percept binding" (linking of fragmentary sensory data into unified constructs), learning, and memory, since stimulation at high frequency can produce synaptic strengthening and enhance neuronal synchrony via long-term potentiation[63] and spike-timing-dependent plasticity.[64,65]

By contrast, the very HFOs (>400 Hz) appear to be a biomarker for epilepsy.[66–68] Bragin et al. identified HFOs (100–500 Hz, which they termed "fast ripples") in both epileptic patients and rats made epileptic by kindling or intrahippocampal kainate injection,[69] and postulated that these discharges were pathological and mechanistically associated with epilepsy. Evidence in favor of the concept of pathological HFOs (pHFOs) includes: (1) that they are found in epileptic animals only adjacent to the epileptogenic lesion in the lesioned hippocampus, EC, and DG, not on the contralateral side,[69] (2) that bursts of HFO activity are temporally associated with the onset of seizure activity in both animals[69] and humans,[70] (3) that they were not seen in rats that had an epileptogenic insult (status epilepticus) but do not develop spontaneous seizures,[69] (4) that in humans, pHFOs were specifically associated with regions that are involved in seizure activity at conventional EEG frequencies, and not seen in areas outside the "epileptic circuit,"[71] and (5) that in patients receiving epilepsy surgery, resection of areas in which pHFOs were recorded was associated with improved epilepsy outcome in both adults[72–75] and children.[76,77] It should be noted, however, that HFOs in the >250 Hz band are also seen in normal sensorimotor cortex, and hence are not always pathological,[78,79] and HFOs associated with epilepsy also occur in the sub-250 Hz frequency range[70,80] or faster than 600 Hz,[81] hence there is not a distinct band of purely pathological frequencies.

Several plausible mechanisms have been proposed for generating HFOs. It is clear that, unlike the electrical fields responsible for EEG in the Berger band frequencies, HFOs are not likely to be produced by the summation of EPSP currents, as most excitatory neurons do not fire at high enough frequency to account for oscillations at >200 Hz, which would require synchronized potentials lasting less than 5 ms. GABA$_A$ receptor-mediated IPSPs are much briefer than EPSPs, and GABAergic inhibitory neurons can sustain burst firing at frequencies up to 200 Hz or faster. HFOs may thus be generated by synchronized IPSPs

---

frequency). These systems typically digitized the signal at 200 Hz, and used low-pass filters to eliminate activity above 70 Hz. The Nyquist theorem states that frequency components can be represented accurately at half of the digital sampling rate, so frequency components above 100 Hz would not be accurately represented, and in the absence of filtering would instead appear as power at lower frequencies due to aliasing.[58] Modern commercial EEG equipment can digitize at up to 1000 Hz, though access to view higher frequencies may be limited by software. Research EEG amplifiers for studies of high-frequency oscillations can digitize at 10 kHz or higher per channel.

with sparse pyramidal cell firing,[19] or alternatively by highly synchronized AP discharges of populations of principal (excitatory) neurons,[81] which appear to be primarily responsible for the higher frequency ("pathological") HFOs.

A prime candidate for generating HFOs in the gamma to ripple range is the PVBCs.[20] Averkin et al.,[20] studying sleep spindle-associated HFOs in the rat hippocampal slice, found that HFOs at high-gamma and ripple frequencies associated with sharp wave-ripple events occurred at spindle troughs. The PVBCs fired at ripple (~200 Hz) and high-gamma (~120 Hz) frequencies in phase with spindle ripple and spindle high-gamma oscillations, respectively. Bursts were centered with millisecond precision at the troughs of spindle waves, in phase with field potential events. In contrast, pyramidal cells fired sporadically and phase shifted relative to the interneurons.

Bursts of APs would have to be highly synchronized to generate HFOs. Bragin et al.,[81] recording from DG granule neurons in pilocarpine-treated epileptic mice, found that these cells showed spontaneous high-frequency spiking that correlated with field potential HFOs at 100–500 Hz, suggesting that pHFOs represent a field of hypersynchronized APs of multiple granule neurons. Synchronization of fast firing within the population of interconnected neurons leads to the formation of an episode of high-frequency population spikes, which is extracellularly recorded as an HFO event. This mechanism requires synchronization on a millisecond time scale, which could be achieved via fast synaptic transmission (e.g., synchronization via basket cell IPSPs, as above), nonsynaptic mechanisms including gap-junction coupling[82,83] (possibly axo-axonal between principal neurons), or ephaptic interactions involving electrical fields and ion gradients between tightly packed parallel dendrites.[84] However, individual neurons cannot fire APs fast enough to account for the frequencies up to 600–800 Hz that have been observed. Possible physiological mechanisms[61] underlying such fast frequencies include out-of-phase firing of distinct neuronal populations due to loss of principal neurons, asymmetric excitatory inputs such that delayed activation of one set of neurons produces a functionally distinct population firing out of phase, functional clustering of neurons due to axonal growth or sprouting, as seen in the DG after chemically induced status epilepticus, or loss of synchrony resulting in pseudorandom firing that summates to a high-frequency field potential oscillation. The latter possibility seems less feasible since out-of-phase activity is more likely to result in phase cancellation, blurring of rhythms, and modulation of amplitude rather than highly synchronized fast oscillations (see Figures 2–7 in Greenfield et al.[85]). Inhibitory mechanisms are also possible for pHFOs. As noted above, PVBC IPSPs can summate to generate HFOs, or synchronize firing of their target principal neuron populations, but these mechanisms would account for oscillations mostly below 200 Hz. Loss of inhibitory interneurons resulting in either functional clustering of distinct populations, or asynchronous pseudorandom firing could theoretically result in higher-frequency pHFOs, as postulated for the excitatory neurons above.

HFOs are of increasing interest in patients with refractory epilepsy requiring intracranial recording as part of the work-up for epilepsy surgery, particularly as an indication of brain regions involved in epileptiform activity, since they can serve as a guide for tailoring the resection to increase the likelihood of a seizure-free outcome.[72,74–77] While it may be possible to record the oscillations in the lower end of the HFO spectrum (up to 200 Hz) with careful use of routine 10–20 scalp electrode placement and appropriate digitization and filtering techniques,[86,87] the significant challenges in recording, analysis, and interpretation prevent their routine use.

2.4 Circuits and Rhythms of Generalized Epilepsies

Until now, we have focused primarily on the mechanisms of focal epileptiform discharges and seizures. The generalized epilepsies are significantly different in both seizure semiology (with the exception of the generalized tonic–clonic seizures that are common to both focal and generalized epilepsies) and underlying pathophysiology. These disorders are primarily of genetic etiology, resulting from known or unknown mutations in ion channels, neurotransmitter receptors, or associated proteins involved in neurotransmission.

2.4.1 Absence Epilepsy and the Thalamocortical Circuit

The model disorder for generalized epilepsies is absence epilepsy, which presents in childhood with episodes of motor arrest and unresponsiveness without loss of tone, associated with the highly stereotyped generalized 3–4 Hz spike-and-wave discharges seen on EEG. The underlying mechanism of this highly rhythmic discharge involves the thalamocortical circuit that relays sensory afferent information to the associated primary cortical regions. This circuit is also responsible for the generation of sleep spindles, the 12–16 Hz oscillations that are characteristic of and define Stage II sleep. Sleep spindles and 3 Hz spike-and-wave have been recorded from the same patient, demonstrating that the circuit is capable of both behaviours in patients with absence epilepsy.[101] Major cell types involved in this circuit include thalamic relay neurons, inhibitory interneurons in the nucleus reticulans thalami, and layer VI cortical neurons.[102] Secondary sensory afferent fibers originating in the cuneate and gracile nuclei (joint position and vibration) and dorsal horn of the spinal cord (touch, pain, temperature) synapse onto thalamic relay neurons in the ventral posterolateral and other thalamic nuclei. Thalamic relay neurons in turn project to layer IV of sensory cortex. The relay neurons also send excitatory fibers to inhibitory neurons in the nucleus reticularis thalami (NRt), which provides reciprocal GABAergic inhibitory connections back onto the relay neurons. This circuit receives feedback excitatory input from layer VI cortical neurons that synapse onto both relay neurons and NRt cells.

The thalamocortical circuit is also modulated by subcortical inputs from a variety of structures, including acetylcholine from the pedunculopontine and laterodorsal tegmental nuclei, histamine from the tuberomammillary nucleus, serotonin from the dorsal raphe nuclei, and norepinephrine from the locus ceruleus. The combination of excitatory glutamatergic activity from the thalamic relay neurons and feedback inhibition from NRt and other GABAergic inhibitory interneurons creates the classic feedback loop essential for generating oscillatory rhythms. There is an additional feature that guarantees that this circuit will oscillate: the presence of low-threshold "T-type" calcium channels in both the relay and NRt neurons.[88–90] These channels open at relatively low depolarized potentials not far above the resting membrane potential, and require hyperpolarization below resting membrane potential to remove inactivation and "reset," which allows them to open again after they have depolarized, opened, and inactivated. The consequence of this biophysical behavior is that they open rapidly as neurons are recovering from hyperpolarization induced by GABAergic inhibition and produce bursts of APs. This creates a strong oscillatory rhythm between the thalamic neurons and NRt neurons, which is then projected by the relay neurons into the overlying cortex.

What is less well understood is how the same circuit is able to generate both the normal 12–16 Hz spindle activity in sleep and the pathological 3 Hz spike-and-wave pattern seen in absence epilepsy. The amplitude and cortical extent of oscillation appear to depend in part on the level of synchrony between relay neurons and NRt neurons, which is regulated by both gap junctions (promoting synchronization) and the degree of cross-inhibition between thalamic reticular neurons (promoting desynchronization).[91] The transition from spindle frequencies to 3 Hz spike-and-wave appears to be related to the type and weight of inhibition from which T-type calcium channel-induced bursting arises. $GABA_A$-receptor-mediated inhibition is both rapid onset and rapidly desensitizing, with postsynaptic potentials lasting 60–90 ms, consistent with the 11–16 Hz frequency of spindle activity, since the frequency of a repetitive discharge will be the inverse of the wave duration. Similarly, metabotropic $GABA_B$ receptor potentials are slower in onset and last around 300 ms, precisely the duration needed for 3 Hz spike-and-wave.[92] In thalamic slice recordings, blocking the fast $GABA_A$ inhibition with bicuculline allows $GABA_B$ currents to predominate, and shifts the frequency of thalamic neuron oscillation from spindle-like 6–10 Hz to 3 Hz, while the slow 3 Hz oscillations are blocked by a $GABA_B$ receptor antagonist.[93] This switch appears to be mediated by cortical hyperexcitability, as changing the corticothalamic input from single stimuli to bursts altered the frequency of thalamic slice activity. Bursts of mock cortical activity switched the slice oscillation from $GABA_A$-mediated spindle waves, with low amounts of burst firing in thalamic neurons, to 3- to 4-Hz $GABA_B$-mediated paroxysms with sustained burst firing in both thalamocortical and GABAergic perigeniculate cells.[94] The precise mechanisms responsible for controlling the frequency and extent of thalamocortical circuit oscillations remain unknown.

The relevance of the thalamocortical circuit to absence epilepsy is further supported by the presence of disease-associated mutations in relevant $GABA_A$ receptor and T-type calcium channel genes. Mutations in the $GABA_A$ receptor γ2 subunit,[95] the CaV2.1 subunit of P/Q-type (presynaptic) voltage-gated calcium channels,[96,97] and the CaV3.2 subunit of T-type calcium channels[98,99] have all been related to childhood absence epilepsy, while no epilepsy-related mutations have been found in two other T-type low-threshold calcium channels, CaV3.1 and CaV3.3.[89] CaV3.1 is expressed in thalamic relay neurons, while CaV3.2 (which has disease-associated mutations) and CaV3.3 are expressed in NRt neurons. This suggests that the NRt cells may play an important role in human absence epilepsy.[89] Ethosuximide, which prevents absence but not generalized tonic–clonic seizures, is a blocker of T-type calcium channels, confirming the pathophysiologic role of this channel and establishing it as a therapeutic target for absence epilepsy. In mice, a variety of mutations in P/Q calcium channels produce animals with (homozygous) phenotypes known as *totterer, leaner, stargazer,* and *lethargic,* all of which have spells of sudden freezing of behavior associated with 5–7 Hz rhythmic spiky discharges that are felt to be the mouse version of the 3 Hz spike-and-wave discharges seen in human absence epilepsy.[89] In humans, however, the genetics of childhood absence epilepsy are complex. There is a 16–45% positive family history in childhood absence epilepsy patients, but penetrance is incomplete, with concordances of 70–85% in monozygotic twins and 33% in first-degree relatives.[100]

2.4.2 Myoclonus and Juvenile Myoclonic Epilepsy

The relationship between myoclonic jerks and cortical spike-and-wave discharges is fraught with difficulties. Myoclonus as a behavior is sometimes categorized as a seizure type, at other times as a movement disorder, depending on the clinical setting.[101] Acute posthypoxic myoclonus is semiperiodic in character, and shows generalized spikes or polyspikes associated with jerks, which can be triggered by sensory stimuli (loud clap, pain, etc.). They likely reflect diffuse cortical injury with loss of inhibition and resulting cortical hyperexcitability, though their generation appears to involve brainstem mechanisms. Complicating the issue, the jerks themselves generate spiky-appearing artifacts, which can be misinterpreted as cortical spikes. This issue can be clarified using short-acting paralytic agents (when the patient is intubated and on a ventilator!) to eliminate the motor/movement artifact component. Chronic posthypoxic myoclonus, known as Lance–Adams syndrome, is a movement disorder in which volitional actions trigger superimposed myoclonic jerks. When jerks occur in the context of seizures, as with juvenile myoclonic epilepsy (JME) or the progressive myoclonic epilepsies, myoclonus is associated with cortical epileptic spike-and-wave or polyspike-and-wave discharges.

JME, which presents in late adolescence with myoclonic jerks and generalized tonic–clonic seizures, is one of the most common and best-studied genetic epilepsies, and understanding the genetic defects can be instructive regarding the underlying pathophysiology. The genetic linkages for JME in affected families include mutations or deletions in: *CACNB4* (the β4 subunit of a voltage-gated calcium channel, the same gene associated with the *lethargic* mouse),[102] *CASR* (an extracellular calcium-sensing G-protein-coupled receptor),[103] *EFC1* (EF-hand domain [C-terminal] containing a calcium-binding protein that increases R-type $Ca_V2.3$ calcium currents,[104] also known as Myoclonin1),[104,105] *GABRA1* (α1 subunit of the $GABA_A$ receptor, found in benzodiazepine-sensitive synaptic $GABA_A$ receptors),[106] and *GABRD* (δ subunit of the $GABA_A$ receptor, found in benzodiazepine-insensitive extrasynaptic $GABA_A$ receptors).[107] The multiplicity of genetic defects that can result in the characteristic JME phenotype and its EEG signature of fast spike-and-wave and polyspike-wave discharges makes it unclear whether mutations alter cortical excitability diffusely, or with particular emphasis on the thalamocortical circuit.

2.4.3 Polyspikes and Generalized Paroxysmal Fast Activity (GPFA)

Polyspikes can be seen as the initial burst of spiky activity associated with the fast (>3 Hz) generalized spike-and-wave discharges seen in generalized epilepsies such as JME. A sustained form of frontally dominant polyspike discharge known as generalized paroxysmal fast activity (GPFA) with discharges at 8–26 Hz (peak frequencies at 12–14 Hz and 22–24 Hz) is generally associated with the tonic seizures seen in epileptic encephalopathies such as Lennox–Gastaut syndrome, but can also be seen in patients with normal cognition and presumed genetic epilepsies.[108]

To explore the physiology underlying fast bursts of spike-and-wave discharges in the generalized epilepsies, Steriade's group (Timofeev et al.)[109] recorded intracellularly from both thalamic reticular neurons and thalamocortical relay cells *in vivo* in cats administered the $GABA_A$ receptor antagonist, bicuculline. Both NRt neurons and thalamocortical relay neurons were hyperpolarized during seizure episodes associated with spike-and-wave or polyspike-wave complexes and relatively depolarized during runs of paroxysmal fast (10–15 Hz) activity suggestive of GPFA. Consistent with the concept that hyperpolarization of thalamic neurons inactivates the low-threshold T-type calcium channel thought to generate high-frequency bursts of spikes, NRt neurons discharged prolonged high-frequency spike bursts synchronously with the spiky component of cortical spike- or polyspike-wave complexes. During the runs of paroxysmal fast activity, they fired single APs, spike doublets, or triplets. In thalamocortical relay cells, the cortical fast runs correlated with EPSPs appearing after short latencies that were compatible with monosynaptic activation through corticothalamic pathways. These data suggest that spike-and-wave, polyspike-wave, and GPFA seizures in this model are of cortical origin. This was confirmed by recording from isolated cortical slabs, in which electrical stimulation within the slab induced seizures with paroxysmal fast runs and spike- and polyspike-wave complexes that were virtually identical to those elicited in animals with intact thalamocortical connections. Hence, generalized seizure patterns induced by blockade of $GABA_A$-mediated inhibition, including spike-and-wave, polyspike-and-wave, and paroxysmal fast activity are all likely generated in the neocortex.

The hyperexcitability of neocortex in the generalized epilepsies may explain the relatively high prevalence of photoparoxysmal responses (about 30% of JME patients).[110] Flash or checkerboard stimulation synchronously and rhythmically activates large portions of primary visual cortex via the massive optic radiations from the lateral geniculate nucleus (visual thalamus), and can trigger either myoclonus or generalized convulsions. By analogy, the synchronizing activity of somatosensory thalamocortical rhythms in sleep may play a similar role in triggering seizure activity in patients with excessive cortical excitability.

The precise physiological effects of epilepsy-associated mutations depend on what brain regions, and which cell types within those regions, express the altered channel subunits or related proteins. While animal models with diffuse disinhibition show cortical hyperexcitability and the ability to sustain seizures independently from the thalamus, it is also plausible that polyspikes may represent a hypersynchronized thalamocortical rhythm generated by the same circuit as sleep spindles and the 3 Hz spike-and-wave discharges seen in absence epilepsy. Indeed, the faster 3–6 Hz periodicity of JME spike-and-wave discharges suggests a tendency toward more rapid cycling of this oscillator. The common observation that both myoclonic and generalized tonic–clonic seizures in JME tend to occur in the early morning and increase with sleep deprivation are features that suggest association with sleep mechanisms and thalamocortical rhythms. Unfortunately (for us but not the patients), the fact that JME is often well-controlled with medication and not readily susceptible to surgical approaches, means that we have few opportunities to study the physiology of human generalized epilepsies using intracranial recordings. However, as more of the genes associated with generalized epilepsies are discovered, animal models incorporating these genes will continue to reveal in ever greater detail the molecular and physiological mechanisms responsible for these syndromes.

References

1. Gewirtz P. On "I know it when I see it". *The Yale Law Journal*. 1996;105(4):1023.

2. Buzsaki G. *Rhythms of the Brain*. Oxford: Oxford University Press; 2006.

3. Grundfest H, Purpura DP. Nature of dendritic potentials and synaptic mechanisms in cerebral cortex of cat. *J Neurophysiol*. 1956;19(6):573–595.

4. Li CL, Jasper H. Microelectrode studies of the electrical activity of the cerebral cortex in the cat. *J Physiol*. 1953;121(1):117–140.

5. Hughes SW, Crunelli V. Thalamic mechanisms of EEG alpha rhythms and their pathological implications. *Neuroscientist*. 2005;11(4):357–372.

6. van Strien NM, Cappaert NL, Witter MP. The anatomy of memory: an interactive overview of the parahippocampal-hippocampal network. *Nat Rev Neurosci*. 2009;10(4):272–282.

7. Heinemann U, Beck H, Dreier JP, et al. The dentate gyrus as a regulated gate for the propagation of epileptiform activity. *Epilepsy Res Suppl*. 1992;7:273–280.

8. Lothman EW, Stringer JL, Bertram EH. The dentate gyrus as a control point for seizures in the hippocampus and beyond. *Epilepsy Res Suppl*. 1992;7:301–313.

9. Krook-Magnuson E, Armstrong C, Bui A, et al. In vivo evaluation of the dentate gate theory in epilepsy. *J Physiol.* 2015;593 (10):2379–2388.

10. Liu YQ, Yu F, Liu WH, He XH, Peng BW. Dysfunction of hippocampal interneurons in epilepsy. *Neurosci Bull.* 2014;30 (6):985–998.

11. Buzsaki G. Theta oscillations in the hippocampus. *Neuron.* 2002;33 (3):325–340.

12. Allen K, Monyer H. Interneuron control of hippocampal oscillations. *Curr Opin Neurobiol.* 2015;31:81–87.

13. Lever C, Wills T, Cacucci F, Burgess N, O'Keefe J. Long-term plasticity in hippocampal place-cell representation of environmental geometry. *Nature.* 2002;416 (6876):90–94.

14. Moser EI, Paulsen O. New excitement in cognitive space: between place cells and spatial memory. *Curr Opin Neurobiol.* 2001;11(6):745–751.

15. Zhang SJ, Ye J, Miao C, et al. Optogenetic dissection of entorhinal-hippocampal functional connectivity. *Science.* 2013;340 (6128):1232627.

16. Csicsvari J, Dupret D. Sharp wave/ripple network oscillations and learning-associated hippocampal maps. *Philos Trans R Soc Lond B Biol Sci.* 2014;369 (1635):20120528.

17. Buzsaki G. Hippocampal sharp wave-ripple: a cognitive biomarker for episodic memory and planning. *Hippocampus.* 2015;25(10):1073–1188.

18. Buzsaki G, Horvath Z, Urioste R, Hetke J, Wise K. High-frequency network oscillation in the hippocampus. *Science.* 1992;256(5059):1025–1027.

19. Ylinen A, Bragin A, Nadasdy Z, et al. Sharp wave-associated high-frequency oscillation (200 Hz) in the intact hippocampus: network and intracellular mechanisms. *J Neurosci.* 1995;15(1 Pt 1):30–46.

20. Averkin RG, Szemenyei V, Borde S, Tamas G. Identified cellular correlates of neocortical ripple and high-gamma oscillations during spindles of natural sleep. *Neuron.* 2016;92(4):916–928.

21. Jadhav SP, Kemere C, German PW, Frank LM. Awake hippocampal sharp-wave ripples support spatial memory. *Science.* 2012;336(6087):1454–1458.

22. Ayala GF, Matsumoto H, Gumnit RJ. Excitability changes and inhibitory mechanisms in neocortical neurons during seizures. *J Neurophysiol.* 1970;33(1):73–85.

23. McCormick DA, Contreras D. On the cellular and network bases of epileptic seizures. *Annu Rev Physiol.* 2001;63(1):815–846.

24. Johnston D, Brown TH. The synaptic nature of the paroxysmal depolarizing shift in hippocampal neurons. *Ann Neurol.* 1984;16 (Suppl):S65–71.

25. Ayala GF. The paroxysmal depolarizing shift. *Prog Clin Biol Res.* 1983;124:15–21.

26. Witte OW. Physiological basis of pathophysiological brain rhythms. *Acta Neurobiol Exp (Wars).* 2000;60(2):289–297.

27. Cooper R, Winter AL, Crow HJ, Walter WG. Comparison of subcortical, cortical and scalp activity using chronically indwelling electrodes in man. *Electroencephalogr Clin Neurophysiol.* 1965;18:217–228.

28. Tao JX, Baldwin M, Hawes-Ebersole S, Ebersole JS. Cortical substrates of scalp EEG epileptiform discharges. *J Clin Neurophysiol.* 2007;24(2):96–100.

29. Reiher J, Beaudry M, Leduc CP. Temporal intermittent rhythmic delta activity (TIRDA) in the diagnosis of complex partial epilepsy: sensitivity, specificity and predictive value. *Can J Neurol Sci.* 1989;16 (4):398–401.

30. Normand MM, Wszolek ZK, Klass DW. Temporal intermittent rhythmic delta activity in electroencephalograms. *J Clin Neurophysiol.* 1995;12(3):280–284.

31. Di Gennaro G, Quarato PP, Onorati P, et al. Localizing significance of temporal intermittent rhythmic delta activity (TIRDA) in drug-resistant focal epilepsy. *Clin Neurophysiol.* 2003;114(1):70–78.

32. Gullapalli D, Fountain NB. Clinical correlation of occipital intermittent rhythmic delta activity. *J Clin Neurophysiol.* 2003;20(1):35–41.

33. Watemberg N, Linder I, Dabby R, Blumkin L, Lerman-Sagie T. Clinical correlates of occipital intermittent rhythmic delta activity (OIRDA) in children. *Epilepsia.* 2007;48(2):330–334.

34. Accolla EA, Kaplan PW, Maeder-Ingvar M, Jukopila S, Rossetti AO. Clinical correlates of frontal intermittent rhythmic delta activity (FIRDA). *Clin Neurophysiol.* 2011;122(1):27–31.

35. Brigo F. Intermittent rhythmic delta activity patterns. *Epilepsy Behav.* 2011;20 (2):254–256.

36. Westmoreland BF, Klass DW, Sharbrough FW. Chronic periodic lateralized epileptiform discharges. *Arch Neurol.* 1986;43(5):494–496.

37. Sen-Gupta I, Schuele SU, Macken MP, Kwasny MJ, Gerard EE. "Ictal" lateralized periodic discharges. *Epilepsy Behav.* 2014;36:165–170.

38. Ali II, Pirzada NA, Vaughn BV. Periodic lateralized epileptiform discharges after complex partial status epilepticus associated with increased focal cerebral blood flow. *J Clin Neurophysiol.* 2001;18 (6):565–569.

39. Garzon E, Fernandes RM, Sakamoto AC. Serial EEG during human status epilepticus: evidence for PLED as an ictal pattern. *Neurology.* 2001;57(7):1175–1183.

40. Hirsch LJ, LaRoche SM, Gaspard N, et al. American Clinical Neurophysiology Society's standardized critical care EEG terminology: 2012 version. *J Clin Neurophysiol.* 2013;30(1):1–27.

41. Fisch BJ, Klass DW. The diagnostic specificity of triphasic wave patterns. *Electroencephalogr Clin Neurophysiol.* 1988;70(1):1–8.

42. van Putten MJ, Hofmeijer J. Generalized periodic discharges: pathophysiology and clinical considerations. *Epilepsy Behav.* 2015;49:228–233.

43. Tjepkema-Cloostermans MC, Hindriks R, Hofmeijer J, van Putten MJ. Generalized periodic discharges after acute cerebral ischemia: reflection of selective synaptic failure? *Clin Neurophysiol.* 2014;125 (2):255–262.

44. San-Juan OD, Chiappa KH, Costello DJ, Cole AJ. Periodic epileptiform discharges in hypoxic encephalopathy: BiPLEDs and GPEDs as a poor prognosis for survival. *Seizure.* 2009;18(5):365–368.

45. Racine RJ. Modification of seizure activity by electrical stimulation. II. Motor seizure. *Electroencephalogr Clin Neurophysiol.* 1972;32(3):281–294.

46. de Curtis M, Gnatkovsky V. Reevaluating the mechanisms of focal ictogenesis: the role of low-voltage fast activity. *Epilepsia.* 2009;50(12):2514–2525.

47. Wendling F, Bartolomei F, Bellanger JJ, Bourien J, Chauvel P. Epileptic fast intracerebral EEG activity: evidence for spatial decorrelation at seizure onset. *Brain.* 2003;126(Pt 6):1449–1459.

48. Timofeev I, Steriade M. Neocortical seizures: initiation, development and cessation. *Neuroscience.* 2004;123 (2):299–336.

49. Jiruska P, de Curtis M, Jefferys JG, et al. Synchronization and desynchronization in epilepsy: controversies and hypotheses. *J Physiol.* 2013;591(4):787–797.

50. Ward AA, Thomas LB. The electrical activity of single units in the cerebral cortex of man. *Electroencephalogr Clin Neurophysiol.* 1955;7(1):135–136.

51. Tankus A. Exploring human epileptic activity at the single-neuron level. *Epilepsy Behav.* 2016;58:11–17.

52. Verzeano M, Crandall PH, Dymond A. Neuronal activity of the amygdala in patients with psychomotor epilepsy. *Neuropsychologia.* 1971;9(3):331–344.

53. Ishijima B, Hori T, Yoshimasu N, Fukushima T, Hirakawa K. Neuronal activities in human epileptic foci and surrounding areas. *Electroencephalogr Clin Neurophysiol.* 1975;39(6):643–650.

54. Fried I, Wilson CL, Maidment NT, et al. Cerebral microdialysis combined with single-neuron and electroencephalographic recording in neurosurgical patients: technical note. *J Neurosurg.* 1999;91 (4):697–705.

55. Schevon CA, Ng SK, Cappell J, et al. Microphysiology of epileptiform activity in

human neocortex. *J Clin Neurophysiol.* 2008;25(6):321–330.

56. Bower MR, Stead M, Meyer FB, Marsh WR, Worrell GA. Spatiotemporal neuronal correlates of seizure generation in focal epilepsy. *Epilepsia.* 2012;53(5):807–816.

57. Matsumoto H, Marsan CA. Cortical cellular phenomena in experimental epilepsy: interictal manifestations. *Exp Neurol.* 1964;9(4):286–304.

58. Chatrian GE, Bickford RG, Uihlein A. Depth electrographic study of a fast rhythm evoked from the human calcarine region by steady illumination. *Electroencephalogr Clin Neurophysiol.* 1960;12(1):167–176.

59. Weiergraber M, Papazoglou A, Broich K, Muller R. Sampling rate, signal bandwidth and related pitfalls in EEG analysis. *J Neurosci Methods.* 2016;268:53–55.

60. Belluscio MA, Mizuseki K, Schmidt R, Kempter R, Buzsaki G. Cross-frequency phase-phase coupling between theta and gamma oscillations in the hippocampus. *J Neurosci.* 2012;32(2):423–435.

61. Jiruska P, Alvarado-Rojas C, Schevon CA, et al. Update on the mechanisms and roles of high-frequency oscillations in seizures and epileptic disorders. *Epilepsia.* 2017;58 (8):1330–1339.

62. Hughes JR. Gamma, fast, and ultrafast waves of the brain: their relationships with epilepsy and behavior. *Epilepsy Behav.* 2008;13(1):25–31.

63. Axmacher N, Mormann F, Fernandez G, Elger CE, Fell J. Memory formation by neuronal synchronization. *Brain Res Rev.* 2006;52(1):170–182.

64. Levy WB, Steward O. Temporal contiguity requirements for long-term associative potentiation/depression in the hippocampus. *Neuroscience.* 1983;8 (4):791–797.

65. Dan Y, Poo MM. Spike timing-dependent plasticity: from synapse to perception. *Physiol Rev.* 2006;86(3):1033–1048.

66. Staba RJ. Normal and pathological high-frequency oscillations. In: Noebels JL, Avoli M, Rogawski MA, Olsen RW, Delgado-Escueta AV, eds., *Jasper's Basic Mechanisms of the Epilepsies.* Oxford: Oxford University Press; 2012:202–212.

67. Frauscher B, Bartolomei F, Kobayashi K, et al. High-frequency oscillations: the state of clinical research. *Epilepsia.* 2017;58 (8):1316–1329.

68. Brazdil M, Pail M, Halamek J, et al. Very high-frequency oscillations: novel biomarkers of the epileptogenic zone. *Ann Neurol.* 2017;82(2):299–310.

69. Bragin A, Engel J, Jr., Wilson CL, Fried I, Mathern GW. Hippocampal and entorhinal cortex high-frequency oscillations (100–500 Hz) in human epileptic brain and in kainic acid-treated rats with chronic seizures. *Epilepsia.* 1999;40(2):127–137.

70. Fisher RS, Webber WR, Lesser RP, Arroyo S, Uematsu S. High-frequency EEG activity at the start of seizures. *J Clin Neurophysiol.* 1992;9(3):441–448.

71. Bragin A, Wilson CL, Staba RJ, et al. Interictal high-frequency oscillations (80–500 Hz) in the human epileptic brain: entorhinal cortex. *Ann Neurol.* 2002;52 (4):407–415.

72. Jacobs J, Zijlmans M, Zelmann R, et al. High-frequency electroencephalographic oscillations correlate with outcome of epilepsy surgery. *Ann Neurol.* 2010;67 (2):209–220.

73. Haegelen C, Perucca P, Chatillon CE, et al. High-frequency oscillations, extent of surgical resection, and surgical outcome in drug-resistant focal epilepsy. *Epilepsia.* 2013;54(5):848–857.

74. Fedele T, Burnos S, Boran E, et al. Resection of high frequency oscillations predicts seizure outcome in the individual patient. *Sci Rep.* 2017;7(1):13836.

75. Holler Y, Kutil R, Klaffenbock L, et al. High-frequency oscillations in epilepsy and surgical outcome: a meta-analysis. *Front Hum Neurosci.* 2015;9:574.

76. Akiyama T, McCoy B, Go CY, et al. Focal resection of fast ripples on extraoperative intracranial EEG improves seizure outcome in pediatric epilepsy. *Epilepsia.* 2011;52 (10):1802–1811.

77. Fujiwara H, Leach JL, Greiner HM, et al. Resection of ictal high frequency

oscillations is associated with favorable surgical outcome in pediatric drug resistant epilepsy secondary to tuberous sclerosis complex. *Epilepsy Res.* 2016;126:90–97.

78. Jones MS, Barth DS. Spatiotemporal organization of fast (>200 Hz) electrical oscillations in rat Vibrissa/Barrel cortex. *J Neurophysiol.* 1999;82 (3):1599–1609.

79. Kandel A, Buzsaki G. Cellular-synaptic generation of sleep spindles, spike-and-wave discharges, and evoked thalamocortical responses in the neocortex of the rat. *J Neurosci.* 1997;17 (17):6783–6797.

80. Worrell GA, Parish L, Cranstoun SD, et al. High-frequency oscillations and seizure generation in neocortical epilepsy. *Brain.* 2004;127(Pt 7):1496–1506.

81. Bragin A, Benassi SK, Kheiri F, Engel J, Jr. Further evidence that pathologic high-frequency oscillations are bursts of population spikes derived from recordings of identified cells in dentate gyrus. *Epilepsia.* 2011;52(1):45–52.

82. Draguhn A, Traub RD, Schmitz D, Jefferys JG. Electrical coupling underlies high-frequency oscillations in the hippocampus in vitro. *Nature.* 1998;394(6689):189–192.

83. Traub RD, Draguhn A, Whittington MA, et al. Axonal gap junctions between principal neurons: a novel source of network oscillations, and perhaps epileptogenesis. *Rev Neurosci.* 2002;13 (1):1–30.

84. Jefferys JG. Nonsynaptic modulation of neuronal activity in the brain: electric currents and extracellular ions. *Physiol Rev.* 1995;75(4):689–723.

85. Greenfield LJ, Geyer JD, Carney PR. *Reading EEGs: A Practical Approach.* Philadelphia: Lippincott Williams & Wilkins; 2010.

86. Andrade-Valenca LP, Dubeau F, Mari F, Zelmann R, Gotman J. Interictal scalp fast oscillations as a marker of the seizure onset zone. *Neurology.* 2011;77(6):524–531.

87. von Ellenrieder N, Andrade-Valenca LP, Dubeau F, Gotman J. Automatic detection of fast oscillations (40–200 Hz) in scalp EEG recordings. *Clin Neurophysiol.* 2012;123(4):670–680.

88. Chen Y, Parker WD, Wang K. The role of T-type calcium channel genes in absence seizures. *Front Neurol.* 2014;5:45.

89. Cheong E, Shin HS. T-type Ca2+ channels in absence epilepsy. *Pflugers Arch.* 2014;466 (4):719–734.

90. Cain SM, Snutch TP. T-type calcium channels in burst-firing, network synchrony, and epilepsy. *Biochim Biophys Acta.* 2013;1828(7):1572–1578.

91. Bal T, McCormick DA. What stops synchronized thalamocortical oscillations? *Neuron.* 1996;17(2):297–308.

92. Blumenfeld H. From molecules to networks: cortical/subcortical interactions in the pathophysiology of idiopathic generalized epilepsy. *Epilepsia.* 2003;44 (Suppl 2):7–15.

93. Kim U, Sanchez-Vives MV, McCormick DA. Functional dynamics of GABAergic inhibition in the thalamus. *Science.* 1997;278(5335):130–134.

94. Blumenfeld H, McCormick DA. Corticothalamic inputs control the pattern of activity generated in thalamocortical networks. *J Neurosci.* 2000;20 (13):5153–5162.

95. Kang JQ, Macdonald RL. The GABAA receptor gamma2 subunit R43Q mutation linked to childhood absence epilepsy and febrile seizures causes retention of alpha1beta2gamma2S receptors in the endoplasmic reticulum. *J Neurosci.* 2004;24 (40):8672–8677.

96. Imbrici P, Jaffe SL, Eunson LH, et al. Dysfunction of the brain calcium channel CaV2.1 in absence epilepsy and episodic ataxia. *Brain.* 2004;127(Pt 12):2682–2692.

97. Jouvenceau A, Eunson LH, Spauschus A, et al. Human epilepsy associated with dysfunction of the brain P/Q-type calcium channel. *Lancet.* 2001;358(9284):801–807.

98. Liang J, Zhang Y, Wang J, et al. New variants in the CACNA1H gene identified in childhood absence epilepsy. *Neurosci Lett.* 2006;406(1–2):27–32.

99. Chen Y, Lu J, Pan H, et al. Association between genetic variation of CACNA1H and childhood absence epilepsy. *Ann Neurol.* 2003;54(2): 239–243.

100. Crunelli V, Leresche N. Childhood absence epilepsy: genes, channels, neurons and networks. *Nat Rev Neurosci.* 2002;3 (5):371–382.

101. Hallett M. Physiology of human posthypoxic myoclonus. *Mov Disord.* 2000;15(Suppl 1):8–13.

102. Escayg A, De Waard M, Lee DD, et al. Coding and noncoding variation of the human calcium-channel beta4-subunit gene CACNB4 in patients with idiopathic generalized epilepsy and episodic ataxia. *Am J Hum Genet.* 2000;66 (5):1531–1539.

103. Kapoor A, Satishchandra P, Ratnapriya R, et al. An idiopathic epilepsy syndrome linked to 3q13.3-q21 and missense mutations in the extracellular calcium sensing receptor gene. *Ann Neurol.* 2008;64 (2):158–167.

104. Suzuki T, Delgado-Escueta AV, Aguan K, et al. Mutations in EFHC1 cause juvenile myoclonic epilepsy. *Nat Genet.* 2004;36 (8):842–849.

105. Medina MT, Suzuki T, Alonso ME, et al. Novel mutations in Myoclonin1/EFHC1 in sporadic and familial juvenile myoclonic epilepsy. *Neurology.* 2008;70(22 Pt 2):2137–2144.

106. Cossette P, Liu L, Brisebois K, et al. Mutation of GABRA1 in an autosomal dominant form of juvenile myoclonic epilepsy. *Nat Genet.* 2002;31(2):184–189.

107. Dibbens LM, Feng HJ, Richards MC, et al. GABRD encoding a protein for extra- or peri-synaptic GABAA receptors is a susceptibility locus for generalized epilepsies. *Hum Mol Genet.* 2004;13 (13):1315–1319.

108. Halasz P, Janszky J, Barcs G, Szucs A. Generalised paroxysmal fast activity (GPFA) is not always a sign of malignant epileptic encephalopathy. *Seizure.* 2004;13 (4):270–276.

109. Timofeev I, Grenier F, Steriade M. Spike-wave complexes and fast components of cortically generated seizures. IV. Paroxysmal fast runs in cortical and thalamic neurons. *J Neurophysiol.* 1998;80 (3):1495–1513.

110. Poleon S, Szaflarski JP. Photosensitivity in generalized epilepsies. *Epilepsy Behav.* 2017;68:225–233.

Chapter 3

Pathology of the Epilepsies

Kamal Shouman and William J. Kupsky

3.1 Introduction

The pathology of epilepsy is a complex and evolving field, reflecting both rapid developments in diagnostic and therapeutic techniques, and the continued difficulties in translating electrical and functional phenomena into traditional categories of morphological disease. A seizure is an acute neurological event due to sudden excessive disorderly discharge of neurons.[1] Lesions that are presumed to cause seizures can be either structural, definable by morphological techniques such as radiology and anatomic pathology, or functional, definable by clinical localization, electrophysiology, and, in some cases, functional imaging defining a focus. Causality is inferred by correlation of morphological findings and location with clinical and electrophysiological data and, in some cases, by the cessation of subsequent seizures after removal of the lesion or focus. Epilepsy is intermittent recurrence of seizures. The finding of structural lesions in some forms of epilepsy suggests and supports causality, but our understanding of the chain between the definable structural lesion and the recurrence of seizures is often less clear.[2] Causality may be particularly difficult to determine in conditions producing multiple structural lesions such as tuberous sclerosis, where one lesion is epileptogenic and other similar lesions are not. Even determining how a particular electrically active focus propagates to evolve into a particular seizure or series of intractable seizures is also incompletely understood. To add to the difficulty, seizures or epilepsy itself can be causal, resulting in progressive brain damage and self-perpetuating seizures, particularly in some forms of temporal lobe epilepsy. Moreover, some treatments for epilepsy themselves have been associated with some forms of brain damage.

Morphologic understanding of the pathology associated with some forms of seizure and epilepsy has come about both through postmortem brain examination and through examination of brain tissues removed at surgery. Advances in neurosurgical technique, coupled with a multidisciplinary approach to evaluation of patients with epilepsy, have led to increasing acquaintance and understanding of various pathological lesions associated with seizures. Types of neurosurgical intervention include classic temporal lobectomy with hippocampectomy for intractable temporal lobe epilepsy, resections of discrete epileptogenic lesions such as tubers and certain types of tumor, and resections of large parts of single or multiple lobes (partial lobectomy or lobectomy) and subtotal or total hemispherectomy for some conditions involving large portions of brain.

Temporal lobectomy with hippocampectomy is used in pediatric and adult populations for treatment of intractable temporal lobe epilepsies. The specimen may include portions of inferolateral normal temporal lobe in addition to the anterior hippocampus. Resection of seizure foci, with or without a well-defined structural lesion is used both in the setting of localizable seizures as well as in some cases of chronic intractable epilepsy. Examples of focal lesions include glial or fibrous scars, malformative lesions such as cortical dysplasias or single tubers, localized Sturge–Weber, vascular malformations, and tumors. Subtotal or total lobectomy can be performed when more extensive pathology or seizure activity is present. Subtotal or total hemispherectomy has been used in some conditions such as Rasmussen encephalitis and hemimegalencephaly or in the presence of widespread malformative or genetic lesions such as tuberous sclerosis and diffuse Sturge–Weber. Functional hemispherectomy or hemispherotomy, however, is replacing anatomic hemispherectomy in many centers.[3] Brain biopsy for diagnosis has also proven useful in some cases of autoimmune encephalitis.

3.2 Techniques for Handling Tissues Resected for Diagnosis or Treatment of Epilepsy

Standard pathological techniques for examination of brain specimens are also applicable to the study of pathology in epilepsy and include examination of formalin-fixed, paraffin-embedded tissues. Important in the evaluation are properly fixed and processed tissues and the ability to orient the specimen and identify the area of epileptogenic interest.[4] Proper orientation and fixation require a container large enough to allow the specimen to remain undistorted and to supply an adequate volume of fixative for the size of the specimen. Large specimens such as lobectomies or hemispherectomies also require adequate duration of fixation to achieve proper tissue preservation. Orientation of the specimen by the surgeon or member of the epilepsy team is essential to correlate areas of epileptogenic activity or epileptic spread with morphological findings. In two-stage surgeries, a diagram of grid electrode activity obtained during the intraoperative recording stage (stage 1) can be provided to guide sampling during the dissection of the resected specimen (stage 2).

In addition to routine hematoxylin and eosin staining of formalin-fixed paraffin-embedded tissue, traditional neuropathological stains such as cresyl violet, Luxol fast blue, and Bielschowsky can be supplemented with a variety of immunohistochemical stains. In our laboratory, commonly employed immunostains included glial fibrillary acidic protein (GFAP), NeuN, phosphorylated neurofilament protein (NFP), synaptophysin, and CD68. GFAP staining is useful in highlighting gliosis. NeuN has largely replaced cresyl violet in demonstrating cerebral cortical architecture. In addition to highlighting axons and axonal architecture, NFP staining assists in identifying dysplastic neurons. Synaptophysin staining of neuropil is useful in assessing structural abnormalities of gray matter such as heterotopias, and CD68, along with other leukocyte markers, helps in highlighting areas of tissue damage or inflammation. Other antibodies useful in particular cases include CD34, useful to assess vascular architecture or to demonstrate the presence of some forms of immature neuroglial cell, and anti-alphaB-crystallin, an astrocytic protein overexpressed in some pathological settings such as balloon cells (see below).

Although formalin-fixed tissues are still the mainstay of diagnosis, banked frozen tissues for adjunct morphological studies or for subsequent molecular or biochemical studies can be useful, particularly in the evaluation of the autoimmune encephalitides or in any unusual case. Frozen tissues are also critical to the researchers seeking a greater understanding of the basic causes of epilepsy and the nature of various epileptogenic pathologies.

Preoperative multidisciplinary conferences that include the epileptologist, neuroradiologist, electrophysiologist, and neuropathologist are very helpful in identifying the foci of greatest pathologic interest and the expected pathological findings. This information can be

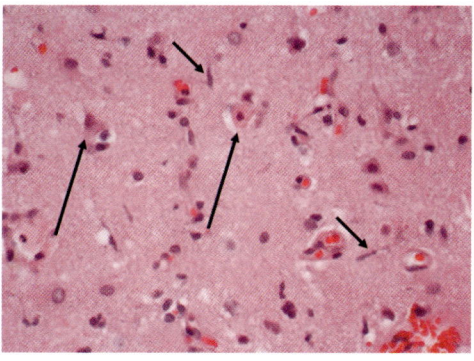

Figure 3.1 Acute neuronal necrosis in cortex from a patient succumbing after prolonged status epilepticus. Note the hypereosinophilic acutely necrotic pyramidal neurons (long arrows) and reactive microglial cells (short arrows).

particularly important in locating areas of cortical dysplasia or lesions such as small tubers or dysembryoplastic neuroepithelial tumors that may produce minimal findings on gross inspection of the resected tissues.

Postmortem examination of brain has also provided insight into pathology associated with epilepsy. In addition to the opportunity to study in situ lesions such as those seen in surgical specimens, examination of the intact brain has provided insight into the consequences of chronic epilepsy or chronic epilepsy therapy on the whole brain in cases such as status epilepticus, autoimmune epilepsies, and antiepileptic drug toxicities (Figure 3.1).

3.3 Hippocampal Sclerosis (Mesial Temporal Sclerosis)

Hippocampal sclerosis (HS), also referred to as medial or mesial temporal sclerosis or Ammon's horn sclerosis, refers to the occurrence of neuronal cell loss and accompanying gliosis in the hippocampus associated with chronic epilepsy, usually temporal lobe epilepsy (TLE). The review by Sommer in 1880, describing atrophied and stiffened hippocampi in brains of autopsied epilepsy patients, is generally regarded as the major work on the subject, and work by many subsequent investigators has clarified the association with temporal lobe epilepsy (TLE) and provided important insights into cause (reviewed in reference 2). In typical cases, the development of HS is associated with an antecedent event, e.g., febrile convulsions in early childhood. Approximately 7% of children with febrile status epilepticus will evolve into hippocampal sclerosis, predicted by visual evidence of hippocampal edema on MRI.

The characteristic pathological findings of HS are usually limited to the hippocampus, in particular hippocampal areas CA1, CA3, and CA4, and consist of loss of pyramidal neurons and gliosis. Although many cases show severe involvement of CA1, CA3, and CA4, the severity and extent of the cell loss and gliosis vary among different patients and include some cases showing global neuronal loss throughout the hippocampus, more limited involvement to particular segments such as area CA4 or fascia dentata, or gliosis without apparent neuronal loss. Many cases are associated with granule cell dispersion (GCD). In some cases, HS is associated with other pathological findings such as focal cortical dysplasia, a tumor or a vascular malformation ("dual pathology") or shows more widespread neuronal loss and gliosis in extra-hippocampal structures.

Various methods and terms for grading and classifying the distribution and severity of the findings have been proposed. The International League Against Epilepsy (ILAE) in 2013 published a classification of hippocampal sclerosis that is becoming widely accepted[5]

Table 3.1 Hippocampal sclerosis: International League Against Epilepsy classification

HS ILAE type	Predominant distribution of neuronal loss	Percentage of neuronal loss	Dentate gyrus	Comments
Type 1	CA1 and CA4	CA1: >80%, CA4: 40–90% Also CA2: 30–50% and CA3: 30–90%	50–60% granule cell loss Can be focal with GCD Any type of granule cell pathology might be present	Most common type: 60–80% Also refers to classic and total HS
Type 2	CA1	80% of pyramidal cells Barely visible cell loss in other sectors	GCD Usually no severe loss of granule cells	Uncommon: 5–10% Atypical type (restriction to CA1)
Type 3	CA4 and DG	CA1: 50% cell loss Moderate cell loss in CA1, CA2, and CA3	35% cell loss	Rare variant: 4–7.4% Probably similar to end folium sclerosis More often associated with a dual pathology like Rasmussen's encephalitis

GCD: granule cell dispersion. Compiled from criteria detailed in reference 5.

(See Table 3.1). While the ILAE classification used NeuN to highlight neuronal loss, a more recent study suggested that use of MAP2, which emphasizes dendritic labeling and neuronal soma, in addition to NeuN, may aid in better classification of equivocal cases of HS< e.g., in differentiating between ILAE type 1 and type 2 HS.

A typical intact hippocampectomy specimen includes the pes hippocampi and anterior body covered by alveus. Atrophy may be apparent grossly as shrinkage or narrowing limited to area CA1. Microscopic neuronal loss is characteristically confined to particular sectors, and evaluation by routine hematoxylin and eosin staining can be supplemented by classic Nissl stains such as cresyl violet or by neuronal immunostaining markers such as NeuN. The presence of chronic gliosis can be subtle but is often easily demonstrated with GFAP immunostaining (Figure 3.2). Gliosis limited to the hippocampal end plate (CA4 region) is occasionally seen, but recent classification excludes this entity from HS.

GCD is commonly encountered in association with HS and refers to alterations in the thickness, packing density, neuronal size, and neuronal orientation of the granular cell layer of the fascia dentata (Figure 3.3). The pathogenesis of GCD is incompletely understood but may represent neurogenesis or aberrant migration of granule cells occurring in the setting of chronic seizure activity, particularly in the young brain.[2,6]

3.4 Glial Scars

Focal injury to the brain and formation of glial or glial and fibrous scars can result from a variety of causes, including perinatal brain injury, head trauma, previous neurosurgical

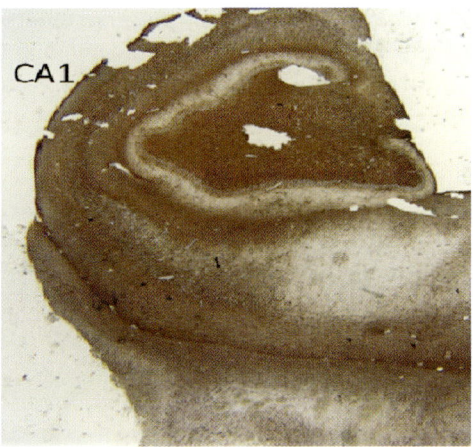

Figure 3.2 GFAP staining shows dense gliosis in areas CA1, CA3, and CA4 with lighter staining elsewhere.

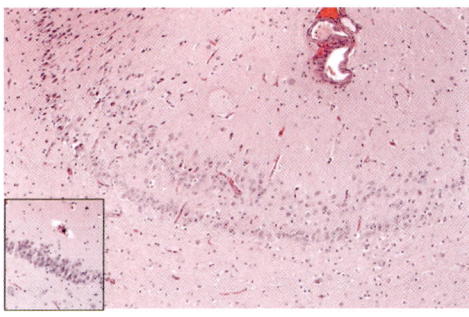

Figure 3.3 Granule cell dispersion shows a bilaminar thickening of the fascia dentata. Inset: Normal fascia dentata consists of a compact granule cell layer.

intervention, infections, infarctions, and other pathological processes. These can cause focal "localization-related" seizures at the time of the injury or later in life, and the seizures can occasionally evolve into intractable epilepsy.[1] Perinatal injury is an important contributor, particularly following vascular events such as infarctions or hemorrhages involving cortex. (Damage occurring early in the immature brain may be associated with secondary malformative lesions such as polymicrogyria or porencephaly.)[7]

3.5 Congenital and Developmental Disorders

Many developmental abnormalities can have seizures or chronic epilepsy as part of their clinical manifestations. Congenital central nervous system abnormalities account for 3.2 to 10% of neonatal seizures.[8,9] These include disorders of neuronal migration such as polymicrogyria and heterotopias, malformations of cortical development and maturation (cortical dysplasias), and genetic diseases affecting cortical development, maturation, and growth, such as hemimegalencephaly and tuberous sclerosis. In some instances, abnormalities of migration and growth occur in the setting of disruptive ("encephaloclastic") events occurring during early development. Polymicrogyric cortex and nodular heterotopias, for example, may be associated with porencephaly, a circumscribed cavitary defect in the cerebral mantle likely arising following a destructive event during earlier cerebral development. While many of these seizure-associated conditions may have widespread brain involvement and epileptiform activity, some produce localized epileptogenic lesions amenable to surgical treatment by resection. In some cases of intractable and debilitating epileptic activity, even conditions showing extensive or bilateral cerebral involvement such as hemimegalencephaly, polymicrogyria, or tuberous sclerosis may benefit from larger-scale resections, including complete lobectomy or hemispherectomy.

Congenital malformations due to abnormalities in neuronal migration, formation of cerebral cortex, and gyration include the agyria/lissencephaly/pachygyria series of malformations, polymicrogyria, and heterotopias.[10] Major malformations with extensive agyria, lissencephaly, or pachygyria represent severe abnormalities of neuronal migration, can occur in both sporadic and familial forms, and are characteristically bilateral and associated with severe neurological deficits and seizures. Surgical treatment with resection is seldom employed in individuals with these severe forms of brain malformation.

Heterotopias are masses of mature neurons and neuropil in subcortical or periventricular locations. Cerebral heterotopias have been divided into nodular and laminar or band heterotopias.[10] Nodular heterotopias occur singly or in groups and may be present in the setting of other malformations, including the agyria/lissencephaly/pachygyria series, polymicrogyria, holoprosencephaly, and encephaloclastic events. The nodules show a variety of cell patterns, including randomly ordered neurons, discrete clusters, and partly laminated arrays. Although heterotopias may be asymptomatic and discovered as incidental findings, some are associated with epilepsy. More extensive heterotopias can occur in syndromic familial forms and be associated with more widespread neurological dysfunction, as well as seizures. Laminar or band heterotopia refers to the occurrence of variable numbers of mature neurons and neuropil forming a relatively demarcated layer underlying normal-appearing cortex (Figure 3.4). In addition to nodular or laminar heterotopia, the occurrence of increased numbers of subcortical neurons has also been reported as a form of "diffuse" heterotopia in some patients with epilepsy. This finding is difficult to distinguish from the finding of subcortical neurons in substantial numbers in some parts of the brain such as the anterior temporal lobe white matter in nonepileptic patients.

Polymicrogyria (PMG) refers to the formation of dyslaminated cortex folded into small gyral-like folds and can occur in widespread symmetrical as well as limited focal

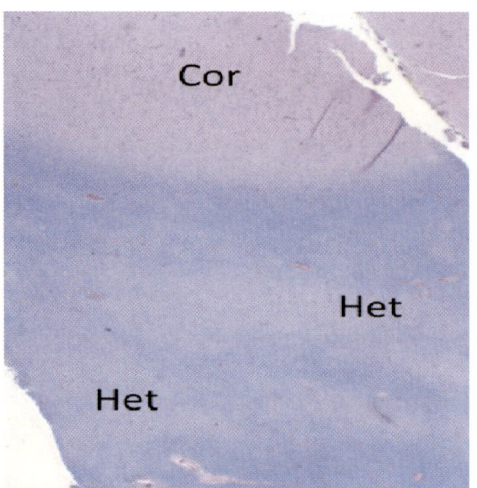

Figure 3.4 Subcortical band heterotopia consists of irregular bands of cortical-type gray matter seen as areas of pale staining (Het) with Luxol fast blue in the white matter underlying the cortex (Cor).

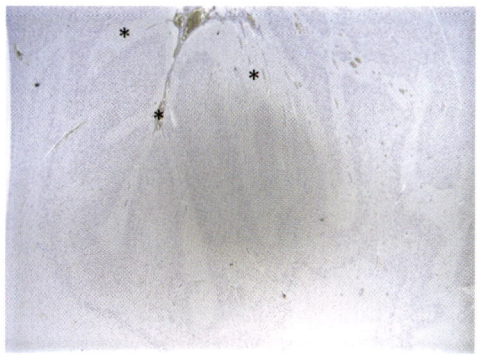

Figure 3.5 Four-layered PMG: low-power photomicrograph shows typical complex undulating patterns of neurons with "fused sulci" (asterisks) on staining with neuronal stains such as cresyl violet.

distributions. Distribution in the middle cerebral artery territory or perisylvian region is common, with bilateral distribution more likely to be syndromic.[11] PMG can be localized to cortex surrounding lesions such as porencephalic cysts and can also be seen as isolated foci in cortex, sometimes along the bottom of a sulcus or in the insular region. The development of PMG has also been associated with intrauterine infections such as cytomegalovirus. The polymicrogyric cortex grossly shows a pebbled or smooth cortical surface and, on sectioning, poor demarcation from underlying white matter and a feather-like pattern of myelinated fiber bundles entering or exiting the cortex in mature well-myelinated brains (Figure 3.5). Microscopically PMG has been classified into unlayered and four-layered patterns. Both patterns show undulation of cell layers into small convolutions and undulation of the hypocellular molecular layer and small leptomeningeal blood vessels, creating the impression of fusion of adjacent small gyri. PMG may coexist with nodular heterotopias in the underlying white matter.

Focal cortical dysplasias (FCDs) are a group of sporadic, epileptogenic, localized abnormalities of cortical architecture and cell appearance, often resembling the lesions of tuberous sclerosis but lacking an association with specific hereditary syndromes. They comprise 12–40% or greater of pathologic findings in surgical epilepsy specimens.[2] Since the original report by Taylor in 1971, various classification schemes have been proposed, including the Palmini and Luders classification, revised in 2004. The recent ILAE classification recognizes three categories (FCD I, II, III) with subtypes in each category.[12] The incidence of the types and subtypes varies among series. FCDs are often associated with chronic intractable seizures of varying semiologies. Lesions may be difficult to recognize or inapparent on CT or MRI imaging studies. Although clinical manifestations are variable, FCD II appears to have a stronger association with intractable epilepsy than FCD I.

FCD I is characterized by abnormalities in cortical architecture encompassing abnormalities of cortical lamination, neuronal orientation, and neuronal size. Lesions may be difficult to recognize by imaging or gross inspection of the resected tissue. Subtypes are based on the pattern of dyslamination (Ia – radial, Ib – tangential, Ic – both). Abnormally large but otherwise normal-appearing neurons (hypertrophic neurons) in upper cortical layers are present (Figures 3.6 and 3.7).

FCD II shares pathologic features with tuberous sclerosis lesions and is characterized by dyslamination and cytological dysmorphic features. The presence of dysmorphic neurons, showing varying combinations of abnormal size, shape, orientation, dendritic patterns, and cytoplasmic and nuclear structure, characterizes FCD IIa (Figures 3.8 and 3.9).

Table 3.2 The three-tiered ILAE classification system of focal cortical dysplasia (FCD)

ILAE FCD type	Definition	Subtypes			
Type I	Isolated lesions of dyslamination of the neocortex microscopically identified in one or multiple lobes	Type Ia: radial dyslamination	Type Ib: tangential dyslamination	Type Ic: both radial and tangential	
Type II	Isolated lesion characterized by cortical dyslamination and dysmorphic neurons	Type IIa: without balloon cells		Type IIb: with balloon cells	
Type III	Cortical lamination abnormalities associated with another principal lesion	Type IIIa: in combination with HS	Type IIIb: with epilepsy-associated tumors	Type IIIc: found adjacent to vascular malformations	Type IIId: in association with epileptogenic lesions acquired in early life (i.e., traumatic injury, ischemic injury or encephalitis)

FCD Type III NOS: if clinically/radiologically suspected principal lesion is not available for microscopic inspection. Compiled from criteria presented in reference 12.

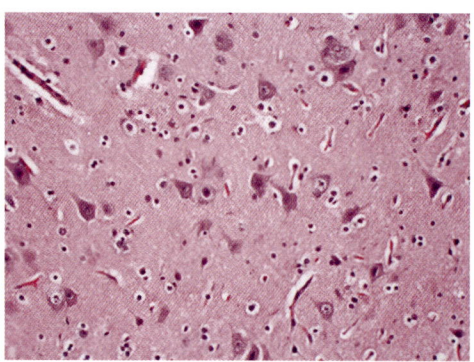

Figure 3.6 FCD with neuronal cytomegaly is characterized by abnormally large (hypertrophic) but otherwise appropriately formed and oriented neurons. Hematoxylin and eosin stain.

The additional presence of balloon cells, dysmorphic cells with a generally globoid appearance, homogeneous astrocyte-like cytoplasm, and variable immunohistochemical profile, characterizes FCD IIb (Figures 3.10 and 3.11). FCD III encompasses abnormalities in cortical lamination associated with other pathologic entities such as HS, tumor, vascular malformations, or acquired lesions.

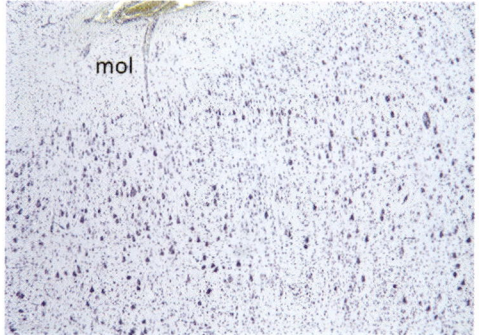

Figure 3.7 In FCD type 1b, the normal six-layered pattern is obscure and large neurons are distributed in all cortical layers, including the molecular layer (mol) instead of remaining confined to cortical layer 5 (cresyl violet stain).

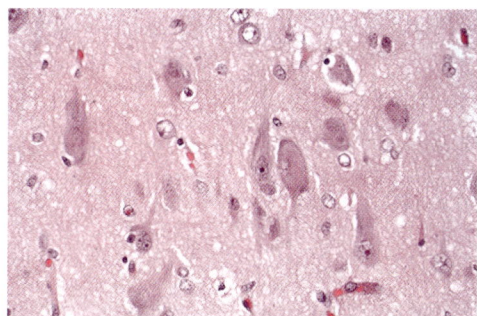

Figure 3.8 FCD IIa. Dysplastic neurons are often abnormally large and vary in size, shape, cytoplasmic appearance and orientation.

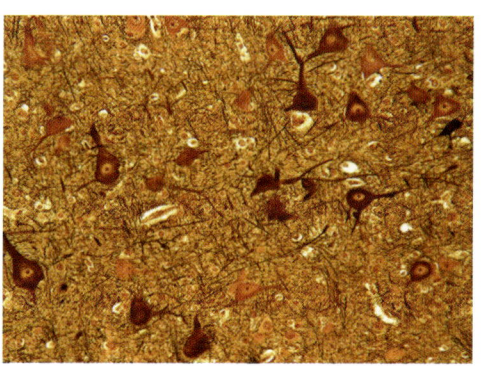

Figure 3.9 Bielschowsky staining emphasizes the coarsened irregular processes and dysplastic features such as increased cellular content of neurofilaments.

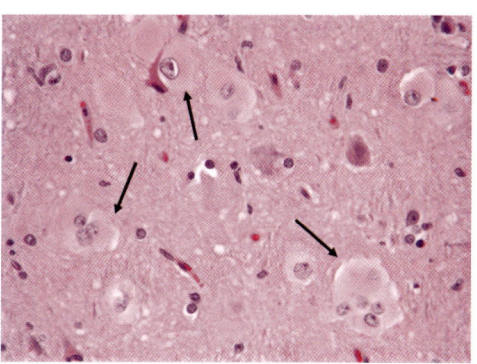

Figure 3.10 FCD IIb is characterized by balloon cells (arrows), large globoid cells with abundant astrocyte-like cytoplasm.

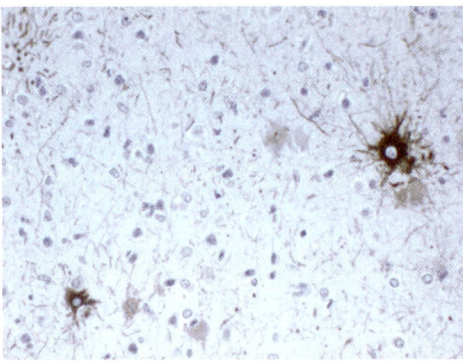

Figure 3.11 Balloon cells may be highlighted with alpha B-crystallin immunostaining, which also demonstrates coarse glial-like cytoplasmic processes.

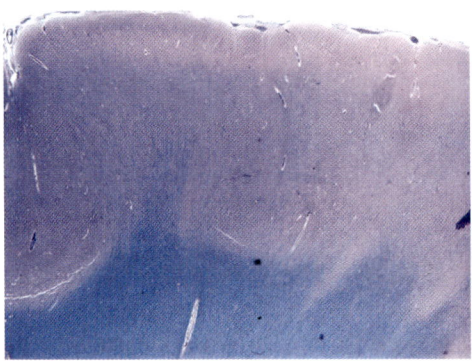

Figure 3.12 Low-power microscopic section confirms the irregular cortical thickness and lack of normal boundaries between cortex and white matter. Wispy bundles of myelinated axons resemble the gray and white matter border in cases of polymicrogyria (Luxol fast blue/H&E, 20×.)

Hemimegalencephaly is a major malformation characterized by asymmetry of the cerebral hemispheres, with one hemisphere larger than the other and showing widespread dysplasia. The malformation occurs in several settings, including in association with systemic conditions such as Proteus syndrome, hypomelanosis of Ito, and tuberous sclerosis, as a rare form referred to as total hemimegalencephaly (also involving the ipsilateral brainstem and cerebellum) and as a sporadic form.[13] The rare sporadic form of widespread cerebral cortical dysplasia chiefly involves one cerebral hemisphere and is characterized by the presentation of intractable seizures in early life. The specific pathological findings vary with the type and distribution of the abnormalities in the brain. In typical cases, the enlarged hemisphere shows expanded gyri with a variably abnormal pattern of gyration, thickening of the cortical ribbon, and poor demarcation of gray and white matter (Figure 3.12). Microscopically the involved cortex appears dysplastic with variations in cell density and lamination and cytological abnormalities in both neurons and glial cells. These may include abnormally large and dysplastic neurons, gliosis, calcifications, and dysplastic glial cells, including balloon cells identical to those seen in FCD IIb and in tuberous sclerosis (see below). The abnormalities may involve the hippocampus and other medial temporal lobe structures as well as neocortex.

Tuberous sclerosis complex (TSC) is an autosomal dominant disorder related to mutations in TSC1 and TSC2 genes (mapped to chromosomes 9q34 and 16p13, respectively). The disease is characterized by the formation of hamartomatous masses (tubers) in the brain involving the cerebral cortex, white matter, or subependymal regions;

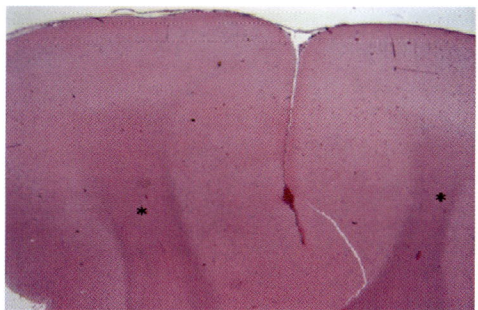

Figure 3.13 Tubers in two adjacent gyri show poor demarcation of cortex and white matter and pallor (*) in subcortical and intragyral white matter due to reduction in normal axonal density.

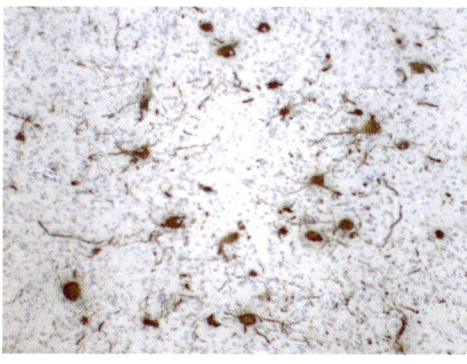

Figure 3.14 Alpha B-crystallin shows a loose aggregate of dysplastic "balloon" cells and cell processes in gliotic subcortical white matter.

a low-grade neoplasm (subependymal giant cell astrocytoma – SEGA) arising along the cerebral ventricles; and a variety of other hamartomatous and other lesions in other organs.[14] The number and clinical significance of the lesions varies greatly from individual to individual, but involvement of the brain is usually predominant. Both cortical tubers and cortex around tubers may be epileptogenic and result in intractable seizures.[15] Surgical treatment for intractable seizures can vary from resection of a single electrically active tuber to partial lobectomy to major resections such as hemispherectomy in occasional cases of extensive disease or multiple epileptogenic foci. Although considered low grade, resection of SEGA may be performed when the SEGA is associated with epilepsy or shows rapid growth, blocks the ventricular system causing hydrocephalus, or impinges on vital structures.

Cortical tubers are relatively discrete masses, whose gross appearance and firm texture in the unfixed brain led to the designation "tuberous sclerosis (TS)." Although typically circumscribed, tubers are often associated with microscopic abnormalities such as scattered dysplastic cells in the adjacent cortex, as well as abnormalities in the underlying white matter, often extending to the subependymal region. Grossly, tubers appear as areas of gyral expansion with poor demarcation from surrounding gray and white matter along with white discoloration and rubbery firmness, due to the dense gliosis ("sclerosis"). Lesions may contain few or many microcalcifications. The cortical tubers are characterized by obscuration of normal cortical lamination and frank dyslamination with dysplastic and often cytomegalic neurons (Figure 3.13). Balloon cells (similar to those seen in FCD IIb) are characteristic (see Figure 3.10) and are easily demonstrated with immunostaining for alpha B-crystallin (Figure 3.14). The dysplastic neurons and balloon cells often trail out radially

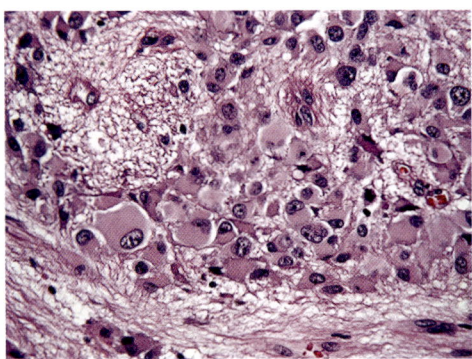

Figure 3.15 Subependymal giant cell astrocytoma is composed of characteristic large cells from a patient with a tumor in the frontal horn similar to cells within the tuber or in FCD IIb.

into the underlying white matter, but occasionally occur in discrete tumor-like aggregates. The axonal density in the white matter underlying the tuber is reduced. In the tubers themselves, the background density is increased, due to dense fibrillary gliosis, which contributes to the discrete appearance and texture of the tuber. Subependymal tubers, sometimes referred to as "candle guttering," consist of similar cellular aggregates, often balloon cells, in a gliotic background along the ependymal surfaces.

SEGA is the most common neoplasm in the CNS in patients with tuberous sclerosis, occurring in 5–15% of confirmed TS cases, and is a slowly growing tumor composed of large "ganglionic" astrocytes resembling the balloon cells[16] (Figure 3.15). The prevalence of SEGA has been reported to vary from 6 to 19%. SEGA tumors most commonly arise in the walls of the frontal horns of the lateral ventricles near the foramen of Monro, are sharply demarcated from surrounding tissues, and may become calcified. The tumor cells are usually immunoreactive for S-100 protein and alpha B-crystallin, but demonstrate variable immunoreactivity for GFAP. The WHO grade 1 designation reflects the typically low cell proliferation rate and indolent clinical behavior in most cases.

3.6 Sturge–Weber Syndrome

Sturge–Weber syndrome or encephalofacial angiomatosis is a sporadic neurocutaneous syndrome characterized by congenital angiomatous vascular malformations involving the skin in the territory of the trigeminal nerve (cranial nerve V), the eye, and small or large portions of the ipsilateral cerebral hemisphere.[17] The cutaneous lesion is the characteristic "port wine" nevus. The cerebral lesion consists of masses of small tortuous venous channels in the subarachnoid space of the leptomeninges, imparting a red-purple discoloration to the brain surface (Figure 3.16). The presence of the vessels is associated with progressive damage to the underlying cortex and white matter, probably resulting from vascular flow effects that produce neuronal loss and gliosis of the affected areas.[15] Calcifications accumulate within the cortex and, to a lesser extent, the white matter, eventually forming a relatively dense layer that can follow the undulations of the cortex and even be visualized on imaging studies (Figure 3.17). Occasional cases are associated with other malformations such as disorders of cortical structure and migrational defects. The progressive cortical damage is associated with the development of focal neurological deficits and seizures progressing to intractable epilepsy. Surgical resection of epileptogenic areas and gliotic calcified cortex can be effective in reducing seizures. Recently, a genetic defect has been

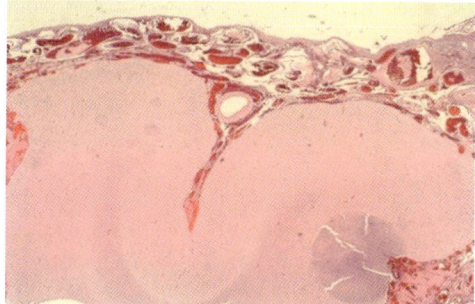

Figure 3.16 Low-power photomicrograph of resected cortex shows a layer of closely packed, thin-walled blood vessels in the subarachnoid space.

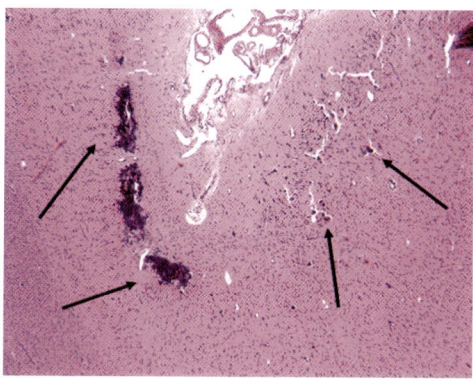

Figure 3.17 Calcifications are visible even under low magnification as basophilic densities (arrows) and often follow the contours of the cortex.

identified in the guanine nucleotide binding protein Q polypeptide (*GNAQ*) gene and appears to be a somatic activating mutation.[18]

3.7 Neoplasms Associated with Epilepsy

Seizures can be associated with almost any neoplasm in the brain and are often the presenting manifestation of a neoplasm in a patient with no previous history of epilepsy.[19] In addition to metastatic tumors, primary brain tumors commonly causing seizures include glioblastomas, astrocytomas, and oligodendrogliomas, along with the occasional meningioma. In most cases, individuals with these tumors have no prior history of seizure. Several less common primary neuroectodermal tumors, however, have a close and presumably causal association with epilepsy, frequently early-onset, long-term, and intractable. These tumors are most commonly encountered in children or younger adults and are usually slowly growing tumors that often show neuronal differentiation and directly involve the cerebral cortex, in particular, parts of the temporal lobe.[20] The close association with chronic epilepsy has led to the proposed term "long-term epilepsy-associated tumors" (LEATs) and suggestions for future directions in clinicopathologic correlation and treatment approaches.[21] Tumors in this category include gangliocytomas and gangliogliomas, dysembryoplastic neuroepithelial tumor (DNT), extraventricular neurocytomas, and variant forms of astrocytoma such as SEGA (see Section 3.5) and pleomorphic xanthoastrocytoma (PXA). Detailed summaries of the pathological features of these neoplasms are included in the 2016 update of the World Health Organization Classification of Brain Tumors.[21]

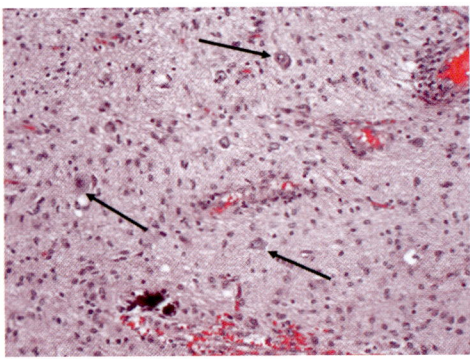

Figure 3.18 Ganglioglioma consists of a mixture of moderately large, mildly pleomorphic neurons (arrows), astrocytes, blood vessels with sparse perivascular mononuclear inflammation, and occasional calcifications (H&E, 100×).

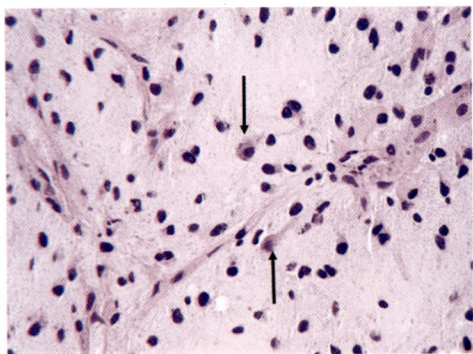

Figure 3.19 High-power photomicrograph consists of loosely arranged, small, oligodendroglial-like cells in a mucoid background. Scattered neurons (arrows) are seen, often "floating" in the mucoid matrix.

Gangliocytomas and gangliogliomas are well-differentiated, slowly growing neoplasms composed, respectively, of mature-appearing dysplastic neurons or an intermixture of mature-appearing dysplastic neurons and neoplastic glial cells, the latter usually showing astrocytic features. Both tumor types occur most frequently in children or younger adults with a history of epilepsy and preferentially occur in the temporal lobe. Gangliocytomas and gangliogliomas are often discrete, solid or cystic tumors and contain variably prominent components of connective tissue fibers, calcifications, and mononuclear inflammation (Figure 3.18). Most tumors behave indolently and are graded WHO grade 1. Rare gangliogliomas with anaplastic features, usually in the glial component, are considered WHO grade 3.

Dysembryoplastic neuroepithelial tumor (DNT), WHO grade 1, is a slowly growing glioneuronal neoplasm that most commonly arises in supratentorial cortex, particularly in the medial temporal lobe, and is associated with early-onset drug-resistant epilepsy. The tumors typically show a multinodular growth pattern and a cystic component. The finding of deformations in the calvarial bone overlying superficially located tumors may reflect the chronic course of the tumor. The tumor exhibits several histological patterns, termed simple and complex, with some cases showing a more diffuse growth pattern.[22] The characteristic "specific glioneuronal element" consists of loosely arranged oligodendroglial-like cells, arranged in a microcystic mucoid matrix, and generally normal-appearing neurons, often seen within the microcysts ("floating neurons") (Figure 3.19). The neurons may represent entrapped normal cortical neurons. The mucoid matrix stains with

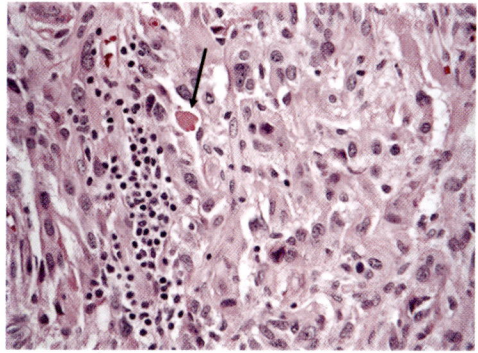

Figure 3.20 Microscopic examination of PXA shows a solid cellular tumor composed of pleomorphic astrocyte-like cells with coarse processes and, in many instances, vacuolated cytoplasm. Eosinophilic granular bodies (arrow) and mononuclear inflammation are common (H&E, 200X).

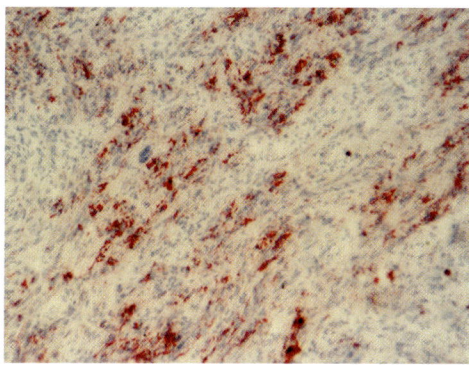

Figure 3.21 Staining with oil red O shows abundant lipid in tumor cell cytoplasm and in macrophages.

Alcian blue. The oligodendroglial-like cells may express glial markers such as S-100 protein, but are usually negative for GFAP. Neighboring cortex may contain scattered microscopic clusters of tumor contributing to the multinodular growth pattern. The complex form shows more heterogeneous morphology, often overlapping with patterns seen in astrocytomas. Tumors may contain prominent capillaries and calcifications. Staining for oncofetal antigen CD34 is frequently positive in parts of the tumor or adjacent dysplastic cortex in the absence of a distinct ganglion cell component. DNTs usually show a low proliferation rate with markers such as Ki-67.

PXA, WHO grade 2 (rare anaplastic form, WHO grade 3), usually occurs in children and young adults with a history of chronic seizures.[20] It forms a largely solid, occasionally cystic tumor involving the superficial cortex and overlying leptomeninges in the cerebrum, most commonly in the temporal lobe. PXA is composed of masses of highly pleomorphic astrocyte-like cells, ranging from giant and multinucleate cells to smaller spindle-shaped cells (Figure 3.20). Most tumors contain eosinophilic granular bodies, a variably prominent background of connective tissue fibers, and collections of mononuclear inflammatory cells. Vacuolated cells due to the presence of cytoplasmic lipid droplets and foamy macrophages containing lipid are characteristic (Figure 3.21). In addition to staining for GFAP and S-100 protein, PXA cells may express neuronal markers such as synaptophysin and neurofilament protein and are characteristically immunoreactive for CD34. The presence of BRAF V600E mutation is characteristic.[23]

3.8 Inflammatory Conditions

Named after neurosurgeon Theodor Rasmussen, who described this entity with his colleagues in 1958,[24] Rasmussen encephalitis (RE) is a rare, sporadic, inflammatory syndrome characterized by progressive destruction of the cerebral cortex in one cerebral hemisphere and most commonly arising in childhood.[25] Although the etiology is unknown, RE is thought to be autoimmune, based on the finding of inflammation by cytotoxic T cells, but specific autoantibodies have not been reliably identified and the process does not appear to be arrested by immunotherapies.[26] In many cases, RE progresses from an early "prodromal" stage of scattered seizures to an active or "acute" stage of increasing, treatment-refractory seizures (epilepsia partialis continua).[2] Seizures are lateralized to the involved hemisphere, and unilateral neurological deficits develop as areas of cortex are destroyed. Over months, the disease inevitably progresses to an "end" stage with lower seizure activity and fixed deficits. Anatomical or functional cerebral hemispherectomy is used to control seizures. Early-stage lesions are characterized by lymphocytic inflammation, particularly CD8-immunoreactive T cells, in the cerebral cortex and overlying leptomeninges, along with microglial activation, microglial nodules, and neuronophagia in the cortex (Figure 3.22). In later stages, with progressive loss of neurons and gliosis, the inflammation subsides, and the cortex is reduced to a thinned spongy layer of residual glial cells and small blood vessels. In hemispherectomy specimens removed during active disease, areas of active cortical inflammation and destruction are frequently intermixed with normal cortex, cortex showing sparse early inflammation, and areas of atrophic spongiotic "burnt out" cortex (Figure 3.23). Brain biopsy is sometimes used to confirm the presence of active inflammation when hemispherectomy is being contemplated for treatment of suspected RE. The findings of T lymphocytic inflammation and microglial nodules in the absence of a recognizable infectious agent such as a virus are supportive of the diagnosis of RE, though not specific. Currently, no marker for RE is available for diagnostic confirmation.

Pathological examination of brain tissues can also contribute to the diagnosis of the rare autoimmune encephalitides that produce epilepsy. These have included encephalitis associated with systemic neoplasms such as carcinoma of the lung (paraneoplastic encephalitis) and encephalitis occurring in the absence of an underlying neoplasm (non-paraneoplastic encephalitis). Recent awareness and advances in immunological and other diagnostic techniques have identified a growing group of cases of encephalitis associated with a variety of antibodies in both the pediatric and adult populations.[27,28] Both groups

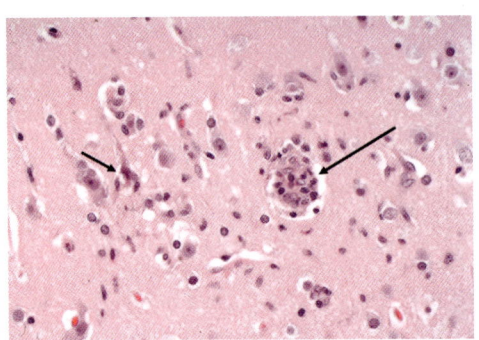

Figure 3.22 High-power photograph from a cortical biopsy in a child with confirmed RE shows diffuse microglial activation, a microglial nodule (long arrow), sparse lymphocytic inflammation, and necrotic neurons surrounded by microglial cells (short arrow) (H&E, 200×).

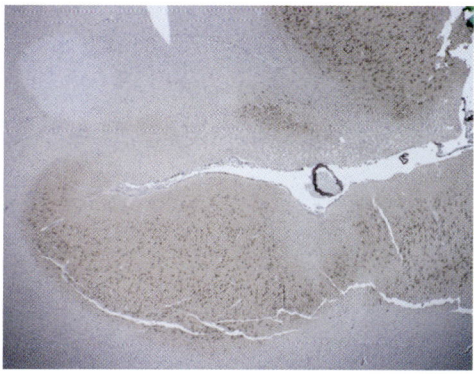

Figure 3.23 A low-power view of involved cortex stained for NeuN shows patchy areas of severe cortical neuronal loss and atrophy alternating with better preserved foci. NeuN, 20× original magnification.

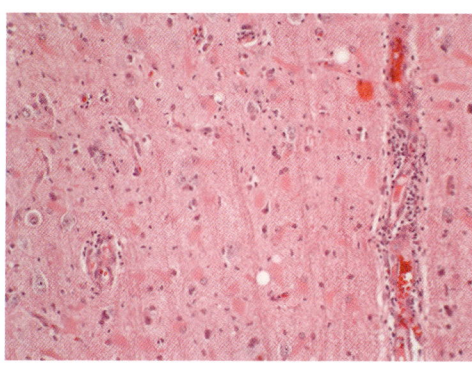

Figure 3.24 Biopsy of cerebral cortex shows marked neuronal loss, astrocytosis, diffuse microglial activation, and perivascular collections of lymphocytes. H&E, 200× original magnification.

include patients who typically present with a subacute onset of neurological symptoms, including psychiatric and behavioral symptoms, alterations in cognition, and seizures, and then progress to severe seizures and status epilepticus. Reported cases have identified serum antibodies against neuron-associated markers such as GAD, NMDA receptor subunits, and voltage-gated potassium channels, which support the diagnosis of an autoimmune encephalitis, though the precipitating factors are poorly understood. As in the case of RE, the examination of affected areas of cortex shows a non-specific pattern of cortical neuronal destruction with microglial nodules and lymphocytic inflammation (Figure 3.24).

3.9 Conclusion

The pathology of epilepsy includes a diverse collection of lesions ranging from glial scars and developmental errors to unusual neoplasms and complex developmental and genetic conditions. The small sample of readily identifiable structural lesions illustrated in this chapter merely scratches the surface and, in many cases probably only identifies one link in the complex chain of events that translates neuronal dysfunction into the chronic clinical condition of intractable epilepsy. The development and introduction of increasingly sophisticated techniques in neuroimaging and molecular genetics will undoubtedly aid both in the identification of more links in the chain and the nature of the connections between them.

Acknowledgements

The authors wish to thank the many members of the epilepsy team at the Children's Hospital of Michigan and the other hospitals of the Detroit Medical Center and Wayne State University School of Medicine who have contributed over many years to the pathology examples illustrated here.

References

1. Scharfman HE. Epilepsy. In: Zigmond MJ, Rowland LP, Coyle JT, eds., *Neurobiology of Brain Disorders: Biological Basis of Neurological and Psychiatric Disorders*. Waltham, MA: Academic Press; 2015:236–261.

2. Thom M, Sisodiya S. Epilepsy. In: Love S, Perry A, Ironside JW, Budka H, eds., *Greenfield's Neuropathology*. 9th edn. Boca Raton, FL: CRC Press; 2015:683–739.

3. Marras CE, Granata T, Franzini A, et al. Hemispherotomy and functional hemispherectomy: indications and outcome. *Epilepsy Res*. 2010;89(1):104–112.

4. Blumcke I, Aronica E, Miyata H, et al. International recommendation for a comprehensive neuropathologic workup of epilepsy surgery brain tissue: a consensus Task Force report from the ILAE Commission on Diagnostic Methods. *Epilepsia*. 2016;57(3):348–358.

5. Blumcke I, Thom M, Aronica E, et al. International consensus classification of hippocampal sclerosis in temporal lobe epilepsy: a Task Force report from the ILAE Commission on Diagnostic Methods. *Epilepsia*. 2013;54(7):1315–1329.

6. Blumcke I, Kistner I, Clusmann H, et al. Towards a clinico-pathological classification of granule cell dispersion in human mesial temporal lobe epilepsies. *Acta Neuropathol*. 2009;117(5):535–544.

7. Squier W. Grey matter lesions. In: Golden J, Harding BN, eds., *Developmental Neuropathology*. Basel, Switzerland: ISN Neuropath Press; 2004:171–175.

8. Loman AM, ter Horst HJ, Lambrechtsen FA, Lunsing RJ. Neonatal seizures: aetiology by means of a standardized work-up. *Eur J Paediatr Neurol*. 2014;18 (3):360–367.

9. Ronen GM, Penney S, Andrews W. The epidemiology of clinical neonatal seizures in Newfoundland: a population-based study. *J Pediatr*. 1999;134(1):71–75.

10. Barkovich AJ, Guerrini R, Kuzniecky RI, Jackson GD, Dobyns WB. A developmental and genetic classification for malformations of cortical development: update 2012. *Brain*. 2012;135(Pt 5):1348–1369.

11. Barkovich AJ. Current concepts of polymicrogyria. *Neuroradiology*. 2010;52 (6):479–487.

12. Blumcke I, Thom M, Aronica E, et al. The clinicopathologic spectrum of focal cortical dysplasias: a consensus classification proposed by an ad hoc Task Force of the ILAE Diagnostic Methods Commission. *Epilepsia*. 2011;52(1):158–174.

13. Mirzaa GM, Poduri A. Megalencephaly and hemimegalencephaly: breakthroughs in molecular etiology. *Am J Med Genet C Semin Med Genet*. 2014;166C (2):156–172.

14. Islam MP, Roach ES. Tuberous sclerosis complex. *Handb Clin Neurol*. 2015;132:97–109.

15. Stafstrom CE, Staedtke V, Comi AM. Epilepsy mechanisms in neurocutaneous disorders: tuberous sclerosis complex, neurofibromatosis type 1, and Sturge-Weber syndrome. *Front Neurol*. 2017;8:87.

16. Adriaensen ME, Schaefer-Prokop CM, Stijnen T, et al. Prevalence of subependymal giant cell tumors in patients with tuberous sclerosis and a review of the literature. *Eur J Neurol*. 2009;16 (6):691–696.

17. Comi AM. Sturge-Weber syndrome. *Handb Clin Neurol*. 2015;132:157–168.

18. Shirley MD, Tang H, Gallione CJ, et al. Sturge-Weber syndrome and port-wine

stains caused by somatic mutation in GNAQ. *N Engl J Med.* 2013;368 (21):1971–1979.

19. Erturk Cetin O, Isler C, Uzan M, Ozkara C. Epilepsy-related brain tumors. *Seizure.* 2017;44:93–97.

20. Soffietti R, Ruda R, Reardon D. Rare glial tumors. *Handb Clin Neurol.* 2016;134:399–415.

21. Blumcke I, Aronica E, Urbach H, Alexopoulos A, Gonzalez-Martinez JA. A neuropathology-based approach to epilepsy surgery in brain tumors and proposal for a new terminology use for long-term epilepsy-associated brain tumors. *Acta Neuropathol.* 2014;128 (1):39–54.

22. Chassoux F, Daumas-Duport C. Dysembryoplastic neuroepithelial tumors: where are we now? *Epilepsia.* 2013;54 (Suppl 9):129–134.

23. Ida CM, Rodriguez FJ, Burger PC, et al. Pleomorphic xanthoastrocytoma: natural history and long-term follow-up. *Brain Pathol.* 2015;25(5):575–586.

24. Rasmussen T, Olszewski J, Lloyd-Smith D. Focal seizures due to chronic localized encephalitis. *Neurology.* 1958;8(6): 435–445.

25. Bien CG, Granata T, Antozzi C, et al. Pathogenesis, diagnosis and treatment of Rasmussen encephalitis: a European consensus statement. *Brain.* 2005;128(Pt 3):454–471.

26. Varadkar S, Bien CG, Kruse CA, et al. Rasmussen's encephalitis: clinical features, pathobiology, and treatment advances. *Lancet Neurol.* 2014;13 (2):195–205.

27. Brenton JN, Goodkin HP. Antibody-mediated autoimmune encephalitis in childhood. *Pediatr Neurol.* 2016;60:13–23.

28. Bauer J, Bien CG. Neuropathology of autoimmune encephalitides. *Handb Clin Neurol.* 2016;133:107–120.

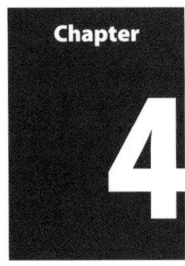

Classifications of Seizures and Epilepsies

Anthony L. Fine, Elaine C. Wirrell, and
Katherine C. Nickels

4.1 Epidemiology of Pediatric Epilepsy

Epilepsy is amongst the most common of neurological disorders seen in children, with incidence rates ranging from 33.3–82 cases per 100,000 per year.[1–4] The incidence is highest in the first year of life, and decreases in the teen years. Epilepsy is clearly focal in onset in approximately two-thirds of pediatric cases and generalized in onset in one-quarter.[4] Approximately half of children have no known etiology.[4]

Population-based studies have shown a relatively favorable long-term outcome in pediatric epilepsy, with nearly two-thirds achieving seizure freedom for longer than 3–5 years, and nearly half achieving seizure remission (seizure freedom off antiepileptic drugs).[5–9] In most cases, response to therapy is achieved early in the course of epilepsy. Two years after diagnosis, 53–57% of children achieve seizure freedom for a minimum of 12 months.[10,11] Conversely, intractable epilepsy is seen in 10–20% of children by two years,[9,10] and half of those children continue to have refractory seizures long term. Achievement of early remission however, does not always guarantee favorable long-term outcome, particularly in children with focal epilepsy. Berg et al. found that 26% of patients presenting to an epilepsy surgical center had achieved a prior remission of at least twelve months.[12] Similarly, a follow-up study of children with new-onset temporal lobe epilepsy found that one-third, who either had ongoing seizures at last follow-up, or had undergone resective surgery, had previously achieved a remission lasting at least one year.[13]

Table 4.1 summarizes predictors of intractability in pediatric epilepsy. One of the most robust predictors is *epilepsy syndrome*. In a long-term follow-up of children with "symptomatic generalized epilepsy," which included West syndrome, Lennox–Gastaut and myoclonic atonic epilepsy, 24% had died and 53% continued to suffer from intractable seizures.[14] Of survivors, 88% had intellectual disability and only 13% were living independently.[15] Poor outcome is also noted in children with lesional focal epilepsy. Long-term follow-up studies have shown that 69–100% of such children either have medically intractable epilepsy at final follow-up or had undergone resective surgery.[13,16] Approximately one-third of children with focal epilepsy have no identified cause found for their seizures. Prognosis in this group is significantly better than those with known lesions, with 55–67% achieving terminal remission off antiepileptic drugs and only 7% developing intractable epilepsy.[17,18] Similarly, intractability rates are low in childhood and juvenile absence epilepsy[19] and juvenile myoclonic epilepsy.[20] In the benign focal epilepsies, remission always occurs.[21]

Another very significant predictor is underlying etiology. Increasingly, genetic etiologies are being identified, many of which are highly associated with early onset, intractable epilepsy, including ARX, CDKL5, STXBP1, SCN8A, and PCDH19. Other genetic etiologies

Table 4.1 Summary of intractability

	Consistently reported in studies		Inconsistently reported in studies
Intractability	**Seizure frequency or type** • High initial seizure frequency • Focal seizures or multiple seizure types • Neonatal seizures • Age of onset >12 years **Epilepsy syndrome** • Symptomatic generalized epilepsy* **Physical exam** • Intellectual disability • Neurological deficits on exam **Investigations** • Temporal lobe epilepsy, especially with hippocampal atrophy or hippocampal sclerosis • Cortical dysplasia **Response to treatment** • Failure to respond within first year • Failure to respond to first drug		**History** • History of febrile seizures • History of status epilepticus **Investigations** • Epileptiform discharges on EEG • Focal slowing on EEG

Includes West syndrome, Lennox–Gastaut, Dravet syndrome

have a more varied, and not necessarily intractable phenotype, including SCN1A missense mutations, SCN1B, SCN2A, DEPDC5, and Trisomy 21. While structural abnormalities portend poorer outcome, the specific type is important, with higher rates of intractability in cases with cortical dysplasia, mesial temporal sclerosis and dual pathology, as opposed to encephalomalacia.[16]

4.2 Why is Classification Important?

Epilepsy classification provides a framework for diagnosis. Epilepsy in children comprises a diverse group of etiologies and syndromes. While the primary goal of classification is to improve clinical epilepsy care, accurate classification is also important for epidemiological reasons.

4.2.1 Clinical

Classification based on seizure and epilepsy type allows one to identify the most likely type(s) of etiology or syndrome and target investigations to these areas. Using such a framework increases the likelihood of finding a precise diagnosis in a more cost-effective manner with fewer investigations for the patient.

Reaching a precise diagnosis is essential to inform treatment recommendations and in the design of potential research trials evaluating new therapies. Medications which can be very effective for one type of epilepsy are ineffective, or may even exacerbate others. While sodium channel agents are often useful for focal epilepsies, they exacerbate Dravet syndrome and many types of genetic generalized epilepsies. Increasingly, precision therapies are being identified based on specific etiologies. Stiripentol, when used in combination with valproic acid and clobazam has unique efficacy in Dravet syndrome,[22] and children with SCN2A encephalopathy respond well to high-dose phenytoin.[23] Certain metabolic disorders have very specific therapies, which not only improve seizure control but also neurocognitive outcomes.[24] For example, in children with glucose transporter deficiency due to SLC2A1, a ketogenic diet therapy affords seizure control and improves development. Patients with focal cortical dysplasias are typically medically intractable, but have a high likelihood of seizure freedom with resective surgery. Those with autoimmune epilepsies respond favorably to immunomodulatory therapy, with better outcomes with more prompt onset of therapy.[25]

Specific diagnoses and syndromes also inform prognosis. Many early-onset, severe epilepsies are highly correlated with cognitive decline,[26] due in part to epileptic encephalopathy, and in certain cases prompt initiation of precision therapy may improve neurocognitive outcome. Examples include early initiation of vigabatrin in children with tuberous sclerosis.[27,28] Specific etiologies and syndromes are highly predictive of pharmacoresistance (e.g. Lennox–Gastaut syndrome, Dravet syndrome, malformations of cortical development, mesial temporal sclerosis) whereas in others, seizures are usually easily controlled (e.g. benign focal epilepsies of childhood, childhood absence epilepsy). Finally, many pediatric epilepsies are self-limited and are typically outgrown by adolescence (e.g. benign focal epilepsies, childhood absence epilepsy) even if seizures are initially challenging to control (myoclonic atonic epilepsy).

4.2.2 Epidemiological

Accurate classification of epilepsies is also important for epidemiologic reasons. Correlating specific phenotypes in a particular region or population may provide clues to underlying etiology, which may be potentially modifiable. Numerous studies have documented clusters of new-onset seizure disorders due to various infectious agents and toxins.[29,30] Identification of such etiologies will allow health care dollars to be targeted for possible preventative strategies as well as ensuring adequate resources to care for affected individuals.

4.3 Historical Review of Epilepsy Classification

The concept of classifying epileptic seizures was initiated by Professor H. Gastaut as part of the Commission on Classification of the International League Against Epilepsy (ILAE) in the 1969 report "Clinical and electroencephalographical classification of epileptic seizures."[31] This seminal publication prompted a proposal for worldwide adoption of an international classification of epilepsies, not just seizures, the following year.[32]

This was followed in 1981 by a proposal to revise the clinical and electroencephalographic classification of epileptic seizures, due to better abilities to classify seizures provided by newer diagnostic techniques.[33] However, the 1981 International Classification of Epileptic Seizures described only individual seizure types, whereas clear descriptions of epileptic syndromes were needed for communication among physicians, researchers, and for hospital documentation. Therefore, the Proposal for Revised Classification of Epilepsies and Epileptic Syndromes (ICES) was published in 1989 and became the standard for classifying seizures, epilepsies, and epileptic syndromes.[34] Epileptic syndromes were defined by clinical signs and symptoms, including seizure types, age at onset, and precipitating factors, as well as outcome in some. It was made clear that syndromes did not always have common etiologies or outcomes.[34]

Etiologies were also defined as idiopathic, symptomatic, or cryptogenic. The idiopathic localization-related epilepsies were those that occurred during childhood in children with normal neuroimaging, normal development, normal neurologic exam, and normal EEG background activity. There could be a family history of benign epilepsy and the etiology was presumed to be genetic. Examples include benign childhood epilepsy with centrotemporal spikes and childhood epilepsy with occipital paroxysms. Symptomatic localization-related epilepsies include those with a known or suspected structural cause. Those with a presumed symptomatic cause, but with no structural abnormalities identified on neuroimaging, were classified as cryptogenic.[34]

Similarly, the generalized epilepsies were classified as idiopathic, cryptogenic/symptomatic, and symptomatic. Those with idiopathic generalized epilepsies were characterized as having all seizures being initially generalized with generalized discharges on EEG in the setting of normal EEG background activity and without other neurologic abnormalities on exam or imaging. The cause was presumed to be genetic and examples include childhood absence epilepsy, juvenile absence epilepsy, and juvenile myoclonic epilepsy. The symptomatic generalized epilepsies were typically characterized by multiple different generalized seizure types associated with bilateral discharges, but also asymmetric and focal discharges. Furthermore, the background EEG could also be abnormal, including slowing. There were also associated clinical and radiologic signs of diffuse encephalopathy. If no clear etiology was identified, these could also be classified as generalized cryptogenic epilepsy. Examples include West syndrome and Lennox Gastaut syndrome.[34] Although the 1989 proposed classification scheme remained the standard, and is still used by many who care for patients with epilepsy, the concepts upon which it is based predate modern diagnostic tools such as MRI and the majority of current genetic testing. Therefore, in 2010 the ILAE presented the Revised Terminology and Concepts for Organization of Seizures and Epilepsies.[35] Like its 1989 predecessor, this classification scheme also looked at mode of seizure onset, specific seizure types, electroclinical components of epilepsy syndromes, as well as outcome and etiology, when known. In addition, minimal changes were made to the pre-existing list of epilepsy syndromes. However, substantial changes were proposed.

Neonatal seizures were no longer classified separately. Epileptic spasms were identified as a specific seizure type and included infantile spasms. The concepts of generalized and partial/localization-related seizures were altered due to increased understanding of seizures occurring due to hyperexcitability and synchrony of neurons within networks, rather than specific areas of neocortex.[36] Generalized seizures, rather than being presumed to involve the entire cortex at onset symmetrically, were conceptualized to having onset within and rapidly engaging bilateral networks, but not necessarily the entire cortex. Generalized seizures can appear to have focal features and be asymmetric, but the lateralization is inconsistent. The term "partial seizures" was felt to be imprecise, especially "simple partial" and "complex partial." Therefore, seizures arising within a network limited to one hemisphere were termed "focal seizures."[35]

Further classification into simple and complex partial seizures was replaced by a recommendation that focal seizures be described by their features, including awareness, motor and autonomic features, sensory or psychic phenomena, and evolution to bilateral convulsive seizure. It was recommended that seizures described as impairments in awareness/consciousness be specifically recognized and the term "dyscognitive features" was used.[35]

The classification of epilepsies was also revised and the terms idiopathic, symptomatic, and cryptogenic were discarded and replaced by more specific etiological categories including genetic, structural/metabolic, or unknown.[35]

4.4 Introduction to the 2017 ILAE Classification of Seizure Types and Epilepsies

In 2017, the ILAE Classification Task Force published new proposals for classification of seizure types and classification of the epilepsies.[37,38]

The newly proposed classification scheme is described as a multilevel classification with three levels of classification (Figure 4.1). While diagnosis at all three levels is preferable, it is recognized that this is not always possible, due to a wide variety of diagnostic resources around the world, or due to incomplete understanding of an individual's epilepsy.[38] The first level of classification is the seizure type – focal, generalized, or unknown onset. The second level is the epilepsy type – generalized, focal, combined generalized and focal, or unknown, based on clinical and EEG findings. The third level is diagnosing a specific epilepsy syndrome, based on clinical features, seizure types, EEG, and imaging. Furthermore, etiology and comorbidities should be identified at each level, if possible. This classification scheme is summarized in Figure 4.1 and described in detail below.[38,39]

4.4.1 Classification of Seizure Types

The 2017 ILAE Operational Classification of Seizure Types begins with stratification into focal versus generalized seizure onset.[37,40] In certain circumstances, seizure onset is unknown due to unwitnessed or unclear initial onset of the seizure and additional information is required for classification. As part of the updated classification schema, the level of detail specified is up to the classifier (clinician, researcher, patient, family member, etc.) and the seizure description can stop at any level.

Rather than a tiered approach to seizure classification, the most recent categorization relies upon the provider/classifier's familiarity and comfort with seizure classification to select

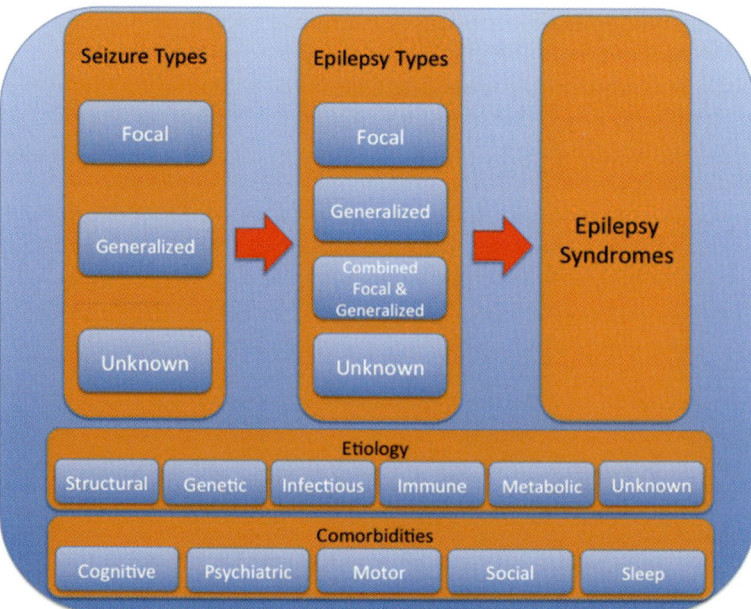

Figure 4.1 Summary of 2017 classification scheme, Framework for Classification of the Epilepsies. (Adapted with permission from: Scheffer, I., et al., ILAE classification of the epilepsies: Position paper of the ILAE Commission for Classification and Terminology. Epilepsia, 2017; 58(4): 512–521, copyright John Wiley and Sons 2017.)

Seizure classification based on updated 2017 ILAE classification[1]

I. Classification of generalized-onset seizures

Motor	Generalized tonic–clonic
	Tonic
	Clonic
	Myoclonic
	Myoclonic–atonic
	Myoclonic–tonic
	Myoclonic–tonic–clonic
	Epileptic spasms
Nonmotor	Absence (typical, atypical)
	Absence with eyelid myoclonia
	Absence with myoclonus

II. Classification of focal-onset seizures

Motor	Tonic
	Clonic
	Tonic–clonic
	Myoclonic
	Atonic
	Epileptic spasms
Nonmotor	Behavioral arrest
Awareness	Automatisms
	Retained awareness (aware)
	Impaired awareness

III. Classification of unknown-onset seizures

Motor	Epileptic spasms
Nonmotor	Behavioral arrest
Unclassified onset	

which information to include. The new classification aims to enhance communication between those who provide routine care for patients with epilepsy and those less familiar with this disorder, and to reflect our current and increasing understanding of the epilepsies.[41]

Generalized-onset seizures engage bilateral or bihemispheric cortical networks at seizure initiation versus focal-onset seizures, which begin within a localized cortical network within one hemisphere. Generalized-onset seizures can be further classified into motor or non-motor onset. The level of awareness is not included as it is assumed that awareness is impaired in the majority of generalized-onset seizures. Nonmotor seizures are considered absence seizures. Classification of generalized-onset seizures is outlined in Table 4.2.

Seizures of focal onset can be further subclassified based on additional features seen at seizure initiation (see box). Level of awareness should be specified if known. A seizure in a patient who retains awareness of self and environment during the entire event would be classified as a focal seizure with retained awareness (or focal aware seizure). If awareness were to be lost at any time during the seizure, then it would be classified as a focal impaired awareness seizure. Awareness is an important feature to note as it has anatomic and pathophysiologic implications (seizure onset/spread) as well as lifestyle and social implications for patient counseling (i.e. seizure safety, bathing, cooking, driving, etc.).[42,43]

Further subdivision can be made based on motor and nonmotor findings seen at seizure onset. Seizures should be named based on the earliest seen motor or nonmotor finding. If awareness is not known then motor or nonmotor onset findings can be used for naming and awareness excluded. Seizures that begin with focal onset but then spread to involve other cortical networks are classified as focal to bilateral tonic–clonic (compared to the previous classification of partial or focal with secondary generalization).

For focal seizures with multiple signs and symptoms, classification is based on the most prominent initial feature at seizure onset. Often there may be several features associated with the focal seizure that aid in seizure description, but are not necessary for classification. Additional "free text" descriptors are encouraged to provide more information regarding seizure anatomic basis, behavioral characteristics, and etiology (Table 4.2).[35,44]

Seizures of unknown onset are termed "unclassified" with the hope that future information will allow classification of that seizure; or if further details are known, then it can be described as unknown onset with additional features such as motor, nonmotor, tonic–clonic, or epileptic spasms (Table 4.2). The term unknown onset should only be used until further information is apparent for continued classification. In these instances, classification should be held until additional corroborating information is available such as additional history, video-electroencephalogram data, or neuroimaging findings.

With the updated 2017 ILAE seizure classification, there is added terminology and updates to previously used terminology. Updated seizure type classification with updated terminology based on prior ILAE classifications can be found in Table 4.4.

The terminology used in the classification can be abridged so that when the next term used to describe the seizure supersedes the prior term, the prior term would be assumed. For example, a focal motor clonic seizure can also be described as a focal clonic seizure, as the term motor is inherent in that descriptor (i.e., clonic). Another example would be an individual who has altered awareness with oral and hand automatisms at seizure onset – this would be classified as a focal impaired awareness nonmotor automatism seizure (or focal impaired awareness automatism seizure).

4.4.2 Classification of Epilepsy Type

The 2017 ILAE revised classification of the epilepsies was developed to work in concert with the 2017 revision on classification of seizures. Epilepsy classification guides patient care, including choice of antiseizure medications, prediction of medical comorbidities, and prognostication.[38]

Once seizure onset has been established, then the epilepsy type may be classified. Generalized epilepsy, focal epilepsy, combined generalized and focal epilepsy, and unknown epilepsy are the categories included in this classification tier. The specific category may be determined on clinical grounds with electroencephalographic information providing supporting evidence.

Patients with generalized epilepsy would be expected to have seizures within the generalized seizure onset category, including absence, atonic, myoclonic, tonic, clonic, and tonic–clonic, etc. (Table 4.2). The interictal EEG should demonstrate generalized spike and wave discharges, although focal interictal discharges can be seen in idiopathic generalized epilepsies.[45–47] Patients with focal epilepsy can present with a wide variety of focal

Table 4.2 Descriptors of focal onset seizures[6,7]

Automatisms	Eye blink Orofacial Hand picking Foot pedaling, kicking Vocalization
Autonomic	Cardiovascular (asystole, bradycardia, tachycardia, palpitations) Diaphoresis Flushing Gastrointestinal symptoms (nausea, emesis) Respiratory change Pallor Piloerection
Emotional	Agitation Anger Anxiety Crying (dacrystic) Fear Laughter (gelastic) Joy Paranoia
Cognitive	Acalculia Aphasia Déjà vu Dissociation Hallucination Illusions Jamais vu Memory impairment Neglect Impaired responsiveness
Motor	Dystonic posturing Fencer's posturing Jacksonian march Versive
Sensory	Auditory Gustatory Olfactory Somatosensory Vestibular Visual

onset seizures (Table 4.2). The interictal EEG typically demonstrates focal epileptiform abnormalities, although, depending on the seizure onset zone, if interictal discharges are not readily detected this should not dissuade from diagnosis in this category, as it can be difficult to record focal ictal or interictal discharges in some focal epilepsies. For instance, seizures of focal onset may have rapid propagation to involve bilateral cortical networks,

Updated seizure type classification and terminology based on 2017 ILAE classification[1,6]

Seizure type		Classification	Description
Focal onset seizure	Motor	Focal tonic	Sustained muscle contraction
		Focal clonic	Rhythmic, repetitive jerking of a muscle group
		Focal tonic–clonic	Tonic contraction followed by clonic muscle activity.
		Focal myoclonic	Sudden brief muscle contraction (<100 ms)
		Focal atonic	Sudden loss of muscle tone without preceding tonic or myoclonic component
		Hyperkinetic	Agitated thrashing or leg pedaling movements. To replace hypermotor. Often described in autosomal dominant nocturnal frontal lobe epilepsy with hyperkinetic frontal lobe seizures
		Focal onset bilateral tonic–clonic	Focal onset seizure (motor or nonmotor) which then spreads to involve bilateral cortical networks causing bilateral tonic–clonic activity. Replaces terms partial seizure with secondary generalization and focal seizure evolving to bilateral convulsive/tonic–clonic seizure
	Nonmotor	Automatisms	Nonpurposeful motor activity that may resemble voluntary movement and usually occurs with impaired awareness. Examples include chewing, picking, hand fumbling
		Autonomic	Seizure causing impairment in autonomic nervous system (cardiovascular, gastrointestinal, vasomotor, thermoregulation)
		Behavioral arrest	A pause in activity
		Cognitive	Seizure that affects higher cognitive functions (language, memory, spatial planning, praxis). Examples of symptoms include aphasia, apraxia, neglect, déjà vu, jamais vu, illusions, or hallucinations. Previous term was psychic seizure
		Emotional	Seizure with predominant emotional component. Emotions can include fear, anger, joy, etc. Additionally can be applied to manifestations of dacrystic (crying) or gelastic (laughter) seizures
Generalized onset	Motor	Myoclonic–atonic	Myoclonic jerk followed by atonic seizure with loss of tone. Previously classified as myoclonic–astatic (also known as Doose syndrome)
		Myoclonic–tonic–clonic	Myoclonic jerk followed by a tonic–clonic seizure. As described in patients with juvenile myoclonic epilepsy
	Nonmotor	Absence with eyelid myoclonia	Absence with jerking up of eyelids and upward eye deviation. Often precipitated by eye closure. Eyelid myoclonia can also occur without loss of awareness. Seen in Jeavons syndrome
Focal and generalized onset	Motor	Epileptic spasms	Sudden flexion, extension or mixed extension-flexion of limbs and trunk, typically occurring in clusters. Motor activity is more sustained than myoclonus

becoming bilateral tonic–clonic seizures that may appear to demonstrate diffuse onset at seizure initiation.[48] Similarly, focal hyperkinetic impaired awareness seizures in nocturnal frontal lobe epilepsy (sleep-related hyperkinetic epilepsy) often have onset obscured by muscle artifact on electroencephalogram.[49–51] A new category, combined generalized and focal epilepsy, is for patients with both focal and generalized onset seizures. These patients may have both focal and generalized discharges on EEG. Unknown epilepsy type is an additional category when there is not enough information for further classification. If there is insufficient data to classify the patient's seizure type, then the epilepsy type will also be unknown.

4.4.3 Classification of Syndrome

Following classification of seizure type, the next step in classification is characterization of the patient's syndrome. An epilepsy syndrome is a distinctive clinical entity that can be reliably identified by a cluster of electroclinical characteristics, including age at onset, seizure type(s), EEG characteristics (both background and epileptiform abnormalities), and etiology, as well as other associated factors such as neurocognitive delay, neurological examination abnormalities, or imaging changes.[35] The educational ILAE website www.epilepsydiagnosis.org, provides an excellent resource for the diagnosis of epilepsy syndromes, and contains parameters for diagnosis, as well as videos of specific seizure types and images of characteristic EEG findings. Table 4.3 consists of epilepsy syndromes presently recognized by the International League Against Epilepsy.

Many epilepsy syndromes have clear implications for etiology, treatment, and prognosis. Certain syndromes are highly correlated with a single specific cause (i.e., SCN1A mutation in Dravet syndrome), whereas others may be caused by a diverse group of genetic, structural, or metabolic etiologies, such as West syndrome or Lennox–Gastaut syndrome. Increasingly, drug trials in pediatric epilepsy are focusing on efficacy in defined syndromes. Randomized, controlled trials have documented the efficacy of hormonal treatment and vigabatrin in West syndrome,[52] of add-on clobazam, rufinamide, topiramate, lamotrigine, and felbamate in Lennox–Gastaut syndrome,[53] and of add-on stiripentol in Dravet syndrome.[22]

Syndrome identification also, in many cases, informs prognosis regarding both seizures and long-term neurocognitive function. For example, many early-onset syndromes such as early myoclonic encephalopathy, West syndrome, Dravet syndrome, and Lennox–Gastaut syndrome are associated with life-long, intractable epilepsy, significant cognitive impairment, and increased mortality.[54–56] In others, such as myoclonic atonic epilepsy and epilepsy with continuous spike and wave during sleep (CSWS), early seizure control can be challenging, and cognitive concerns can initially be seen, but long-term outcome can still be reasonably favorable in some cases.[57,58] In the genetic generalized epilepsies, including childhood absence epilepsy, juvenile absence epilepsy, and juvenile myoclonic epilepsy, seizures are typically controlled and cognitive outcomes are reasonably favorable. However, higher rates of learning disability, executive dysfunction and attention disorders, as well as poorer long-term psychosocial outcomes may be seen.[59,60] Finally, in the benign focal epilepsies of childhood, such as Panayiotopoulos syndrome or benign epilepsy with centrotemporal spikes, patients may have subtle neurocognitive deficits during the active stage of their epilepsy, but remission always occurs and long-term social prognosis is excellent.[61,62]

Table 4.3 Epilepsy syndromes

Typical Age at Onset	Epilepsy Syndrome
Neonatal period	Benign familial neonatal epilepsy Early myoclonic encephalopathy Early infantile epileptic encephalopathy (Ohtahara syndrome)
Infancy	Epilepsy of infancy with malignant migrating seizures West syndrome Myoclonic epilepsy in infancy Benign infantile epilepsy Benign familial infantile epilepsy Dravet syndrome Myoclonic encephalopathy in nonprogressive disorders
Childhood	Genetic epilepsy with febrile seizures plus Panayiotopoulos syndrome Benign epilepsy with centrotemporal spikes Autosomal dominant nocturnal frontal lobe epilepsy Late onset childhood occipital epilepsy (Gastaut type) Myoclonic atonic epilepsy Lennox–Gastaut syndrome Epileptic encephalopathy with continuous spike-and-wave (CSWS) Landau–Kleffner syndrome Childhood absence epilepsy Epilepsy with myoclonic absences
Adolescence–adult	Juvenile absence epilepsy Juvenile myoclonic epilepsy Epilepsy with generalized tonic–clonic seizures alone Progressive myoclonic epilepsies Autosomal dominant epilepsy with auditory features Other familial temporal lobe epilepsies
Less specific age relationship	Familial focal epilepsy with variable foci Reflex epilepsies

For many epilepsy syndromes that are due to a diverse group of etiologies, prognosis can be further clarified by defining the underlying etiology. Many genetic (e.g., CDKL5, STXBP1), metabolic (e.g., POLG1) or structural (e.g., diffuse lissencephaly/pachygyria) etiologies result in diffuse brain dysfunction with profound, premorbid intellectual disability that remains severe even if seizures are ultimately controlled.

While epilepsy syndromes are much more commonly identified in children than in adults, a clear epilepsy syndrome can only be defined in just over one-quarter of children.[4] Furthermore, some syndromes may evolve over time to other syndromes. For example, in the severe, early-onset epilepsy syndromes, approximately 30% evolve over time to other syndromes, including one-third of children with West syndrome who evolve to Lennox–Gastaut.[14] Evolution from Panayiotopoulos syndrome to benign epilepsy with centrotemporal spikes[63] and from childhood absence to juvenile myoclonic epilepsy[64] has also been reported.

4.4.4 Classification of Etiology

As previously noted, the terms idiopathic, symptomatic, and cryptogenic are imprecise and should no longer be used to decribe epilepsy cause.[41] The current proposal classifies etiology into genetic, structural, metabolic, infectious, immune, and unknown categories. In certain cases, etiology may fall into two or more categories, such as the patient with tuberous sclerosis complex who has a structural etiology related to a genetic cause. Furthermore, etiology does not portend a specific epilepsy syndrome or prognosis. There can be considerable heterogeneity in the phenotypic presentation of different etiologies.[41] Previously, structural and metabolic epilepsies were classified together and immune etiologies were not specifically classified.[35]

Genetic epilepsies are those in which a genetic mutation directly causes a disorder and epilepsy is considered to be a core symptom of that disorder. Given the advances in molecular techniques, there are more potential causative mutations being identified in patients with epilepsy. It is important to understand that gene mutations can be associated with a variety of electroclinical epileptic syndromes and electroclinical syndromes can be associated with different genetic mutations. For example, mutations in the potassium channel KCNQ2 are associated with benign familial neonatal epilepsy (BNFE), early infantile epileptic encephalopathy (Ohtahara syndrome), and KCNQ2 encephalopathy, which are all associated with neonatal onset epilepsy. BNFE is an autosomal dominant inherited epilepsy syndrome characterized by frequent, brief, asymmetric tonic seizures during the first 3–6 days of life. However, children with BNFE are expected to have normal development, as well as seizures that respond to treatment and spontaneously remit. Ohtahara syndrome and KCNQ2 encephalopathy are early-onset epileptic encephalopathies that are associated with pharmacoresistant seizures and profound intellectual disability.[65–67] Furthermore, the genetic mutations in these syndromes are often de novo. Therefore, we should not assume genetic etiology is inherited.[38]

Often, the specific genetic change is not known, but rather is presumed based on family history suggestive of an autosomal dominant disorder, clinical research in populations with the same electroclinical syndrome that suggests a genetic basis, or identification of a de novo single gene change or copy number variant of major effect through molecular genetics.

The previously termed idiopathic generalized epilepsies (IGEs), which include childhood absence epilepsy, juvenile absence epilepsy, juvenile myoclonic epilepsy, and generalized tonic–clonic seizures alone, likely would be better described as genetic generalized epilepsies. While the term "idiopathic" has been removed from the current proposed classification scheme, this specific group of epilepsies is so well known as the IGEs that the ILAE Task Force has determined that IGE can be used to describe these four syndromes, although genetic generalized epilepsy can be used when a genetic cause is highly suspected.[38]

Structural abnormalities seen on neuroimaging, along with electroclinical assessment that supports seizures emanating from the structural abnormality, are necessary to define an epilepsy as being due to a structural etiology. These imaging abnormalities can be acquired, such as stroke or infection, or genetic, such as tuberous sclerosis complex. It is important to identify structural causes so that surgical resection can be considered carefully if medical treatments fail.[38] Furthermore, specific associations have been made for some structural etiologies that often respond to surgical resection/disconnection. These include mesial temporal lobe epilepsy with hippocampal sclerosis, Rasmussen syndrome, elastic seizures with hypothalamic hamartoma, and hemiconvulsion-hemiplegia epilepsy.[35,38]

Epilepsy of metabolic etiology refers to known or presumed metabolic disorders with diffuse manifestations throughout the body. Seizures are a core symptom of the disorder and the metabolic epilepsy results directly from this disorder. Metabolic disorders can be due to a genetic cause, such as glucose transporter deficiency, but can also be acquired, as in cerebral folate deficiency. Identification of a metabolic etiology is essential because some metabolic disorders have specific effective therapies and early implementation thereof may improve developmental and seizure outcomes.[38] Furthermore, it is important to understand that epilepsy due to metabolic causes can be associated with early-onset epileptic encephalopathies, but can also present during adulthood with variable phenotypes.[24,68]

Infections are the most common cause of epilepsy throughout the world. The seizures should be directly due to a known infection with which seizures are commonly associated, such as meningitis, encephalitis, and neurocysticercosis. This can also include congenital infections, including Zika virus and cytomegalovirus. This does not refer to acute seizures occurring in the setting of the infection, but rather the subsequent epilepsy with unprovoked seizures that occurs after the infection. Infections can also cause structural changes.[38] Furthermore, infections can initially be latent, only to cause epilepsy later, such as subacute sclerosing panencephalitis (SSPE).[69]

Immune epilepsies are a newer concept that also present a potentially treatable cause of epilepsy and encephalopathy, if the cause is identified, through targeted immunotherapy. The seizures must directly result from an immune disorder for which seizures are a core symptom. Examples include anti-NMDA (*N*-methyl-D-aspartate) receptor and anti-LGI1 encephalitis. These can affect both children and adults and must not be forgotten in children with acute onset seizures and encephalopathy.[70] Furthermore, the presenting features can differ between adults and children. In adults with NMDA-receptor encephalitis, the presenting symptoms are often psychiatric in nature, such as depression, anxiety, or psychosis, and later the development of seizures. In adults, there is often an underlying neoplasm, such as an ovarian teratoma in women. In children, the presenting symptoms are typically orofacial dyskinesias and an encephalopathy with seizures. In children, an underlying neoplasm is very rare.[71,72]

In cases where no etiology is found, the term "unknown" should be used to describe the etiology, rather than "cryptogenic." Cryptogenic often was "presumed symptomatic," but this has been the subject of debate, especially regarding expected outcome.[18] Furthermore, the degree to which a cause can be identified is dependent upon the resources available for testing, which are variable.[38]

4.4.5 Identification of Comorbidities

It is increasingly recognized that epilepsy is a disorder with manifestations that clearly extend well beyond seizures.[73] Comorbidities such as behavior changes, intellectual disabilities, learning disorders, psychological/psychiatric diseases, social disturbances, and sleep disorders are also an integral part of their disease (Table 4.4).[74,75] Comorbidities are not due to seizures and medications alone. They are also due to underlying etiology, age of epilepsy onset, epilepsy syndrome, seizure location, and possibly epileptiform abnormalities.[76] Therefore, the findings should be viewed as additional symptoms of epilepsy as a disease. Furthermore, comorbidities are so prevalent that it was recommended that we no longer

Table 4.4 Epilepsy comorbidities

Comorbidity type	Comorbidity
Cognitive	Intellectual disability Specific learning impairments Decreased working memory Slowed processing speed Nonverbal, visuospatial memory disorders Verbal memory deficit Attention deficit hyperactivity disorder Autism spectrum disorder
Psychiatric	Executive dysfunction Behavior problems Anxiety Depression Oppositional-defiant disorder Ictal psychosis
Motor	Fine motor dexterity difficulties Developmental coordination disorder Reduced psychomotor speed
Social	Impaired social cognition Reduced recognition of faces, emotional facial expressions Underemployment Social isolation Alcohol abuse Unplanned pregnancy Reduced independence
Sleep	Poor sleep quality Insomnia – sleep onset and maintenance Excessive daytime sleepiness Sleep-related breathing disorders

use the term "benign" when describing epilepsies that are typically responsive to medications and resolve in adolescence, such as benign epilepsy with centrotemporal spikes and childhood absence epilepsy. To use this term would fail to bring attention to the learning disabilities, depression, anxiety, psychosocial concerns, and other issues that children experience.[39] Thus, in the new classification scheme it is recommended that comorbidities be considered at each level of classification, so they can be identified and managed.[38]

4.4.6 Other Important Concepts and Terms in the Classification of Pediatric Epilepsy

The term epileptic encephalopathy applies to epilepsies with encephalopathic features that may present or worsen after onset of epilepsy. This means that ongoing epileptic activity adversely impacts cognition and behavior, above and beyond what can be ascribed to the underlying etiology, if one is present (e.g., cortical dysplasia). Inherent to this concept is that amelioration of epileptiform activity has the potential to improve the developmental consequences of the disorder. There are clear cases in which obvious cognitive decline parallels onset of frequent seizures and interictal discharges, and where resolution of the epileptiform abnormalities correlates with improved development. Examples of such cases include infants with West syndrome of unknown cause treated with ACTH, or Landau–Kleffner syndrome treated with high-dose steroids. However, in other cases, the exact relationship between neurocognitive delay and frequent seizures and/or interictal discharges can be challenging to determine, particularly in the presence of diffuse brain disorders, that even in the absence of seizures are associated with severe delay.

The 2017 Epilepsy Classification[38] suggests broadening of this terminology to include both developmental and/or epileptic encephalopathy, to emphasize that both the underlying etiology and the epileptic process may independently impact development. Acceptable terms include epileptic encephalopathy, developmental encephalopathy, or developmental epileptic encephalopathy. The term "gene name" encephalopathy (e.g., *KCNQ2* encephalopathy) can be used when a genetic mutation of major effect is identified. These terms replace the previous term "symptomatic generalized epilepsy," which should no longer be used.

The terms *benign*, *malignant*, and *catastrophic* have been used in the past to describe the natural history of epilepsy. Epilepsies were previously classified as "benign" if they were expected to spontaneously resolve with age and were not previously believed to be associated with other neuropsychological disease. Epilepsies, often early onset, which did not respond to antiseizure medications, were classified as "catastrophic." However, such terms are imprecise given the frequent association with comorbidities for all epilepsy types and inappropriate due to the emotional connotation. These terms have been replaced with more descriptive ones, such as *self-limited* (to denote epilepsies where spontaneous remission is likely), *pharmacoresponsive* (for those in which there is high likelihood of rapid control with medication), and *pharmacoresistent* (for cases that are medically intractable).[35]

4.5 Conclusions

Epilepsy is comprised of a diverse group of etiologies and syndromes which result in seizures as well as associated comorbidities. Accurate classification is paramount to: (1) target investigations in a cost-effective manner, (2) inform the choice of optimal therapy in order to maximize seizure control and minimize adverse effects, and (3) provide accurate long-term prognosis for families.

References

1. Adelow C, Andell E, Amark P, et al. Newly diagnosed single unprovoked seizures and epilepsy in Stockholm, Sweden: first report from the Stockholm Incidence Registry of Epilepsy (SIRE). *Epilepsia*. 2009;50 (5):1094–1101.

2. Camfield CS, Camfield PR, Gordon K, Wirrell E, Dooley JM. Incidence of epilepsy in childhood and adolescence: a population-based study in Nova Scotia from 1977 to 1985. *Epilepsia*. 1996;37(1):19–23.

3. Freitag CM, May TW, Pfafflin M, Konig S, Rating D. Incidence of epilepsies and epileptic syndromes in children and adolescents: a population-based prospective study in Germany. *Epilepsia*. 2001;42 (8):979–985.

4. Wirrell EC, Grossardt BR, Wong-Kisiel LC, Nickels KC. Incidence and classification of new-onset epilepsy and epilepsy syndromes in children in Olmsted County, Minnesota from 1980 to 2004: a population-based study. *Epilepsy Res.* 2011;95(1–2):110–118.

5. Brorson LO, Wranne L. Long-term prognosis in childhood epilepsy: survival and seizure prognosis. *Epilepsia.* 1987;28(4):324–330.

6. Camfield P, Camfield C. Childhood epilepsy: what is the evidence for what we think and what we do? *J Child Neurol.* 2003;18(4):272–287.

7. Sillanpaa M, Schmidt D. Natural history of treated childhood-onset epilepsy: prospective, long-term population-based study. *Brain.* 2006;129(Pt 3):617–624.

8. Berg AT, Rychlik K, Levy SR, Testa FM. Complete remission of childhood-onset epilepsy: stability and prediction over two decades. *Brain.* 2014;137(Pt 12):3213–3222.

9. Wirrell EC, Wong-Kisiel LC, Mandrekar J, Nickels KC. What predicts enduring intractability in children who appear medically intractable in the first 2 years after diagnosis? *Epilepsia.* 2013;54(6):1056–1064.

10. Berg AT, Shinnar S, Levy SR, et al. Defining early seizure outcomes in pediatric epilepsy: the good, the bad and the in-between. *Epilepsy Res.* 2001;43(1):75–84.

11. Arts WF, Geerts AT, Brouwer OF, et al. The early prognosis of epilepsy in childhood: the prediction of a poor outcome. The Dutch study of epilepsy in childhood. *Epilepsia.* 1999;40(6):726–734.

12. Berg AT, Langfitt J, Shinnar S, et al. How long does it take for partial epilepsy to become intractable? *Neurology.* 2003;60(2):186–190.

13. Spooner CG, Berkovic SF, Mitchell LA, Wrennall JA, Harvey AS. New-onset temporal lobe epilepsy in children: lesion on MRI predicts poor seizure outcome. *Neurology.* 2006;67(12):2147–2153.

14. Camfield P, Camfield C. Long-term prognosis for symptomatic (secondarily) generalized epilepsies: a population-based study. *Epilepsia.* 2007;48(6):1128–1132.

15. Camfield C, Camfield P. Twenty years after childhood-onset symptomatic generalized epilepsy the social outcome is usually dependency or death: a population-based study. *Dev Med Child Neurol.* 2008;50(11):859–863.

16. Dhamija R, Moseley BD, Cascino GD, Wirrell EC. A population-based study of long-term outcome of epilepsy in childhood with a focal or hemispheric lesion on neuroimaging. *Epilepsia.* 2011;52(8):1522–1526.

17. Berg AT, Testa FM, Levy SR. Complete remission in nonsyndromic childhood-onset epilepsy. *Ann Neurol.* 2011;70(4):566–573.

18. Wirrell EC, Grossardt BR, So EL, Nickels KC. A population-based study of long-term outcomes of cryptogenic focal epilepsy in childhood: cryptogenic epilepsy is probably not symptomatic epilepsy. *Epilepsia.* 2011;52(4):738–745.

19. Wirrell E, Camfield C, Camfield P, Dooley J. Prognostic significance of failure of the initial antiepileptic drug in children with absence epilepsy. *Epilepsia.* 2001;42(6):760–763.

20. Camfield CS, Camfield PR. Juvenile myoclonic epilepsy 25 years after seizure onset: a population-based study. *Neurology.* 2009;73(13):1041–1045.

21. Wirrell EC. Benign epilepsy of childhood with centrotemporal spikes. *Epilepsia.* 1998;39(Suppl 4):S32–41.

22. Chiron C, Marchand MC, Tran A, et al. Stiripentol in severe myoclonic epilepsy in infancy: a randomised placebo-controlled syndrome-dedicated trial. STICLO Study Group. *Lancet.* 2000;356(9242):1638–1642.

23. Howell KB, McMahon JM, Carvill GL, et al. SCN2A encephalopathy: a major cause of epilepsy of infancy with migrating focal seizures. *Neurology.* 2015;85(11):958–966.

24. Pearl PL. Amenable treatable severe pediatric epilepsies. *Semin Pediatr Neurol.* 2016;23(2):158–166.

25. Toledano M, Britton JW, McKeon A, et al. Utility of an immunotherapy trial in evaluating patients with presumed autoimmune epilepsy. *Neurology.* 2014;82 (18):1578–1586.

26. Berg AT, Zelko FA, Levy SR, Testa FM. Age at onset of epilepsy, pharmacoresistance, and cognitive outcomes: a prospective cohort study. *Neurology.* 2012;79 (13):1384–1391.

27. Bombardieri R, Pinci M, Moavero R, Cerminara C, Curatolo P. Early control of seizures improves long-term outcome in children with tuberous sclerosis complex. *Eur J Paediatr Neurol.* 2010;14(2):146–149.

28. Cusmai R, Moavero R, Bombardieri R, Vigevano F, Curatolo P. Long-term neurological outcome in children with early-onset epilepsy associated with tuberous sclerosis. *Epilepsy Behav.* 2011;22 (4):735–739.

29. Shrivastava A, Kumar A, Thomas JD, et al. Association of acute toxic encephalopathy with litchi consumption in an outbreak in Muzaffarpur, India, 2014: a case-control study. *Lancet Glob Health.* 2017;5(4): e458–e466.

30. Torres JR, Falleiros-Arlant LH, Duenas L, et al. Congenital and perinatal complications of chikungunya fever: a Latin American experience. *Int J Infect Dis.* 2016;51:85–88.

31. Gastaut H. Classification of the epilepsies: proposal for an international classification. *Epilepsia.* 1969;10(Suppl):14–21.

32. Gastaut H. Clinical and electroencephalographical classification of epileptic seizures. *Epilepsia.* 1970;11 (1):102–113.

33. Commission on Classification and Terminology of the International League Against Epilepsy. Proposal for revised clinical and electroencephalographic classification of epileptic seizures. *Epilepsia.* 1981;22(4):489–501.

34. Commission on Classification and Terminology of the International League Against Epilepsy. Proposal for revised classification of epilepsies and epileptic syndromes. *Epilepsia.* 1989;30(4): 389–399.

35. Berg AT, Berkovic SF, Brodie MJ, et al. Revised terminology and concepts for organization of seizures and epilepsies: report of the ILAE Commission on Classification and Terminology, 2005–2009. *Epilepsia.* 2010;51(4):676–685.

36. Engel J, Jr. Report of the ILAE classification core group. *Epilepsia.* 2006;47 (9):1558–1568.

37. Fisher RS, Cross JH, French JA, et al. Operational classification of seizure types by the International League Against Epilepsy: Position Paper of the ILAE Commission for Classification and Terminology. *Epilepsia.* 2017;58 (4):522–530.

38. Scheffer IE, Berkovic S, Capovilla G, et al. ILAE classification of the epilepsies: Position Paper of the ILAE Commission for Classification and Terminology. *Epilepsia.* 2017;58(4):512–521.

39. Scheffer IE, French J, Hirsch E, et al. Classification of the epilepsies: new concepts for discussion and debate – Special Report of the ILAE Classification Task Force of the Commission for Classification and Terminology. *Epilepsia Open.* 2016;1(1–2):37–44.

40. Fisher RS, Cross JH, D'Souza C, et al. Instruction manual for the ILAE 2017 operational classification of seizure types. *Epilepsia.* 2017;58(4):531–542.

41. Berg AT, Scheffer IE. New concepts in classification of the epilepsies: entering the 21st century. *Epilepsia.* 2011;52 (6):1058–1062.

42. Blumenfeld H, Meador KJ. Consciousness as a useful concept in epilepsy classification. *Epilepsia.* 2014;55 (8):1145–1150.

43. Luders H, Amina S, Bailey C, et al. Proposal: different types of alteration and loss of consciousness in epilepsy. *Epilepsia.* 2014;55(8):1140–1144.

44. Blume WT, Luders HO, Mizrahi E, et al. Glossary of descriptive terminology for ictal semiology: report of the ILAE Task

Force on Classification and Terminology. *Epilepsia.* 2001;42(9):1212–1218.

45. Seneviratne U, Cook M, D'Souza W. Focal abnormalities in idiopathic generalized epilepsy: a critical review of the literature. *Epilepsia.* 2014;55(8):1157–1169.

46. Lombroso CT. Consistent EEG focalities detected in subjects with primary generalized epilepsies monitored for two decades. *Epilepsia.* 1997;38(7):797–812.

47. Ferrie CD. Idiopathic generalized epilepsies imitating focal epilepsies. *Epilepsia.* 2005;46 (Suppl 9):91–95.

48. Holmes MD, Brown M, Tucker DM. Are "generalized" seizures truly generalized? Evidence of localized mesial frontal and frontopolar discharges in absence. *Epilepsia.* 2004;45(12):1568–1579.

49. Yeh SB, Schenck CH. Sporadic nocturnal frontal lobe epilepsy: A consecutive series of 8 cases. *Sleep Sci.* 2014;7(3):170–177.

50. Oldani A, Zucconi M, Ferini-Strambi L, Bizzozero D, Smirne S. Autosomal dominant nocturnal frontal lobe epilepsy: electroclinical picture. *Epilepsia.* 1996;37 (10):964–976.

51. Tinuper P, Bisulli F. From nocturnal frontal lobe epilepsy to sleep-related hypermotor epilepsy: a 35-year diagnostic challenge. *Seizure.* 2017;44:87–92.

52. O'Callaghan FJ, Edwards SW, Alber FD, et al. Safety and effectiveness of hormonal treatment versus hormonal treatment with vigabatrin for infantile spasms (ICISS): a randomised, multicentre, open-label trial. *Lancet Neurol.* 2017;16(1):33–42.

53. Montouris GD, Wheless JW, Glauser TA. The efficacy and tolerability of pharmacologic treatment options for Lennox-Gastaut syndrome. *Epilepsia.* 2014;55(Suppl 4):10–20.

54. Riikonen R. Long-term outcome of West syndrome: a study of adults with a history of infantile spasms. *Epilepsia.* 1996;37 (4):367–372.

55. Genton P, Velizarova R, Dravet C. Dravet syndrome: the long-term outcome. *Epilepsia.* 2011;52(Suppl 2):44–49.

56. Kim HJ, Kim HD, Lee JS, et al. Long-term prognosis of patients with Lennox-Gastaut

syndrome in recent decades. *Epilepsy Res.* 2015;110:10–19.

57. Caraballo RH, Chamorro N, Darra F, Fortini S, Arroyo H. Epilepsy with myoclonic atonic seizures: an electroclinical study of 69 patients. *Pediatr Neurol.* 2013;48(5):355–362.

58. Van Bogaert P. Epileptic encephalopathy with continuous spike-waves during slow-wave sleep including Landau-Kleffner syndrome. *Handb Clin Neurol.* 2013;111:635–640.

59. Wirrell EC, Camfield CS, Camfield PR, et al. Long-term psychosocial outcome in typical absence epilepsy: sometimes a wolf in sheeps' clothing. *Arch Pediatr Adolesc Med.* 1997;151(2):152–158.

60. Baykan B, Martinez-Juarez IE, Altindag EA, Camfield CS, Camfield PR. Lifetime prognosis of juvenile myoclonic epilepsy. *Epilepsy Behav.* 2013;28(Suppl 1):S18–24.

61. Bouma PA, Bovenkerk AC, Westendorp RG, Brouwer OF. The course of benign partial epilepsy of childhood with centrotemporal spikes: a meta-analysis. *Neurology.* 1997;48(2):430–437.

62. Camfield CS, Camfield PR. Rolandic epilepsy has little effect on adult life 30 years later: a population-based study. *Neurology.* 2014;82(13):1162–1166.

63. Caraballo R, Cersosimo R, Medina C, Fejerman N. Panayiotopoulos-type benign childhood occipital epilepsy: a prospective study. *Neurology.* 2000;55(8):1096–1100.

64. Wirrell EC, Camfield CS, Camfield PR, Gordon KE, Dooley JM. Long-term prognosis of typical childhood absence epilepsy: remission or progression to juvenile myoclonic epilepsy. *Neurology.* 1996;47(4):912–918.

65. Allen NM, Mannion M, Conroy J, et al. The variable phenotypes of KCNQ-related epilepsy. *Epilepsia.* 2014;55(9):e99–105.

66. Kato M, Yamagata T, Kubota M, et al. Clinical spectrum of early onset epileptic encephalopathies caused by KCNQ2 mutation. *Epilepsia.* 2013;54(7):1282–1287.

67. Weckhuysen S, Mandelstam S, Suls A, et al. KCNQ2 encephalopathy: emerging phenotype of a neonatal epileptic

encephalopathy. *Ann Neurol.* 2012;71 (1):15–25.

68. Nordli DR, Jr., De Vivo DC. Classification of infantile seizures: implications for identification and treatment of inborn errors of metabolism. *J Child Neurol.* 2002;17(Suppl 3):3S3–7; discussion 3S8.

69. Campbell C, Levin S, Humphreys P, Walop W, Brannan R. Subacute sclerosing panencephalitis: results of the Canadian Paediatric Surveillance Program and review of the literature. *BMC Pediatr.* 2005;5 (1):47.

70. Vezzani A, Fujinami RS, White HS, et al. Infections, inflammation and epilepsy. *Acta Neuropathol.* 2016;131(2):211–234.

71. Britton JW. Autoimmune epilepsy. In: Pittock SJ, Vincent A, eds., *Handbook of Clinical Neurology.* Vol 133. Cambridge, MA: Elsevier; 2016:219–245.

72. Suleiman J, Dale RC. The recognition and treatment of autoimmune epilepsy in children. *Dev Med Child Neurol.* 2015;57 (5):431–440.

73. Jensen FE. Epilepsy as a spectrum disorder: implications from novel clinical and basic neuroscience. *Epilepsia.* 2011;52 (Suppl 1):1–6.

74. Fisher RS, van Emde Boas W, Blume W, et al. Epileptic seizures and epilepsy: definitions proposed by the International League Against Epilepsy (ILAE) and the International Bureau for Epilepsy (IBE). *Epilepsia.* 2005;46(4):470–472.

75. Ismayilova V, Demir AU, Tezer FI. Subjective sleep disturbance in epilepsy patients at an outpatient clinic: a questionnaire-based study on prevalence. *Epilepsy Res.* 2015;115:119–125.

76. Nickels KC, Zaccariello MJ, Hamiwka LD, Wirrell EC. Cognitive and neurodevelopmental comorbidities in paediatric epilepsy. *Nat Rev Neurol.* 2016;12(8):465–476.

Electro-clinical Syndromes and Epilepsies in the Neonatal Period, Infancy, and Childhood

Jules E. C. Constantinou

5.1 Introduction

Apart from age of presentation, the electro-clinical syndromes are elaborated by a distinctive and recognizable set of features including the type of seizure(s) and the electrographic traits which aggregate together.[1] Imaging findings can be considered. Neurodevelopmental and psychiatric comorbidities of varying degree are often associated. Causation may be included in the classification system. According to the 2017 position paper of the ILAE Commission for Classification and Terminology, the etiology of epilepsy may be structural, genetic, infectious, metabolic, or immune. Causation may also be unknown (formerly cryptogenic).[2] Idiopathic and self-limited (formerly benign) epilepsies occur in children with a normal neurological examination and normal neuro-imaging, in whom there may be a familial predisposition. The term idiopathic (as opposed to genetic) is still preferred by some in respect of four well-recognized idiopathic generalized epilepsy syndromes (IGEs): childhood absence epilepsy (CAE), juvenile absence epilepsy (JAE), juvenile myoclonic epilepsy (JME), and generalized tonic–clonic seizures alone (formerly generalized tonic–clonic seizures on awakening). Although monogenic or more complex genetic or environmental susceptibility factors may be implicated in these epilepsies, the mechanisms are not always fully elucidated. The attribution to genetic causation may incorrectly suggest a high rate of inheritance. Benign focal epilepsies, such as benign or childhood epilepsy with centrotemporal spikes (CECTS) and the occipital lobe epilepsies of Panayiotopoulos and Gastaut are, again according to the position paper, termed self-limited as the term benign does not seem to fully address the developmental impact of these transient epilepsies.[2] The epileptic encephalopathies, recognized as a distinct category, comprise a polymorphous group of epilepsy syndromes in which the epileptic activity itself contributes to cognitive and behavioral impairments above and beyond what might be expected from the underlying pathology alone.[1] There is abundant epileptiform activity and inherently there is the idea that limiting or suppressing the activity will improve the neurodevelopmental outlook.

5.2 Epilepsy Syndromes of the Neonate and of Infancy

5.2.1 Self-Limited Familial Neonatal Epilepsy and Self-Limited Neonatal Seizures

Self-limited familial neonatal epilepsy (SLFNE), previously benign familial neonatal seizures, is an autosomal dominant disorder which is recognized by the timing of onset, the seizure type, and the family history.

The seizures usually start in the first week in otherwise healthy newborn babies; 80% of cases present on day 2 or 3 of life. In babies who are preterm, seizure onset does not occur until the baby is conceptionally at term.[3]

There are frequent brief tonic seizures with shifting left or right predominance that are typically accompanied by tachycardia and a short apnea. There follows a clonic phase, beginning with a small vocalization and chewing movements, which captures the oculo-facial muscles and the limbs either in a focal or generalized manner.[4] Pure clonic seizures are rare.

The interictal electroencephalogram (EEG) may be normal or may show focal or multifocal sharp transients or theta pointu (see below). There are never marked background abnormalities, such as suppression or suppression burst (SB). During the seizures, there is generalized ictal flattening followed by focal or generalized spikes and waves which last as long as the seizure (59–155 s).[5]

The seizures generally remit by 4 months, although seizures can persist in some infants until 18 months of age. There are no guidelines for treatment but most children are given phenobarbital for 2–6 months.[6] Epilepsy, which is almost always easily controlled, develops later in about 11%. Some children will develop the phenotype of CECTS.[5]

In most families with SLFNE, there is a mutation of the potassium channel subunit gene *KCNQ2*. Mutations in *KCNQ3* are reported in a few families.[3] *KCNQ2* and *KCNQ3* form a heteromeric potassium channel responsible for stabilizing neuronal excitability by means of the M current. The penetrance of the mutations is about 85%.

Self-limited neonatal seizures (SLNS) or benign (idiopathic) neonatal seizures have been referred to as "fifth day fits." The seizures begin between day 4 and day 6 of life in 90%.[5] The seizures consist of unilateral or bilateral migratory clonic movements of the limbs and the face lasting 1–3 min. Apnea is noted in about one-third of seizures. Tonic seizures do not happen. Clustering of the seizures even to the point of status epilepticus is typical.

The interictal EEG is usually normal or near normal. There is often theta pointu alternant, which consists of runs of sharp theta that alternate asynchronously from side to side and contain admixed sharp waves.[5] Theta pointu is, however, a nonspecific finding that can also occur in other conditions in which neonatal seizures can develop, such as hypocalcemia, meningitis, and subarachnoid hemorrhage.

Self-limited neonatal seizures are not associated with a family history and the diagnosis is one of exclusion that relies on the elimination of other causes of neonatal encephalopathy. Acute seizures are treated with phenobarbital, benzodiazepines, or phenytoin, but treatment does not seem to have a consistent impact on the duration of the seizures.[6] Treatment with antiseizure medications beyond the acute phase is not necessary as the seizures quickly dissipate.

5.2.2 Self-Limited Familial and Nonfamilial Infantile Epilepsy

Self-limited familial infantile epilepsy (SLFIE), or benign familial infantile seizures, is another age-dependent and highly penetrant autosomal dominant disorder occurring in well babies. The age of onset is between 4 and 8 months. Seizures remit in the second year of life.

Seizures typically cluster over 1–3 days with up to 8–10 episodes a day. During seizures, there is slow head and eye deviation to one side, diffuse hypertonia and cyanosis, which is followed by limb jerks that begin on one side and become bilateral and occur synchronously or asynchronously. The side of head and eye deviation may change from seizure to seizure.[7] Interictal EEG is normal except during a cluster of seizures, when lateralized slow waves and spikes are noted in the occipitoparietal areas. Ictal recording shows focal onset in these regions.[8]

The majority of cases of self-limited familial infantile epilepsy carry a mutation of the gene for proline-rich transmembrane protein (*PRRT2*).[9] *PRRT2* is also associated with later-onset paroxysmal kinesiogenic dyskinesia. The co-segregation of infantile seizures and movement disorder is termed infantile convulsions with choreoathetosis. Individuals in a kindred are not necessarily subject to both types of attack.[3]

In addition to self-limited familial neonatal and infantile epilepsy, molecular studies do separate a third autosomal dominant focal epilepsy of the first year of life. Self-limited (benign) familial neonatal-infantile seizures presents at an intermediate age, between 2 and 3 months of age. A mixture of neonatal and infantile onsets may be seen in some families. Posterior focal seizure onset predominates.[10] There is a missense mutation in *SCN2A*, which encodes the alpha subunit of the voltage-gated sodium channel.

There are also nonfamilial forms of self-limited infantile epilepsy, previously benign partial epilepsy in infancy. There is greater variability in the age of presentation and seizures begin from 3–20 months of age. There are clusters of seizures with staring, oral automatisms, and mild convulsive movements. Ictal EEG may show temporal rather than parieto-occipital onset.[7] Apparently generalized convulsive seizures may also occur on the basis of evolution from a focal seizure. Like self-limited familial infantile epilepsy, the nonfamilial form of infantile epilepsy is also associated with time-limited seizure susceptibility.

5.2.3 Ohtahara Syndrome and Early Myoclonic Encephalopathy

Ohtahara syndrome (OS) or early infantile epileptic encephalopathy, and early myoclonic encephalopathy (EME) are rare syndromes which constitute the earliest expression of the age-related epileptic encephalopathies.[11]

Both OS and EME share characteristics of onset in the newborn period or in early infancy (before 3 months of age), frequent brief seizures which are refractory to treatment, neurological abnormalities including lethargy, coma, and low tone, and a SB pattern on EEG. The SB is persistent over at least 2 weeks (as distinct from other causes of transient SB).[12]

The syndromes are separated in terms of differences in seizure type. Tonic spasms are the cardinal feature of OS and erratic myoclonia and focal seizures prevail in EME. There are also differences in the morphology, duration, and evolution of the SB pattern. The majority of cases of OS are associated with structural brain anomalies, while the EME is mostly associated with metabolic disorders.[13]

The tonic spasms of OS are similar to those of West syndrome (WS) although there are differentiating features, including the occurrence of the tonic spasms both in the awake and sleep states. Spasms may be generalized and symmetric or lateralized. Spasms which last less than 10 s occur singly and in clusters. Seizure frequency is high and there may be from 10–300 seizures in a day in 10–20 clusters.[14]

Partial seizures with variable focality occur in 30–50% of cases. Myoclonic seizures are rare and erratic myoclonia does not occur.[15]

Myoclonia, which is erratic and fragmentary, is the core symptom of EME. The myoclonia consists of twitching that is restricted to a small area and randomly shifts from the eyelids to the corner of the mouth to the distal extremities.[11] Focal seizures occur in 80% of cases and often occur very frequently, more than several dozen times a day.[12] Symptoms may include apnea, eye deviation, migratory clonic seizures, and asymmetric tonic seizures. Tonic spasms may appear later in the evolution of EME at between 3 and 4 months of age.

The EEG in OS shows a SB pattern that consists of 1–3 s bursts of high-voltage hypsarrhythmic (150–350 μV) slow waves separated by 2–5 s stretches of diffuse background suppression (less than 10 μV). Multifocal spikes are prominent within the bursts of activity. The regularity and periodicity of the bursts and the prominence of multifocal spikes within the bursts of activity distinguish the SB pattern of OS from the SB pattern occurring as a nonspecific finding in newborns with severe brain injury.[14]

The SB pattern in OS is classically noted in both the awake and sleep states and there is no wake–sleep differentiation. In contrast, SB in EME is not continuous and is more distinct in deep sleep. Epochs of suppression are longer, lasting 3–10 s. SB in EME may not be evident at presentation and repeat EEG with capture of sleep may be necessary to establish the diagnosis.[11]

Most cases of OS relate to structural brain anomalies and particularly severe cortical lesions, which may be asymmetric.[14] Cortical dysplasias, cerebral migration disorders, hemimegalencephaly, porencephaly, agenesis of the corpus callosum, and dentato-olivary dysplasia are among the reported etiologies. Causation is, however, heterogeneous and a metabolic (including nonketotic hyperglycinemia) or genetic substrate is possible. Mutations in the syntaxin binding protein 1 (STXBP 1) and Aristaless-related homeobox (ARX), and cyclin-dependent kinase like-5 (CDKL-5) are recognized causes of OS and also of WS.[16]

Focal structural brain abnormalities are not frequently observed in EME. EME is most often associated with metabolic causes of which non-ketotic hyperglycinemia may be the most common. Organic acidemias, pyridoxine dependency, Zellweger syndrome, and molybdenum cofactor deficiency are reported.[17]

The evolution of OS and EME differs. In OS, there is typically an age-linked transition from OS to WS to Lennox-Gastaut syndrome (LGS) suggesting a close relationship between these three syndromes. SB transforms into hypsarrhythmia at 3–6 months of age and hypsarrhythmia transforms to generalized slow spike waves (SSWs) at about 12 months of age.[12] In EME, the sleep activated SB pattern persists into childhood, although transient atypical hypsarrhythmia may develop between 3–5 months of age.

There is considerable overlap between OS and EME and both syndromes may be thought of as part of a continuum. Brainstem dysfunction is presumed to generate the tonic seizures, which occur early in OS and late in EME. It is possible that brainstem dysfunction is more prominent and develops earlier in OS. Brainstem dysfunction may also serve an important role in the transformation to WS.[13]

The prognosis of OS/EME is guarded. Treatment is extremely challenging. Pyridoxine, valproate, zonisamide, benzodiazepines, and adrenocorticotropic hormone (ACTH) may be given, but are of limited efficacy. Success with a ketogenic diet is reported in OS but not in EME.[11] Vigabatrin may exacerbate EME. Resective surgery is possible in some babies with OS.

5.2.4 Epilepsy of Infancy with Migrating Focal Seizures

Epilepsy of infancy with migrating focal seizures is a very rare devastating epileptic encephalopathy of infancy. The main features include a first phase in the first 6 months of life consisting of only sporadic focal seizures with autonomic features and a second phase during which near continuous migratory polymorphic focal seizures develop. The neurodevelopmental trajectory is characterized by stagnation associated with microcephaly.[18,19]

The herald seizures typically begin in infancy and only rarely in the newborn period. Seizures are focal clonic or tonic with rapid secondary generalization and there are frequent autonomic changes such as apnea, flushing, and cyanosis.[18]

In the second phase (between 1 and 12 months, mean 4 months), there are intractable seizures during which seizures arise independently, sequentially, and sometimes in an overlapping fashion from both hemispheres.[20] Seizures occur in clusters of 5–30 seizures several times a day or can be near continuous.

EEG shows a complex status epilepticus consisting of waxing and waning and migratory multifocal ictal patterns typically in the theta–alpha range in the rolandic regions and in the theta–delta range over the posterior quadrants. Occipital seizures coincide with lateral deviation of the head and eyes, rolandic seizures with contralateral clonic or tonic jerks, temporal lobe seizures with oro-alimentary automatisms and flushing, and frontal seizures with bilateral limb hypertonia.[18]

The seizures are typically very difficult to control and most antiseizure medications are ineffective. Sustained seizure freedom has been reported on treatment with stiripentol, clonazepam, and levetiracetam in combination.[21]

The cause of most cases of epilepsy of infancy with migrating focal seizures is not known. Some cases have been associated with a gain of function mutation affecting *KCNT1*, which encodes a sodium-activated potassium channel.[19]

5.2.5 West Syndrome

West syndrome (WS) is an epileptic encephalopathy of infancy that comprises three elements including: (1) a unique seizure type, the infantile spasm (IS), which typically occur in clusters, (2) an EEG pattern of hypsarrhythmia, and (3) developmental arrest or regression.[22] Each of the elements of the triad is not always present.[23] Spasms may occur singly; hypsarrhythmia is not always present and developmental arrest is variable.

The incidence of WS ranges from 2–3.5/10,000 live births.[24] There is a slight male predominance. The peak age of onset is between 3 and 7 months and the majority (90%) of cases present before 1 year of age. Onset after 18 months is rare.[25]

Infantile spasms are time limited. Even without treatment, the spasms abate in from one-half and two-thirds of children before 3 years of age and in 90% of children before the age of 5.[26] Other seizure types often follow and 20–50% will develop LGS.[23]

A cryptogenic (cause unknown) etiology accounts for about 20% of cases.[27] Development is normal or near normal before the development of the spasms and investigation is unrevealing. Disappearance of social smile, loss of visual regard, and autistic withdrawal is often noted with the onset of the spasms.[28]

Spasms are symptomatic in 80%, occurring in babies with developmental delay and brain abnormalities. In the United Kingdom Infantile Spasms Study (UKISS), the most common etiologies identified were hypoxic-ischemic encephalopathy (10%), malformations of cortical development (8%), stroke (8%), chromosomal, especially Down's syndrome (8%), tuberous sclerosis complex (7%), and periventricular leukomalacia or hemorrhage (5%).[29]

Brain magnetic resonance imaging (MRI) shows causal abnormalities in half of the infants with new onset spasms.[30] Genetic testing which includes array comparative genomic hybridization (aCGH) followed by an epilepsy gene panel provides a diagnosis in about 40% of the remaining infants in whom causation is not readily apparent after clinical examination and MRI of the brain.

Infantile spasms are sudden, brief, bilateral, salaam-like or jack-knife contractions, involving the neck, trunk, and extremities, which may be flexor, extensor, or mixed. Each spasm consists of a quick phasic component with a rhombus or half rhombus appearance of less than 1–2 s, which may occur in isolation or may be followed by a less intense, longer tonic component lasting up to 10 s.[27]

Subtle spasms may consist simply of a slight head nod or a shoulder shrug and may be easily missed.[26] Other symptoms of a subtle spasm may include isolated eye movements, yawning, facial grimacing, and grasping.[23] Misdiagnosis is common and spasms may be dismissed as colic, an unduly prominent Moro reflex or atypical behaviors, resulting in a delay in treatment.

The classic tendency for spasms to cluster is an important diagnostic clue. Clusters of between 3 and 20 seizures over periods of 1–10 min occur several times a day and typically on awakening or before sleep.[31] A crescendo–decrescendo variation in spasm intensity is often noted through the cluster. Irritability or lethargy is evident after the cluster.

Spasms are usually symmetric. Asymmetric and asynchronous spasms are associated with symptomatic etiology and may be seen in the setting of bilateral asymmetric cortical lesions.[32] Focal features within the cluster of spasms, such as unilateral eye deviation or fisting of one hand, may also suggest a contralateral cortical focus.[27]

Hypsarrhythmia, the well-recognized interspasm EEG feature of WS, consists of a disorganized background of asynchronous, arrhythmic, very high voltage slow waves. There are admixed multifocal spikes that "shift from moment to moment" and are often posterior predominant.[26] Hypsarrhythmia is most prominent in nonrapid eye movement (NREM) sleep and is greatly attenuated in rapid eye movement (REM) sleep. Prolonged EEG is recommended to detect the hypsarrhythmia.

There are many symmetric variations of hypsarrhythmia, some of which include increased interhemispheric synchronization and increased periodicity that do not seem to correlate with prognosis.[26] Hypsarrhythmia that is not symmetric is associated with symptomatic etiology[33] and a worse outcome.[34] A persistent focus of abnormal discharge points towards a concordant focal lesion.[35]

Paroxysmal fast activity (PFA) is the prototypical ictal EEG signature of the IS. PFA without a slow wave is characteristic of subtle spasms, whereas motor spasms are associated with a diffuse slow wave (often containing a vertex positive component) that occurs with or without PFA.[32,34] The PFA typically over-rides the ascending portion of the slow wave. Asymmetric PFA is over-represented in the symptomatic group.

The goals for optimal treatment of IS include cessation of the spasms, normalization of the EEG in cryptogenic cases, and abolition of the hypsarrhythmia in symptomatic cases.[36] The response to treatment is "all-or-none," rather than graded, and this correlates with a good developmental outcome.

The evidence-based practice parameter of the American Academy of Neurology and the Child Neurology Society concludes that ACTH, as well as vigabatrin, are useful for the short-term treatment of IS.[36] ACTH or oral steroids, as opposed to vigabatrin, are preferred in cryptogenic IS because of an association with an improved developmental outcome. A shorter interval from onset of spasms to treatment initiation may improve long-term neurodevelopmental outcome.[37]

The dose and duration of treatment with ACTH is a subject of debate, as is the question of whether oral steroids are just as effective.[22] In randomized controlled trials, the response rate to natural or synthetic ACTH varies from 42–87%.[24] High-dose ACTH (150 IU/day) is not necessarily more efficacious than low dose ACTH (20-40 IU/day).[38] Short-duration treatment is associated with fewer side effects.

Vigabatrin, in a dose of between 50–150 mg/kg/day, is considered a drug of first choice in children with IS and tuberous sclerosis.[39] Vigabatrin may also be more effective than ACTH in infants with perinatal hypoxic-ischemic encephalopathy.[40] Periodic ophthalmologic evaluation is critical because of the association with constriction of visual fields and retinal toxicity in children on treatment with vigabatrin.[41] The frequency of retinal toxicity in childhood is uncertain. In one study, only 1 of 16 children treated in infancy developed vigabatrin-related visual loss when evaluated at school age.[42] Treatment with vigabatrin has also been associated with reversible regions of signal change affecting the thalami, basal ganglia, brainstem, and corpus callosum.[43]

UKISS, a prospective multicenter study, showed that cessation of spasms was more likely in infants treated with synthetic ACTH or high-dose prednisolone versus vigabatrin (73% versus 54%).[44] Those with no identified etiology who were assigned hormonal treatment had better development at 12–14 months and at 4 years of age.[45,46]

A proposed mechanism for IS postulates an interaction of cortical and subcortical structures, including the brainstem and the lenticular nuclei. The idea is that IS may be focally generated and that generalization occurs in a manner that is specific to the infant brain.[47] In babies with intractable cryptogenic IS, fluorodeoxyglucose-positron emission tomography (FDG-PET) scan may identify a single region of hypometabolism, which may reflect a previously undetected area of MRI-negative focal cortical dysplasia. Resective surgery results not only in seizure control but also in an improved developmental outcome.[48]

The prognosis of IS is determined by the cause and the best prognosis is in those with cryptogenic IS. Mental retardation is reported to occur in 85–90% of those with symptomatic spasms and in 70–80% of those with cryptogenic spasms.[49] In one study, only one-third of cryptogenic cases were cognitively impaired.[50] As already mentioned, 20–50% will develop LGS or other seizure types.[23] Adverse prognostic factors include symptomatic causation, early onset (less than 3 months), pre-existing seizures other than spasms, asymmetric EEG, and relapse after initial response to treatment.[51]

5.2.6 Dravet Syndrome

Dravet syndrome (DS), formerly severe myoclonic epilepsy of infancy (severe MEI), is the paradigm of how the syndromic approach has facilitated the uncovering of genetic mechanisms in a particular epilepsy. Between 70% and 80% of patients have a mutation of the SCN1A sodium channel, which is usually de novo. Truncation mutations make up 40% of the mutations and may be associated with an earlier age of presentation.[52] Missense mutations, which make up another 40% of the mutations, have been associated with a more severe phenotype when located within the pore-forming region of the sodium channel.[53] Genotype–phenotype correlations are, however, not consistently followed.

In the United States, the incidence of DS has been estimated at 1 in 15,700.[54] Despite the rarity of DS, the syndrome is eminently recognizable because of a characteristic age-linked cascade of different seizures types.

The onset is almost always before 1 year of age (peak 5–8 months) with a prolonged (10–90 min) generalized or unilateral clonic seizure that is typically triggered by fever.[55]

Recurrent, frequent, and prolonged seizures set in within 2 weeks to 2 months of onset. Febrile (sometimes with only mild fever) and afebrile seizures occur. Seizures may be provoked by immunizations, hot baths, or a minor infection. Alternating laterality of the hemi-clonic seizures, even within the same seizure, is typical in DS.[56]

Other seizure types appear between 1 and 4 years of age. These include myoclonic seizures, which typically occur before 2 years, atypical absence seizures, and focal impaired awareness seizures with prominent automatisms, which occur after 2 years.[57]

Convulsive seizures, either unilateral or generalized, remain prominent and are often followed by unilateral Todd's paresis. Convulsive status epilepticus occurs in up to three-quarters of cases.[58] Hyperthermia continues to trigger seizures. Other triggers include flashing lights, visual patterns, bathing, eating, and overexertion.[57]

Myoclonic seizures may be massive or erratic. Massive myoclonia, which occurs in about three-quarters of the patients, involves mostly the axial muscles.[56] The myoclonia varies in intensity and occurs singly or in brief clusters. More intense myoclonia may result in the dropping of an object or uncommonly in a fall, while less intense myoclonus may result in just a head nod. Erratic or segmental myoclonia, which affects about one-third, affects the facial or distal muscles causing subtle muscle twitches. In contrast to massive myoclonia, erratic myoclonia is not associated with generalized spike and slow wave activity.

Myoclonic seizures may occur in the few hours after waking or before a convulsive seizure, or sometimes near constantly.[55] Sudden changes to ambient lighting may bring on myoclonic seizures. Twenty-five percent of children engage in self-stimulating behaviors, such as waving a hand in front of the eyes or staring at patterns such as grids and checkered fabric.[59]

Atypical absence seizures are often accompanied by myoclonic phenomena such as eye fluttering, head nodding, and forehead myoclonic jerks.[60] Obtundation or nonconvulsive status occurs in about 40% of cases and consists of fluctuating confusion associated with erratic perioral and distal myoclonic jerks over several hours.[61]

Tonic seizures are exceedingly rare in DS and this feature, together with the occurrence of prominent myoclonic seizures permits differentiation from LGS.[61] Typical absence seizures and epileptic spasms are also probably exclusionary.

Myoclonic seizures, it is important to note, are not invariably expressed in DS and may be absent (borderline severe MEI). Borderline and core forms of DS, however, share the same genetic basis and outcome.

The EEG is usually normal in the first year of life. Interictal epileptiform abnormalities become increasingly prominent between the second and fifth year of life and typically consist of brief paroxysms of generalized, frontocentral dominant, fast polyspikes, which are induced by eye closure.[62] Photosensitivity and pattern sensitivity occurs in about half the children. Fragmentary multifocal spikes are also noted. Myoclonic seizures are associated with generalized spike/polyspike and wave discharges at more than 3 Hz.

DS is associated with a characteristic neurodevelopmental outlook. Development is normal in the first year of life but begins to stagnate between 1 and 4 years of age. The severity of the delay may relate to the severity of the epilepsy.[63] Hyperactivity and autistic spectrum features become apparent. There are fine motor delays and eye–hand coordination is poor.[55] Hypotonia, crouch gait, and ataxia occur in 60% and 20% develop pyramidal signs.

In adults with DS, cognitive impairment is the rule and only a very few are able to live independently. Seizures are less frequent and less severe. Sleep-related secondarily generalized convulsive seizures predominate. Fever sensitivity persists, but is not as prominent. Cerebellar features, including ataxia, dysarthria, intention tremor, and eye-movement disorder, become more prominent.[64] Extrapyramidal signs may also be noted. Kyphosis, kyphoscoliosis, and claw feet may develop. There is debate with regard to the relative contribution of the epileptic encephalopathy and of the genetic mutation to the cognitive and motor deterioration.

One notable characteristic of DS is a high mortality rate of between 10% and 18%.[60] Acute encephalopathy with status epilepticus accounts for about 30% of the deaths.[65] Sudden unexpected death in epilepsy patients (SUDEP) accounts for about 50% of the mortality and there are two peaks, one in infancy and another after 18 years. There is no clear evidence that the high incidence of SUDEP can be directly related to the sodium channelopathy.

Complete seizure control is difficult to achieve in children with DS. Elimination or significant reduction of episodes of convulsive and nonconvulsive status epilepticus is critical because of their association with a worse developmental outcome. Clobazam and valproic acid are considered optimal first-line medications, while stiripentol and topiramate are good second-line treatments.[57] Lamotrigine (LTG), oxcarbazepine, carbamazepine, phenytoin, and vigabatrin should be avoided because of a potential for seizure exacerbation.

5.2.7 Febrile Seizures Plus or Genetic Epilepsy with Febrile Seizures Plus

Genetic epilepsy with febrile seizures plus (GEFS+) is inherited as an autosomal dominant disorder with variable penetrance. Variability of the epilepsy phenotype within the same family is characteristic.[66]

About one-third of affected family members have febrile seizures only. The predisposition to febrile seizures extends beyond the usual age of extinction of febrile seizures at 5 to 6 years and even into adolescence.[67] About one-third develop occasional afebrile generalized tonic–clonic seizures in childhood, which usually remit in the teenage years. The remaining third develop a polymorphous epilepsy and there may be other seizure types, including absence, myoclonic, or atonic seizures.[68] DS does occur rarely in GEFS+ kindreds, but most DS cases are de novo and are not part of a GEFS+ family.[69]

Focal seizures also occur in GEFS+. These may include temporal lobe seizures, which on rare occasions are not preceded by febrile seizures, and also hemi-clonic seizures.

In contrast to DS, only 10% of patients with GEFS+ carry a mutation of *SCN1A*. Rare mutations of *SCN1B* are identified. There are also reports of a mutation in the gamma-2 subunit gene (*GAB-RG2*) of the GABA$_A$ receptor.[68]

5.2.8 Myoclonic Epilepsy of Infancy

Myoclonic epilepsy of infancy (MEI, formerly benign myoclonic epilepsy) is an uncommon syndrome that presents in normal infants between 6 months and 3 years of age. A family history of epilepsy or febrile seizures occurs in about 30%.[70]

MEI is characterized purely by myoclonic seizures. The myoclonic seizures occur, usually singly, many times a day. Occasionally seizures may occur in brief pseudo-rhythmic clusters.[71] Seizures happen in wakefulness and in light sleep.[72] The myoclonic seizures are not favored by awakening and this allows separation from IS. Myoclonic seizures may be reflex-induced by unexpected touch or sound stimulation in some patients.[73]

The myoclonic seizures involve the arm and the head and this results in a head drop and an upper-outward movement of the arms.[70] The jerks are frequently asynchronous and are not always generalized.[74] Falls occur in about one-fifth of patients.[73]

IS is different from myoclonic seizures in that IS is more intense. IS can involve strong flexion of the whole body and this is never observed in MEI.[70]

The interictal EEG is often completely normal while awake and asleep. Synchronous or asynchronous low-amplitude focal spike waves restricted to the frontocentral regions and the vertex may be seen.[74] The myoclonic seizures are associated with 3–4 Hz generalized spike/polyspike activity often preceded by anterior predominant spike and wave.[71] Ictal discharges may be bilaterally synchronous or asynchronous.[75] Subtle seizures may be associated with bilateral frontocentral spike waves with shifting asymmetry, the epileptiform nature of which may not be readily appreciated.

The focal, asymmetric, and asynchronous component of the myoclonic seizures may reflect a manifestation of age-dependent hyperexcitability of the motor cortex.[75]

It is important to highlight features that distinguish MEI from myoclonic atonic epilepsy of Doose (MAE). It should be remembered that MAE rarely presents before 3 years of age. In MAE, seizures do not occur in the drowsy sleep transition. Falls are also more frequent in MAE. Spike wave and polyspike wave bursts are often more numerous in MAE and are often grouped in long bursts.[70]

Benign nonepileptic myoclonus in an infant with normal development is another important differential diagnostic consideration. Serial video-EEG in the awake and asleep states is normal even when episodes of myoclonus are captured.

In MEI, valproate is the most effective medication and early control of the myoclonic seizures, which often run a limited course, may optimize the cognitive outlook. In some children isolated generalized tonic–clonic seizures develop in the long term. There are occasional reports of evolution into juvenile myoclonic epilepsy or absence seizures with or without eyelid myoclonia (EM).[75] The developmental outcome is not as favorable as previously suggested. Mild to moderate cognitive impairments, specific learning disabilities, and attentional disorders develop in about one-third of the children.[71]

5.3 Epilepsy Syndromes of Childhood

5.3.1 Childhood Absence Epilepsy (CAE)

This idiopathic generalized epilepsy which generally presents between 3 and 8 years of age (peak 6 to 7 years of age), constitutes 10–17% of all childhood epilepsies.[76] The incidence is 6.3–8.0/100,00 of children aged 0–15 years. There is a preponderance in girls.

The hallmark seizure type is the typical absence seizure. Children are subject to very frequent and sometimes dozens of absences a day so that the term pyknolepsy (derived from the Greek pyknos, which means frequent or dense) may be applied. Although generalized tonic–clonic seizures were said to occur in about 10% of children with childhood absence epilepsy (CAE) in the 1989 International League Against Epilepsy classification,[77] a more restrictive schema in which generalized tonic–clonic seizures hardly ever occur in true pyknolepsy has been proposed.[78] True CAE or pyknolepsy, which should be distinguished from juvenile absence epilepsy, can be conceptualized as a self-limited maturational epilepsy with a good tendency to remission when strict criteria are applied.

Absence seizures are brief and of sudden onset. They consist of an arrest of activity, staring, and profound impairment of awareness and responsiveness. There is no aura. Most children become still and will completely stop activity. Reactive automatisms, however, may occur and the child may sometimes continue a preictal activity such as walking or eating. Slight confusion may occur after the seizure but there is no prolonged postictal period.

The average duration of the absence seizure in CAE has been reported at 9.4 s in one study[79] and 12.4 s in another.[80] Seizures lasting less than 4 s or more than 30 s are not characteristic of CAE.

Eye opening is very often noted when the eyes are closed at the start of an absence, but is not invariable.[79] There may be brief upward drifting of the eyes. Eyelid movements of 3 Hz are generally not sustained. Pallor is common. Slight tonic or clonic movements may occur in the first second or two of the absence seizure, but atonic falls never occur. Incontinence of urine is unusual.[81]

Mild myoclonic features affecting the eyes, eyebrows, and eyelids may occur in the first few seconds of the typical absence seizure. Prominent EM, perioral myoclonia, and rhythmic massive limb jerking during the active stage of the absence are not seen in CAE.[78]

Oral automatisms such as lip-smacking, mouthing, chewing, and swallowing occur in more than 60% of absences. The occurrence of oral automatisms relates to the length of the absence and these automatisms are especially prominent when the absences last more than 16 s.[82] Limb automatisms such as scratching or picking with the hands and fingers may also occur. Automatisms are particularly frequent during absences induced by hyperventilation.[83]

In children with active CAE, the procedure of hyperventilation almost always induces an absence. Indeed, the failure to provoke an absence after 3 to 5 min of hyperventilation at the bedside calls the diagnosis into question. The maneuver can also be used to monitor the clinical response to treatment.

The electrographic signature of typical absence seizures consists of spontaneous and hyperventilation-activated trains of bilateral, anterior dominant, synchronous and symmetric, rhythmical single- or double-spike, and slow wave activity at a repetition rate of 3 Hz (not less than 2.7 Hz and not greater than 4 Hz).[81] A discharge frequency of up to 4 Hz may be noted in the opening second of the burst. After that the 3 Hz discharge is very regular, almost metronomic, and there is a consistent relationship between the well-modulated spikes and the slow waves. A gradual reduction in frequency occurs towards the end of the burst.

Interictally, there is a normal background. Occipital intermittent rhythmic delta (OIRDA) is seen in about one-third of children.[79] OIRDA consists of runs of rhythmic, sinusoidal, and occasionally notched 3 Hz delta across the occipital head regions. The OIRDA blocks with eye opening and is enhanced by drowsiness and hyperventilation.[84] The presence of OIRDA has been associated with a good prognosis.[85]

Fragments of generalized spike and slow wave discharges, which may be disorganized and may exhibit a polyspike component, lasting less than 2 s, occur frequently in drowsiness and sleep.[79] The activity is not necessarily generalized and there are typically no associated clinical symptoms.

Electrographic exclusion criteria for the diagnosis of CAE, according to the 2005 proposal of the ILAE, include the presence of multiple spikes (more than three), fragmentation of the discharge, and irregular, arrhythmic spike and multiple spike discharges with marked variability in the intradischarge frequency. Predominant brief discharges of less than 4 s also counter against a diagnosis of CAE.[86] Mild or no impairment of consciousness during the spike and slow wave burst is another exclusion criterion, as is the provocation of clinical seizures by photic or sensory stimuli.

CAE is associated with remission in 56–84% of cases.[87–89] The application of the strict exclusion criteria described above identifies a relatively homogenous CAE group with an especially high rate of remission (81%).[88] Remission is more likely in those with a good response to the initial seizure medication and juvenile myoclonic epilepsy (JME) may follow in those with unremitting absences.[90]

Remission of the epilepsy occurs from 2 to 5 years after onset such that seizure medications can be successfully withdrawn.[91] Only a few children with CAE (7%) still have seizures after 12 to 17 years of follow-up.[89]

A nonpyknoleptic pattern of the absence seizures, or the subsequent development of myoclonic or generalized tonic–clonic seizures (GTCS), predicts a less favorable outcome.[92] Older age at onset, failure of treatment response at 16 to 20 weeks and shortest burst duration early in the course of the epilepsy may forecast the subsequent development of GTCS early in the course of the epilepsy and may indicate an overlap diagnosis of juvenile absence epilepsy (JAE) rather than one of CAE.[93]

Absence seizures are treated because of the idea that frequent absences may undermine cognition, learning, and attention. Ethosuximide (ESM) is the treatment of choice, and sodium valproate and LTG are also considered first-line medications.[39] Carbamazepine, vigabatrin, gabapentin, and tiagabine may exacerbate absences and are contraindicated.

A seminal prospective multicenter study compared valproate (VPA), ESM, and LTG in the treatment of 446 children with CAE.[94] ESM and VPA were more effective than LTG in achieving seizure control. Treatment failure was not infrequent and was defined in terms of lack of seizure control (24% of the subjects, most often in the LTG group) or in terms of intolerable side effects to medication (22% of the subjects).

A secondary outcome of the study was the finding that VPA adversely affects attention more than either ESM or LTG. The importance of considering both cognitive and seizure outcome in choosing optimal therapy was highlighted.

There is increasing recognition that CAE may be associated with cognitive differences and an adverse psychosocial outcome. Attention deficits occur in about one-third of children with CAE.[95] Attention deficits often persist, even though seizure freedom has been attained. There is an impact on memory, executive function, and academic achievement. Parental assessment does not reliably detect the attentional difficulties. Watchful cognitive and behavioral evaluation is necessary. Young adults with CAE are more likely to have repeated a grade at school and to need special educational assistance. There are high rates of work, social, and emotional difficulties.[96]

5.3.2 Epilepsy with Myoclonic Absences

Myoclonic absences are the defining seizure type in this rare epilepsy, which is considered an absence epilepsy with the special feature of myoclonus.

Loss of awareness during the seizures does not extend through the entire duration of the EEG discharge and is typically not as profound as in CAE. Myoclonic jerks rhythmically affect the shoulders, arms, and legs. There is progressive elevation of the upper limbs owing to concomitant progressive tonic contraction.[97] Perioral myoclonia may be seen, but eyelid twitching is seldom noted. The myoclonus and the tonic contraction may be asymmetric or unilateral (despite the presence of a generalized EEG discharge), and this may result in jerky rotation of the head and trunk.

The seizures, which last from 10 to 60 s, are longer than those of CAE, occurring with pyknoleptic frequency, often on awakening, and are provoked by hyperventilation. The ictal EEG shows bilateral, symmetric, and synchronous 3 Hz spike and slow wave patterns that cannot be distinguished from those of CAE.[78]

In the pure form of epilepsy with myoclonic absence, the myoclonic absences are the only or dominant seizure type. Remission of the epilepsy is more likely and intellectual function is not impaired when remission occurs rapidly. Treatment with high-dose valproate is recommended.

In another group of children, the myoclonic absences are associated with other seizure types, especially generalized tonic–clonic seizures, which occur frequently. The prognosis is less favorable.

5.3.3 Self-Limited (Benign) Focal Epilepsies of Childhood

The self-limited focal epilepsies are characterized by focal onset seizures in the absence of a structural brain abnormality. The group includes CECTS, childhood (formerly benign) epilepsy with centrotemporal spikes (CECTS) or benign rolandic epilepsy and also the self-limited occipital epilepsies of childhood including the early-onset Panayiotopoulos syndrome (PS) and the later-onset syndrome of Gastaut: childhood occipital epilepsy-Gastaut type (COE-G.)

5.3.3.1 Childhood (Benign) Epilepsy with Centrotemporal Spikes (CECTS) or Benign Rolandic Epilepsy (BRE)

CECTS, or BRE, is the most common epilepsy syndrome of childhood and accounts for about 15% of childhood epilepsies. The incidence is 10–20/100,000 of children aged 0–15 years.[98] CECTS presents between 1 and 14 years of age and 75% of cases start between 7 and 10 years of age.[99] There is a preponderance in boys with a male:female ratio of 3:2.[100]

The hallmark seizures of CECTS are focal and include in descending order of frequency: oropharyngolaryngeal symptoms (OPLS) (53% of patients), speech arrest (40%), hypersalivation (30%), and hemifacial sensory motor symptoms (30%).[101]

The OPLS seizures are the most distinctive. There are unilateral sensory symptoms, described as tingling, prickling, or freezing, and less commonly numbness, which affect the corner of the mouth, the teeth, gums, tongue, and the pharynx and larynx.

Motor symptoms include grunting, gurgling, guttural, and choking vocalizations that often bring the seizures to attention.[102] When there is speech arrest, there is severe dysarthria and the child is unable to speak. Gestures may be used to communicate.

Hemifacial seizures typically involve the lower lip and there may be spread to the ipsilateral hand. Motor symptoms, which are usually the more prominent, comprise clonic contractions of the angle of the mouth sometimes with ipsilateral tonic deviation of the mouth. Sensory symptoms consist of numbness at the corner of the mouth.[101]

When the arm is involved it is mostly with clonic jerks and a Jacksonian march is rare. The lower limb is infrequently affected, but in younger children the seizures are less localized and may involve the entire half of the body.[103]

Hypersalivation or sialorrhea, thought to reflect a true autonomic manifestation and not simply frothing, is another distinctive feature of BRE. Hypersalivation may accompany seizures with OPLS, speech arrest, and hemifacial symptoms.

Awareness and recollection are retained in more than half of the children (58%) and the children are often able to describe the episodes after the seizure. Progression to hemi-convulsion or generalized tonic–clonic seizures occurs in about half the cases.[104]

The seizures of CECTS are characteristically sleep related. Seizures occur in the drowsy sleep transition (20%), in the middle of the night (25%), on waking or in the 2 hours before waking (35%).[105] The seizures occur only in sleep in about half of the children. Seizures may occur in sleep and in the awake state in the others. The seizures in the awake state are typically focal and generalized convulsions hardly ever occur when awake. In a very few children, seizures may occur only in the awake state.[106]

The diagnosis is confirmed by EEG, which shows drowsy- and sleep-activated centro-temporal (or more accurately central) sharp waves or less frequently centrotemporal spikes (CTS). In 70% of patients the discharges arise from C5/C6 (half way between C3/C4 and P7/P8 in the low central supra-sylvian region near the junction of the rolandic area and the Sylvian fissure). In the remaining 30%, the discharges arise mostly from C3/C4 (high central supra-sylvian region).[104,107] Orofacial involvement is common in the low central group, while hand involvement is observed in the high central group.[107]

The sharp waves or spikes are typically high amplitude (often more than 200 μV) diphasic and blunted. Small spikes may also occur. The negative peak of the centrotemporal spike is preceded by a small positive wave and there is a subsequent slow wave that is smaller than the negative peak.[108]

Classically, there is horizontal or tangential dipole formation. In clinical practice, this is best demonstrated with referential EEG, which shows negativity at C3/C4 and P7/P8, together with positivity across the frontal electrodes (FP1/FP2, F7/F8, and F3/F4). A single and stable source dipole with negativity in the central regions and positivity in the frontal regions is demonstrated with dipole EEG analysis, functional MRI and magnetoencephalo-graphy (MEG).[109–111]

There is marked activation of the CTS in sleep and they occur only in sleep in about a third of cases. The discharges often occur in brief series at 1.5 to 3 Hz. The focus is unilateral in 60% and may be found ipsilateral or contralateral to the symptomatic side.[112] Synchronous or asynchronous bilateral spikes occur in 40% and may shift from side to side from one EEG to the other. The discharges may also occur in other regions, especially in the frontal and occipital regions. The spikes dissipate within 6 months to 6 years.[106]

CTS occur in 2–3% of normal children of school age, and the vast majority (90%) do *not* develop clinical seizures.[113] There is no correlation whatsoever between the frequency and persistence of the discharges and the frequency and severity of seizures, and indeed the prognosis for remission. Rolandic spikes may also occur in other disorders such as Rett syndrome, fragile X syndrome, and focal cortical dysplasia.[104]

Seizures are generally infrequent in those children with CTS who do manifest seizures. A quarter of patients have only a single seizure and half have less than five seizures. Only 8% have 20 seizures or more.[114]

Remission occurs in virtually all children; in 92% by age 12 and in 99.8% by age 18.[115] Remission happens regardless of whether seizures occur infrequently or very frequently, and even in the presence of treatment resistance, which happens in 20% of patients.[116] The EEG discharges usually resolve after clinical remission of the epilepsy and the persistence of epileptiform abnormalities does not mitigate against the possibility of successful withdrawal of antiseizure medication.[105]

Treatment with antiseizure medication is generally not advocated unless the seizures occur in the daytime, are particularly frequent at night, or cause anxiety for the child or parent. Oxcarbazepine, carbamazepine, levetiracetam, and to a lesser extent gabapentin or LTG, are often prescribed.[117] Consideration of withdrawal of seizure medications can be given after 1 or 2 years of seizure freedom.

Rarely, treatment may be associated with exacerbation of the electrographic anomalies and the clinical seizures, culminating in status epilepticus or continuous spike waves of slow sleep.[118] This paradoxical response is more likely in the setting of rolandic spike waves, as opposed to the more typical sharp wave discharges.[119] Some authors recommend a trial of valproate in BRE to avert this rare complication.

There is increased understanding that transient mild cognitive impairments, which are predominantly language based, are frequent when CECTS is active. The impairments may include reading disorders and language impairment, and a disorder of speech motor control, which is also termed speech sound disorder.[120] Onset of the seizures before 8 years of age, a high frequency of seizures, and multifocal EEG spikes are all risk factors.[121] The question of whether or not seizure medications can modify the cognitive burden is moot.[122]

5.3.3.2 Panayiotopoulos Syndrome (PS)

Expert consensus defines PS as a "benign (self-limited) age-related focal seizure disorder characterized by seizures that are often prolonged, with predominantly autonomic symptoms, and by an EEG that shows shifting or multiple foci, often with occipital predominance."[123] Early-onset benign childhood epilepsy, at one time a synonym for PS, does not appreciate the broad pathophysiologic spectrum of PS, which implicates much more than just the occipital cortex.[124]

Three-quarters of cases present between 3 and 6 years of age (range 1 to 14 years, mean 4.7 years).[99] In the original cohort of Panayiotopoulos, the prevalence was about 13% in children aged 3 to 6 years with one or more afebrile seizure.[125] In a prospective study from Argentina, PS occurred with about half the frequency of CECTS.[124]

Autonomic seizures and autonomic status epilepticus are the chief clinical manifestations of PS.[99] The so-called emetic triad consisting of nausea, retching, and vomiting occurs in 74% of the seizures. Vomiting can be severe and repetitive and intravenous hydration may be necessary.[101] In a few cases, there is only nausea and retching, and emesis does not arise.[126] Other autonomic manifestations may occur in the sequence, either at onset, together with the abdominal symptoms, or later in the evolution of the seizure. There may be pallor (less often cyanosis or flushing), pupillary dilatation and less frequently constriction, irregularity of breathing and tachycardia, elevation of temperature, and incontinence of urine and less often of feces.[123,127]

In at least one-fifth of seizures, there are unusual syncopal-like manifestations, which may be the only expression of the seizure.[128] The child becomes totally unresponsive and flaccid for periods of between 1 or 2 minutes to half an hour.

In 90% of cases, definitive seizure symptoms begin after the onset of vomiting and autonomic symptoms. The child is interactive at the outset of the seizure but becomes confused either gradually or suddenly. Awareness can rarely be maintained. There is deviation of the eyes and often the head to one side (60%). The eyes may open wide. Speech arrest (8–13%), visual hallucinations (6–10%), and nystagmus (1%) are uncommon.[99] Only 40% of the seizures terminate with brief hemi-convulsions or generalized convulsions.

Two-thirds of the seizures occur in sleep. The seizures are usually of more than 10 minutes in duration; 44% of seizures last more than 30 minutes and sometimes many hours, consistent with an autonomic status epilepticus.[123,126] There are no neurologic sequelae. Seizures may vary markedly in terms of duration and semiologic characteristics, even in the same child.

The EEG is characterized by sleep-activated, high-amplitude, sharp, slow wave complexes, which are similar in morphology to those of CECTS. Occipital complexes, suppressed by eye opening, are the most frequent, but are not present in about one-third of patients. The occipital paroxysms may occur in brief rhythmic series at 1 to 4 Hz. Frontal and centrotemporal sharp waves also occur. The discharges typically shift from one region to the other and from one side to the other on repeat EEG. Serial EEG may, however, fail to detect any interictal epileptiform abnormalities in about 1 in 5 cases.[129]

Cloned-like spikes have been observed in 19% of cases. There are repetitive multifocal spikes occurring concurrently, which propagate to the frontal head regions suggesting the occurrence of generalized discharges or of secondary bilateral synchrony. The primary spike generator, which may be small or hard to detect, is predominantly posterior and precedes the other spikes by a few milliseconds.[130]

The EEG findings, as in CECTS, do not predict the clinical course of the epilepsy. One-quarter of patients are subject to just one seizure and another half suffer between two and five seizures.[127] A very few have more than 10 seizures, but even in those children with very frequent seizures, there is an excellent tendency to remission. Remission generally occurs within 1–2 years of onset, but 10% of patients are subject to seizures for a longer period of time.[99] A fifth of the patients develop age-related CECTS and less often occipital seizures of the Gastaut type, but these seizures also remit.[126]

Rectal or nasal benzodiazepines are frequently administered for rescue treatment. Treatment with prophylactic seizure medication is often not necessary unless the seizures are frequent and disabling. If preventive seizure medication is necessary, many authorities recommend trials of oxcarbazepine, carbamazepine, levetiracetam, or valproate.[101] There are reports of occasional exacerbation of seizures by carbamazepine.[131]

5.3.3.3 Childhood Occipital Epilepsy-Gastaut Type (COE-G)

COE-G is a rare, but well-recognized syndrome, which comprises only 2–7% of the self-limited focal epilepsies of childhood.[132] Most cases present between 8 and 11 years of age.[99]

Visual ictal symptoms and interictal occipital spikes that are brought on by eye closure are the signature features. Elementary visual hallucinations are frequently the first (82%) and sometimes the only (18%) seizure manifestation.[132] The elementary hallucinations, which are always stereotypic in the same patient, consist of flashing lights or multicolored circular patterns that appear in the periphery, become larger, and spread to the other side. Ictal amaurosis, typically sudden and complete, is the second most common visual symptom. Complex visual hallucinations such as faces and figures, and visual illusions (micropsia, macropsia, palinopsia, and metamorphopsia) are almost always preceded by elementary visual symptoms and occur in only 10% of cases.[101]

As the seizures evolve, there is progression to deviation of the eyes, which is often forceful and tonic, in about 70% of cases. Ipsilateral head version is associated. Ocular flutter and repetitive eye closure occur in 10% of patients, usually when consciousness is affected and just before evolution into convulsion.[99] Hemi-clonic seizures develop in 41% of patients and generalized tonic–clonic seizures in 8%.[103] Progression to a temporal lobe seizure is uncommon and may suggest symptomatic etiology. Postictal headache sometimes with nausea or vomiting occurs in about one-half the patients.

Most children with COE-G are subject to frequent brief visual seizures, which present several times a day or a few times a week. Convulsive seizures are much less frequent, occurring once a month to once a year or less frequently.

The interictal EEG typically shows reactive occipital paroxysms, similar to those of PS, in 80% of patients. The occipital spikes may, however, be unreactive to eye closure and eye opening in 12%.[132] The occipital spikes are typically potentiated by sleep and concomitant CTS may be activated. In comparison to PS, extra-occipital discharges occur less frequently.

Photic stimulation may activate occipital spikes and generalized spikes in photo-sensitive patients and may result in occasional visual and motor seizures.[133] There may be some overlap with photosensitive occipital lobe epilepsy, which is considered a distinct syndrome by the ILAE.

High-resolution MRI is recommended because structural occipital lobe epilepsy may present in a similar way to COE-G.

In contrast to BRE and PS, COE-G is NOT associated with an almost universal tendency to remission and the prognosis is more difficult to forecast. Seizures remit in 50–60% of patients within 2–4 years of onset. EEG abnormalities persist after the clinical resolution of seizures in about one-third.[99,133] Seizures often respond to treatment with carbamazepine but 40–50% of patients will continue to have visual seizures and infrequent convulsive episodes.

5.3.4 Autosomal Dominant Nocturnal Frontal Lobe Epilepsy

Autosomal dominant nocturnal frontal lobe epilepsy (ADNFLE) is characterized by clusters of brief, stereotypical seizures occurring in sleep. It was in ADNFLE that the first epilepsy gene, CHRNA4, was discovered.

There are familial and sporadic forms of nocturnal frontal lobe epilepsy (NFLE), which share the same clinical features. Familial ADNFLE, accounting for one-third of cases, exhibits Mendelian autosomal dominant inheritance and a variable penetrance of between 30% and 100%.[134] There is marked variation of clinical severity within a pedigree.

Gene mutations are uncovered in about 20% of patients with familial NFLE. Three genes encoding gain-of-function mutations in the neuronal acetyl choline receptor (CHRNA4, CHRNB2, and CHRNA2) have been implicated. Mutations in KCNT1, the gene associated with migrating focal seizures of infancy, and DEPDC5, originally associated with familial focal epilepsy with variable foci, have also been detected.[135]

The mean age of onset of the epilepsy is between 8 and 11.5 years. The seizures occur from sleep at any time, typically in clusters, with a mean of eight seizures each night. Seizures may occasionally occur during the day at times of poor seizure control or in continuation of a cluster through the night in about one-third of patients.[136]

The seizures are of variable duration and complexity, even in the same patient. The most common feature is hyperkinetic with frenetic bimanual and bipedal automatisms with a thrashing and sometimes tremulous, choreiform, athetoid, or ballistic quality.[137] Repetitive body rocking, rolling, or pelvic thrusting may happen. There may be vocalizations includ-ing screaming, the shouting of obscenities, or laughing. There are rapidly changing move-ments of the limbs. Brief asymmetric tonic–dystonic posturing is the second most common feature. Seizures are of 20 s to 2 min in duration.[138]

Seizures may be accompanied by a sensation of choking or shortness of breath. There are often associated autonomic phenomena. Tachycardia occurs with seizure onset in 90% of patients. Awareness is often retained during the seizures and may cause the child to be fearful of falling asleep. The mistaken diagnosis of parasomnia or conversion disorder may be given.[136]

Episodic nocturnal wandering occurs in about 40% of patients and lasts 1–3 min. The patient may get out of bed and ambulate. Screaming vocalizations and bizarre dystonic movements may occur. Differentiation from sleep walking can be very difficult, even for the sleep specialist and epileptologist.[137]

Brief paroxysmal arousals constitute another seizure type in NFLE. These are recurrent, sometimes pseudo-periodic, abrupt arousals from NREM sleep lasting less than 20 s. Motor patterns, which accompany the seizures, include eye opening, head raising, and movements of the trunk and arms.[138] The attacks may coincide with K-complexes of stage 2 sleep.

Interictal EEG is often normal. The ictal EEG is also often normal and an ictal electrographic pattern is identified in only 40–88% of patients.[136] The seizures occur in NREM sleep, mainly in stage 2 sleep, and may be initiated from a sleep spindle. Ictal electrographic patterns when noted consist of unilateral or bilateral 8–11 Hz spikes or theta activity or diffuse attenuation.

In the presence of a normal ictal EEG, semiologic characteristics may distinguish NFLE from a parasomnia. Hyperkinetic automatisms such as kicking, cycling, or rocking are specific to NFLE.

Verbal interaction and failure to arouse fully after the episode are in keeping with a diagnosis of parasomnia. Complex behaviors such as sitting, standing, or walking, which are associated with fear, occur both in NFLE and in parasomnias.[137]

Carbamazepine or oxcarbazepine is an effective treatment in low doses in many patients. Seizures are resistant to drug treatment in about 30% of patients, especially in those with more frequent and complex attacks.[134] There are anecdotal reports of benefit from treatment with acetazolamide or a nicotine patch.[138]

5.3.5 Lennox–Gastaut Syndrome (LGS)

LGS is categorized as a childhood-onset epileptic encephalopathy consisting of a triad of: (1) multiple seizure types including tonic seizures, atypical absences, and drop attacks, (2) paroxysms of fast activity (PFA and generalized slow spike wave discharges (SSW) at less than 2.5 Hz) on EEG, and (3) cognitive and behavioral abnormalities.[1]

There is limited consensus as to the minimum features necessary to make the diagnosis when one or more of these factors is lacking. Each of the seizure types is not necessarily present in every patient, especially at the onset.[139] SSW is not specific. Tonic seizures are considered a prerequisite feature for the diagnosis. Caution is necessary in ascribing a definite diagnosis because of the serious long-term implications.

The peak age of presentation is between 3 and 5 years of age (range 1 to 8 years) and the epilepsy is five times more common in boys.[140] LGS accounts for between 1% and 10% of childhood epilepsies.[141] The incidence is 1–2/100,000.

Three-quarters of cases are symptomatic.[142] The causes, which are similar to those of WS, include perinatal hypoxic-ischemic encephalopathy, congenital vascular insults, malformations of cortical development, tuberous sclerosis, Down's syndrome, and brain tumor and radiotherapy. LGS evolves from WS in 33%[140] to 65%[143] of cases.

In the cryptogenic (cause unknown) group, which accounts for about 25% of cases, there is no identifiable cause, MRI is normal and development is within normal limits before the onset of the seizures.

Tonic seizures are the distinguishing and most frequent seizure type, but are often not evident at the onset of the epilepsy.[144] The tonic seizures may occur in the awake state, but are markedly activated in sleep. The clinical changes are often subtle and the frequency of the tonic seizures is often clinically underestimated.

Minimal tonic seizures may consist simply of briefly sustained sursum deviation of the eyes, opening of the eyes and jaw, a tight facial grimace, slight neck flexion, a small vocalization, and respiratory changes.[145] Other autonomic features are prominent and include tachycardia, facial flushing, dilated pupils, and urinary incontinence (tonic-autonomic seizures).[146]

More intense tonic seizures may involve the axial muscles or nearly the entire body. The arms may raise in a semi-flexed or extended position. Prolonged tonic seizures (>10 s) may culminate in vibratory tremors (tonic-vibratory seizures).[142]

On EEG, the tonic seizures are associated with a variably initiating slow wave followed by generalized flattening or desynchronization. Fast rhythms at 15 to 25 Hz that gradually increase in amplitude as the seizure evolves may be superimposed. A recruiting rhythm at 10 to 15 Hz, which is high amplitude from the start of the seizure, may also be seen[147].

Atypical absence seizures are the second most common seizure type and occur in about two-thirds of patients. Atypical absences are similar to typical absences in that there is brief loss of awareness, but there may be clouding of consciousness (obnubilation) rather than complete loss of interaction.[148] The onset and offset are often not readily apparent. Drooling, changes in postural tone, and eyelid and perioral myoclonia may accompany the absences. The absences may be very difficult to recognize, especially in a child with severe cognitive impairment and video-EEG monitoring is necessary to measure the frequency of the absences.[149]

Atypical absences are most reliably distinguished from typical absences by the frequency of the concomitant generalized spike and slow wave discharge, which is at 1.5 to 2.5 Hz (SSW) rather than at 3 Hz. The ictal discharge is difficult to separate from the interictal SSW, but the ictal pattern is higher amplitude and is more rhythmic and sustained. Occasionally, PFA at 10–20 Hz may be admixed.[150]

Drop attacks, the third most frequent type of seizure, are present in about one-half of patients. Drop attacks consist of a split-second loss of posture resulting in a sudden fall either forwards or backwards. The drop may affect just the head (head drop) or the whole body. Injuries affecting especially the face and head are common. Drop attacks are not pathognomonic for LGS and may be seen in other epilepsy syndromes, especially myoclonic atonic epilepsy of Doose.[151]

Drop attacks may be the result of a variety of seizure types, including atonic, myoclonic–atonic, myoclonic, and tonic. Pure atonic seizures, in contrast to prevailing notions, are rare in LGS. In one study, atonic seizures were responsible for only 2 of 48 recorded drops.[152] Indeed, the majority of falls in LGS seem to reflect brief tonic seizures associated with increases in tone affecting agonist and antagonist muscles, especially of the trunk and the hips.[152,153] This results in a loss of balance, which causes the fall.

The ictal EEG associated with drop seizures is varied. Tonic seizures are associated with slight flattening or desynchronization or with PFA. Atonic seizures coincide with the slow wave component of a generalized polyspike wave complex.[142]

Associated, but not defining, seizure types in LGS may include focal seizures, generalized tonic–clonic seizures, and myoclonic seizures.

Nonconvulsive status epilepticus complicates the course of the epilepsy in as many as two-thirds of patients.[141] Absence status consists of continuous or near continuous atypical absences.

There is a mild and insidious clouding of interaction and confusion, which may last hours to days and can be difficult to recognize.[144] Brief tonic seizures may be superimposed. EEG correlates consist of near continuous SSW containing brief bursts of generalized polyspikes.[145]

The cardinal interictal EEG feature of LGS is SSW on a slow background. Individual sharp waves in the sharp and slow wave complexes are typically, but not always, broad based and are of 70 to 200 ms in duration. There is an aftercoming sinusoidal slow wave of 300 to 500 ms.[154] The frequency of the SSW may vary between 1 to 4 Hz, but is generally at 1.5 to 2.5 Hz. In contrast to the very regular 3 Hz discharge of CAE, the discharges are characteristically irregular in frequency, amplitude, and morphology, often within the same burst. Slow waves are not always preceded by a spike or sharp wave. Shifting asymmetry is common and persisting asymmetry may suggest the possibility of a unilateral hemisphere lesion.[142]

Another characteristic of the SSW pattern of LGS is its abundance. Bursts with unclear onset and offset may wax and wane over long periods. There may not be any distinct clinical concomitants such that the differentiation between ictal and interictal patterns is obscured.[139] Clinically apparent absences are, however, always associated with a SSW burst.[144]

Bursts of PFA at 10 to 20 Hz, noted especially in NREM sleep, are another hallmark and perhaps a necessary feature for the diagnosis of LGS.[155] Bursts without appreciable ictal evolution or recruitment, lasting 1–9 s, may recur every few seconds.[156] Clinical concomitants are not easily appreciated, but polygraphic recording may frequently elaborate subtle changes, such as brief apnea or axial contraction.[146]

LGS is associated with a poor outcome. Less than 10% achieve freedom from seizures in adulthood.[141] Seizure frequency does decrease in adolescence but daily or weekly seizures continue in two-thirds of cases.[147] A previous history of WS, onset before 3 years of age, high seizure frequency, and long periods of exacerbation, episodes of status epilepticus, persistence of a slow background and SSW augur an adverse prognosis.[157]

Tonic seizures and drop attacks often persist into adulthood, but atypical absences often subside. The SSW continues in about one-third of patients and another one-third develop multifocal spikes with or without generalization.[158]

LGS is associated with severe intellectual and psychiatric disability. Cognitive impairment is increasingly evident with the passage of time. Although 30–50% of patients are affected at the presentation of the epilepsy, 70–80% are affected after 4 years.[159] There may be associated autistic spectrum features and difficulties with behavior regulation are common. The prognosis for independent living is guarded.[159]

LGS is drug resistant in 90% of cases.[160] Polytherapy is almost always obligatory, rather than "rational," and there is a balance between the need to control seizures and the need to avoid side effects. Additive side effects may result in sedation, behavioral disturbance, and exacerbation of seizures.[161]

Valproate is the most commonly prescribed medication and is considered first line by many even in the absence of level I or II evidence. Six seizure medications including LTG, topiramate, felbamate, rufinamide, clobazam, and clonazepam are approved by the US Food and Drug Administration (FDA) on the basis of blinded prospective trials.[161]

Nondrug treatments include a ketogenic diet, vagus nerve stimulation (VNS), and corpus callosotomy (CC). A recent meta analysis comparing CC and VNS showed that CC is significantly more effective in achieving a >50% and a >75% reduction in drop seizures. Patients in the analysis were more likely to be free of drop seizures if they underwent CC (48% versus 22.8% with VNS), but the differences were not significant.[162]

5.3.6 Epilepsy with Myoclonic–Atonic Seizures (Doose Syndrome)

Epilepsy with myoclonic–atonic (myoclonic astatic) seizures (EMAS) or Doose syndrome can be difficult to differentiate from LGS, myoclonic epilepsy of infancy (MEI), and atypical CECTS or pseudo-Lennox syndrome.

Doose syndrome accounts for 1–2% of childhood epilepsies and the incidence is about 1/10,000 children.[163] The epilepsy characteristically presents in previously typically developing children between 2 to 6 years of age. About three-quarters of cases occur in boys.[59] There may be a family history of epilepsy in 15–30%.

Doose syndrome is characterized by multiple seizure types, including myoclonic, atonic, and myoclonic–atonic seizures.[164] The myoclonic–atonic seizures, which are necessary for the diagnosis, consist of a loss of muscle tone preceded by a short myoclonia. Drop attacks occur in about 64% of patients. Generalized tonic–clonic seizures and episodes of absence or myoclonic status may occur.

The tonic seizures characteristic of LGS, are only occasionally seen in Doose syndrome. Tonic seizures while awake occur only in LGS. Infrequent sleep-related tonic seizures may, however, occur late in the presentation of Doose syndrome, which runs an unfavorable course.[164]

The EEG background is typified by rhythmical parietally accentuated 4–7 Hz theta, which develops early in the course of the epilepsy, and although similar to a drowsy rhythm, is expressed when the child is alert.[165] The posterior awake background and intrinsic sleep architecture are preserved. Occipital 4 Hz activity may occur and is blocked by eye opening.

Spikes, irregular spikes, and polyspikes first appear in sleep. In children with myoclonic–atonic seizures there are generalized 2–3 Hz spike and waves. Fast and irregular polyspike and waves and spike and waves are prominent should myoclonic seizures dominate the epilepsy at a given time.[165] Photosensitivity with 4–7 Hz spike wave complexes may be noted in some patients.

These EEG features separate Doose syndrome from LGS in which there is background slowing and in which slower (2–2.5 Hz) spike wave runs occur for long periods.[163] Multifocal spikes and sleep-related PFA are not anticipated in Doose syndrome.

Doose syndrome is heterogeneous. In 50–89% of patients, there is permanent remission of the epilepsy within 3 years of onset.[166] In most, the seizures are readily controlled with antiseizure medications (especially valproic acid), which can be successfully withdrawn in a few years. In a few cases, Doose syndrome is severe and over time cannot be distinguished from LGS.[144]

5.3.7 Atypical Childhood Epilepsy with Centrotemporal Spikes/Pseudo-Lennox Syndrome

The onset of seizures is typically between 2 and 7 years of age. A period of typical rolandic seizures is followed by the development of drop attacks after about 18 months.[167] The course of the epilepsy is characterized by active periods with multiple falls punctuated by periods of marked seizure quiescence, sometimes lasting several months.[139] It is suggested that the syndrome can sometimes reflect typical CECTS, which is modified by medication toxicity.

The EEG shows central spikes identical to those of BRE, but there are also very frequent spike wave complexes that occur bisynchronously across the frontocentral head regions.[144] There is no PFA and tonic seizures do not occur.

The syndrome is important to identify. Although seizures are difficult to treat at times of seizure exacerbation, most patients have spontaneous remission of seizures at puberty.[133]

5.3.8 Epilepsy with Eyelid Myoclonia (Jeavons Syndrome)

The diagnostic criteria for epilepsy with eyelid myoclonia (EEM), previously Jeavons syndrome, consist of a triad including: (1) eyelid myoclonia (EM) with or without absence, (2) eye-closure-induced seizures/EEG paroxysms, and (3) photosensitivity.[168] EEM may be thought of as an idiopathic generalized epilepsy syndrome, which usually presents between 6 and 8 years of age (range 2–14 years) and more commonly affects girls.[168] There is often a delay in diagnosis because the EM may be mistaken for a tic or habit.[169]

The EM, which is the main seizure type, consists of a marked jerking or flutter of the eyelids together with jerky upward deviation of the eyes and retropulsion of the head. The rapid blinking contrasts with the slight, poorly sustained flicker of the eyelids which may occur in a typical absence.[170] The EM may occur in isolation (EM without absence) or may be associated with mild impairment of consciousness (EM with absence). Absence seizures alone do not occur in EEM.

The EM may be associated with mild myoclonia restricted to the eyebrows, head, and shoulders.[171] Massive myoclonia is, however, considered exclusionary by some authors.[169] It is suggested that EM seizures may occur as an overlap phenomenon in other idiopathic generalized epilepsy syndromes such as juvenile myoclonic epilepsy (JME).[172] EM may also occur in epilepsies of unknown causation or that are structural-metabolic.[170] Significant cognitive impairment, neurologic abnormalities on examination, an abnormal MRI, and an abnormal EEG background suggest symptomatic rather than idiopathic causation.

In EEM, EM seizures, which last 3–6 s, occur in a pyknoleptic pattern. The majority of the seizures occur after slow eye closure (not random eye blinking) in uninterrupted light. The induction of seizures by eye closure is abolished in the dark. There is also sensitivity to both flickering and nonflickering light (in contrast to other photic epilepsies that are sensitive only to flickering light).[168] Self-induction of seizures may occur infrequently.

Eyelid myoclonic status epilepticus happens in one-fifth of patients. The EMs occur repetitively but discontinuously over 40 to 60 min.[170] Generalized tonic–clonic seizures are usually infrequent and may be triggered by sleep deprivation, alcohol, television and video game exposure, and inappropriate choice of medication.

The ictal EEG correlate of EM consists of brief (1–6 s, average 2–3 s) runs of generalized irregular spike wave and polyspike slow waves at 3 to 6 Hz, which are most likely to occur after eye closure in a well-lit room. Photosensitivity occurs in all untreated patients, is masked or modified by medication, and decreases with age.[168] The discharges may show frontal or posterior predominance. Posterior spikes or "spiky" alpha may precede the generalized spikes.[173] This lends credence to the concept of a systemic epilepsy that includes pathways from the occipital to the frontal cortex that are modulated through reciprocal thalamo-cortical connections.[171]

EEM is a lifelong disorder. The EM persists into adulthood and is notoriously recalcitrant to treatment. It occurs several times a day often without apparent absence or EEG concomitants.[78] EM is considered a myoclonic as opposed to an absence epilepsy and drugs with antimyoclonic properties, such as valproate, levetiracetam, zonisamide, and benzodiazepines are recommended.[169] LTG may be associated with an exacerbation of myoclonic jerks.

5.3.9 Epileptic Encephalopathy with Continuous Spike-and-Wave During Sleep/Landau–Kleffner Syndrome (Acquired Epileptic Aphasia)

Electrical status epilepticus in sleep (ESES) refers to an electrographic finding consisting of profound activation of epileptiform activity in sleep, while the terms continuous spike and wave during slow wave sleep (CSWS) and Landau-Kleffner syndrome (LKS) refer to the clinical epileptic encephalopathy associated with ESES.[174] In LKS, the epileptiform disturbance affects the posterior temporal regions and is associated with auditory agnosia and regression of language. CSWS preferentially involves the frontal regions and is associated with more global loss of skills.[175]

LKS presents between 3 and 8 years (peak 4–5 years) of age, typically in children with previously normal or near normal language. A verbal auditory agnosia (an inability to understand verbal and nonverbal sounds) underpins a progressive and sometimes fluctuating loss of language over days to months. There are difficulties of articulation, word retrieval, and fluency, with perseverations and neologisms.[176] In severe cases, mutism may develop. The child may seem deaf and may not appreciate the significance of sounds such as the telephone ringing or door knocking.[177] Behavioral and attentional disorders are common.

Clinical seizures are not present in 20–30% of children with LKS and in those with seizures, the seizures are generally infrequent and easy to control.[175] Atypical absence, focal clonic, or generalized tonic–clonic seizures predominate.[178] Seizures generally subside by 15 years of age.[179]

The prognosis of the aphasia is variable and residual deficits in adulthood may range from a mild to moderate language disorder to almost no verbal ability.[178] Onset before 5 years of age and longstanding EEG abnormalities are adverse prognostic factors. Fluctuations in the aphasia may imply a more favorable prognosis.[180]

CSWS presents between 1 and 14 years (mean 4–8 years). In contrast to LKS, which is typically non-lesional, MRI may demonstrate a structural lesion such as polymicrogyria or a porencephalic cyst in 30–50% of cases of CSWS.[174]

There is a pervasive spectrum of neurodevelopmental deterioration that includes cognitive impairment, learning disorder, and hyperactivity.[181] There are impairments of short-term memory and temporospatial skills and attention. Fluctuating mostly expressive aphasia occurs and there is preservation of receptive language. There may also be declines in fine and gross motor abilities in the form of dyspraxia, ataxia, or dystonia, which may be unilateral.[182]

Seizures, first occurring between 3 and 5 years of age, are the presenting symptom in 80% of children with CSWS. Initially, seizures tend to occur infrequently in sleep and are unilateral about 50% of the time. The seizures may mimic those of BRE. Unilateral status epilepticus occurs in 6%.[183]

There is a marked increase in the type and frequency of seizures when ESES appears 2 to 3 years after seizure onset, and this coincides with the time of neurodevelopmental regression; 70% of patients develop daily seizures. Unilateral motor seizures are now rare. Atonic seizures resulting in falls and atypical absences increase in frequency, sometimes culminating in absence status.[184] The absence of tonic seizures, which are not a feature of CSWS, facilitates distinction from LGS.

The clinical seizures in CSWS remit in puberty as the ESES resolves, even in those with a structural brain anomaly.[185] There is residual cognitive morbidity in the majority. In about half, there are residual deficits that preclude independent living.[184] Normal language and intelligence is seen in only 10–44%.[174]

In wakefulness, the EEG shows focal or multifocal frontotemporal or centrotemporal (CSWS) or posterior temporal spikes (LKS) often with associated generalized spike waves. In some, the discharges may call to mind those of CECTS. The presence of fast spikes or of background asymmetry may suggest structural pathology.[177]

ESES is recognized by the marked potentiation of epileptiform discharges in NREM sleep that results in a near continuous pattern of generalized, irregular slow spike and waves at 1.5–2.5 Hz. The epileptiform activity occupies a significant proportion (classically more than 85%) of the sleep state record, although some authors accept a lower spike and wave index.[181] ESES dissipates in REM sleep.

The discharges are frontocentral or frontotemporal dominant in CSWS and posterior temporal dominant in LKS.[174] Unilateral or more focal subcontinuous paroxysmal discharges may also occur and may alternate with generalized activity in the same patient.[177]

ESES runs a self-limited course and disappears 3 to 4 years after onset at about 11 years of age.[181] An ESES duration of more than 2 years has been associated with worse prognosis.

The aim of treatment in LKS/CSWS is not just to control seizures, but to eliminate the ESES as promptly as possible.[186] Phenytoin, carbamazepine, and phenobarbital may result in clinical and electrographic deterioration. Valproate, benzodiazepines, ethosuximide, and levetiracetam may result in some improvement.[177]

Treatment with steroids/ACTH is associated with improvement in three-quarters of cases.[187] ESES often relapses when steroids are withdrawn and long-term treatment may be necessary. Intermittent 3–4-week cycles of high-dose rectal diazepam can result in temporary remission.[188] Treatment with daily maintenance clobazam or clonazepam may be associated with more sustained benefits. Improvement in language after multiple subpial transection has been reported in some children with highly refractory LKS.[189]

5.4 Conclusion

In any child with seizures, recognition of the epilepsy syndrome facilitates discourse between medical professionals and families about the expected course of the epilepsy in the child, about appropriate investigation and treatment, whether or not there is a potential for remission, and what the cognitive outlook might be. For the epileptologist, the classification provides a common glossary that enables exchange of ideas for the advancement of knowledge about epilepsy especially in the fields of genetics, epileptic mechanisms, and advanced imaging.[190]

References

1. Berg AT, Berkovic SF, Brodie MJ, et al. Revised terminology and concepts for organization of seizures and epilepsies: report of the ILAE Commission on Classification and Terminology, 2005–2009. *Epilepsia*. 2010;51(4):676–685.

2. Scheffer IE, Berkovic S, Capovilla G, et al. ILAE classification of the epilepsies: position paper of the ILAE Commission for Classification and Terminology. *Epilepsia*. 2017;58(4):512–521.

3. Scheffer IE, Harkin LA, Dibbens LM, Mulley JC, Berkovic SF. Neonatal epilepsy syndromes and generalized epilepsy with febrile seizures plus (GEFS+). *Epilepsia*. 2005;46(Suppl 10):41–47.

4. Hirsch E, Velez A, Sellal F, et al. Electroclinical signs of benign neonatal familial convulsions. *Ann Neurol*. 1993;34 (6):835–841.

5. Plouin P, Neubauer BA. Benign familial and non-familial neonatal seizures. In: Bureau M, Genton P, Dravet C, et al., eds., *Epileptic Syndromes in Infancy, Childhood and Adolescence*. 5th edn. Montrouge, France: John Libbey Eurotext; 2012:77–88.

6. Yamamoto H, Okumura A, Fukuda M. Epilepsies and epileptic syndromes starting in the neonatal period. *Brain Dev*. 2011;33 (3):213–220.

7. Specchio N, Vigevano F. The spectrum of benign infantile seizures. *Epilepsy Res*. 2006;70(Suppl 1):S156–167.

8. Vigevano F. Benign familial infantile seizures. *Brain Dev*. 2005;27(3):172–177.

9. Zara F, Specchio N, Striano P, et al. Genetic testing in benign familial epilepsies of the first year of life: clinical and diagnostic significance. *Epilepsia*. 2013;54(3):425–436.

10. Berkovic SF, Heron SE, Giordano L, et al. Benign familial neonatal-infantile seizures: characterization of a new sodium channelopathy. *Ann Neurol*. 2004;55 (4):550–557.

11. Beal JC, Cherian K, Moshe SL. Early-onset epileptic encephalopathies: Ohtahara syndrome and early myoclonic encephalopathy. *Pediatr Neurol*. 2012;47 (5):317–323.

12. Ohtahara S, Yamatogi Y. Epileptic encephalopathies in early infancy with suppression-burst. *J Clin Neurophysiol*. 2003;20(6):398–407.

13. Djukic A, Lado FA, Shinnar S, Moshe SL. Are early myoclonic encephalopathy (EME) and the Ohtahara syndrome (EIEE) independent of each other? *Epilepsy Res*. 2006;70(Suppl 1):S68–76.

14. Ohtahara S, Yamatogi Y. Ohtahara syndrome: with special reference to its developmental aspects for differentiating from early myoclonic encephalopathy. *Epilepsy Res*. 2006;70 (Suppl 1):S58–67.

15. Mizrahi EM, Milh M. Early severe neonatal and infantile epilepsies. In: Bureau M, Genton P, Dravet C, et al., eds., *Epileptic Syndromes in Infancy, Childhood and Adolescence*. 5th edn. Montrouge, France: John Libbey Eurotext; 2012:89–98.

16. Pavone P, Spalice A, Polizzi A, Parisi P, Ruggieri M. Ohtahara syndrome with emphasis on recent genetic discovery. *Brain Dev*. 2012;34(6):459–468.

17. Gursoy S, Ercal D. Diagnostic approach to genetic causes of early-onset epileptic encephalopathy. *J Child Neurol*. 2016;31 (4):523–532.

18. Coppola G. Malignant migrating partial seizures in infancy: an epilepsy syndrome of unknown etiology. *Epilepsia*. 2009;50 (Suppl 5):49–51.

19. McTague A, Appleton R, Avula S, et al. Migrating partial seizures of infancy: expansion of the electroclinical, radiological and pathological disease spectrum. *Brain*. 2013;136(Pt 5):1578–1591.

20. Marsh E, Melamed SE, Barron T, Clancy RR. Migrating partial seizures in infancy: expanding the phenotype of a rare seizure syndrome. *Epilepsia*. 2005;46(4):568–572.

21. Merdariu D, Delanoe C, Mahfoufi N, Bellavoine V, Auvin S. Malignant migrating partial seizures of infancy

controlled by stiripentol and clonazepam. *Brain Dev.* 2013;35(2):177–180.

22. Trevathan E. Infantile spasms and Lennox-Gastaut syndrome. *J Child Neurol.* 2002;17 (Suppl 2):2S9–2S22.

23. Pavone P, Striano P, Falsaperla R, Pavone L, Ruggieri M. Infantile spasms syndrome, West syndrome and related phenotypes: what we know in 2013. *Brain Dev.* 2014;36 (9):739–751.

24. Pellock JM, Hrachovy R, Shinnar S, et al. Infantile spasms: a U.S. consensus report. *Epilepsia.* 2010;51(10):2175–2189.

25. Riikonen R. Epidemiological data of West syndrome in Finland. *Brain Dev.* 2001;23 (7):539–541.

26. Hrachovy RA, Frost JD, Jr. Infantile epileptic encephalopathy with hypsarrhythmia (infantile spasms/West syndrome). *J Clin Neurophysiol.* 2003;20 (6):408–425.

27. Fusco L, Chiron C, Trivisano M, Vigevano F, Chugani HT. Infantile spasms. In: Bureau M, Genton P, Dravet C, et al., eds., *Epileptic Syndromes in Infancy, Childhood and Adolescence.* 5th edn. Montrouge, France: John Libbey Eurotext; 2012:99–113.

28. Kramer U, Sue WC, Mikati MA. Focal features in West syndrome indicating candidacy for surgery. *Pediatr Neurol.* 1997;16(3):213–217.

29. Osborne JP, Lux AL, Edwards SW, et al. The underlying etiology of infantile spasms (West syndrome): information from the United Kingdom Infantile Spasms Study (UKISS) on contemporary causes and their classification. *Epilepsia.* 2010;51 (10):2168–2174.

30. Wirrell EC, Shellhaas RA, Joshi C, et al. How should children with West syndrome be efficiently and accurately investigated?: results from the National Infantile Spasms Consortium. *Epilepsia.* 2015;56 (4):617–625.

31. Dulac O. What is West syndrome? *Brain Dev.* 2001;23(7):447–452.

32. Fusco L, Vigevano F. Ictal clinical electroencephalographic findings of spasms

in West syndrome. *Epilepsia.* 1993;34 (4):671–678.

33. Drury I, Beydoun A, Garofalo EA, Henry TR. Asymmetric hypsarrhythmia: clinical electroencephalographic and radiological findings. *Epilepsia.* 1995;36(1):41–47.

34. Gaily E, Liukkonen E, Paetau R, Rekola R, Granstrom ML. Infantile spasms: diagnosis and assessment of treatment response by video-EEG. *Dev Med Child Neurol.* 2001;43 (10):658–667.

35. Oka M, Kobayashi K, Akiyama T, Ogino T, Oka E. A study of spike-density on EEG in West syndrome. *Brain Dev.* 2004;26 (2):105–112.

36. Mackay MT, Weiss SK, Adams-Webber T, et al. Practice parameter: medical treatment of infantile spasms. Report of the American Academy of Neurology and the Child Neurology Society. *Neurology.* 2004;62 (10):1668–1681.

37. Wilmshurst JM, Gaillard WD, Vinayan KP, et al. Summary of recommendations for the management of infantile seizures: task force report for the ILAE Commission of Pediatrics. *Epilepsia.* 2015;56 (8):1185–1197.

38. Hrachovy RA, Frost JD, Jr., Glaze DG. High-dose, long-duration versus low-dose, short-duration corticotropin therapy for infantile spasms. *J Pediatr.* 1994;124 (5 Pt 1):803–806.

39. Wheless JW, Clarke DF, Carpenter D. Treatment of pediatric epilepsy: expert opinion, 2005. *J Child Neurol.* 2005;20 (Suppl 1):S1–56; quiz S59–60.

40. Vigevano F, Cilio MR. Vigabatrin versus ACTH as first-line treatment for infantile spasms: a randomized, prospective study. *Epilepsia.* 1997;38(12):1270–1274.

41. Brodie SE. Screening for vigabatrin (Sabril®) retinal toxicity in children. *Ophthalmic Genet.* 2011;32(4):193–195.

42. Gaily E, Jonsson H, Lappi M. Visual fields at school-age in children treated with vigabatrin in infancy. *Epilepsia.* 2009;50 (2):206–216.

43. Pearl PL, Vezina LG, Saneto RP, et al. Cerebral MRI abnormalities associated

with vigabatrin therapy. *Epilepsia.* 2009;50 (2):184–194.

44. Lux AL, Edwards SW, Hancock E, et al. The United Kingdom Infantile Spasms Study comparing vigabatrin with prednisolone or tetracosactide at 14 days: a multicentre, randomised controlled trial. *Lancet.* 2004;364(9447):1773–1778.

45. Lux AL, Edwards SW, Hancock E, et al. The United Kingdom Infantile Spasms Study (UKISS) comparing hormone treatment with vigabatrin on developmental and epilepsy outcomes to age 14 months: a multicentre randomised trial. *Lancet Neurol.* 2005;4(11):712–717.

46. Darke K, Edwards SW, Hancock E, et al. Developmental and epilepsy outcomes at age 4 years in the UKISS trial comparing hormonal treatments to vigabatrin for infantile spasms: a multi-centre randomised trial. *Arch Dis Child.* 2010;95 (5):382–386.

47. Chugani HT. Pathophysiology of infantile spasms. *Adv Exp Med Biol.* 2002;497:111–121.

48. Chugani HT, Shewmon DA, Shields WD, et al. Surgery for intractable infantile spasms: neuroimaging perspectives. *Epilepsia.* 1993;34(4):764–771.

49. Wong M, Trevathan E. Infantile spasms. *Pediatr Neurol.* 2001;24(2):89–98.

50. Kivity S, Lerman P, Ariel R, et al. Long-term cognitive outcomes of a cohort of children with cryptogenic infantile spasms treated with high-dose adrenocorticotropic hormone. *Epilepsia.* 2004;45(3):255–262.

51. Kossoff EH. Infantile spasms. *Neurologist.* 2010;16(2):69–75.

52. Marini C, Scheffer IE, Nabbout R, et al. The genetics of Dravet syndrome. *Epilepsia.* 2011;52(Suppl 2):24–29.

53. Meisler MH, Kearney JA. Sodium channel mutations in epilepsy and other neurological disorders. *J Clin Invest.* 2005;115(8):2010–2017.

54. Wu YW, Sullivan J, McDaniel SS, et al. Incidence of Dravet syndrome in a US population. *Pediatrics.* 2015;136(5): e1310–1315.

55. Dravet C. The core Dravet syndrome phenotype. *Epilepsia.* 2011;52(Suppl 2):3–9.

56. Arzimanoglou A. Dravet syndrome: from electroclinical characteristics to molecular biology. *Epilepsia.* 2009;50(Suppl 8):3–9.

57. Wirrell EC, Laux L, Donner E, et al. Optimizing the diagnosis and management of Dravet syndrome: recommendations from a North American consensus panel. *Pediatr Neurol.* 2017;68:18–34 e13.

58. Oguni H, Hayashi K, Awaya Y, Fukuyama Y, Osawa M. Severe myoclonic epilepsy in infants – a review based on the Tokyo Women's Medical University series of 84 cases. *Brain Dev.* 2001;23(7):736–748.

59. Guerrini R, Aicardi J. Epileptic encephalopathies with myoclonic seizures in infants and children (severe myoclonic epilepsy and myoclonic-astatic epilepsy). *J Clin Neurophysiol.* 2003;20 (6):449–461.

60. Gataullina S, Dulac O. From genotype to phenotype in Dravet disease. *Seizure.* 2017;44:58–64.

61. Dravet C, Bureau M, Oguni H, Cokar O, Guerrini R. Dravet syndrome (severe myoclonic epilepsy in infancy). In: Bureau M, Genton P, Dravet C, et al., eds., *Epileptic Syndromes in Infancy, Childhood and Adolescence.* 5th edn. Montrouge, France: John Libbey Eurotext; 2012:125–156.

62. Bureau M, Dalla Bernardina B. Electroencephalographic characteristics of Dravet syndrome. *Epilepsia.* 2011;52(Suppl 2):13–23.

63. Wolff M, Casse-Perrot C, Dravet C. Severe myoclonic epilepsy of infants (Dravet syndrome): natural history and neuropsychological findings. *Epilepsia.* 2006;47(Suppl 2):45–48.

64. Genton P, Velizarova R, Dravet C. Dravet syndrome: the long-term outcome. *Epilepsia.* 2011;52(Suppl 2):44–49.

65. Sakauchi M, Oguni H, Kato I, et al. Mortality in Dravet syndrome: search for risk factors in Japanese patients. *Epilepsia.* 2011;52(Suppl 2):50–54.

66. Scheffer IE, Berkovic SF. Generalized epilepsy with febrile seizures plus: a genetic disorder

with heterogeneous clinical phenotypes. *Brain*. 1997;120(Pt 3):479–490.

67. Camfield P, Camfield C. Febrile seizures and genetic epilepsy with febrile seizures plus (GEFS+). *Epileptic Disord*. 2015;17 (2):124–133.

68. Scheffer IE, Zhang YH, Jansen FE, Dibbens L. Dravet syndrome or genetic (generalized) epilepsy with febrile seizures plus? *Brain Dev*. 2009;31(5):394–400.

69. De Jonghe P. Molecular genetics of Dravet syndrome. *Dev Med Child Neurol*. 2011;53 (Suppl 2):7–10.

70. Dravet C, Bureau M, Genton P. Benign myoclonic epilepsy of infancy: electroclinical symptomatology and differential diagnosis from the other types of generalized epilepsy of infancy. *Epilepsy Res Suppl*. 1992;6:131–135.

71. Zuberi SM, O'Regan ME. Developmental outcome in benign myoclonic epilepsy in infancy and reflex myoclonic epilepsy in infancy: a literature review and six new cases. *Epilepsy Res*. 2006;70(Suppl 1): S110–115.

72. Hirano Y, Oguni H, Funatsuka M, Imai K, Osawa M. Differentiation of myoclonic seizures in epileptic syndromes: a video-polygraphic study of 26 patients. *Epilepsia*. 2009;50(6):1525–1535.

73. Auvin S, Pandit F, De Bellecize J, et al. Benign myoclonic epilepsy in infants: electroclinical features and long-term follow-up of 34 patients. *Epilepsia*. 2006;47 (2):387–393.

74. Darra F, Fiorini E, Zoccante L, et al. Benign myoclonic epilepsy in infancy (BMEI): a longitudinal electroclinical study of 22 cases. *Epilepsia*. 2006;47(Suppl 5):31–35.

75. Caraballo RH, Flesler S, Pasteris MC, et al. Myoclonic epilepsy in infancy: an electroclinical study and long-term follow-up of 38 patients. *Epilepsia*. 2013;54 (9):1605–1612.

76. Matricardi S, Verrotti A, Chiarelli F, Cerminara C, Curatolo P. Current advances in childhood absence epilepsy. *Pediatr Neurol*. 2014;50 (3):205–212.

77. Commission on Classification and Terminology of the International League Against Epilepsy. Proposal for revised classification of epilepsies and epileptic syndromes. *Epilepsia*. 1989;30(4):389–399.

78. Panayiotopoulos CP. Absence epilepsies. In: Engel J, Pedley TA, eds., *Epilepsy: A Comprehensive Textbook*. Philadelphia: Lippincott-Raven; 1998:2327–2346.

79. Sadleir LG, Farrell K, Smith S, Connolly MB, Scheffer IE. Electroclinical features of absence seizures in childhood absence epilepsy. *Neurology*. 2006;67(3):413–418.

80. Panayiotopoulos CP, Obeid T, Waheed G. Differentiation of typical absence seizures in epileptic syndromes: a video EEG study of 224 seizures in 20 patients. *Brain*. 1989;112(Pt 4):1039–1056.

81. Medina MT, Bureau M, Hirsch E, Panayiotopoulos CP. Childhood absence epilepsy. In: Bureau M, Genton P, Dravet C, et al., eds., *Epileptic Syndromes in Infancy, Childhood and Adolescence*. 5th edn. Montrouge, France: John Libbey Eurotext; 2012:277–296.

82. Penry JK, Porter RJ, Dreifuss RE. Simultaneous recording of absence seizures with video tape and electroencephalography. A study of 374 seizures in 48 patients. *Brain*. 1975;98 (3):427–440.

83. Sadleir LG, Scheffer IE, Smith S, Connolly MB, Farrell K. Automatisms in absence seizures in children with idiopathic generalized epilepsy. *Arch Neurol*. 2009;66 (6):729–734.

84. Riviello JJ, Jr., Foley CM. The epileptiform significance of intermittent rhythmic delta activity in childhood. *J Child Neurol*. 1992;7 (2):156–160.

85. Guilhoto LM, Manreza ML, Yacubian EM. Occipital intermittent rhythmic delta activity in absence epilepsy. *Arq Neuropsiquiatr*. 2006;64(2A):193–197.

86. Panayiotopoulos CP, Engel J, Jr. Childhood absence epilepsy. http://www.medlink.com/article/childhood_absence_epilepsy. Accessed March 15, 2019.

87. Wirrell EC, Camfield CS, Camfield PR, Gordon KE, Dooley JM. Long-term

prognosis of typical childhood absence epilepsy: remission or progression to juvenile myoclonic epilepsy. *Neurology.* 1996;47(4):912–918.

88. Grosso S, Galimberti D, Vezzosi P, et al. Childhood absence epilepsy: evolution and prognostic factors. *Epilepsia.* 2005;46 (11):1796–1801.

89. Callenbach PM, Bouma PA, Geerts AT, et al. Long-term outcome of childhood absence epilepsy: Dutch Study of Epilepsy in Childhood. *Epilepsy Res.* 2009;83(2–3):249–256.

90. Wirrell E, Camfield C, Camfield P, Dooley J. Prognostic significance of failure of the initial antiepileptic drug in children with absence epilepsy. *Epilepsia.* 2001;42 (6):760–763.

91. Koutroumanidis M, Bourvari G, Tan SV. Idiopathic generalized epilepsies: clinical and electroencephalogram diagnosis and treatment. *Expert Rev Neurother.* 2005;5 (6):753–767.

92. Trinka E, Baumgartner S, Unterberger I, et al. Long-term prognosis for childhood and juvenile absence epilepsy. *J Neurol.* 2004;251(10):1235–1241.

93. Shinnar S, Cnaan A, Hu F, et al. Long-term outcomes of generalized tonic-clonic seizures in a childhood absence epilepsy trial. *Neurology.* 2015;85(13):1108–1114.

94. Glauser TA, Cnaan A, Shinnar S, et al. Ethosuximide, valproic acid, and lamotrigine in childhood absence epilepsy. *N Engl J Med.* 2010;362(9):790–799.

95. Masur D, Shinnar S, Cnaan A, et al. Pretreatment cognitive deficits and treatment effects on attention in childhood absence epilepsy. *Neurology.* 2013;81 (18):1572–1580.

96. Wirrell EC, Camfield CS, Camfield PR, et al. Long-term psychosocial outcome in typical absence epilepsy: sometimes a wolf in sheeps' clothing. *Arch Pediatr Adolesc Med.* 1997;151(2):152–158.

97. Bureau M, Tassinari CA. Myoclonic absences and absences with myoclonias. In: Bureau M, Genton P, Dravet C, et al., eds., *Epileptic Syndromes in Infancy and Childhood and Adolescence.* 5th edn.

Montrouge, France. John Libbey Eurotext, 2012:297–304.

98. Larsson K, Eeg-Olofsson O. A population based study of epilepsy in children from a Swedish county. *Eur J Paediatr Neurol.* 2006;10(3):107–113.

99. Panayiotopoulos CP, Michael M, Sanders S, Valeta T, Koutroumanidis M. Benign childhood focal epilepsies: assessment of established and newly recognized syndromes. *Brain.* 2008;131(Pt 9):2264–2286.

100. Ma CK, Chan KY. Benign childhood epilepsy with centrotemporal spikes: a study of 50 Chinese children. *Brain Dev.* 2003;25(6):390–395.

101. Panayiotopoulos CP, Bureau M, Caraballo RH, Bernardina DB, Valeta T. Idiopathic focal epilepsies in childhood. In: Bureau M, Genton P, Dravet C, et al., eds., *Epileptic Syndromes in Infancy, Childhood and Adolescence.* 5th edn. Montrouge, France: John Libbey Eurotext; 2012:218–254.

102. Parakh M, Katewa V. A review of the not so benign- benign childhood epilepsy with centrotemporal spikes. *J Neurol Neurophysiol.* 2015;6:314.

103. Guerrini R, Pellacani S. Benign childhood focal epilepsies. *Epilepsia.* 2012;53(Suppl 4):9–18.

104. Panayiotopoulos CP. *Benign Childhood Partial Seizures and Related Epileptic Syndromes.* London: John Libbey; 1999.

105. Arzimanoglou A, Guerrini R, Aicardi J, eds. *Aicardi's Epilepsy in Children.* 3rd edn. Philadelphia: Lippincott Williams & Wilkins; 2004.

106. Lerman P. Benign childhood epilepsy with centro temporal spikes (BECTS). In: Engel J, Pedley TA, Aicardi J, eds., *Epilepsy: A Comprehensive Textbook.* Philadelphia: Lippincott-Raven; 1998:2307–2314.

107. Legarda S, Jayakar P, Duchowny M, Alvarez L, Resnick T. Benign rolandic epilepsy: high central and low central subgroups. *Epilepsia.* 1994;35 (6):1125–1129.

108. Luders H, Lesser RP, Dinner DS, Morris HH, III. Benign focal epilepsies of

childhood. In: Luders H, Lesser RP, eds., *Epilepsy: Electroclinical Syndromes.* London: Springer-Verlag; 1987:303–346.

109. Jung KY, Kim JM, Kim DW. Patterns of interictal spike propagation across the central sulcus in benign rolandic epilepsy. *Clin Electroencephalogr.* 2003;34 (3):153–157.

110. Boor R, Jacobs J, Hinzmann A, et al. Combined spike-related functional MRI and multiple source analysis in the non-invasive spike localization of benign rolandic epilepsy. *Clin Neurophysiol.* 2007;118(4):901–909.

111. Huiskamp G, van Der Meij W, van Huffelen A, van Nieuwenhuizen O. High resolution spatio-temporal EEG-MEG analysis of rolandic spikes. *J Clin Neurophysiol.* 2004;21(2):84–95.

112. Holmes GL. Benign focal epilepsies of childhood. *Epilepsia.* 1993;34(Suppl 3): S49–61.

113. Cavazzuti GB, Cappella L, Nalin A. Longitudinal study of epileptiform EEG patterns in normal children. *Epilepsia.* 1980;21(1):43–55.

114. Loiseau P, Beaussart M. The seizures of benign childhood epilepsy with Rolandic paroxysmal discharges. *Epilepsia.* 1973;14 (4):381–389.

115. Bouma PA, Bovenkerk AC, Westendorp RG, Brouwer OF. The course of benign partial epilepsy of childhood with centrotemporal spikes: a meta-analysis. *Neurology.* 1997;48(2):430–437.

116. Loiseau P, Duche B, Cordova S, Dartigues JF, Cohadon S. Prognosis of benign childhood epilepsy with centrotemporal spikes: a follow-up study of 168 patients. *Epilepsia.* 1988;29(3):229–235.

117. Coppola G, Franzoni E, Verrotti A, et al. Levetiracetam or oxcarbazepine as monotherapy in newly diagnosed benign epilepsy of childhood with centrotemporal spikes (BECTS): an open-label, parallel group trial. *Brain Dev.* 2007;29(5):281–284.

118. Lerman P. Seizures induced or aggravated by anticonvulsants. *Epilepsia.* 1986;27 (6):706–710.

119. Parmeggiani L, Seri S, Bonanni P, Guerrini R. Electrophysiological characterization of spontaneous and carbamazepine-induced epileptic negative myoclonus in benign childhood epilepsy with centro-temporal spikes. *Clin Neurophysiol.* 2004;115 (1):50–58.

120. Clarke T, Strug LJ, Murphy PL, et al. High risk of reading disability and speech sound disorder in rolandic epilepsy families: case-control study. *Epilepsia.* 2007;48 (12):2258–2265.

121. Bulgheroni S, Franceschetti S, Vago C, et al. Verbal dichotic listening performance and its relationship with EEG features in benign childhood epilepsy with centrotemporal spikes. *Epilepsy Res.* 2008;79(1):31–38.

122. Shields WD, Snead OC, 3rd. Benign epilepsy with centrotemporal spikes. *Epilepsia.* 2009;50(Suppl 8):10–15.

123. Ferrie C, Caraballo R, Covanis A, et al. Panayiotopoulos syndrome: a consensus view. *Dev Med Child Neurol.* 2006;48 (3):236–240.

124. Martinovic Z. The new ILAE report on classification and evidence-based commentary on Panayiotopoulos syndrome and autonomic status epilepticus. *Epilepsia.* 2007;48 (6):1215–1216.

125. Panayiotopoulos CP. Vomiting as an ictal manifestation of epileptic seizures and syndromes. *J Neurol Neurosurg Psychiatry.* 1988;51(11):1448–1451.

126. Panayiotopoulos CP. *Panayiotopoulos Syndrome: A Common and Benign Childhood Epileptic Syndrome.* Eastleigh, England: John Libbey; 2002.

127. Covanis A. Panayiotopoulos syndrome: a benign childhood autonomic epilepsy frequently imitating encephalitis, syncope, migraine, sleep disorder, or gastroenteritis. *Pediatrics.* 2006;118(4):e1237–1243.

128. Oguni H, Hayashi K, Imai K, et al. Study on the early-onset variant of benign childhood epilepsy with occipital paroxysms otherwise described as early-onset benign occipital seizure susceptibility syndrome. *Epilepsia.* 1999;40 (7):1020–1030.

129. Dura Trave T, Yoldi Petri ME, Gallinas Victoriano F. Panayiotopoulos syndrome: epidemiological and clinical characteristics and outcome. *Eur J Neurol*. 2008;15 (4):336–341.

130. Leal AJ, Nunes S, Dias AI, et al. Analysis of the generators of epileptic activity in early-onset childhood benign occipital lobe epilepsy. *Clin Neurophysiol*. 2007;118 (6):1341–1347.

131. Kikumoto K, Yoshinaga H, Oka M, et al. EEG and seizure exacerbation induced by carbamazepine in Panayiotopoulos syndrome. *Epileptic Disord*. 2006;8 (1):53–56.

132. Caraballo RH, Cersosimo RO, Fejerman N. Childhood occipital epilepsy of Gastaut: a study of 33 patients. *Epilepsia*. 2008;49 (2):288–297.

133. Sanchez Fernandez I, Loddenkemper T. Pediatric focal epilepsy syndromes. *J Clin Neurophysiol*. 2012;29(5):425–440.

134. Ferini-Strambi L, Sansoni V, Combi R. Nocturnal frontal lobe epilepsy and the acetylcholine receptor. *Neurologist*. 2012;18 (6):343–349.

135. Tinuper P, Bisulli F, Cross JH, et al. Definition and diagnostic criteria of sleep-related hypermotor epilepsy. *Neurology*. 2016;86(19):1834–1842.

136. Picard F, Scheffer IE. Genetically determined focal epilepsies. In: Bureau M, Genton P, Dravet C, et al., eds., *Epileptic Syndromes in Infancy, Childhood and Adolescence*. 5th edn. Montrouge, France: John Libbey Eurotext; 2012:349–361.

137. Tinuper P, Bisulli F. From nocturnal frontal lobe epilepsy to sleep-related hypermotor epilepsy: a 35-year diagnostic challenge. *Seizure*. 2017;44:87–92.

138. Combi R, Dalpra L, Tenchini ML, Ferini-Strambi L. Autosomal dominant nocturnal frontal lobe epilepsy – a critical overview. *J Neurol*. 2004;251(8):923–934.

139. Arzimanoglou A, French J, Blume WT, et al. Lennox-Gastaut syndrome: a consensus approach on diagnosis, assessment, management, and trial methodology. *Lancet Neurol*. 2009;8 (1):82–93.

140. Trevathan E, Murphy CC, Yeargin-Allsopp M. Prevalence and descriptive epidemiology of Lennox-Gastaut syndrome among Atlanta children. *Epilepsia*. 1997;38 (12):1283–1288.

141. Hancock EC, Cross JH. Treatment of Lennox-Gastaut syndrome. *Cochrane Database Syst Rev*. 2013(2):CD003277.

142. Markand ON. Lennox-Gastaut syndrome (childhood epileptic encephalopathy). *J Clin Neurophysiol*. 2003;20(6):426–441.

143. Camfield P, Camfield C. Long-term prognosis for symptomatic (secondarily) generalized epilepsies: a population-based study. *Epilepsia*. 2007;48 (6):1128–1132.

144. Camfield PR. Definition and natural history of Lennox-Gastaut syndrome. *Epilepsia*. 2011;52(Suppl 5):3–9.

145. Dulac O, N'Guyen T. The Lennox-Gastaut syndrome. *Epilepsia*. 1993;34(Suppl 7): S7–17.

146. Chatrian GE, Lettich E, Wilkus RJ, Vallarta J. Polygraphic and clinical observations on tonic-autonomic seizures. *Electroencephalogr Clin Neurophysiol Suppl*. 1982(35):101–124.

147. Crumrine PK. Lennox-Gastaut syndrome. *J Child Neurol*. 2002;17 (Suppl 1):S70–75.

148. Gastraut H, Roger J, Soulayrol R, et al. Childhood epileptic encephalopathy with diffuse slow spike-waves (otherwise known as "petit mal variant") or Lennox syndrome. *Epilepsia*. 1966;7(2):139–179.

149. Crespel A, Gelisse P, Nikanorova M, Ferlazzo E, Genton P. Lennox-Gastaut syndrome. In: Bureau M, Genton P, Dravet C, et al., eds., *Epileptic Syndromes in Infancy, Childhood and Adolescence*. 5th edn. Montrouge, France: John Libbey Eurotext; 2012:189–216.

150. Yaqub BA. Electroclinical seizures in Lennox-Gastaut syndrome. *Epilepsia*. 1993;34(1):120–127.

151. Camfield P, Camfield C. Epileptic syndromes in childhood: clinical features, outcomes, and treatment. *Epilepsia*. 2002;43(Suppl 3):27–32.

152. Ikeno T, Shigematsu H, Miyakoshi M, et al. An analytic study of epileptic falls. *Epilepsia*. 1985;26(6):612–621.

153. Egli M, Mothersill I, O'Kane M, O'Kane F. The axial spasm – the predominant type of drop seizure in patients with secondary generalized epilepsy. *Epilepsia*. 1985;26 (5):401–415.

154. Markand ON. Slow spike-wave activity in EEG and associated clinical features: often called 'Lennox' or "Lennox-Gastaut" syndrome. *Neurology*. 1977;27(8):746–757.

155. Zupanc ML. Clinical evaluation and diagnosis of severe epilepsy syndromes of early childhood. *J Child Neurol*. 2009;24(8 Suppl):6S–14S.

156. Blume WT. Pathogenesis of Lennox-Gastaut syndrome: considerations and hypotheses. *Epileptic Disord*. 2001;3 (4):183–196.

157. Genton P, Dravet C. Lennox-Gastaut syndrome. In: Engel J, Pedley TA, eds. *Epilepsy: A Comprehensive Textbook*. Philadelphia: Lippincott-Raven; 1998:2355–2366.

158. Ohtahara S, Ohtsuka Y, Kobayashi K. Lennox-Gastaut syndrome: a new vista. *Psychiatry Clin Neurosci*. 1995;49(3): S179–183.

159. VanStraten AF, Ng YT. Update on the management of Lennox-Gastaut syndrome. *Pediatr Neurol*. 2012;47(3):153–161.

160. Bourgeois BF, Douglass LM, Sankar R. Lennox-Gastaut syndrome: a consensus approach to differential diagnosis. *Epilepsia*. 2014;55(Suppl 4):4–9.

161. Ostendorf AP, Ng YT. Treatment-resistant Lennox-Gastaut syndrome: therapeutic trends, challenges and future directions. *Neuropsychiatr Dis Treat*. 2017;13:1131–1140.

162. Lancman G, Virk M, Shao H, et al. Vagus nerve stimulation vs. corpus callosotomy in the treatment of Lennox-Gastaut syndrome: a meta-analysis. *Seizure*. 2013;22 (1):3–8.

163. Kelley SA, Kossoff EH. Doose syndrome (myoclonic-astatic epilepsy): 40 years of progress. *Dev Med Child Neurol*. 2010;52 (11):988–993.

164. Oguni H, Fukuyama Y, Tanaka T, et al. Myoclonic-astatic epilepsy of early childhood – clinical and EEG analysis of myoclonic-astatic seizures, and discussions on the nosology of the syndrome. *Brain Dev*. 2001;23(7):757–764.

165. Neubauer BA, Hahn A, Doose H, Tuxhorn I. Myoclonic-astatic epilepsy of early childhood – definition, course, nosography, and genetics. *Adv Neurol*. 2005;95:147–155.

166. Guerrini R, Mari F, Dravet C. Idiopathic myoclonic epilepsies in infancy and early childhood. In: Bureau M, Genton P, Dravet C, et al., eds., *Epileptic Syndromes in Infancy, Childhood and Adolescence*. 5th edn. Montrouge, France: John Libbey Eurotext; 2012:157–173.

167. Kramer U. Atypical presentations of benign childhood epilepsy with centrotemporal spikes: a review. *J Child Neurol*. 2008;23 (7):785–790.

168. Panayiotopoulos CP. Syndromes of idiopathic generalized epilepsies not recognized by the International League Against Epilepsy. *Epilepsia*. 2005;46(Suppl 9):57–66.

169. Striano S, Capovilla G, Sofia V, et al. Eyelid myoclonia with absences (Jeavons syndrome): a well-defined idiopathic generalized epilepsy syndrome or a spectrum of photosensitive conditions? *Epilepsia*. 2009;50(Suppl 5):15–19.

170. Caraballo RH, Fontana E, Darra F, et al. A study of 63 cases with eyelid myoclonia with or without absences: type of seizure or an epileptic syndrome? *Seizure*. 2009;18 (6):440–445.

171. Nar Senol P, Tezer FI, Saygi S. Eyelid myoclonia seizures in adults: an alternate look at the syndrome paradox. *Epilepsy Behav*. 2015;45:265–270.

172. Destina Yalcin A, Forta H, Kilic E. Overlap cases of eyelid myoclonia with absences and juvenile myoclonic epilepsy. *Seizure*. 2006;15(6):359–365.

173. da Conceicao PO, Guaranha MS, Uchida CG, et al. Blinking and eyelid myoclonia:

characteristics and correlations of eyelid movements. *Seizure*. 2015;24:12–16.

174. Nickels K, Wirrell E. Electrical status epilepticus in sleep. *Semin Pediatr Neurol*. 2008;15(2):50–60.

175. Smith MC, Hoeppner TJ. Epileptic encephalopathy of late childhood: Landau-Kleffner syndrome and the syndrome of continuous spikes and waves during slow-wave sleep. *J Clin Neurophysiol*. 2003;20 (6):462–472.

176. Tuft M, Arva M, Bjornvold M, Wilson JA, Nakken KO. Landau-Kleffner syndrome. *Tidsskr Nor Laegeforen*. 2015;135 (22):2061–2064.

177. Tassinari CA, Cantalupo G, Dalla Bernadina B, et al. Encephalopathy related to status epilepticus during slow wave sleep (ESES) including Landau-Kleffner syndrome. In: Bureau M, Genton P, Dravet C, et al., eds., *Epileptic Syndromes in Infancy, Childhood and Adolescence*. 5th edn. Montrouge, France: John Libbey Eurotext; 2012:255–275.

178. Stefanatos G. Changing perspectives on Landau-Kleffner syndrome. *Clin Neuropsychol*. 2011;25(6):963–988.

179. Smith MC. Landau-Kleffner syndrome and continuous spike and waves during slow sleep. In: Engel J, Jr., Pedley TA, eds., *Epilepsy: A Comprehensive Textbook*. Philadelphia: Lippincott-Raven; 1998:2367–2377.

180. Shimada T, Takemiya T, Sugiura H, Yamagata K. Role of inflammatory mediators in the pathogenesis of epilepsy. *Mediators Inflamm*. 2014;2014:901902.

181. Loddenkemper T, Fernandez IS, Peters JM. Continuous spike and waves during sleep and electrical status epilepticus in sleep. *J Clin Neurophysiol*. 2011;28(2):154–164.

182. Hughes JR. A review of the relationships between Landau-Kleffner syndrome, electrical status epilepticus during sleep, and continuous spike-waves during sleep. *Epilepsy Behav*. 2011;20(2):247–253.

183. Sanchez Fernandez I, Loddenkemper T, Peters JM, Kothare SV. Electrical status epilepticus in sleep: clinical presentation and pathophysiology. *Pediatr Neurol*. 2012;47(6):390–410.

184. Tassinari CA, Rubboli G, Volpi L, et al. Encephalopathy with electrical status epilepticus during slow sleep or ESES syndrome including the acquired aphasia. *Clin Neurophysiol*. 2000;111(Suppl 2): S94–S102.

185. Guerrini R, Genton P, Bureau M, et al. Multilobar polymicrogyria, intractable drop attack seizures, and sleep-related electrical status epilepticus. *Neurology*. 1998;51(2):504–512.

186. Smith MC, Spitz MC. Treatment strategies in Landau-Kleffner syndrome and paraictal psychiatric and cognitive disturbances. *Epilepsy Behav*. 2002;3(5S):24–29.

187. Buzatu M, Bulteau C, Altuzarra C, Dulac O, Van Bogaert P. Corticosteroids as treatment of epileptic syndromes with continuous spike-waves during slow-wave sleep. *Epilepsia*. 2009;50(Suppl 7):68–72.

188. De Negri M, Baglietto MG, Battaglia FM, et al. Treatment of electrical status epilepticus by short diazepam (DZP) cycles after DZP rectal bolus test. *Brain Dev*. 1995;17(5):330–333.

189. Morrell F, Whisler WW, Smith MC, et al. Landau-Kleffner syndrome. Treatment with subpial intracortical transection. *Brain*. 1995;118(Pt 6):1529–1546.

190. Wolf P. Basic principles of the ILAE syndrome classification. *Epilepsy Res*. 2006;70(Suppl 1):S20–26.

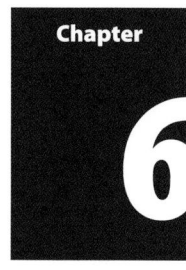

Familial Electro-clinical Syndromes and Epilepsies in Adolescence to Adulthood

Elie Abdelnour, Monisha Sachdev, and Mohamad Mikati

6.1 Autosomal Dominant Epilepsy with Auditory Features (ADEAF)

6.1.1 Introduction/Epidemiology

Autosomal dominant epilepsy with auditory features (ADEAF), also referred to as autosomal dominant lateral temporal epilepsy (ADLTE), is one type of familial temporal lobe epilepsy.

6.1.2 Clinical Presentation

Seizure semiology: ADEAF manifests as focal seizures, typically associated with an auditory aura that ranges from humming and ringing to auditory hallucinations in more severe cases. Spells are infrequent, may be triggered by specific auditory inputs (such as a phone ringing), and are usually well controlled with a standard antiepileptic regimen. Most patients also experience receptive aphasia during the episode, despite intact consciousness. It is important to note that auditory features or receptive aphasia are necessary in order to establish a diagnosis of ADEAF, characteristically related to a localization of discharges in the lateral temporal area. Visual auras have also been described in isolation or preceding a generalized tonic–clonic seizure. Auras may sometimes affect other somatosensory elements such as olfaction, and in some cases may manifest as motor or autonomic symptoms. The majority of patients also experience secondarily generalized seizures.

Age of onset/prognosis: This condition has been reported in a range of patient ages, between 4 and 50 years old, with a predominance during adolescence, and usually follows a mild course under appropriate therapy.

6.1.3 Diagnostic Evaluation

EEG: Interictal EEG recordings reveal focal temporal lobe epileptic discharges in up to two-thirds of patients. Ictal signals typically originate from the mid-temporal and temporal or fronto-temporal regions of the brain.

MRI: ADEAF is typically not associated with any structural abnormality on MRI, in contrast to other familial focal epilepsy syndromes, such as autosomal dominant nocturnal frontal lobe epilepsy. Mesial temporal sclerosis has been reported in a few cases.[1]

Associated genetic mutations: Up to 50% of familial ADEAF are linked to a loss-of-function mutation in *LGI1* (Leucine-rich glioma-inactivated protein 1), a protein involved in autoimmune limbic encephalitis, and also the first discovered epilepsy-associated non-ion channel gene.[2] While the majority of genetic etiologies are attributed to *LGI1* mutations, another pathogenic gene, *RELN*, has recently been described in a number of families.[3,4] Although no significant clinical difference was observed between the two phenotypes, individuals carrying the *RELN* mutation were found to have a higher rate of lateral temporal discharges on EEG when compared to *LGI1*.[4] Both these genetic components contribute to the majority of ADEAF cases, and are screened for when a diagnosis of ADEAF is suspected.

Autosomal dominant epilepsy with auditory features	
Major features	Focal epilepsy with auditory symptoms and/or receptive aphasia
Associated symptoms	N/A
Mean age of onset	Adolescence
Differential diagnosis	ADNFLE, FMTLE, FPEVF
EEG	Interictal discharges (up to 2/3)
Associated genes	*LGI1*, *RELN*
Management	Standard antiepileptic regimen

6.2 Autosomal Dominant Nocturnal Frontal Lobe Epilepsy (ADNFLE)

6.2.1 Introduction/Epidemiology

Autosomal dominant nocturnal frontal lobe epilepsy (ADNFLE) is a relatively common focal epilepsy syndrome with an autosomal dominant inheritance pattern. It has a high penetrance (70%), and high variability in manifestation and severity between different affected family members.

6.2.2 Clinical Presentation

Seizure semiology: Seizures consist of hyperkinetic elements (which could have a variety of manifestations, such as frantic lower extremity movements and pelvic thrusting) and dystonia, with retained awareness. They occur predominantly during sleep, at an average frequency of eight episodes a night, clustered over 1–2 hours, and typically last less than a minute. Some patients experience nonspecific auras prior to the motor seizure. Sleep deprivation and stress are common triggering factors. Half the patients suffering from this type of seizure can secondarily generalize.

Associated symptoms: A few patients may also present with mild intellectual disability and some form of behavioral abnormality, ranging from irritability and aggressiveness (adolescence), to personality disorders and depressive features (adults). These symptoms occur more often in patients carrying a mutation in *KCNT1*, a gene coding for a sodium-gated potassium channel. Psychosis has been reported in a few severe cases.

Age of onset/prognosis: Age of onset is typically 8–11.5 years of age, with up to 80% of cases manifesting before 20 years of age.[5] As patients reach early adulthood, seizure frequency and severity tend to decrease.

6.2.3 Diagnostic evaluation

EEG: This is often unrevealing in ADNFLE, as interictal sleep findings can be normal or show infrequent epileptiform discharges, and ictal recordings may be obscured by movement artifacts.

MRI: Normal in the majority of cases. However, some recently reported ADNFLE-causing gene mutations were associated with focal cortical dysplasia on MRI.

Associated genetic mutations: Several gene mutations have been identified and linked to ADNFLE; 10–15% of the patients have mutations in the *CHRNA2* or *CHRNB2* genes, which code for neuronal acetylcholine receptor subunits. PET imaging with an acetylcholine receptor agonist revealed increased uptake in the mesencephalon and thalamus, and decreased uptake in the prefrontal region.[6] It is still not clear if the prefrontal findings contribute to the frontal seizures, or are a consequence of seizure-induced damage to the area. *KCNT1* mutations have been reported in a number of families with ADNFLE, characterized by a more severe ADNFLE phenotype and prevalent intellectual disability.[7] Some mutations, such as *KCNT1* (encodes a sodium-gated potassium channel) and *DEPDC5* (encodes DEP domain containing protein 5), were consistently found to be associated with ADNFLE, and are thus currently included in genomic screening when a diagnosis of ADNFLE is suspected.

Management: Carbamazepine has shown the most benefit in ADNFLE patients, completely suppressing seizures in up to 70% of patients. Seizures may persist for a few years, but usually decrease with age, and may cease around 40–50 years of age, even after discontinuation of antiepileptic drugs (AEDs). In the case of *KCNT1* mutations, patients may benefit from precision therapies. Some, but not all, of these patients respond to quinidine, a drug that has been shown in vitro to correct the gain of function resulting from the mutation.[8] Individuals resistant to pharmacotherapy may benefit from vagal nerve stimulation (VNS).[9]

Autosomal dominant nocturnal frontal lobe epilepsy	
Major features	Nocturnal motor focal, often dystonic seizures with retained awareness
Associated symptoms	Mild cognitive and behavioral abnormalities
Mean age of onset	10 years old
Differential diagnosis	Parasomnias, paroxysmal kinesigenic dyskinesia, restless leg syndrome
EEG	Stage 2 non-REM abnormalities
Associated genes	CHRNA, CHRNB, KCNT1, DEPDC5
Management	Carbamazepine, quinidine (KCNT1), zonisamide (CHRNA4)

6.3 Familial Focal Epilepsy with Variable Foci (FFEVF)

6.3.1 Introduction/Epidemiology

Familial focal epilepsy with variable foci (FFEVF) describes an entity whereby individuals within the same family have seizures originating from various cortical foci, but each individual only has one specific type of focal seizure. FFEVF cannot be diagnosed at the individual level, but rather reflects the semiology and inheritance patterns of the individual's pedigree.

6.3.2 Clinical Presentation

Seizure semiology: FFEVF does not present with a specific seizure pattern, which makes diagnosis tricky, especially in smaller families. Age of onset, seizure frequency and severity, cortical foci, and drug response vary between individuals. Nevertheless, a higher rate of frontal and temporal events has been observed, and these are generally well controlled on standard AEDs. When the abnormality originates from the frontal lobe, seizures are typically infrequent, but with a higher rate of secondary generalization and EEG abnormalities. When temporal, FFEVF can be confused with FMTLE, especially in the context of a small family, where the absence of symptoms in close relatives sways the diagnosis away from FFEVF.

Age of onset: Varies from infancy to adulthood.

Associated symptoms: A few rare cases have been documented to be associated with psychiatric and cognitive features.

6.3.3 Diagnostic Evaluation

EEG: The same variability is seen in EEG recordings, as interictal focal findings may be seen, that are consistent with each case's seizure pattern, but different within various family members.

MRI: Neuroimaging is generally not revealing, except for a few cases with focal lesions, such as focal cortical dysplasia detected on MRI.

Associated genetic mutations: Despite an extensive phenotypic diversity, multiple studies have mapped FFEVF to chromosome 22q12, later found to be the locus for the *DEPDC5* gene. After its discovery, *DEPDC5* has been linked to a number of focal epilepsy syndromes such as ADNFLE. More recently, mutations in *NPRL2* and *NPRL3* genes have also been described in a number of FFEVF families. Both *DEPDC5* and the *NPRL* genes act on the same downstream pathway, that eventually leads to inhibition of the mTOR pathway. Mutation of either genes leads to mTOR upregulation, which predisposes to the development of cortical lesions and subsequent focal epilepsy.[10]

Familial focal epilepsy with variable foci	
Major features	Various types of focal seizures in individuals of the same family
Associated symptoms	Psychiatric and cognitive dysfunction
Mean age of onset	Variable
Differential diagnosis	ADNFLE, FMTLE, FPEVF
EEG	Consistent with focal seizure pattern
Associated genes	*DEPDC5, NPRL2, NPRL3*
Management	Standard antiepileptic regimen, surgery

6.4 Familial Mesial Temporal Lobe Epilepsy (FMTLE)

6.4.1 Introduction/Epidemiology

Although most cases are due to mesial temporal sclerosis lesions and thus qualify as "acquired" epilepsy syndrome, a subset of familial mesial temporal lobe epilepsy (FMTLE) cases have been described.

6.4.2 Clinical Presentation

Seizure semiology: Individuals presenting with FMTLE can be categorized into two major groups. The first follows a benign course, consisting of infrequent focal seizures originating in the mesial temporal lobe, easily controlled on standard AED regimen, rarely secondarily generalizing, and occasionally associated with psychic disturbances and autonomic symptoms, such as déjà vu and nausea. The second group is comparatively more severe, with a higher association with hippocampal sclerosis, more resistance to standard antiepileptic therapy, and usually preceded by a history of febrile convulsions during infancy.

Age of onset: Individuals in the second group also have an earlier seizure onset (as early as 10-year-old, versus adolescence/early adulthood in the first group).

6.4.3 Diagnostic Evaluation

EEG: Whereas the milder form reveals no abnormality on EEG, the more severe form classically shows interictal temporal discharges.

Associated genetic mutations: FMTLE has in large part a polygenic inheritance and multifactorial etiology. It has been hypothesized that multiple familial genetic variants predispose family members to the hippocampal damage seen in MTLE.[11] Pathogenic variants of the *DEPDC5* gene have been detected in a few families.[12]

Management: Response to standard AEDs ranges from 5–15%, with the higher response rate corresponding to the milder initial clinical presentation. When hippocampal sclerosis is associated with MTLE, surgical intervention can lead to complete seizure cessation. More recently, thermal ablation of mesial temporal lesions has offered an efficient, more tolerable, and less invasive alternative to surgical intervention, eliminating disabling seizures in almost 65% of patients presenting with intractable MTLE.[13] However, current data indicate that the chance of seizure freedom is likely to be less than that achieved after temporal lobectomy.

Familial mesial temporal lobe epilepsy	
• **Major features**	Mesial temporal lobe seizures (mild and severe form)
• **Associated symptoms**	Psychic and autonomic disturbances (mild form)
• **Mean age of onset**	Adolescence/early adulthood (mild), or 1st-3rd decade (severe)
• **Differential diagnosis**	ADNFLE, ADEAF
• **EEG**	Normal (mild) or interictal temporal discharges (severe)
• **Associated genes**	N/A
• **Management**	Standard AED, lobectomy, laser thermal ablation

6.5 Genetic Generalized Epilepsy

The category of genetic generalized epilepsy (GGE), formerly known as idiopathic generalized epilepsy, is a category of genetic adolescence-onset epilepsy syndromes that consists of the following subgroups: juvenile absence epilepsy (JAE), juvenile myoclonic epilepsy (JME), and epilepsy with generalized tonic–clonic seizures (EGTCS). These subclassifications are mainly based on clinical presentation and EEG findings. Although clinically different, they share some genetic components, and similar clinical features, such as response to AEDs. In fact, an overlap between disease entities is often seen in affected individuals, with some transitioning from childhood absence epilepsy (CAE) to JME, and many exhibiting several generalized tonic–clonic (seizures GTCs) throughout their lifetime. The classification of GGE was subject to much debate within the scientific community, with some believing it is a spectrum with a common biological etiology and fluid boundaries between phenotypes, while others argue for a more discrete categorization into several definite entities.[14] Currently, the most recent ILAE classification defined EGCTS, JAE, and JME as separate entities under the label of GGE.

6.5.1 Juvenile Absence Epilepsy

Introduction/epidemiology: JAE is a fairly common cause of genetic generalized epilepsy.

6.5.1.1 Clinical Presentation

Seizure semiology: JAE is characterized by typical absence seizures during adolescence, in otherwise healthy individuals. The spell consists of brief sudden arrest in activity, impaired consciousness, without loss of tone, lasting less than 10 seconds, with spells typically triggered by hyperventilation. Automatisms such as lip smacking are often associated with the episode. The nature and very brief duration of absence spells make the diagnosis delicate, as they can go unnoticed for months to years. Other types of seizures may occur, such as GTCs, GTCs on awakening, and myoclonic seizures. As compared to CAE, automatisms occur at a higher rate and consciousness is less impaired.

Age of onset/prognosis: The main distinguishing factors is, however, age of onset, with JAE typically manifesting around puberty, while CAE is restricted to childhood. Around 10–11 years of age, there seems to be an overlap, and distinction between the two phenotypes becomes more difficult.

6.5.1.2 Diagnostic Evaluation

EEG: EEG findings are similar to typical absence seizures, with bilateral ictal spike-and-wave discharges at a frequency of 3–4 Hz (but of longer duration than in CAE) with a normal background. Focal EEG features such as slow-wave and epileptiform discharges are seen in a few cases, which may lead to misdiagnosis and inappropriate therapy.[15]

MRI: An unremarkable MRI has been a key feature of all GGEs. However, with the current technological advances in neuroimaging, recent evidence has demonstrated variable volumetric thalamic changes in GGEs.[16] When it comes to JAE in particular, subtle volumetric changes have also been reported, although no consensus has been reached as to what specific brain regions are most affected. Recent studies have consistently detected subtle volumetric changes in a JAE cohort in the medial frontal cortex, anterior cingulate cortex, and mesial temporal lobe.[17]

Management: Even though only a few clinical trials have looked at JAE in particular, a good response to ethosuximide and valproate, the standard therapy for absence, has been reported. As previously mentioned, those who did not experience any GTCs had a better outcome than those who did. Lamotrigine is a well-studied and established therapy, often used as first line in JAE.[18] Other AEDs that have been studied such as carbamazepine, oxcarbazepine, and phenytoin were actually shown to be detrimental and are contraindicated for JAE patients. Complete resolution of seizures has been reported in 15–37% of patients, with a higher likelihood in those without a history of prior GTCs. Almost half of patients who do not remit progress to juvenile myoclonic epilepsy (JME).

Juvenile absence epilepsy	
Major features	Absence seizures
Associated symptoms	N/A
Mean age of onset	Adolescence/Puberty
Differential diagnosis	CAE, JME
EEG	Ictal discharges, 3–4 Hz
Associated genes	
Management	Ethosuximide, valproate, lamotrigine

6.5.2 Juvenile Myoclonic Epilepsy

Introduction/epidemiology: Juvenile myoclonic epilepsy (JME), or Janz syndrome, is a common GGE, representing around 4–9% of adolescents suffering from epilepsy, and 25–30% of all GGEs. JME seems to preferentially affect females.

6.5.2.1 Clinical Presentation

Seizure semiology: Patients present with the characteristic triad of myoclonic jerks, GTCs, and absence seizures, and are otherwise healthy. Myoclonia is essential for diagnosis and manifests in all JME patients, but only rarely in isolation, as most cases also exhibit GTCs. The absence spells are not as common as myoclonic jerks and GTCs, and when they occur, they usually precede JME onset by 5 years. In fact, these initial absence spells may lead to a diagnosis of JAE, until the individual grows up and experiences his first generalized or myoclonic seizure. The hallmark myoclonic seizures consist of predominantly upper extremity bilateral myoclonic jerks, occurring as a single or repetitive event, with retained consciousness. Lower extremity involvement may occur, but is uncommon and usually leads to falls. Episodes typically occur within the first hour of awakening, and can be triggered by sleep deprivation and photic stimulation. Reflex seizures have also been reported to occur, whereby electrographic seizures with or without jerks are triggered by various forms of mental activity such as mathematical calculations and higher cognitive tasks, a phenomenon exclusive to JME also known as praxis induction. JME may progress into GTCs, and in most cases, a diagnosis of JME is not reached until GTCs have developed.

Age of onset: A broad range of 8–26 years of age has been reported as age of onset, even though most cases are diagnosed during adolescence, between 12 and 18 years of age.

Associated symptoms: Although the majority of JME patients have normal cognitive development, a number of patients exhibit frontal lobe dysfunction such as verbal and cognitive impairment. A few patients also manifest peculiar personality traits such as impulsiveness, emotional instability, and immaturity.

6.5.2.2 Diagnostic Evaluation

EEG: EEG findings usually consist of 3–6 Hz polyspike waves with frontal predominance on awakening, with a normal background. Ictal findings that correlate with myoclonus consist of fast polyspikes at a variable frequency.

MRI: Neuroimaging in JME has characteristically been normal in the past, yet technological advances in the past decade allowed detection of subtle gray matter changes in the mesial frontal cortex and thalamus, as well as callosal morphology.[19] Such changes have also been linked to the psychiatric and behavioral patterns seen in many JME patients.[20] Occipital lobe involvement has been reported in cases with photosensitivity.[21] White matter changes have also been documented in the temporo-parietal region.[22]

Associated genetic mutations: The following causative genes have been described so far: *EFHC1*, *GABRA1*, and *CLCN2*. However, to date, JME is considered to have a polygenic and multifactorial etiology in most patients.

Management: Valproate has shown superiority in the most recent clinical trials, with response rates as high as 80%.[23] When valproate is contraindicated, and in women of childbearing age, second-line therapy includes levetiracetam, topiramate, and lamotrigine. Antiepileptic drugs like carbamazepine, oxcarbazepine, and phenytoin may aggravate the patient's condition. Most studies demonstrated a favorable outcome on appropriate therapy. Patients who experienced absence spells at onset, GTCs, longer myoclonic episodes, or unsuccessful poly-medication were less likely to achieve seizure control or seizure freedom. Recently, drug-resistance has also been associated with cases that exhibit praxis induction.[24] The majority of JME patients require life-long therapy, while up to 25% achieve seizure freedom off medications.

Juvenile myoclonic epilepsy	
• Major features	Myoclonic jerks on awakening
• Associated symptoms	Personality trait changes
• Age of onset (years)	12 – 18
• Differential diagnosis	Isolated convulsions, CAE, JAE, PME
• EEG	Spike or polyspike waves, 4–6 Hz in frequency, on awakening
• Associated genes	*EFHC1, GABRA1, CLCN2*
• Management	Valproate, levetiracetam

6.5.3 Epilepsy with Generalized Tonic–Clonic Seizures Alone

6.5.3.1 Introduction/Epidemiology

Epilepsy with generalized tonic–clonic seizures alone (EGTCS), was initially called grand mal seizures on awakening upon its first description by Dr Janz in 1962. It is a subsyndrome of the genetic generalized epilepsies, and affects men and women of various ages.

6.5.3.2 Clinical Presentation

Seizure semiology: Patients suffer from generalized tonic–clonic seizures, typically within minutes/hours of waking up. Episodes are triggered by alcohol consumption, sleep deprivation, and photic stimulation. Although classified as a separate entity by the ILAE, there is continuing debate about whether it should rather be part of JME because of their similar triggering factors, similar EEG findings, and response to AEDs.

Age of onset: Age of onset for EGTCS varies broadly, manifesting in individuals as young as 6 and as old as 35. Prognosis is variable as well, and most patients will require AEDs throughout their lifetime.

6.5.3.3 Diagnostic Evaluation

EEG: EEG findings consist of generalized spike wave or polyspike wave discharges, exacerbated by sleep deprivation and during sleep.

MRI: MRI is typically normal.

Management: In the absence of a solid clinical trial for EGTCS, standard AED therapy for JME is applied and has similar response rate as in JME patients. Avoidance of known triggers is helpful.

Epilepsy with generalized tonic–clonic seizures	
• Major features	Generalized tonic–clonic seizures on awakening
• Associated symptoms	
• Age of onset (years)	6 – 35
• Differential diagnosis	Isolated convulsions, CAE, JAE, JME
• EEG	Generalized spike wave or polyspike
• Associated genes	CLCN2
• Management	Standard antiepileptic regimen

6.6 Progressive Myoclonic Epilepsy

Progressive myoclonic epilepsy (PME) is a group of epilepsy syndromes that often start in adolescence, and develop common features including myoclonic seizures and various rates of neurologic decline. Diagnosis is challenging in its early stages, as a number of more common conditions have similar presentations, but as the disease advances and neurologic function starts deteriorating, PME becomes evident. PME is subclassified into several categories, depending on the specific genetic etiologies.

6.6.1 Neuronal Ceroid Lipofuscinoses

The largest in the PME family, neuronal ceroid lipofuscinoses (NCL), or Batten disease, is a group of progressive neurodegenerative syndromes that all share as a common feature intracellular lipofuscin accumulation, an auto-fluorescent pigment involved in many neurodegenerative disease processes such as Alzheimer's and Parkinson's disease. In the US, incidence ranges around 1.6–2.4 per 100,000. With the medical field rapidly shifting towards a genetic-oriented approach, NCL is now classified into 14 groups, with 14 different underlying genetic components (*CLN1* to *CLN14*). All but CLN4 follow an autosomal recessive inheritance pattern. The various clinical presentations are summarized in Table 6.1.

6.6.1.1 Clinical Presentation

CLN1 disease, also called infantile NCL or Haltia–Santavuori disease, presents in infants at 6 months of age with hypotonia and irritability, with rapid development of myoclonic seizures and later loss of vision (lipofuscin also accumulates in the retina leading to optic atrophy). Affected individuals may also experience other types of seizures and have a poor prognosis, with children experiencing cognitive and motor decline and usually dying by the age of 10 years. EEG findings consist of loss of sleep spindles, followed progressively by background abnormality and attenuation, until reaching isoelectric EEG by age 3 years due to neuronal degeneration. Photosensitivity is characteristic of CLN1. MRI reveals cerebral atrophy and thalamic and periventricular hyperintensity. CLN1 is caused by a mutation in *PPT1*. A minority of pathogenic variants have been reported in rare cases of late-infantile and juvenile NCL.

CLN2 disease, also called late-infantile NCL or Jansky–Bielschowsky disease, presents in children between 2 and 4 years of age with various seizure types ranging from myoclonic early on, to tonic–clonic, atonic, and atypical absence spells. Ataxia is typically an early symptom of CLN2, while retinopathy and visual impairment occurs in a more advanced disease stage. Seizures precede neurodevelopmental decline and myoclonic ataxia. Later, regression occurs progressively, leading to a vegetative state and eventual death, usually in adolescence. EEG findings consist of slowed background with generalized epileptiform discharges, and spikes may be elicited in the occipital region by photic stimulation. MRI reveals cerebral atrophy that is more pronounced in the infratentorial area. CLN2 is caused by a mutation in *TPP1*. A minority of pathogenic variants have been reported in rare cases of juvenile NCL.

CLN3 disease, also called juvenile NCL or Spielmeyer–Sjögren disease, presents in children between 4 and 10 years of age with gradual visual impairment and neurocognitive decline. Ocular abnormalities are usually the earliest sign of CLN3, as epilepsy and extrapyramidal symptoms manifest later on, during adolescence. Death typically occurs by the second or third decade of life. Some individuals also develop psychiatric disturbances. EEG findings consist of background slowing and generalized spike-and-slow-wave discharges exacerbated by sleep. MRI is normal until age 10, after which progressive cerebral and cerebellar atrophy starts occurring. CLN3 is caused by a mutation in *CLN3*.

CLN4 disease, also called adult NCL, presents in adults starting at age 30 as myoclonic seizures with visual auras. A few patients have been reported to present with cognitive

Table 6.1 NCL types and characteristics

Disorder	Gene	Age of onset (years)	Clinical presentation	EEG	MRI
CLN1	*PPT1*	0.5–1	Visual impairment, seizures	- Loss of sleep spindles - 2 years: background abnormalities - 3 years: isoelectric	Cerebral atrophy, thalamic and periventricular hyperintensity
CLN2	*TPP1*	2–4	Ataxia, visual impairment, seizures	- Background slowing - Occipital discharges elicited by photic stimulation	Cerebral atrophy
CLN3	*CLN3*	4–10	Visual and cognitive impairment, seizures, psychiatric disturbances	- Background slowing - Spike-slow-wave exacerbated by sleep	Cerebral and cerebellar atrophy after age 10
CLN4	*DNAJC5*	30	Seizures, cognitive deficits	- Fast spike wave - Exacerbated by photic stimulation	Cerebral and cerebellar atrophy
CLN5	*CLN5*	4–7	Visual and cognitive impairment, seizures, motor deterioration	- Occipital discharges elicited by photic stimulation	Cerebellar atrophy, thalamic hypointensity, periventricular hyperintensity
CLN6	*CLN6*	3–5	Visual impairment, seizures, ataxia, motor impairment	- Background slowing - Occipital discharges elicited by photic stimulation	Cerebral and cerebellar atrophy
CLN7	*MFSD8*	2–7	Visual impairment, seizures, motor impairment	- Background slowing - Multifocal sharp waves	Occipital lobe atrophy

Table 6.1 (cont.)

Disorder	Gene	Age of onset (years)	Clinical presentation	EEG	MRI
CLN8	CLN8	3–6 (LINCL) 5–10 (Northern epilepsy)	Visual impairment, seizures, motor impairment	- Background slowing - Focal and non focal epileptiform activity	Cerebral and cerebellar atrophy
CLN9	Unknown	4–10	Similar to CLN3	Similar to CLN3	Similar to CLN3
CLN10	CTSD	Congenital, late infantile or adult form	Congenital: microcephaly, respiratory failure, increased tone		Frontal cerebral and cerebellar atrophy
CLN11	GRN	15–50	Visual impairment, seizures, ataxia	- Background slowing - Occipital discharges elicited by photic stimulation	Cerebellar atrophy
CLN12	ATP13A2	4–10	Seizures, ataxia, psychiatric disturbances, EPS	- Diffuse slowing	Globus pallidus atrophy, followed by diffuse cerebral atrophy
CLN13	CTSF	15–50	Bulbar symptoms, EPS, behavioral and cognitive abnormalities, motor impairment		Cerebral and cerebellar atrophy
CLN14	KCTD7	0.5–1	Visual impairment, cognitive and motor abnormalities	- Generalized epileptiform discharges - Photosensitivity	

deficits and extrapyramidal symptoms. Adult onset NCL was historically labeled as Kufs disease. Nowadays, NCL is classified based on the genetic mutations involved, rather than on age of onset. Previously known as Kufs type B, CLN4 is the only PME to have an autosomal dominant inheritance pattern. Contrary to previously described syndromes, ophthalmologic findings are unremarkable and blindness does not occur. It follows a natural course of around 12 years from onset of symptoms to death. EEG findings consist of generalized fast spike-wave with paroxysmal discharges in response to photic stimuli. CLN4 is caused by a mutation in *DNAJC5*.

CLN5 disease, also called variant late infantile NCL or Finnish variant, presents in children between 4 and 7 years of age with motor deterioration, gradual visual and cognitive impairment, as well as myoclonic spells, with a mortality range between 13 and 35 years of age. EEG findings are similar to CLN2, with occipital epileptiform spikes elicited by photic stimulation. MRI findings consist of cerebellar atrophy, thalamic hypointensity, and periventricular hyperintensity. CLN5 is caused by a mutation in *CLN5*.

CLN6 disease, also called early juvenile NCL, presents in children between 3 and 5 years of age with visual impairment (50% of patients), with later development of ataxia, seizures, and motor impairment. It was previously known as Kufs disease type A, before the new genetic-based classification of NCL was established. CLN6 has a very poor prognosis, with most patients not surviving beyond the age of 12. EEG findings are similar to CLN2, with background slowing and occipital epileptiform discharges elicited by photic stimulation. MRI findings consist of cerebral and cerebellar atrophy. CLN6 is caused by a mutation in *CLN6*.

CLN7 disease, also called late infantile NCL or Turkish variant, presents in children between 2 and 7 years of age with psychomotor deterioration and/or seizures, followed by cognitive impairment, myoclonus, and visual failure at a more advanced stage. CLN7 is caused by a mutation in *MFSD8*.

CLN8 disease, also called late-infantile variant NCL or Northern epilepsy, can present in two ways, depending on the pathogenic variant of *CLN8* involved; it either manifests as intractable epilepsy, with cognitive and visual impairment in children 5 to 10 years old, or as developmental delay, with later myoclonic seizures between 3 and 6 years of age. CLN8 is caused by a mutation in *CLN8*.

CLN9 disease has only been described in two families, with a manifestation similar to CLN3. No gene has been identified yet as disease-causing.

CLN10 disease manifests as a congenital, late-infantile or adult onset NCL. The congenital form presents as multiple neonatal complications such as microcephaly, respiratory failure, and hypertonicity. CLN10 is caused by a mutation in *CTSD*.

CLN11 disease was described in a family with gradual visual impairment, seizures, and ataxia. EEG was similar to CLN2 in having occipital-dominant epileptiform discharges, and MRI findings consisted of cerebellar atrophy, consistent with the clinical presentation. CLN11 is due to a mutation in *GRN*.

CLN12 disease was described in a family with ataxia, myoclonic spells, and psychiatric disturbances early in adolescence, later developing extrapyramidal symptoms (akinesia, rigidity, dysarthria). Compared to most other NCL syndromes, the retina and vision are spared. CLN12 is due to a mutation in *ATP13A2*.

CLN13 disease, an adult-onset NCL previously part of the Kufs disease type B category, presents with neurobehavioral and cognitive abnormalities, often accompanied by motor impairment, bulbar symptoms, and extrapyramidal symptoms. CLN13 is due to a mutation in *CTSF*.

CLN14 disease was described in a family with visual impairment, cognitive and motor decline, and early mortality. CLN14 is due to a mutation in *KCTD7*.

6.6.2 Unverricht–Lundborg Disease

Unverricht–Lundborg disease, also called Baltic myoclonus or EPM1A, is the prototype and most common form of progressive myoclonic epilepsy syndromes. It is prevalent in Mediterranean populations and in Finland.

6.6.2.1 Clinical Presentation

Seizure semiology: Early manifestations include myoclonus, which, if severe enough, may develop into tonic–clonic seizures. Myoclonic spells are typically triggered by action, sensory stimuli, or physiological and physical stressors, and are often drug resistant. Phenytoin has even proven to worsen myoclonus.[25]

Associated symptoms: Cognitive development is initially unaffected, but later it slowly declines over time.

Age of onset/prognosis: Age of onset is between 8 and 13 years of age (mean of 10). Despite a wide intrafamilial variability in clinical severity, symptoms tend to progress in the first few years after onset, and typically stabilize during early adulthood.

6.6.2.2 Diagnostic Evaluation

EEG: Recordings reveal diffuse slowed background, and anteriorly predominating spike-wave epileptiform discharges 3–5 Hz in frequency, with marked photosensitivity. Sporadic focal (often occipital) spikes are sometimes detected.

MRI: Neuroimaging studies helped establish the cerebellar and brainstem atrophy in the disease process.[26]

Associated genetic mutations: EPM1A has been consistently linked to mutations in *CSTB*, a gene on chromosome 21 which codes for cystatin B. Testing for such a mutation is now part of the screening process in patients suspected to have EPM1A. Mutations in *PRICKLE1* gene have been linked to a similar phenotype, EPM1B, characterized by earlier disease onset and more severe symptomatology.

6.6.3 Lafora Disease

Lafora disease, or EPM2, is an autosomal recessive PME, so-called because of the presence of intracellular Lafora body inclusions in the brain, among other tissues. It is prevalent in Mediterranean populations and southern India, but is still relatively rare.

6.6.3.1 Clinical Presentation

Seizure semiology: Early manifestations include myoclonus and generalized seizures. Myoclonic spells are typically triggered by action, photic stimuli, or physiological and physical stressors. Almost half the patients experience focal occipital seizures that manifest as transient loss of vision, visual hallucinations, or migraine with visual aura. Spells are typically attenuated, with standard AED regimen, but almost never completely eradicated.

Associated symptoms: Headaches often accompany the initial manifestation. Visual hallucinations may follow, and have been linked to both epileptic and psychiatric etiology.[27] Progressive cognitive impairment, behavioral changes, and cerebellar ataxia are commonly described.

Age of onset/prognosis: Age of onset is between 8 and 18 years of age (mean age of 14), and death occurs 2–10 years from disease onset in most reported cases.

6.6.3.2 Diagnostic Evaluation

EEG: Recordings reveal interictal epileptiform discharges, with marked photosensitivity, in a normal or slightly slowed background. Occipital discharges responsible for the visual symptoms are characteristic.

MRI: Neuroimaging is typically not revealing, with the exception of a few cases where functional studies revealed hypometabolism in the occipital region. At a later stage, brain MRI may reveal cortical changes, as the seizures and myoclonus progress and become intractable.

Pathological features: The presence of PAS inclusion bodies on skin biopsy helps confirm the diagnosis.

Associated genetic mutations: Lafora disease has been linked to mutations in *EPM2A* and *EPM2B*, which code for laforin and malin respectively, two elements involved in glycogen metabolism regulation pathways. Mutation of either gene on genetic screening is necessary for diagnosis.

PME type 3, due to a mutation in *KCTD7*, presents with early onset myoclonic spells (prior to 2 years of age), followed by progressive neurological decline.

PME type 4 is due to a mutation in *SCARB2/LIMP2*, a gene coding for lysosomal membrane protein. Also known as action-myoclonus renal-failure syndrome, PME 4 presents, as the name implies, with renal failure associated with action myoclonus, that develops from tremors and ataxia. It typically starts in teenagers, and spells are typically easily controlled with standard AED regimen.

PME type 5, due to mutations in *PRICKLE2*, presents with myoclonic spells, as well as impairment of vision, movement, and cognition.

PME type 6 has been associated with mutations in *GOSR2* gene. Also known as North Sea PME, PME 5 presents prior to 2 years of age with ataxia, later followed by myoclonic spells at age 6. Progression of the disease leads to ambulation impairment in the early teenage years.

PME type 7 has been associated with mutations in *KCNC1*, a gene coding for potassium channels specifically found in GABAergic interneurons. PME 7 presents in adolescence with severe myoclonic and in some cases tonic–clonic spells, with progressive ambulation and cognitive decline.

PME type 8, due to mutations in *CESR1*, similarly presents in adolescence with myoclonic and tonic–clonic spells, followed by gradual cognitive decline.

References

1. Klein KM, Pendziwiat M, Cohen R, et al. Autosomal dominant epilepsy with auditory features: a new LGI1 family including a phenocopy with cortical dysplasia. *J Neurol.* 2016;263(1):11–16.

2. Boillot M, Huneau C, Marsan E, et al. Glutamatergic neuron-targeted loss of LGI1 epilepsy gene results in seizures. *Brain.* 2014;137(Pt 11):2984–2996.

3. Michelucci R, Pasini E, Nobile C. Lateral temporal lobe epilepsies: clinical and genetic features. *Epilepsia.* 2009;50 (Suppl 5):52–54.

4. Michelucci R, Pulitano P, Di Bonaventura C, et al. The clinical phenotype of

autosomal dominant lateral temporal lobe epilepsy related to reelin mutations. *Epilepsy Behav.* 2017;68:103–107.

5. Picard F, Baulac S, Kahane P, et al. Dominant partial epilepsies: a clinical, electrophysiological and genetic study of 19 European families. *Brain.* 2000;123 (Pt 6):1247–1262.

6. Picard F, Bruel D, Servent D, et al. Alteration of the in vivo nicotinic receptor density in ADNFLE patients: a PET study. *Brain.* 2006;129(Pt 8):2047–2060.

7. Heron SE, Smith KR, Bahlo M, et al. Missense mutations in the sodium-gated potassium channel gene KCNT1 cause severe autosomal dominant nocturnal frontal lobe epilepsy. *Nat Genet.* 2012;44 (11):1188–1190.

8. Mikati MA, Jiang YH, Carboni M, et al. Quinidine in the treatment of KCNT1-positive epilepsies. *Ann Neurol.* 2015;78 (6):995–999.

9. Carreno M, Garcia-Alvarez D, Maestro I, et al. Malignant autosomal dominant frontal lobe epilepsy with repeated episodes of status epilepticus: successful treatment with vagal nerve stimulation. *Epileptic Disord.* 2010;12(2):155–158.

10. Weckhuysen S, Marsan E, Lambrecq V, et al. Involvement of GATOR complex genes in familial focal epilepsies and focal cortical dysplasia. *Epilepsia.* 2016;57 (6):994–1003.

11. Leventer RJ, Jansen FE, Mandelstam SA, et al. Is focal cortical dysplasia sporadic? Family evidence for genetic susceptibility. *Epilepsia.* 2014;55(3):e22–26.

12. Ishida S, Picard F, Rudolf G, et al. Mutations of DEPDC5 cause autosomal dominant focal epilepsies. *Nat Genet.* 2013;45(5):552–555.

13. Jermakowicz WJ, Kanner AM, Sur S, et al. Laser thermal ablation for mesiotemporal epilepsy: analysis of ablation volumes and trajectories. *Epilepsia.* 2017;58 (5):801–810.

14. Beghi M, Beghi E, Cornaggia CM, Gobbi G. Idiopathic generalized epilepsies of adolescence. *Epilepsia.* 2006;47(Suppl 2):107–110.

15. Japaridze G, Kasradze S, Lomidze G, et al. Focal EEG features and therapeutic response in patients with juvenile absence and myoclonic epilepsy. *Clin Neurophysiol.* 2016;127(2):1182–1187.

16. Seneviratne U, Cook M, D'Souza W. Focal abnormalities in idiopathic generalized epilepsy: a critical review of the literature. *Epilepsia.* 2014;55(8):1157–1169.

17. Tondelli M, Vaudano AE, Ruggieri A, Meletti S. Cortical and subcortical brain alterations in juvenile absence epilepsy. *Neuroimage Clin.* 2016;12:306–311.

18. Bergey GK. Evidence-based treatment of idiopathic generalized epilepsies with new antiepileptic drugs. *Epilepsia.* 2005;46 (Suppl 9):161–168.

19. Anastasopoulou S, Kurth F, Luders E, Savic I. Generalized epilepsy syndromes and callosal thickness: differential effects between patients with juvenile myoclonic epilepsy and those with generalized tonic-clonic seizures alone. *Epilepsy Res.* 2017;129:74–78.

20. Paulus FM, Krach S, Blanke M, et al. Fronto-insula network activity explains emotional dysfunctions in juvenile myoclonic epilepsy: combined evidence from pupillometry and fMRI. *Cortex.* 2015;65:219–231.

21. Aydin-Ozemir Z, Terzibasioglu E, Altindag E, Sencer S, Baykan B. Magnetic resonance spectroscopy findings in photosensitive idiopathic generalized epilepsy. *Clin EEG Neurosci.* 2010;41(1):42–49.

22. Kim SH, Lim SC, Kim W, et al. Extrafrontal structural changes in juvenile myoclonic epilepsy: a topographic analysis of combined structural and microstructural brain imaging. *Seizure.* 2015;30:124–131.

23. Yacubian EM. Juvenile myoclonic epilepsy: challenges on its 60th anniversary. *Seizure.* 2017;44:48–52.

24. Uchida CG, de Carvalho KC, Guaranha MS, et al. Phenotyping juvenile myoclonic epilepsy. Praxis induction as a biomarker of

unfavorable prognosis. *Seizure.* 2015;32:62–68.

25. Iivanainen M, Himberg JJ. Valproate and clonazepam in the treatment of severe progressive myoclonus epilepsy. *Arch Neurol.* 1982;39(4):236–238.

26. Koskenkorva P, Khyuppenen J, Niskanen E, et al. Motor cortex and thalamic atrophy in Unverricht-Lundborg disease: voxel-based morphometric study. *Neurology.* 2009;73(8): 606–611.

27. Andrade DM, del Campo JM, Moro E, Minassian BA, Wennberg RA. Nonepileptic visual hallucinations in Lafora disease. *Neurology.*

7 Distinctive Constellations and Other Epilepsies

Ashley E. Thomas, Wolfgang G. Muhlhofer, and
Jerzy P. Szaflarski

7.1 Introduction

The International League Against Epilepsy recently published an updated classification that better reflects our understanding of epilepsies and their mechanisms.[1] This chapter discusses specific epilepsy syndromes, epilepsies that are not associated with a specific age of onset, reflex epilepsies, and the main etiologic groups described in the updated classification, including structural, genetic, infectious, metabolic, and immune mediated.

7.2 Distinctive Constellations: Mesial Temporal Lobe Epilepsy with Hippocampal Sclerosis, Gelastic Seizures with Hypothalamic Hamartoma, and Rasmussen Syndrome

Mesial temporal lobe epilepsy with hippocampal sclerosis, gelastic seizures with hypothalamic hamartoma, and Rasmussen syndrome are three excellent examples of how unique electroclinical and imaging characteristics are tied to a very specific and fundamentally different etiology and brain pathology. Yet, the commonality is that their prompt recognition and surgical treatment have a great influence on seizure control, cognitive development, and prevention of secondary kindling of unaffected brain regions due to recurrent seizure activity.

7.2.1 Mesial Temporal Lobe Epilepsy with Hippocampal Sclerosis

Temporal lobe epilepsy (TLE) is the most frequent form of medically refractory focal epilepsy. Among TLE, mesial temporal lobe epilepsy with hippocampal sclerosis (mTLE-HS) is a well-characterized entity that associates electroclinical features of seizures originating from the mesial and/or limbic structures of the temporal lobe (mainly the hippocampus and amygdala) with pathological changes of the hippocampus.[2,3] The current US prevalence of drug-resistant mTLE-HS is 0.51–0.66 cases per 1000 people, and the incidence is 3.1–3.4 cases per 100,000 people per year. Based on a US population of 324 million, as many as 143,000–191,000 patients in the USA suffer from medically refractory mTLE-HS.[4] There has been an ongoing discussion whether there is an overall decrease in incidence of mTLE-HS,[5] which might be related to better pre-, peri-, and postnatal care, better treatment of bacterial and viral infections and febrile convulsions, established vaccination programs, and more successful seizure control with second- and third-generation antiseizure medications.[5]

A fairly typical course of mTLE-HS can be recognized in the majority of patients. This includes a prolonged febrile seizure at an early age followed by a latent period of several years prior to the onset of focal seizures (mainly isolated auras without impaired awareness) in mid-to-late childhood. Periods of seizure remission of up to 2 years during adolescence or early adulthood are possible.[6] Then, it typically progresses to elaborate seizures, progressive treatment resistance, and cognitive (mainly short-term memory) difficulties.[7,8]

Mesial temporal lobe seizures usually last 90–120 s. Auras at the beginning of a seizure are very common, with the abdominal-visceral "epigastric rising" sensation being the most specific for mesial temporal onset seizures.[7,8] Autonomic auras (e.g., widened pupils, palpitations, arrhythmias, goose-flesh pimples, and pallor/rubor), psycho-affective auras (e.g., fear and anxiety), and experiential auras (e.g., déjà vu (an illusion of familiarity) and jamais-vu (an illusion of strangeness)), being in a "dream-like" state, premonition, or a sense of depersonalization) are also commonly reported. Less frequent auras are sensory or sensorial symptoms like tingling, pain, or a sensation of constriction of extremities, which are sometimes vague, often bilateral, or not consistently lateralized.[7–9] Auras are absent in approximately 10% of cases, which might be due to a peri-ictal memory dysfunction resulting in retrograde amnesia.[10]

Mesial temporal lobe seizures tend to evolve over 1 to 2 mins, frequently with partial awareness at onset that is followed by loss of awareness with an initially motionless stare and then automatisms, which are typically oro-alimentary (e.g., lip-smacking, chewing, and swallowing), vocal (spontaneously or as a reaction to external stimulation) or gestural (e.g., fumbling, fidgeting, repetitive motor actions, and undressing). The automatisms can be accompanied by motor signs such as contralateral dystonic posturing, which may reflect involvement of the basal ganglia. Some types of automatisms, like running or pedaling may be due to an early spread to the frontal lobes. A typical association of ipsilateral manual automatisms and dystonic posturing of the contralateral hand is frequently encountered in temporal lobe seizures originating from the mesial structures.[7,11] An early, relatively casual head turn is often ipsilateral to the mesial temporal focus (patient looking "into the seizure focus"), whereas a forced, versive head turn and eye deviation to the contralateral side occur later on, as the seizure spreads.[12] Postictal confusion and headache are common after a temporal lobe seizure, and language disruption, if it occurs, is a useful lateralizing sign indicative of seizure origin from the dominant temporal lobe.[13] Postictal nose-rub/wipe is commonly seen in temporal lobe epilepsy and in 90% of cases is ipsilateral to the seizure focus.[14]

Many causative factors, including perinatal hypoxia, tumors, trauma, autoimmune-mediated inflammation, and genetic influences have been considered as possible etiologies of HS.[15,16] A past medical history of complicated febrile seizures (febrile status epilepticus with a cluster of seizures within a 24 hour period or prolonged febrile convulsions lasting longer than 10 minutes and/or the presence of focal, lateralizing features during or right after the seizure)[17] is seen in up to 80% of cases of mTLE-HS.

The process of sclerosis and distribution of neuronal loss can vary from one patient to another.[18] A recent consensus classification, validated through the Neuropathology Taskforce of the ILAE, created a semiquantitative scheme that allows actual correlations between clinical histories, postsurgical outcomes, and neuropathological findings.[19] It is a four-tiered classification system based on hematoxylin and eosin staining and NeuN immunohistochemistry that differentiates "HS type 1" (with severe neuronal loss and gliosis predominantly in CA1 and CA4 regions), from "HS type 2" and "HS type 3" (with CA1- and CA4-predominant neuronal loss, respectively) and "No HS – Gliosis only" which has been misclassified as HS in the past. ILAE HS type 1 is considered the "typical

HS" that is present in about 49–72% of the cases, while HS types 2 and 3 are considered "atypical HS," reported in about 4–10% of the cases. No HS – Gliosis only makes up about 20% of cases.[2,20] These histopathologic types have been associated with postoperative outcomes, with HS type 1 having the best surgical prognosis.[21] The different types of HS may be a manifestation of distinct pathways of epileptogenesis leading to different clinical findings and outcomes. HS type 1 is more frequently associated with a history of initial precipitating insult, such as febrile seizures before age 5 as well as earlier seizure onset, while HS types 2 and 3 are more common in patients with more frequent secondarily generalized seizures and a positive family history of epilepsy.[2,20,22]

Routine electroencephalography (EEG) in patients with mTLE-HS can be normal or show nonspecific temporal slowing or interictal epileptiform discharges, but prolonged EEG-monitoring sessions typically reveal abnormalities.[23] Interictal EEG frequently shows anterior or mid-temporal epileptiform discharges ipsilateral to the focus, best observed in the fronto-temporal scalp electrodes, or in more specific surface electrodes exploring the temporal lobe (e.g., FT9/10). These changes are usually ipsilateral to HS, but may be bilateral in some cases.[23] Moreover, temporal intermittent rhythmic delta activity (TIRDA) seen in some patients is a relatively specific finding for mTLE.[24] Ictal EEG may be unremarkable in approximately 60% at the clinical onset of the seizure (typically characterized by an isolated aura), but lateralized build-up of rhythmic temporal alpha or theta activity within 10–30 s of clinical onset occurs in up to 80% of patients and tends to be relatively well lateralizing and a prognostic marker for a good surgical outcome.[23] However, in 13% of patients, the ictal pattern on scalp EEG can be falsely lateralized (contralateral to the actual seizure onset zone), as determined by subsequent depth EEG recordings and curative surgery. Hence the ictal pattern should always be interpreted in conjunction with the interictal EEG, and clinical and imaging findings.[25]

Magnetic resonance imaging (MRI) has become one of the most utilized tools for noninvasive diagnosis of HS (confirmed with histopathology) and the presence of HS on MRI has proven to be a strong predictor for a favorable postsurgical outcome.[26] The classical MRI findings consist of a noticeable hippocampal atrophy, increased signal intensity of the hippocampal structures on T2-weighted FLAIR sequence, and disruption of the internal, three-layered architecture of the hippocampus on T2-weighted coronal sequences.[26] There is a rapidly growing body of literature on automated analysis of gray and white matter atrophy patterns in mTLE-HS patients. For example, machine-learning methods used to distinguish between TLE patients with and without HS on MRI showed that in addition to hippocampal volume (which is commonly used in regular visual analysis of MRIs[27]), alterations in cortical thickness, surface area, volume, and curvature of the cortex in the inferior frontal and anterior–inferior temporal regions could contribute to a classification accuracy of up to 81% in identifying even subtle cases of HS on MRI.[28]

Fluorodeoxyglucose-positron emission tomography (FDG-PET) studies are of diagnostic and prognostic value in mTLE patients with normal MRI.[29] Hypometabolic patterns on FDG-PET have been shown to correlate with the epileptogenic zone[30] and ictal propagation patterns.[31] In mTLE patients, hypometabolism restricted to temporal pole, antero-mesial, and antero-lateral temporal regions has been related to favorable surgical outcome,[32] while hypometabolism affecting any extratemporal regions (such as the ipsilateral posterior periventricular, mesial frontal, perisylvian, and contralateral fronto-insular regions) has been shown to correlate with a suboptimal or poor outcome.[33] These findings are concordant with electroclinical features reflecting the organization of the epileptogenic zone and the preferential spread pathways, but are independent of the structural abnormalities detected on MRI.[33,34] As such, FDG-PET imaging findings should be taken into consideration when counseling mTLE patients about the success rate of epilepsy surgery. The current evidence does not support the prognostic importance of single-photon emission computed tomography (SPECT) in patients undergoing temporal lobe surgery.[26]

7.2.2 Gelastic Seizures and Hypothalamic Hamartoma

The term gelastic seizures (GS) is derived from the Greek word "gelos" meaning "mirth or laughter."[35] GS are characterized by either a sudden pressure to laugh or an uncontrollable outburst of laughter without any apparent cause, during which consciousness is usually maintained.[36] With a prevalence of 0.8% among patients in epilepsy monitoring units, GS are a rare entity. Hypothalamic hamartomas are present in up to one-third of patients with GS, even though GS are a relatively common clinical presentation of hypothalamic hamartoma (HH).[37] The remainder of cases are felt to be associated with a more widespread epileptic network that frequently involves the temporal and frontal lobes – specifically the basal temporal as well as the mesial, orbito-frontal, and anterior cingulate structures.[38] Less common origins of GS are parietal, multifocal, or undetermined.[37] Small case series indicate that GS in the absence of an HH overall have a more benign natural cause and appear to respond very well to treatment with anticonvulsants such as carbamazepine.[39]

Hypothalamic hamartomas are rare congenital, non-neoplastic lesions located in the small hypothalamic area between the infundibular stalk and the mammillary bodies. They are usually sporadic, but can rarely be associated with the autosomal dominant Pallister–Hall syndrome or other somatic mutations in the *GLI3* gene on chromosome 7p13.[40,41] The incidence of HH is estimated to be from 1–2/100,000 to 1/1,000,000 and their prevalence in patients with focal epilepsy is 1/200,000.[42,43] Yet, GS associated with HH represent the most common disease model of human subcortical epilepsy.[41,44] It is widely accepted that HHs are intrinsically epileptogenic, which leads to the development of seizures and epilepsy; depth electrodes placed into the HH tissue identified the epileptogenic zone within the lesion[45,46] and direct electrical stimulation of intralesional electrodes can evoke a typical GS.[45] Imaging studies including ictal SPECT and FDG-PET showed increased perfusion and metabolism of the HH at the time of a GS.[47,48] Lastly, a selective resection or disconnection of the HH can result in immediate disappearance of GS in the majority of the patients.[49,50]

Isolated GS are frequently the initial seizure type of HH and typically appear in early infancy.[36] Over time focal seizures with impaired awareness and secondary generalized seizures can develop in up to 75% of the cases, which is thought to be related to kindling of the cortical structures that are connected via the hypothalamic output pathway (mainly temporal and frontal lobe).[41,44] These seizures often become refractory to treatment with anticonvulsants, neurostimulation, or dietary measures.[41,51] In up to 40% of the pediatric onset epilepsies due to HH, there are cognitive and behavioral problems (including oppositional defiant disorder, attention-deficit/hyperactivity disorder, conduct disorder, speech/learning impairment, and anxiety and mood disorders), precocious puberty, and even the development of an epileptic encephalopathy (similar to a symptomatic generalized epilepsy or Lennox–Gastaut-like syndrome).[43,52,53] Thereby, the expression and severity of the epilepsy syndrome and its comorbidities appear to be, at least in part, related to the size and location of the HH,[36,54–56] the duration of epilepsy,[55] and an early (typically surgical) intervention.[51,57] As epilepsy associated with HH becomes medically refractory in up to 95% of cases, surgical resection and/or a tissue-destructive disconnection procedure of the hypothalamic lesion is considered to be the most promising treatment.[58]

There are various classification systems for HH, all of which are based on descriptive (macroscopic) anatomical findings, and the recommended surgical approach that looks at the localization of the HH (tuber cinereum versus mamillary bodies), its type of attachment (pediculate versus sessile), the extent of hypothalamic displacement caused by the HH (missing versus marked), and the actual size of the HH (small versus large).[59,60] Sessile HHs (in particular those broadly attached to the tuber cinereum or mammillary bodies) are thought to be more epileptogenic[46,61] and mainly associated with generalized epilepsy, cognitive, behavioral, and psychiatric disorders, while pedunculated HHs are more related to endocrine disturbances such as precocious puberty. HHs can be uni- or bilateral, with bilateral HHs carrying poor surgical prognosis.[54,56]

Interictal scalp EEG may show focal or multifocal (mostly frontal and/or temporal), generalized epileptiform discharges (typically slow spike and slow wave complexes) and/or generalized paroxysmal fast activity. Ictal patterns include electrodecremental (in particular during "pure" GS which are likely related to subcortical seizure activity) and generalized EEG patterns. Hence, scalp EEG findings can be misleading and falsely localizing, suggesting a limited value of scalp EEG in the study of these patients.[62]

Histologically, HH consist of islands of small, interconnected mature interneurons that respond to gamma-aminobutyric acid (GABA), easily synchronized via gap junctions,[63] and have an intrinsic "pacemaker-like" firing behavior.[64] These neurons are intermixed with glial cells and sparse, large, pyramidal-shaped neurons. In contrast to the small interneurons, these large neurons do not have a spontaneous electric activity but have excitatory projections to the thalamus and hypothalamus. Further, they are immature, which makes them excitatory to the typically inhibitory neurotransmitter GABA.[65] The proximity of both neuron populations within the HH is thought to constitute the "functional unit" for ictogenesis in the HH from which the abnormal electrical activity spreads rostrally via the fornices and mammillothalamic tracts, dorsally to the areas of the neighboring limbic system, and caudally to the brainstem where it can induce physiological and psychophysiological manifestations of laughter attacks.[66]

On MRI, HH are located in the tuber cinereum and third ventricle/inferior hypothalamus and appear isointense to gray matter on T1-weighted images and either iso- or hyperintense to gray matter on T2-weighted sequences.[67] HHs associated with epilepsy consistently attach to the posterior hypothalamus in the immediate vicinity of the mammillary bodies, which might indicate that connections to limbic circuitry via the fornices and mammillothalamic tracts may play an important role in epileptogenesis in GS patients with HH.[44,68]

7.2.3 Rasmussen Syndrome

Rasmussen syndrome (RS) is a rare neuroinflammatory disease (Rasmussen encephalitis) characterized by intractable seizures and unilateral brain atrophy.[69] RS is mostly a disease of children, starting around 6 years of age, with an age range from 1 to 14 years and disease onset before the age of 10 years in about 85% of the cases. Adolescent and adult cases comprise approximately 10%, and there is no gender, geographic, or ethnic predominance.[70–72] Well-defined diagnostic criteria for RS include a combination of the electroclinical presentation and characteristic imaging features as described in the consensus statement from 2005.[73] In the differential diagnosis for RS, other clinical entities such as mitochondrial encephalopathy with lactic acidosis and stroke-like events, focal cortical dysplasia, tuberous sclerosis complex, cerebral tumors, or primary CNS vasculitis should be taken into account.[74]

The natural course of RS is characterized by three stages.[72,75] The first is the prodromal stage, which can last months to years and typically consists of no or only mild hemiparesis and infrequent focal seizures with or without impaired awareness. EEG and MRI are often normal in this stage. As a result, early diagnosis of RS can be difficult.[76] The acute second stage is characterized by frequent and commonly treatment-resistant focal seizures that originate from one or sometimes multifocal regions within one hemisphere.[70,77] Typically, these are focal motor seizures in the form of arrhythmic clonic activity of one upper extremity with or without involvement of the head.[70,77] Secondary generalized seizures are noted in 42 to 61% of cases.[70] Focal motor status epilepticus, also called epilepsia partialis continua (EPC) develops within 1 year of seizure onset in about 50–83% of cases.[70,75] This presentation goes along with a progressive hemiparesis of the affected limb in up to 94.4%. Hemianopsia, language dysfunction (particularly with involvement of the dominant hemisphere), and cognitive decline may also be part of the clinical presentation. Finally, there is the residual or "burned out" stage, which includes fixed neurologic deficits and medically intractable epilepsy.

Typically, RS patients progress through the different disease stages in a linear fashion, but patients with a relapsing remitting course going on for multiple years has been described.[78] While young patients in their first decade of life tend to have a more explosive onset that can skip the prodromal phase,[79] adolescent or adult onset RS tends to present with a less aggressive course[80] and unusual features such as temporal or occipital lobe involvement, bilateral involvement (which is very rare), or absence of EPC.[81–84] Atypical presentations of RS without seizures include unilateral movement disorders including hemiathetosis or hemidystonia.[85] Young patients are also more likely to have "dual pathology," which refers to the presence of typical findings of RS alongside alternative epileptogenic pathologies, such as focal cortical dysplasias, tumors, and cortical tubers, being the most commonly reported.[79,86] The pathogenesis of "dual pathology" in RS is disputed but theorized to occur in one of two ways: frequent seizures secondary to a pre-existing lesion lead to a breakdown of the blood–brain barrier and allow the entrance of inflammatory factors leading to stereotypic encephalitis, or frequent seizures from RS-related inflammation contribute to dysplastic neurogenesis.[79] Anatomical or functional hemispherectomy provides long-term seizure-free outcome in 70–80% and cognitive improvement in >90% of RS patients with medically intractable epilepsy.[72,73]

The EEG findings in RS are dynamic and stage dependent. During the initial stage, the EEG may be normal in up to 20% of cases.[87] Within months of seizure onset there is almost always persistent, high-amplitude delta slowing and focal epileptiform discharges over the affected hemisphere, while the unaffected hemisphere typically exhibits normal background.[87] Independent epileptiform discharges over the nonaffected hemisphere emerge in 25% of patients within 6 months and in 62% within 3–5 years from seizure onset. They are a marker of impending cognitive decline rather than bihemispheric disease and should raise the consideration of a more definitive, surgical treatment.[72,87]

Ictal patterns are not always present, particularly EPC, which does not necessarily have an EEG correlate.[88] Therefore, a normal EEG, especially early in the disease course, does not preclude a diagnosis of RS.

The examination of the resected brain tissue in patients with RS shows multifocal cortical inflammation, neuronal loss, and gliosis.[89] An area of pronounced cortical damage is often surrounded by normal cerebral cortex or milder stages of inflammation, which explains why a biopsy can be misleading or falsely negative.[72] Activated brain-resident macrophages (microglia), as well as "nodules" and perivascular cuffing of cytotoxic (CD8+) T-lymphocytes leading to neuronal death and neuronophagia, suggest that the active stage of RS is a primarily T-cell-mediated process.[75,90] However, the factors involved in triggering the inflammatory process are unclear.

MRI of the brain has an essential role in the diagnosis and follow-up of RS, as MRI changes have been found to be concordant with the pathological staging.[75] Early imaging changes (within the first four months of disease onset) can sometimes include focal cortical swelling followed by relatively common hyperintense signal changes on FLAIR and T2-weighted sequences, which typically affect cortical and subcortical regions and, to a lesser extent, deep gray matter structures (such as the basal ganglia).[91] The signal changes can be heterogeneous in distribution and fluctuate over time, related to seizure frequency or the presence of EPC.[92] With disease progression, cortical atrophy within the affected hemisphere, primarily in the perisylvian and fronto-insular region, is present in 100% of the cases.[75,92] Frequently, there is also atrophy of the ipsilateral basal ganglia, specifically, the head of the caudate and putamen.[72,93] Although RS does not typically involve abnormal parenchymal contrast enhancement, an initial contrast-enhanced study should be performed to rule out alternative etiologies along with consideration of non-contrast CT scan of the head to rule out the presence of calcifications.[79] No formal recommendations exist to guide monitoring with MRI, but loose guidelines suggest repeating MRIs every 6–12 months.[79] There might be a potential utility of diffusion tensor imaging tractography to recognize subtle atrophic changes.[94] In addition, automated quantitative analyses of volumetric T1 MRI sequences reliably distinguished RS patients from healthy controls and epilepsy patients without RS by identifying a specific gray matter atrophy pattern primarily affecting the insula and frontal lobe region.[95] FDG-PET shows diffuse unilateral cerebral hypometabolism that might manifest when MRI atrophy is still at a minimum, and hypometabolism of the contralateral cerebellar hemisphere may be seen owing to crossed cerebellar diaschisis.[96] In rare cases, PET hypermetabolism can indicate ictal regions of affected brain.[97]

7.3 Epilepsies with Less-Specific Age Relationship: Familial Focal Epilepsy with Variable Foci and Reflex Epilepsies

The new terminology and concepts were meant to improve organization and reflect advances in our understanding of epilepsies. Electroclinical syndromes include a complex of clinical features, EEG changes, and other signs and symptoms that are specific for a particular disorder. Many types of epilepsy do not fit precise electroclinical syndromes, but do encompass distinct constellations based on specific lesions or other causes. Epilepsies that are not associated with a specific age of onset, such as familial focal epilepsy with variable foci and reflex epilepsies, are discussed in this section.

7.3.1 Familial Focal Epilepsy with Variable Foci

Familial focal epilepsy with variable foci (FFEVF) is a rare autosomal dominant focal-onset epilepsy with variable penetrance that includes affected family members with focal seizures emanating from a specific cortical location – temporal, frontal, centroparietal, or occipital lobe; within a member but not within the family, seizure onset remains constant.[98,99] Loss-of-function mutations in the gene for DEPDC5 (DEP domain containing protein 5) have been found on chromosome 22q12.[100] Mutations in *DEPDC5* may play a role in neuronal signal transduction,[101] rather than ion channel function, as seen in other forms of genetic epilepsies, which may account for the variable presentation seen in FFEVF.[99] About 60–86% of patients will have focal to bilateral tonic–clonic seizures. Age of onset varies from 2 months to 43 years, with a median age of onset at 10 years. Neuroimaging, development, and intelligence are usually normal.[98] Interictal EEG may be normal or may show frontal, central, and/or temporal spikes and spike–wave complexes.[102] EEG severity varies significantly in different individuals and does not correlate with seizure frequency. Healthy family members may also have an EEG epileptiform focus,[98] thus indicating that this could be a marker for this disorder. Treatment includes the use of antiseizure drugs (ASDs) indicated for focal seizures. There is significant variability among family members in their symptoms and treatment response ranging from asymptomatic individuals to treatment-resistant seizures.

7.3.2 Reflex Epilepsy

Generalized or focal seizures in reflex epilepsy (RE) are consistently evoked by a specific stimulus or activity. The temporal relationship has yet to be defined, but it is generally thought that the evoking stimulus or activity occurs concurrently with or immediately prior to the seizure. Reflex seizures can be a part of a larger epilepsy syndrome or can occur in isolation. Reflex epilepsy is diagnosed when all seizures are evoked by a specific stimulus or activity.[103] It has been suggested that reflex seizures are the result of an interaction between the underlying predisposition for seizures and the precipitating event. Some make this distinction with the term "seizure facilitators," which indirectly increase seizure likelihood by sensitizing the central nervous system to some stimulus, and "seizure evokers," which directly and consistently result in a seizure within seconds.[104] Nonreflex precipitation occurs when there are factors that may generally lower the seizure threshold, but there is no consistent pattern or temporal relationship, such as fever, sleep deprivation, and stress.[103] Reflex seizures are thought to arise from areas of cortical hyperexcitability, which overlap with regions normally involved with cognition, motor, or sensory stimulation. Precipitating stimuli for reflex seizures can be categorized as simple (e.g., photosensitive, gustatory, and audiogenic) or complex stimuli (e.g., hot water, musicogenic, and complex visual). Reflex epilepsies are typically named for the stimulus that causes the seizure.

7.3.2.1 Visually Induced Seizures

Seizures can be evoked by several different types of visual stimuli. Photosensitivity, seen in 0.3–3% of the population, is an abnormal brain response whereby epileptiform activity is provoked by photic or pattern stimulation.[105] Photosensitivity is found in up to 5% of people with epilepsy and is twice as common in women.[106] It is also more prevalent in children, decreases in the third decade of life, and may disappear thereafter in 25–30% of patients.[107] Photosensitivity is highly heritable, possibly autosomal dominant with reduced penetrance, although no specific gene has been identified.[108] Photosensitivity is found in many epilepsy syndromes,[109] but is commonly seen in patients with idiopathic generalized epilepsy (IGE), especially juvenile myoclonic epilepsy (JME), with 40–90% of patients reporting photosensitivity.[107,109] The photoparoxysmal response includes spike, spike and wave, or slow-wave patterns on the EEG.[105] Intermittent photic stimulation is often used to reproduce this response, and frequencies in the 15–25Hz range are the most provocative.[110] Photosensitivity in patients with IGE has been shown to require occipital cortical hyper-excitability and abnormal neuronal synchronization in both functional MRI (fMRI)[111] and magnetoencephalography (MEG)[112] studies. Photosensitive seizures are typically generalized and can include absences, symmetric or asymmetric jerking of the arms or whole body, negative myoclonus, and subtle eyelid myoclonus with or without loss of consciousness.[113] Focal seizures can also be provoked by visual stimuli, particularly in patients with cerebral palsy, brain malformations, or ischemic occipital lesions,[114] and prolonged exposure can lead to generalized tonic–clonic seizures.[107] In patients with idiopathic photosensitive occipital lobe epilepsy, seizures are primarily focal, consisting of visual hallucinations and blurring, followed by epigastric discomfort/vomiting and ictal headache.[115] Seizures can also be induced by other forms of visual stimuli, such as television/video games and geometric patterns. Pattern sensitivity, as seen in escalator steps, striped wallpaper, or clothing, is the second most common cause of visually induced seizures after flashing lights.[114]

7.3.2.2 Reading Epilepsy

Reading epilepsy is a rare, benign, nonprogressive syndrome that includes seizures provoked by reading. Other language-related activities such as speaking or writing may also trigger seizures.[106,116] The average age of onset is in adolescence, but ranges from 10–40 years.[109,116] There is a family history of reading epilepsy in some cases.[107] Seizures typically involve oral and facial muscles that are involved in speech production; however, reading aloud is not required to trigger a seizure. Seizures can be divided into the typical and atypical variants.[116] In the typical form of reading epilepsy, orofacial and jaw myoclonus appears after a certain amount of reading, which may or may not spread to the upper limb and body. Patients may also experience ocular symptoms, such as blinking or eye movements. In the atypical form of reading epilepsy, visual hallucinations, blurred vision, movement of letters on the page, and words becoming incomprehensible have been noted, accompanied by dyslexia or alexia. In either form, continued reading may result in seizure propagation and evolution into a generalized tonic–clonic seizure. EEG is frequently normal, however left (dominant) hemisphere or bilateral epileptiform discharges have been noted.[107] Structural imaging such as computerized tomography (CT) or MRI is typically normal. Ictal SPECT hyperperfusion in the left temporal, left occipitoparietal, and bilateral frontal regions have been noted.[117] Functional MRI displayed changes in the left motor and premotor areas during clinical seizures.[118]

7.3.2.3 Audiogenic and Musicogenic Epilepsy

Both audiogenic and musicogenic seizures are triggered by sounds in the environment. Audiogenic seizures are evoked within seconds by sudden, simple sounds.[119] This is in contrast to musicogenic epilepsy, which includes seizures that are triggered by complex music, frequently melodic or harmonic with complex features, and may require several minutes of stimulation to evoke a seizure.[119,120] The musical complexity of the sound and longer latency suggest a cognitive or emotional aspect to the trigger, and most patients have a specific type of music or piece of music that is their trigger.[121] Musicogenic seizures are extremely rare, with an estimated prevalence of 1 case per 10,000,000 people.[122] The average age of onset is 28 years, and women are slightly more affected than men.[121] Seizure semiology is similar to that of temporal lobe onset, whereby the patient will experience behavioral arrest, oral/manual automatisms, and possible secondary generalization. The latency to seizure onset is typically within several minutes, although some patients may have spontaneous seizures as well.[119] EEG findings suggest localization to the right temporal lobe in a majority of cases.[121] Functional MRI, ictal SPECT, and FDG-PET have localized musicogenic seizures to the right temporal lobe.[119,121,123] It has been suggested that there is activation of more diffuse networks involving the limbic system, and simple activation of Heschel's gyrus is inadequate to generate these seizures. Musicogenic epilepsy occurs more often in musically talented people, with musicians making up 43% of patients in one study, suggesting that patients with more elaborate musical abilities may be at higher risk for developing musicogenic seizures.[121] Most cases of musicogenic epilepsy are nonlesional; however, trauma, demyelinating lesions, cerebrovascular disease, and a nonspecific cerebellar syndrome have been reported as causes.[120] Musicogenic seizures can be treated by behavioral methods such as stimulus avoidance, however ASDs may be required, and surgical interventions can be used in refractory cases.

7.3.2.4 Hot-Water Epilepsy

Hot-water epilepsy (HWE) is known for seizures that are precipitated by hot water poured over the head, although some patients may have seizures caused by pouring hot water during a body bath; seizures occur typically within seconds to minutes of exposure to stimulus. Children are more frequently affected, and males are more affected than females by about 2.5:1.[124] Seizures are generally focal onset with loss of awareness and may or may not secondarily generalize. Seizure semiology has been described as including behavioral arrest and dazed look, sense of fear, irrelevant speech, and visual and auditory hallucinations with complex automatisms.[125] Primary generalized tonic–clonic seizures have been reported in up to one-third of cases. Interictal EEG is typically normal, but temporal epileptiform discharges have been reported. Ictal EEG recordings are uncommon, however findings include left temporal rhythmic delta activity, sharp and slow waves in the left hemisphere, and bilateral spikes.[125] Imaging is typically unremarkable. Ictal SPECT scans demonstrated increased uptake in the mesial temporal structures and hypothalamus on the left.[125] HWE is generally felt to be benign and self-limited, however treatment with ASDs may be necessary in some patients.

7.3.2.5 Eating Epilepsy

Seizures triggered by eating are rare and occur in 1/1000–1/2000 of all patients with epilepsy.[126] Seizures are typically complex partial, however generalized seizures have been reported, particularly atypical absences.[127] Seizures are stereotyped for each patient, but may differ between patients. They frequently occur shortly after beginning to eat and usually do not recur during the same meal.[127] Brain imaging may be normal, however malformations of cortical development have also been reported.[109]

7.3.2.6 Startle Epilepsy

Startle seizures include axial tonic or hemitonic seizures (and rarely atonic seizures) that are triggered by a sudden and unexpected stimulus (usually auditory). Seizures typically consist of a startle response followed by axial tonic or hemitonic posture and are often associated with autonomic phenomena as well.[109,128] People frequently have an exaggerated startle response at baseline, and large brain lesions are often noted on imaging, such as perinatal hypoxic injury, schizencephaly, or focal cortical dysplasias, which involve the sensorimotor and premotor cortex.[107,109] Functional MRI suggests that startle-induced seizures could be generated by the mesial fronto-parietal network, with the supplementary motor area postulated to be involved in generating seizures.[129,130] Reflex myoclonic epilepsy in infancy is a self-limited startle epilepsy in infants characterized by myoclonus with generalized spikes and polyspike and wave complexes, which can be induced by sudden auditory or tactile stimuli.[131]

7.3.2.7 Other Reflex Epilepsies

Somatosensory stimulations can lead to reflex seizures, particularly when certain skin regions are involved, such as the head and back. Examples of these include rubbing epilepsy (caused by skin friction), auricular epilepsy (caused by contact with the external ear), and tooth-brushing epilepsy. Seizure semiology varies from myoclonic jerks to somatomotor or somatosensory seizures with Jacksonian propagation and occasional secondary generalization.[109] Brain imaging frequently reveals a lesion in the parietal cortex or supplementary motor area.[109]

7.4 Epilepsies with Structural, Metabolic, Infectious, and Inflammatory Causes

The strength of the ILAE's new classification is that it includes the etiology at each step of the diagnostic path, with six etiologic groups identified because of their potential treatment implications. These etiologies are structural, genetic, infectious, metabolic, immune, and unknown.[1] In this section we specifically focus on the structural, metabolic, infectious, and inflammatory etiologies of epilepsies with the understanding that the epilepsy may have more than one etiology – for example, in a patient with tuberous sclerosis complex (TSC) there is a structural abnormality (e.g., cortical dysplasia or subependymal nodules), but the etiology is also genetic as it relates to genes encoding hamartin and tuberin.[132] Or, a patient with mitochondrial encephalopathy, lactic acidosis, and stroke-like symptoms (MELAS) may have triple etiology of their seizures – genetic, lesion (stroke), and encephalopathy.[133] Thus, identification of etiology in patients with seizures and epilepsy may have important prognostic and treatment implications.[134]

7.4.1 Epilepsies with Structural Etiology

In patients with new-onset seizures, identification of a lesion may have important implications for long-term prognosis. A recently published evidence-based guideline concluded that patients with a first unprovoked seizure have approximately twice the chance of seizure recurrence if a lesion is identified.[135] In such cases, the provider may take more aggressive treatment approach when compared to a similar patient whose initial structural imaging is normal. Further, a recent study indicated that recurrence of seizures and transition into chronic epilepsy may be predicted by functional imaging.[136] Once chronic epilepsy develops, treatment responsiveness may depend on the presence or absence of a lesion and a lesion type.[137] Decisions regarding treatment may also be driven by the presence of structural abnormalities, as identification of a lesion provides a potential target for surgical treatment and may affect epilepsy surgery outcome.[134]

7.4.1.1 Brain-Tumor-Related Epilepsy

Up to 5% of new-onset epilepsy is related to brain tumors, the incidence of which increases after the age of 45.[138] Seizures are the first symptom of a brain tumor in 20–40% of patients, with an additional 20–45% of patients developing seizures during the course of their disease.[139] Patients with brain tumors constitute 10–30% of patients with treatment-resistant epilepsies. Tumors vary in their epileptogenicity from relatively high in diffuse low-grade tumors like gangliogliomas and dysembrioplastic neuroepithelial tumors to relatively low epileptogenicity in high-grade tumors like anaplastic glioma and glioblastoma multiforme.[140,141] In one study of 1028 patients, epilepsy was a positive uni- and multivariate prognostic factor for survival, with the prevalence of epilepsy at 49% in patients with glioblastoma, 69% in patients with anaplastic gliomas, and 85% in patients with low-grade gliomas.[142] Epileptic foci are thought to develop in the cortex that surrounds the tumor/lesion, and worsening of brain-tumor-related epilepsy (BTRE) typically raises worries of tumor progression or recurrence. BTRE is typically resistant to treatment with ASDs but may respond to antitumor medications or surgical management.[143] In patients treated surgically, the outcome may be better when "epilepsy surgery" with epileptogenic zone mapping/resection is performed rather than simple lesionectomy,[144] since the lesion does not correspond to the epileptogenic focus in up to one-third of these patients. This is probably due to another area of the brain generating paroxysmal activity via secondary epileptogenesis.[145] Finally, of importance to patients with BTRE is that the use of ASDs can lead to increased adverse events and lower quality of life.[139]

Risk for developing seizures and epilepsy can be inferred by the location of the tumor.[143] While a majority of patients with supratentorial tumors have seizures, less than 10% of patients with infratentorial tumors have seizures. Further, involvement of the cortex in the peritumoral tissue infers greater than 60% risk of having seizures versus less than 30% in tumors that are noncortical or deep-seated. There is an increased incidence of seizures in patients with peri-Rolandic lesions and in patients with dual pathology (e.g., tumor and hippocampal sclerosis).[143]

Glial Tumors

In general, glial tumors are divided into oligodendrogliomas and astrocytomas, including glioblastoma multiforme, which constitute the majority of glial tumors. Up to 50% of patients with glial tumors have seizures/epilepsy. Glial tumors are typically slow growing and are the most epileptogenic.[143] For example, up to 90% of patients with oligodendrogliomas have seizures, while seizure incidence in glioblastoma multiforme is typically less than 50%; presentation with seizures is usually considered a good prognostic factor.[140,142] The mechanism of epileptogenesis in peritumoral epilepsy is likely multifactorial including micro- and macroscopic changes. In patients with slow-growing tumors, there is gradual deafferentiation of the cortex causing denervation hypersensitivity[146] and resulting in changes in the peritumoral tissue including inflammation,[147] overexpression of excitatory neurotransmitters such as glutamate, and possible down-regulation of GABA.[143] Metabolic changes in the peritumoral tissue have also been observed including increased levels of N-acetyl aspartate, acidosis, and focal disruption in the blood–brain barrier.[148,149] Epilepsy is considered the final common pathway in the course of various brain lesions that affect the brain.

Glioneuronal Tumors

1. *Dysembryoplastic neuroepithelial tumors* (DNETs) are microscopically defined as tumors that contain specific glioneuronal elements with oligodendrocyte-like cells arranged around axons in columns, which causes them sometimes to be mistaken for other types of tumors, such as hamartomas or low-grade gliomas. These tumors typically arise in children and young adults and have the highest rates of seizures, which are frequently difficult to treat medically, but are quite amenable to surgical resection if not located in eloquent cortex.[140] They may have focal cortical dysplasia (FCD) type IIB or type III present in the surrounding peritumoral tissue or be associated with HS (HS+). Their most frequent location is temporal, and surgical resection gives greater than 80% chance of seizure freedom when temporal lobectomy is performed. However, seizure freedom is substantially lower in patients who receive simple lesionectomy.[150] If the patient is seizure-free with standard ASDs, observation rather than resection may be warranted as tumor growth and/or progression is typically not a major concern.

2. *Gangliogliomas* are histologically benign and well-differentiated neuroepithelial tumors that contain dysplastic neuronal elements (ganglion cells) with some cytological or architectural abnormalities. Some neoplastic cells may also be present, which explains the small chance of malignant anaplastic transformation. While they represent the relative minority of brain tumors (approximately 1% of all tumors), they are frequently present in patients with epilepsy. There is increased presence of gangliogliomas in temporal and frontal lobes, but they can occur anywhere in the central nervous system, including the spinal cord. They can be surrounded by FCD or associated with hippocampal sclerosis. In one study of 24 patients with gangliogliomas, 16 presented with signs of increased intracranial pressure and 12 with epilepsy.[151] In this study, more than 80% of patients with preoperative seizures were seizure-free at >1 year after resection. Similar results were observed in another study.[152]

3. *Gangliocytomas* are slowly growing tumors that contain dysplastic ganglion cells only. These tumors are typically benign (or low grade), and they are relatively rare. Gangliocytomas can occur anywhere in the central nervous system, but when they arise from the cerebellum, they constitute a distinct entity called Lhermitte–Duclos disease and may present with symptoms and signs of obstructive hydrocephalus and unilateral weakness, tremor, diplopia, or other neurological symptoms. Seizures may be part of the presentation if the lesion is cortically based.[153]

Meningioma

Meningiomas constitute about 30% of brain tumors in adults and are considered pathologically the most benign intracranial tumors. Approximately 40% of patients present with seizures prior to meningioma resection, and overall up to 60% of patients with meningiomas have seizures during the course of their disease (up to 20% develop seizures after resection). Prefrontal tumors, tumors with severe peritumoral edema, and tumors with cortical involvement are most frequently associated with seizures.[154] The risk of seizures may also be increased in patients with parietal meningiomas.[155] Surgical resection is typically curative of seizures (up to 90% are seizure-free), but many may develop new types of seizures, especially if the resection is complicated by prolonged retraction, vascular injury, peritumoral edema, incomplete resection, or if the tumor is located in the parietal lobe.[154]

Metastatic Tumors

Metastatic brain tumors are more common than primary brain tumors, but are less likely to cause seizures.[156] It is estimated that 10–20% of patients with systemic cancer will develop seizures and that seizures will constitute approximately 5% of all neurological complications of cancer.[157] Metastases are frequently found at the gray–white matter junction in watershed areas. In cases of neoplastic meningitis, seizures occur in approximately 15% of these patients, with the majority of cases due to lymphoma or leukemia. About 50% of seizures in patients with systemic cancer can be attributed to metastasis and the other 50% to causes other than metastases – such as metabolic disturbances, cancer treatments, and non-neoplastic conditions like brain abscesses.[158] The types of cancer that most frequently metastasize to the brain are lung, skin (melanoma), colon, and renal cancers. Children are reported to have a higher incidence of seizures than adults, with most seizures occurring in those with acute leukemia. Seizures can also be related to spread of the disease or to the side effects of treatments.

7.4.1.2 Cerebrovascular Disease

Cerebrovascular disease has long been recognized as a risk factor for seizures at all ages.[159,160] While cortical strokes are typically considered ictogenic, white-matter injury may also result in seizures.[161] The incidence of seizures is higher in children than in adults, which is thought to be related to the immaturity of the neural networks that results in imbalances between excitation and inhibition, leading to a heightened susceptibility to develop seizures at younger ages.[159,162] Similarly, while in adults the incidence of seizures after stroke increases with age, the proportion of younger adults with seizures after stroke is higher than that of older patients. Many children with pre- or perinatal injury and epilepsy develop epileptic spasms, which are a long-term predictor of epilepsy severity.[163] In these patients, the presence of epilepsy and the severity of the disability increase the risk of early mortality. In some patients with clearly unilateral injury, epilepsy surgery may play a role (hemispherectomy or functional hemispherectomy).

Prenatal, Perinatal, and Postnatal Insults

Prenatal, perinatal, and early postnatal strokes frequently result in cerebral palsy that is associated with seizures and epilepsy.[164] One study showed that 67% of children with perinatal stroke had seizures/epilepsy after 6 months of life, but in one-third seizures have later resolved.[165] Presence of a lesion on prenatal ultrasound and family history of epilepsy predicted the development of poststroke seizures in this age group. In another population-based study of children aged 0–18 years, the incidence of acute seizures in the setting of stroke (ischemic or hemorrhagic) was 58% after adjusting for age and type of stroke.[159] This study calculated the relative risk of seizures after stroke to be approximately 18 times higher in children than in the elderly. Finally, a study of children with delayed presentation of perinatal stroke examined the association of epilepsy at time of last follow-up with initial presentation with seizures, infantile spasms, radiographic findings, and initial abnormal EEG.[163] In this study, presentation with infantile spasms was associated with moderate-to-severe epilepsy at follow-up. Overall, the incidence of seizures in children with cerebral insults is relatively high when compared with adults; this is likely a result of more severe brain injury and/or of higher susceptibility to develop sezures/epilepsy.

Hypoxic-Ischemic Encephalopathy

Perinatal or postnatal hypoxic-ischemic injury typically results in chronic neurological disability and increased mortality and, together with other static injuries, is frequently referred to as "cerebral palsy."[164,166] The incidence of hypoxic-ischemic injury is approximately 0.2% in healthy full-term newborns, but its incidence is much higher in premature births.[167] In hypoxic-ischemic encephalopathy the injury is most severe to the most intensely developing areas of the brain, including the hippocampus. Neuronal injury and death in this and other areas results macroscopically in long-term periventricular encephalomalacia and brain atrophy. The severity of the injury typically correlates with low Apgar scores, with scores at 10 minutes being the most predictive of long-term outcomes.[168] Induced hypothermia has been shown to improve long-term neurological and functional outcomes.[169] Approximately 50–70% of infants with hypoxic-ischemic encephalopathy develop seizures, which along with delayed breathing and administration of chest compressions, are predictors of poor long-term outcomes. In the majority of infants, seizures occur within the first 24 hours.[170] EEG, including amplitude-integrated EEG, may be very helpful in evaluating the severity of the injury and assessing for the presence of seizures.[167,171] After the neonatal period, the presence of neurological deficits, including static hypoxic-ischemic encephalopathy and/or tetraplegia may be predictive of developing epilepsy, especially in patients with large areas of damage or with temporal or frontal damage.[166,172]

Ischemic and Hemorrhagic Stroke in Adults

In adults, similar to children, the presence of ischemic or hemorrhagic stroke predisposes patients to seizures and long-term epilepsy. However, the calculated risk of having seizures after stroke in adults is much lower than in children.[159] The incidence of poststroke seizures is dependent on the presence/absence of risk factors other than stroke and the duration of follow-up. Multiple temporal classifications have been developed over the years, adding to the inconsistency of the reported data. In general, seizures are considered acute if they occur in the first 24 hours of the stroke, early if they occur in the first 7–14 days, and late if they occur thereafter.[160] The incidence and prevalence of seizures and epilepsy are different between patients with ischemic and hemorrhagic strokes. Acute seizures occur in approximately 2.5% of patients with ischemic stroke and approximately 8.5% of patients with hemorrhagic stroke.[160] In one study, patients with seizures had increased mortality when compared with patients who did not have seizures, including a twofold increase in the risk of 30-day mortality after controlling for age, hemorrhagic stroke, presence of heart disease, prior functional status, prior stroke, gender, and race.[160] In studies that assessed the incidence of seizures within the first few weeks after stroke, the incidence was reported to be 4.2–6.1%, with early seizures predicting the development of chronic epilepsy.[160,173,174] Long term, 5–20% of stroke patients develop seizures, with a higher prevalence of epilepsy in patients with hemorrhagic than ischemic strokes.[175] In patients who develop seizures after stroke, their epilepsy is typically easier to control when compared to patients with TLE.[137]

7.4.1.3 Epilepsy in Mitochondrial Disorders

The term mitochondrial disorder refers to the primarily genetically mediated disorders (mitochondrial or nuclear deoxyribonucleic acid (DNA) mutations[176]) that are caused, in general, by primary dysfunction of the mitochondrial respiratory chain resulting in abnormal (e.g., decreased) production of adenosine triphosphatase (ATP) that leads to instability of the cellular membrane.[177] Studies have shown that the proportion of mutated to normal DNA in mitochondria needs to reach a specific threshold in order for the abnormality to be expressed clinically. Metabolically, there is typically elevated lactate in the cerebrospinal fluid and serum, and morphologically, there is mitochondrial proliferation in target tissues (e.g., muscle) seen as "ragged red fibers."[178] In maternal carriers, there is typically a dearth of symptoms, the presence of which may depend on the percentage of mutated DNA. Mitochondrial disorders are single- or multiorgan diseases with presentation at any age. Symptoms or features of the disease depend on whether nuclear or mitochondrial genes are involved and include various combinations of neurological (seizures, encephalopathy, stroke-like symptoms, ataxia, and dementia) and non-neurological symptoms – eye symptoms (ptosis, external ophthalmoplegia, optic atrophy, and retinopathy), muscle problems (proximal myopathy and exercise intolerance), cardiomyopathy (cardiomegaly and septal/ventricular hypertrophy), and endocrinopathy (diabetes mellitus, hypoparathyroidism, adrenal insufficiency, short stature, and hypogonadism).[178] Only those with clinical symptoms of seizures/epilepsy are discussed here (disorders not typically associated with seizures/epilepsy such as Kearns–Sayre syndrome, Leber hereditary optic neuropathy, chronic progressive external ophthalmoplegia, or neurogenic weakness with ataxia and retinitis pigmentosa are not discussed). Therapy in mitochondrial disorders is mostly supportive and aimed at the symptoms present in the individual. Various combinations of vitamin supplements targeting mitochondrial metabolism have been used to provide symptomatic support, but strong evidence for this approach is lacking.[177,179]

Myoclonic Epilepsy with Ragged Red Fibers

Myoclonic epilepsy with ragged red fibers (MERRF) is a progressive myoclonic epilepsy that is associated with myopathy with ragged red fibers, ataxia, and slowly progressive cognitive decline; other features may include photosensitivity, dementia, short stature, hearing loss, and optic atrophy. Rarely, patients may present with multiple lipomas that occur either in isolation or as part of Ekbom syndrome.[178] In the majority of affected individuals, the genetic mutation is in the mitochondrial gene for transfer ribonucleic acid-lysine (tRNA-Lys), which results in decreased cytochrome C oxidase activity. While the typical onset is in childhood through early adulthood, there is variable expression in some families.

Mitochondrial Encephalopathy, Lactic Acidosis and Stroke-Like Symptoms

In patients with mitochondrial encephalopathy, lactic acidosis, and stroke-like symptoms (MELAS), stroke-like episodes typically occur before the age of 40 years and most often in the occipital head regions, resulting in hemianopsia or cortical blindness. These patients usually have fluctuating encephalopathy and seizures at the time of presentation and there is evidence of mitochondrial dysfunction, ragged red fibers, and lactic acidosis.[178] MELAS has been associated with several point mutations, most of which are located in tRNA-Leu (tRNA-leucine), which reduces the activity of complex I of the mitochondrial respiratory chain (NAPDH dehydrogenase–ubiquinone cytochrome C oxidoreductase). The seizures are initially related to metabolic derangements, but later are caused by structural lesions (ischemic strokes) that do not conform to the major vessel distribution.[178] Clinically, these patients also have migraines, weakness, myoclonus, ataxia, hearing loss, and short stature.

Leigh's syndrome

Leigh's syndrome is another name for subacute necrotizing encephalomyclopathy, a rare disorder often precipitated by an illness associated with a febrile seizure or with illness that challenges cellular energy metabolism. Typically, onset is within the first year of life, but prenatal or late-childhood onset has been reported. Clinically, there is psychomotor regression, hypotonia, optic neuropathy or pigmentary retinopathy, progressive external ophthalmoplegia, hearing loss, nystagmus, ataxia, and gastrointestinal and respiratory problems.[180] Some patients with Leigh's syndrome have seizures, although this is not a consistent or prominent feature of this syndrome. The genetic mutation is in the mitochondrial or nuclear subunits of complex I of the mitochondrial respiratory chain.[181] Thus, inheritance can be not only mitochondrial, but also autosomal recessive or X-linked, resulting in variable age and clinical symptoms at the time of presentation.[180]

Alpers Syndrome

Alpers syndrome typically presents between the ages of 2 and 4, but initial symptoms may be delayed until the age of 25 years. It is one of the nuclear polymerase gamma-related disorders inherited in an autosomal recessive pattern.[182] Patients typically present with intractable seizures, hypotonia, episodic neurodegeneration with developmental regression, and liver failure. It is important for patients with Alpers syndrome to avoid valproic acid as it can cause fulminant encephalopathy.[183]

7.4.1.4 Malformations of Cortical Development

Malformations of cortical development (MCDs) are an important cause of epilepsy and developmental delay, and encompass a large spectrum of disorders related to abnormal gray matter development, neuronal migration, and neuronal organization.[184] In general, MCDs are classified into four major groups: MCDs resulting from abnormalities of cell proliferation or apoptosis (e.g., micro-/macrocephaly, hamartomas, and DNET), neuronal migration (e.g., heterotopia and lissencephaly), abnormal cortical organization (polymicrogyria and schizencephaly), and other MCDs (e.g., mitochondrial and peroxisomal disorders).[184] Patients with MCDs are frequently refractory to ASDs, with up to 30% being treatment resistant. They constitute approximately 40% of refractory epilepsy in children and 15–20% in adults.[185] Surgical treatment is often necessary with seizure-free rates dependent on multiple factors, including the extent of resection and location of the lesion, with ~50% of patients becoming seizure-free after temporal resection, but only ~30% after frontal resections. Only the MCDs that have relatively high incidence of seizures are discussed below.

Hemimegalencephaly

Hemimegalencephaly is a congenital unilateral enlargement of a cerebral hemisphere that can be associated with other pathologies, including epidermal nevus syndrome or hypomelanosis of Ito (see also below), and with contralateral cerebellar enlargement in rare cases.[186] These patients present with diverse pathology including cortical dysplasia, white matter abnormalities with abnormal cellular components, polymicrogyria, etc. that may be associated with an asymmetrically enlarged skull.[186] In addition to treatment-resistant seizures in the first few months of life, these patients frequently have neurological deficits including contralateral hemiparesis, developmental delay, and progressive unilateral deterioration of neurologic function with ongoing seizures. In the majority of cases, hemimegalencephaly is present in isolation, but in one study, 47% of cases were associated with known or suspected genetic syndrome such as TSC, hypomelanosis of Ito, or epidermal nevus syndrome.[186] Epilepsy surgery (hemispherectomy or modified hemispherectomy) is frequently performed early and with high seizure-free success rates.

Focal Cortical Dysplasia

A large proportion of children and adults with epilepsy have FCDs. It is estimated that up to 75% of patients with FCDs will have at least one seizure in their lifetime.[187] Seizures may be the first sign of FCD; they typically start early in life, but can occur at any age. FCD type II, especially with multilobar involvement, presents typically earlier in life than FCD type I.[188,189] Usually, patients with FCDs present with focal-onset seizures with secondary generalization, and their seizures frequently occur in clusters. Patients with epilepsy related to FCDs are typically refractory to treatment, as up to 75% continue to have seizures despite several medication trials.[137,185] MRI may be negative on standard review, but newer imaging and data-processing techniques have increased the chance of identifying subtle lesions such as subtle blurring of a gray–white matter junction, cortical thickening, transmantle sign, or bottom of the sulcus dysplasia.[134] Histological classification of FCDs has also evolved. The most recent classification published in 2011[188] divides FCDs into three types, depending on the presence and extent of the areas of abnormal neuronal architecture and/or abnormal cells. FCD type I includes architectural abnormalities only (abnormal radial lamination). FCD type II has abnormal/dysmorphic neurons (FCD type IIA) and balloon cells (FCD type IIB), while FCD type III is associated with a principal lesion, such as hippocampal sclerosis (FCD type IIIA), glial or neuronal tumors (FCD type IIIB), vascular malformations (FCD type IIIC), or other lesions (FCD type IIID). If located in an accessible location, surgical treatment should be considered, with the outcome typically dependent on the completeness of the resection. Scalp EEG will accurately characterize an ictal onset zone in up to 66% of patients. Structural MRI will be positive in up to 70% of patients and FDG-PET may be positive in up to 90% of patients.[189] Up to 50% of patients receive intracranial EEG monitoring prior to resection. Up to 20% of patients with incomplete and 80% of patients with complete resection are seizure-free.[189]

Periventricular Nodular Heterotopia

The term heterotopia refers to normal cells in an abnormal location. It occurs due to a failure of cellular/neuronal migration between the 7th and 16th gestational weeks or a failure of programmed cell death within the periventricular germinal matrix.[190] The etiology can be acquired (e.g., due to infection or injury) or genetic (e.g., X-linked dominant filamin A mutation).[191] Typically, abnormal aggregates of neurons are located along the walls of the lateral ventricle that do not enhance on MRI. In a majority of patients, these are bilateral (75%), with an additional 30% of patients exhibiting subcortical heterotopias and 20% having additional cortical malformations. Clinically, these patients typically have normal development. Seizures occur in up to 80% of these patients with the usual age of onset in adolescence, though later or earlier onset is possible. Seizures are typically mesial temporal or parieto-occipital in onset, but in some patients, they may start exclusively in the heterotopia with later spread to other brain regions.[190] Such variability in onset and spread patterns is likely related to the presence of neuronal connections among the nodules and between the nodules and cortex.[192]

Schizencephaly

This term schizencephaly refers to a cleft in a cerebral hemisphere (bilateral in about 40% of cases) that is partially or completely lined with gray matter that typically extends from the pia to the ependyma.[193] In some cases there is genetic etiology (EMX2), but in the majority of cases, there is no clear reason for the defect, raising the question whether schizencephaly is truly a developmental defect. There are two types of schizencephaly – type I is "closed," which means the clefts are fused, and type II is "open," which means the clefts are separated by cerebrospinal fluid. Open-lip clefts are more frequent in patients with bilateral schizencephaly. The location is parietal in about 70% of cases. The cortex around the cleft may be either normal or abnormal, with polymicrogyria seen frequently; these patients typically have other abnormalities, including subependymal/periventricular heterotopias.[193] Besides epilepsy, patients typically present with hemi- or quadriparesis, cognitive deficits, and language disorders. Epilepsy is present in up to 65% of cases, and it can present as multiple seizure types, including epileptic spasms and focal seizures that are refractory to treatment.

Lissencephaly

Lissencephaly (aka agyria/pachygyria or type I lissencephaly) means "smooth" brain, denoted by the absence of a gyration pattern. Lissencephaly is a migration and motility disorder that constitutes approximately 15% of cortical malformations in childhood.[187] Pathologically, there is abnormally thick cortex with four instead of six layers,[194] diffuse heterotopia, ventriculomegaly, and corpus callosum abnormalities. In the majority of cases, lissencephaly is genetically determined, such as autosomal dominant *LIS1* gene with more anterior rather than posterior pattern of cortical smoothness and more posterior-to-anterior pattern of smoothness in *DCX* (doublecortin) or *ARX* (*aristaless-related homeobox*) gene abnormalities (X-linked dominant).[195] There is a spectrum of severity in *LIS1* mutations with the most severely affected individuals carrying the diagnosis of Miller–Dieker syndrome.[195] DCX typically has more posterior pattern of cortical smoothness while ARX is associated with genital and corpus callosum (midline) abnormalities. Clinically, there is severe intellectual disability, epilepsy with multiple seizure types including epileptic spasms, hypotonia, feeding difficulties, and quadriplegia.

Cobblestone Lissencephaly

Cobblestone lissencephaly (or type II lissencephaly) presents with a relatively smooth brain, but has a pebbled-like appearance caused by leptomeningeal neuronal and glial heterotopias and is associated with dysmyelination, cerebellar dysplasia, and brainstem hypoplasia.[196] This is, as the classic lissencephaly, a neuronal migration and motility disorder, but there is also "overmigration" into the arachnoid space that results in abnormal settlement of the cortical plate and, thus, the cobblestone appearance.[196] It is associated with several genetic abnormalities, including autosomal disorders like Walker–Warburg syndrome or Fukuyama muscular dystrophy. Clinically, these patients typically present with variable combinations of ventriculomegaly, brain stem atrophy, agenesis of the corpus callosum, retinal dysplasia, and muscular defects. Recently, three types of cobblestone lissencephaly were described based on differences in genetic and clinical features.[196] The majority of patients with cobblestone lissencephaly have seizures.

Band Heterotopia (Subcortical Band Heterotopia)

Double cortex syndrome or subcortical band heterotopia is a disorder of later neuronal migration and mobility whereby bands of neurons are located midway between the ependyma and lateral surface.[195] In some patients, there may be a combination of subcortical band heterotopia with lissencephaly. Typically, band heterotopia is X-linked dominant (*DCX* gene mapped to Xq22.3-q23), with only some of the neurons being dysfunctional due to X-inactivation (the unaffected neurons typically migrate normally), but its inheritance can also be autosomal (*LIS1* mapped to 17p13.3). The vast majority of patients with subcortical band heterotopia are females, while the affected males have a more severe phenotype, including classical type I lissencephaly.[197] Thus, affected individuals present with a variable spectrum of symptoms ranging from seizures/epilepsy in an otherwise unaffected individual (typically female) to patients with seizures and severe intellectual disability (typically male). The majority (probably more than 90%) of patients with subcortical band heterotopia have seizures which, in addition to standard ASDs, may be treated with epilepsy surgery.[198]

Polymicrogyria

The term polymicrogyria means "too many, too small gyri" or simply put, an excessive number of small gyri. Pathologically, there is abnormal lamination of the cortex that is either uni- or four-layered.[199] It is a heterogeneous disorder with unclear, possibly migrational, genetic, or nongenetic, etiology. Clinically, presentation will be dependent on the location of the abnormality and its size. Frequently, these abnormalities are present bilaterally in the perisylvian regions (greater than 60%), may be associated with other abnormalities, such as heterotopia, and are associated with congenital pseudobulbar paresis, quadriparesis, language problems, intellectual disability, and seizures. Seizures occur in ~80% of patients with polymicrogyria.[199]

7.4.1.5 Neurocutaneous Syndromes

The term neurocutaneous syndrome refers to conditions that have prominent skin and central nervous system manifestations. Several neurocutaneous conditions are associated with epilepsy and are discussed in this section.

Tuberous Sclerosis Complex

Tuberous sclerosis (Bourneville disease) is a commonly occurring neurocutaneous syndrome that is caused by mammalian target of rapamycin (mTOR) pathway dysregulation, related either to TSC1 (hamartin) or TSC2 (tuberin) gene-inactivating mutations.[200] It is an autosomal dominant syndrome with complete penetrance but variable expression, including a more severe phenotype in men than in women.[201] Pathologically, in the central nervous system, there are cortical tubers at the gray–white matter interface in more than 90% of patients, subependymal nodules projecting into the ventricles, and subependymal giant cell astrocytomas. Brain calcifications are also frequently observed. The peripheral manifestations include renal lesions (angiomyolipomas, renal cell carcinoma, and cysts), skin problems (hypomelanotic patches, facial angiofibromas, and shagreen patches), retinal hamartomas, heart problems (rhabdomyomas and arrhythmias), and lung problems.[132] Progression and prognosis depend on central nervous system involvement and lesion burden; clinically, more than 80% of patients have seizures and more than 90% have intellectual disability. The development of epilepsy and subsequent prognosis depend on the presence or absence of EEG abnormalities and the timing of when they appear; thus EEG can be used as a biomarker for predicting the development of epilepsy.[202]

Sturge–Weber Syndrome

Patients with Sturge–Weber syndrome are typically very easy to recognize due to a facial venous hemangioma (port-wine stain) that co-occurs with leptomeningeal angiomatosis. This is a result of maturation failure of primitive cephalic veins during the first trimester of pregnancy.[203] Better visible on CT than MRI, there is gyriform calcification that has a tram-track appearance. The incidence of central nervous system involvement is highest with lesions encompassing the V1 division of the trigeminal nerve, resulting in a high incidence of epilepsy and intellectual disability. In addition, contralateral to the leptomeningeal abnormality is typically hemiparesis and seizures. Surgical treatment (hemispherectomy) is usually needed to achieve seizure freedom.

Hypomelanosis of Ito

Hypomelanosis of Ito (aka incontinentia pigmenti achromians) is a rare neurocutaneous syndrome with brain abnormalities related to neuronal migration abnormalities. It typically presents in the first year of life with large areas of hypopigmented skin and is associated with neurological signs and symptoms including seizures and intellectual disability as well as many non-neurological manifestations. Central nervous system abnormalities are nonspecific and can include hemimegalencephaly, pachygyria, neuronal abnormalities, heterotopias, porencephaly, arterio-venous malformations (AVMs), lissencephaly, and polymicrogyria. Seizures typically are poorly responsive to medical therapy but may respond to surgery.[204]

Incontinentia Pigmenti

Incontinentia pigmenti is a rare X-linked disorder (Xq28) that presents with variable symptoms of skin (e.g., vesicular and bullous lesions), central nervous, and other systems. Only a minority of patients with incontinentia pigmenti have seizures (10–30%), but seizures may be the first symptom of the disease.[205] Many have intellectual disability, spasticity, and tooth and hair abnormalities, including patches of alopecia.

Neurofibromatosis

Neurofibromatosis type I (NF1) is the most common neurocutaneous syndrome; it is caused by a mutation in the *NF1* tumor-suppressor gene. Presentation is typically non-neurological with various types of skin abnormalities including café au lait patches, freckling in skinfolds, and benign peripheral nerve sheath tumors (neurofibromas), as well as iris Lisch nodules, optic pathway gliomas, and sphenoid wing dysplasias. Seizures and epilepsy occur in less than 10% of patients with NF1.[206] Of importance is that central nervous system lesions may occur at any point in the disease, with ~20% of patients developing a new neuroimaging abnormality at the time of seizure onset. Surgical intervention may be needed for seizure control.[206] There are no good data for seizure incidence/prevalence in patients with NF2, which occurs ~10 times less frequently than NF1.[207]

7.4.1.6 Post-traumatic Epilepsy

Post-traumatic epilepsy (PTE) occurs in about 6% of patients with epilepsy. Frequently, seizures in these patients are difficult to control with standard ASDs.[208] The presence of early and late seizures has a significant effect on subsequent outcomes. Based on numerous studies, patients with moderate or severe traumatic brain injury (TBI) are typically placed on an ASD right after the initial trauma for up to 7 days.[209,210] If seizures do not occur, the ASD is typically weaned with an expectation that seizures will not occur in the future. Post-traumatic seizures and epilepsy can be divided into acute seizures, occurring for up to 1 week after incident trauma, and late seizures, occurring more than 1 week after the trauma.[211] The incidence of early seizures after TBI is reported to be between 2.6% and 16.3%.[211,212] In a population-based cohort, the risk of PTE after a severe TBI was 7.1% at 1 year and 11.5% at 5 years; for a moderate TBI, the risk of PTE was 0.7% at 1 year and 1.6% at 5 years; the risk of PTE was not increased by mild TBI.[213] The majority of post-traumatic epilepsy starts in the first 12–24 months after the initial trauma.[214] Several risk factors for post-traumatic epilepsy have been identified, including severity of the injury and the duration of post-traumatic coma, presence of depressed skull fracture, and intracranial blood.[215] Seizure prevention focuses on treatment with phenytoin for the first week (American Academy of Neurology (AAN) practice guideline), but this approach only decreases the incidence of early seizures and does not affect the incidence of post-traumatic epilepsy.[216] Other treatments, including older ASDs and, more recently, levetiracetam, have not been shown to be effective for prevention of post-traumatic epilepsy. However, levetiracetam may afford better short- and intermediate-term cognitive outcomes.[217,218] In patients who have a single late seizure, the risk of subsequent epilepsy is high, and treatment at this point is suggested with standard ASDs. Up to one-third of patients with post-traumatic epilepsy have evidence of dual pathology (e.g., hippocampal sclerosis), and in those patients, epilepsy surgery may be considered if they are resistant to treatment with ASDs.

7.4.1.7 Vascular Causes of Epilepsy

Overall, the risk of seizures and epilepsy is moderately high in patients with vascular malformations. The highest risk is carried by patients with arterio-venous malformations and cavernous malformations, and the risk of seizures is lowest with capillary telangiectasias.

Arterio-venous Malformation

Arterio-venous malformations (AVMs) are congenital malformations that consist of arteries and veins communicating without the intervening capillaries. Patients typically present with hemorrhage and secondary seizures. Approximately 50% of patients with AVMs are reported to have seizures and epilepsy. The mechanism by which AVMs cause seizures is not very clear, but in one study several factors were predictive of the development of epilepsy, including cortical location of the AVM or the feeder vessel, middle cerebral artery distribution, lack of aneurysm, and presence of varicose drainage.[219] Risk factors for having seizures also include male gender, age younger than 65, large size of AVM, and superficial location of AVM in the temporal or frontal cortex.[220] Treatment, in addition to ASDs, includes surgical resection, embolization, and radiation, which are typically performed to lower the risk of hemorrhage. Predictors of favorable seizure outcomes include short duration of epilepsy, presence of generalized seizures, presence of deep or posterior fossa AVMs, surgical resection or complete obliteration of the AVM.

Cerebral Cavernous Malformation

Cerebral cavernous malformations (cavernomas, CCMs) are masses of tightly arranged thin-walled vessels without any obvious feeding arteries and/or veins that occur in 0.4–0.9% of the population.[221] They are congenital and can be familial, found in patients with CCM 1–3 mutations. Cavernomas have a risk of bleeding, in the range of 1–3% per year, thus perilesional hemosiderin deposits are common on MRI and the likely reason for developing seizures and epilepsy.[222] Seizures are the presenting symptom in ~25% of patients with cavernomas, and epilepsy occurs in about 50% of patients with cavernous malformations. Typically onset is in adulthood, and seizures are often difficult to treat with ASDs, thus surgical treatment is recommended in such cases. Risk factors for epilepsy include supratentorial location, cortical involvement, mesial temporal location, size, and presence of hemosiderin around the cavernoma. Surgical resection (lesionectomy) that includes a wider margin of hemosiderin stain provides better outcome than incomplete resection.[221] Cavernomas may coexist with other pathologies, including hippocampal sclerosis, and in those cases, invasive monitoring and/or resection of cavernoma and of the mesial temporal structures is typically recommended. Predictors of good outcome include small size, lesion located in mesial temporal regions, presence of focal seizures without generalization, and single ictal focus.

Venous Angioma

Venous angiomas are frequently identified incidentally on MRIs obtained for other reasons. They are large parenchymal venous structures with many tributaries that eventually drain into the venous sinuses, and they are frequently difficult to relate to epilepsy.[223] In one large study of over 1000 patients with epilepsy, there were four cases of venous angiomas and in only two of them was there spatial concordance between the location of the lesion and the EEG.[223] Thus, it remains to be determined whether venous angiomas carry an epileptogenic potential.

7.4.2 Epilepsies with Metabolic Etiology

As indicated in the 2017 classification of epilepsies, there is increasing understanding of the spectrum of epilepsies associated with or related to metabolic abnormalities. But again, metabolic epilepsies can have dual etiology such as in porphyria or uremia, where metabolic causes are driven by genetic abnormalities.[1] The spectrum of disorders with known metabolic abnormalities is increasing, and thus, several of these epilepsies need to be discussed in more detail. Evaluation for the presence of metabolic abnormalities will depend on the overall presentation of the patient. Of importance is detailed examination and laboratory testing, including cerebrospinal fluid evaluation. Other testing, such as skin or muscle biopsy, is typically reserved for specific cases – skin biopsy in cases of suspected neuronal ceroid lipofuscinosis or Lafora body disease and muscle biopsy in case of mitochondrial disorders. Neuroimaging may be helpful in directing the diagnostic evaluation since progressive cerebral atrophy is observed in neuronal ceroid lipofuscinosis or white matter abnormalities are observed in several disorders, such as metachromatic leukodystrophy, Canavan disease, or organic acidurias. Magnetic resonance (MR) spectroscopy may provide additional insight if metabolic disorders are suspected, including elevation of lactate in mitochondrial disorders. Of the metabolic disorders, we only discuss here pyridoxine-dependent epilepsy and glucose transporter type-1 deficiency syndrome.

Metabolic disorders may be a reason for seizures not only in children but also in adults. Electrolyte derangements (e.g., hypo- or hypernatremia) may result in seizures. Further, uremic and hepatic encephalopathy (liver transplant) can also result in seizures and status epilepticus, or be a contributing factor in the development of a seizure-like state in cefepime encephalopathy. Seizures may also be seen in dialysis disequilibrium or encephalopathy syndromes. Endocrine disorders are well recognized to be associated with seizures, including glucose abnormalities (hyper- or hypoglycemia), thyroid and pituitary disorders, or hypo- or hyperparathyroidism. Finally, seizures may be present in patients with gastrointestinal disorders, such as celiac sprue (occipital calcifications in 1–2% of patients with celiac sprue) or Whipple disease.

7.4.2.1 Pyridoxine-Dependent Epilepsy

Pyridoxine-dependent epilepsy is an autosomal recessive disorder (ALDH7A1; antiquitin) that typically presents with refractory neonatal seizures associated with unusual EEG with bursts of diffuse and asynchronous high-voltage delta waves with intermixed spikes. There is a deficiency in antiquitin that presents with a variable clinical spectrum, including multisystem pathology.[224] Treatment of the seizures typically uses IV pyridoxine, although patients may respond to standard ASDs and not respond to pyridoxine.

7.4.2.2 Glucose Transporter Type-1 Deficiency Syndrome

Glucose transporter type-1 (GLUT1) deficiency syndrome is an autosomal dominant entity with complete penetrance. It is associated with an *SLC2A1* gene mutation, which results in low cerebrospinal fluid glucose and lactate, but normal serum glucose.[225] Clinically, it is associated with encephalopathy and developmental delay, and seizures occur in approximately 90% of patients. Up to 10% of patients with GLUT1 have a nonepileptic phenotype expressed mainly as a movement disorder. Seizure types are multifocal, myoclonic, and atypical absences, and typically start in the first year of life. EEG is grossly abnormal with multifocal and generalized epileptiform discharges that enhance with fasting, but improve after a meal. Treatment is with the ketogenic diet, as ASDs typically do not work. Valproate should probably be avoided since it inhibits GLUT1 activity and thus decreases glucose transport.

7.4.3 Epilepsies with Infectious Etiology

In general, any infection of the central nervous system can cause seizures in the acute stages, and infections of the central nervous system have some of the highest rates for the development of acute symptomatic seizures and epilepsy.[138,226] For example, patients with viral encephalitis have about 16 times higher chance of developing epilepsy compared to population norms.[226] Rather than discussing each infectious agent, we only focus on some aspects of epilepsies that are due to infections.

7.4.3.1 Perinatal Infections

Perinatal infections are observed relatively infrequently, with the majority of them being TORCH infections (toxoplasmosis, rubella, cytomegalovirus, and herpes simplex virus

(IISV)). Clinically, these patients present with a myriad of symptoms, including micro-cephaly, deafness, chorioretinitis, hepatomegaly, and thrombocytopenia, in addition to the neurological signs of intellectual disability, cerebral palsy, autism, and seizures/epilepsy. Some patients may have a chronic or subclinical course making the diagnosis difficult. The rationale for indiscriminate screening has been questioned because of low yield and high cost.[227]

7.4.3.2 Viral Infections

Aseptic (viral) meningitis and encephalitis are defined as an inflammatory process in the meninges or parenchyma, respectively, due to direct viral infection. Patients typically present with fever, seizures, focal neurological deficits, and behavioral symptoms, including encephalopathy. There are over 100 viruses that can cause encephalitis, many of which have specific geographic predilection.[228] Overall, aseptic meningitis, in contrast to viral enceph-alitis does not increase the risk of later epilepsy.[226] Viral infection may be preceded or associated with typical symptoms of muscle pains, soreness, and general malaise, conjunc-tivitis, rash, and respiratory symptoms. The most common viral encephalitis leading to seizures is HSV, with up to 50% of people with HSV encephalitis presenting with seizures.[228] Of note, in patients with human immunodeficiency virus, seroconversion can be associated with meningitis with encephalopathy and seizures, but this needs to be differentiated from seizures caused by an opportunistic infection, such as toxoplasmosis, brain abscess, lymphoma, or progressive multifocal leukoencephalopathy. Overall, history of viral encephalitis increases the risk of seizures several-fold when compared with the general population.

7.4.3.3 Bacterial Infections

Bacterial meningitis increases the risk of developing epilepsy fourfold (11.5-fold if the patient presents with acute seizures).[229] In addition to focal encephalitis caused by bacterial infection, seizures can also be caused by transformation of that infection into an abscess, empyema, or pyogenic meningitis. Brain abscesses typically present with fever, altered mental status, and focal neurological deficits. Acute symptomatic seizures occur in a high percentage of patients with a bacterial abscess, and the risks of postabscess epilepsy include presence of valvular heart disease and fronto-parietal distribution of the abscess, with most seizures occurring in the first 3 years after the infection.[230] Empyema is a subdural and/or epidural collection of purulent material that, in addition to typical symptoms of infection, can also cause venous thrombosis and resultant venous strokes, leading to the development of focal seizures. Seizures also occur in a high percentage of patients with acute pyogenic meningitis, but the long-term risk of epilepsy in these patients is likely lower than in patients with a focal abscess.

7.4.3.4 Tuberculosis

Central nervous system tuberculosis (CNS TB) is caused by the spread of *Mycobacterium tuberculosis* into the subarachnoid space, resulting in meningoencephalitis or the growth of tuberculoma(s) into the brain parenchyma. In a recent epidemiological study, out of 203 patients diagnosed with encephalitis in England, approximately 5% had CNS TB.[231] While CNS TB is relatively rare in developed countries, the incidence is higher in develop-ing countries where many patients with intracranial lesions have tuberculomas that can appear even after obtaining control of their systemic tuberculosis. In patients with CNS TB, seizures may be the first manifestation of the disease. Treatment includes antitubercular drugs, steroids, ASDs, and shunting/resection if amenable or necessary.

7.4.3.5 Neurocysticercosis

Neurocysticercosis is a parasitic infection of the central nervous system with *Taenia solium*. Cysticerci can be located in the brain parenchyma, ventricular system, spinal cord, or subarachnoid space.[232] Pathologically, there typically is a vesicular stage with live larvae that later may degenerate (colloidal stage) to produce an inflammatory nodule (nodular or granular stage) that may later calcify (parasite is no longer viable); there may be all three stages present in an individual. Depending on its location, the cysticercus may cause edema, gliosis, and hydrocephalus. Neurocysticercosis is the most common cause of adult-onset epilepsy in the developing world, affecting up to 4% of the population and is responsible for up to 30% of all epilepsy cases in endemic areas. Up to 70% of patients with neurocysticercosis develop epilepsy that is frequently the only manifestation of the disease. Clinically, besides seizures, patients have focal deficits, cognitive symptoms, and elevated intracranial pressure. In patients with symptomatic disease, treatment based on the AAN evidence-based guideline is focused on seizures and lowering the activity of the disease with steroids and anticysticercal drugs.[233] Surgical therapy may be an option in patients with a single lesion causing seizures that are resistant to ASDs, and ventricular shunting may be necessary. The presence of seizures prior to initiation of therapy, presence of multiple calcified lesions prior to initiation of therapy, and duration of epilepsy prior to treatment may affect prognosis.

7.4.4 Epilepsies with Inflammatory Etiology

Inflammation in epilepsy has been a focus of intensive research in the last decade, with many studies reporting inflammatory changes in patients with new-onset or chronic epilepsy. Inflammation is now considered one of the main etiologies of epilepsy, especially intractable epilepsies, including status epilepticus,[234,235] and a possible biomarker of disease development and severity.[236] Here we briefly discuss only three conditions with clear immune etiology that are associated with epilepsy: systemic lupus erythematosus, cerebral vasculitis, and sarcoidosis.

7.4.4.1 Systemic Lupus Erythematosus

More than 50% of patients with systemic lupus erythematosus (SLE) develop nervous system manifestations, known as neuropsychiatric lupus. While the mechanisms involved in central nervous system presentation of SLE are not entirely clear, several have been proposed, including antibody-mediated neurotoxicity, vasculopathy due to antiphospholipid antibodies, and cytokine-induced neurotoxicity.[237] When present, the symptoms of neuropsychiatric lupus typically include focal neurological signs, seizures, headaches, strokes, and signs of transverse myelitis, but encephalopathy can also be present, as well as infectious manifestations related to the immunosuppressive therapy often administered to these patients. Up to 20% of patients with cerebral manifestations of SLE have seizures/epilepsy, and their treatment is with standard ASDs that may be aided with immunosuppression, depending on the activity and severity of the disease.[237]

7.4.4.2 Cerebral Vasculitis

Cerebral vasculitis, divided into primary and secondary (e.g., related to connective tissue disease, infections, use of vasoactive drugs, malignancies, or hypersensitivity reactions), can be associated with seizures and epilepsy. Classification may also be based on the size of the involved vessel – such as large-artery (primary – giant cell arteritis or secondary – syphilitic) versus medium- or small-artery vasculitis. In cerebral vasculitis, while ischemia is the main reason for function loss (e.g., stroke), the process is due to inflammation within the vessel wall, a hypercoagulable state caused by proinflammatory cytokines, or changes in the vasomotor tone. Finally, classification may be based on the temporal pattern of disease development – acute, as in seizures, or chronic, as in chorea or myoclonus.[238] In patients with central nervous system vasculitis, seizures are typically, but not always a complication of strokes; less frequently they are the result of a metabolic encephalopathy caused by a systemic process such as renal or hepatic failure associated with the primary disease process.

7.4.4.3 Sarcoidosis

In contrast to a very high incidence of neuropsychiatric lupus in patients with SLE, only 5% of patients with sarcoidosis develop central nervous system involvement. Neurosarcoidosis commonly presents with focal neurologic deficits related to either cranial nerve or cerebral parenchymal involvement. The clinical presentation may be complicated by vasculitis. Seizures and epilepsy occur in up to 20% of patients with neurosarcoidosis, and they are typically well-controlled with ASDs.[239]

References

1. Scheffer IE, Berkovic S, Capovilla G, et al. ILAE classification of the epilepsies: position paper of the ILAE Commission for Classification and Terminology. *Epilepsia.* 2017;58(4):512–521.

2. de Lanerolle NC, Kim JH, Williamson A, et al. A retrospective analysis of hippocampal pathology in human temporal lobe epilepsy: evidence for distinctive patient subcategories. *Epilepsia.* 2003;44 (5):677–687.

3. Noulhiane M, Samson S, Clemenceau S, et al. A volumetric MRI study of the hippocampus and the parahippocampal region after unilateral medial temporal lobe resection. *J Neurosci Methods.* 2006;156(1-2):293–304.

4. Asadi-Pooya AA, Stewart GR, Abrams DJ, Sharan A. Prevalence and incidence of drug-resistant mesial temporal lobe epilepsy in the United States. *World Neurosurg.* 2017;99:662–666.

5. Helmstaedter C, Kurthen M, Lux S, Reuber M, Elger CE. Chronic epilepsy and cognition: a longitudinal study in temporal lobe epilepsy. *Ann Neurol.* 2003;54 (4):425–432.

6. Gomez-Ibanez A, Gasca-Salas C, Urrestarazu E, Viteri C. Clinical phenotypes within non-surgical patients with mesial temporal lobe epilepsy caused by hippocampal sclerosis based on response to antiepileptic drugs. *Seizure.* 2013;22(1):20–23.

7. Engel J, Jr., Williamson PD, Wieser HG. Medial temporal lobe epilepsy with hippocampal sclerosis. In: Engel J, Pedley TA, eds., *Epilepsy: A Comprehensive Textbook.* Philadelphia, PA: Lippincott Williams & Wilkins; 2007:2479–2486.

8. Wieser HG, Epilepsy ICoNo. ILAE Commission Report. Mesial temporal lobe epilepsy with hippocampal sclerosis. *Epilepsia.* 2004;45(6):695–714.

9. Ferrari-Marinho T, Caboclo LO, Marinho MM, et al. Auras in temporal lobe epilepsy with hippocampal sclerosis: relation to seizure focus laterality and post surgical outcome. *Epilepsy Behav.* 2012;24 (1):120–125.

10. Palmini AL, Gloor P, Jones-Gotman M. Pure amnestic seizures in temporal lobe epilepsy. Definition, clinical symptomatology and functional anatomical considerations. *Brain*. 1992;115(Pt 3):749–769.

11. Kotagal P, Bleasel A, Geller E, et al. Lateralizing value of asymmetric tonic limb posturing observed in secondarily generalized tonic-clonic seizures. *Epilepsia*. 2000;41(4):457–462.

12. Loddenkemper T, Kotagal P. Lateralizing signs during seizures in focal epilepsy. *Epilepsy Behav*. 2005;7(1):1–17.

13. Privitera MD, Morris GL, Gilliam F. Postictal language assessment and lateralization of complex partial seizures. *Ann Neurol*. 1991;30(3):391–396.

14. Geyer JD, Payne TA, Faught E, Drury I. Postictal nose-rubbing in the diagnosis, lateralization, and localization of seizures. *Neurology*. 1999;52(4):743–745.

15. Cendes F, Sakamoto AC, Spreafico R, Bingaman W, Becker AJ. Epilepsies associated with hippocampal sclerosis. *Acta Neuropathol*. 2014;128(1):21–37.

16. Vanli-Yavuz EN, Erdag E, Tuzun E, et al. Neuronal autoantibodies in mesial temporal lobe epilepsy with hippocampal sclerosis. *J Neurol Neurosurg Psychiatry*. 2016;87(7):684–692.

17. Cendes F, Andermann F, Gloor P, et al. Atrophy of mesial structures in patients with temporal lobe epilepsy: cause or consequence of repeated seizures? *Ann Neurol*. 1993;34(6):795–801.

18. Thom M. Review: hippocampal sclerosis in epilepsy. A neuropathology review. *Neuropathol Appl Neurobiol*. 2014;40(5):520–543.

19. Blumcke I, Thom M, Aronica E, et al. International consensus classification of hippocampal sclerosis in temporal lobe epilepsy: a task force report from the ILAE Commission on Diagnostic Methods. *Epilepsia*. 2013;54(7):1315–1329.

20. Blumcke I, Pauli E, Clusmann H, et al. A new clinico-pathological classification system for mesial temporal sclerosis. *Acta Neuropathol*. 2007;113(3):235–244.

21. Jardim AP, Neves RS, Caboclo LO, et al. Temporal lobe epilepsy with mesial temporal sclerosis: hippocampal neuronal loss as a predictor of surgical outcome. *Arq Neuropsiquiatr*. 2012;70(5):319–324.

22. Tezer FI, Xasiyev F, Soylemezoglu F, et al. Clinical and electrophysiological findings in mesial temporal lobe epilepsy with hippocampal sclerosis, based on the recent histopathological classifications. *Epilepsy Res*. 2016;127:50–54.

23. Sirin NG, Gurses C, Bebek N, et al. A quadruple examination of ictal EEG patterns in mesial temporal lobe epilepsy with hippocampal sclerosis: onset, propagation, later significant pattern, and termination. *J Clin Neurophysiol*. 2013;30(4):329–338.

24. Reiher J, Beaudry M, Leduc CP. Temporal intermittent rhythmic delta activity (TIRDA) in the diagnosis of complex partial epilepsy: sensitivity, specificity and predictive value. *Can J Neurol Sci*. 1989;16(4):398–401.

25. Dericioglu N, Saygi S. Ictal scalp EEG findings in patients with mesial temporal lobe epilepsy. *Clin EEG Neurosci*. 2008;39(1):20–27.

26. Jones AL, Cascino GD. Evidence on use of neuroimaging for surgical treatment of temporal lobe epilepsy: a systematic review. *JAMA Neurol*. 2016;73(4):464–470.

27. Azab M, Carone M, Ying SH, Yousem DM. Mesial temporal sclerosis: accuracy of NeuroQuant versus neuroradiologist. *Am J Neuroradiol*. 2015;36(8):1400–1406.

28. Rudie JD, Colby JB, Salamon N. Machine learning classification of mesial temporal sclerosis in epilepsy patients. *Epilepsy Res*. 2015;117:63–69.

29. Muhlhofer W, Tan YL, Mueller SG, Knowlton R. MRI-negative temporal lobe epilepsy – what do we know? *Epilepsia*. 2017; 58(5):727–742.

30. Guedj E, Bonini F, Gavaret M, et al. 18FDG-PET in different subtypes of temporal lobe epilepsy: SEEG validation and predictive value. *Epilepsia*. 2015;56(3):414–421.

31. Lee EM, Im KC, Kim JH, et al. Relationship between hypometabolic patterns and ictal scalp EEG patterns in patients with unilateral hippocampal sclerosis: an FDG-PET study. *Epilepsy Res*. 2009;84(2–3):187–193.

32. Dupont S, Semah F, Clemenceau S, et al. Accurate prediction of postoperative outcome in mesial temporal lobe epilepsy: a study using positron emission tomography with 18fluorodeoxyglucose. *Arch Neurol*. 2000;57(9):1331–1336.

33. Chassoux F, Artiges E, Semah F, et al. 18F-FDG-PET patterns of surgical success and failure in mesial temporal lobe epilepsy. *Neurology*. 2017;88(11):1045–1053.

34. Wong CH, Bleasel A, Wen L, et al. The topography and significance of extratemporal hypometabolism in refractory mesial temporal lobe epilepsy examined by FDG-PET. *Epilepsia*. 2010;51(8):1365–1373.

35. Daly DD, Mulder DW. Gelastic epilepsy. *Neurology*. 1957;7(3):189–192.

36. Striano S, Santulli L, Ianniciello M, et al. The gelastic seizures-hypothalamic hamartoma syndrome: facts, hypotheses, and perspectives. *Epilepsy Behav*. 2012;24(1):7–13.

37. Kovac S, Diehl B, Wehner T, et al. Gelastic seizures: incidence, clinical and EEG features in adult patients undergoing video-EEG telemetry. *Epilepsia*. 2015;56(1):e1–5.

38. Gutierrez C, Asadi-Pooya AA, Skidmore CT, et al. Clinical features and postoperative seizure outcome in patients with drug-resistant gelastic seizures without hypothalamic hamartoma. *Epilepsy Behav*. 2016;64(Pt A):90–93.

39. Striano S, Meo R, Bilo L, et al. Gelastic epilepsy: symptomatic and cryptogenic cases. *Epilepsia*. 1999;40(3):294–302.

40. Craig DW, Itty A, Panganiban C, et al. Identification of somatic chromosomal abnormalities in hypothalamic hamartoma tissue at the GLI3 locus. *Am J Hum Genet*. 2008;82(2):366–374.

41. Kerrigan JF, Ng YT, Chung S, Rekate HL. The hypothalamic hamartoma: a model of subcortical epileptogenesis and encephalopathy. *Semin Pediatr Neurol*. 2005;12(2):119–131.

42. Brandberg G, Raininko R, Eeg-Olofsson O. Hypothalamic hamartoma with gelastic seizures in Swedish children and adolescents. *Eur J Paediatr Neurol*. 2004;8(1):35–44.

43. Weissenberger AA, Dell ML, Liow K, et al. Aggression and psychiatric comorbidity in children with hypothalamic hamartomas and their unaffected siblings. *J Am Acad Child Adolesc Psychiatry*. 2001;40(6):696–703.

44. Berkovic SF, Kuzniecky RI, Andermann F. Human epileptogenesis and hypothalamic hamartomas: new lessons from an experiment of nature. *Epilepsia*. 1997;38(1):1–3.

45. Kahane P, Ryvlin P, Hoffmann D, Minotti L, Benabid AL. From hypothalamic hamartoma to cortex: what can be learnt from depth recordings and stimulation? *Epileptic Disord*. 2003;5(4):205–217.

46. Palmini A, Chandler C, Andermann F, et al. Resection of the lesion in patients with hypothalamic hamartomas and catastrophic epilepsy. *Neurology*. 2002;58(9):1338–1347.

47. DiFazio MP, Davis RG. Utility of early single photon emission computed tomography (SPECT) in neonatal gelastic epilepsy associated with hypothalamic hamartoma. *J Child Neurol*. 2000;15(6):414–417.

48. Palmini A, Van Paesschen W, Dupont P, Van Laere K, Van Driel G. Status gelasticus after temporal lobectomy: ictal FDG-PET findings and the question of dual pathology involving hypothalamic hamartomas. *Epilepsia*. 2005;46(8):1313–1316.

49. Ng YT, Rekate HL, Prenger EC, et al. Transcallosal resection of hypothalamic hamartoma for intractable epilepsy. *Epilepsia*. 2006;47(7):1192–1202.

50. Rekate HL, Feiz-Erfan I, Ng YT, Gonzalez LF, Kerrigan JF. Endoscopic surgery for hypothalamic hamartomas causing medically refractory gelastic epilepsy. *Childs Nerv Syst*. 2006;22(8):874–880.

51. Berkovic SF, Arzimanoglou A, Kuzniecky R, et al. Hypothalamic hamartoma and seizures: a treatable epileptic encephalopathy. *Epilepsia.* 2003;44 (7):969–973.

52. Quiske A, Frings L, Wagner K, Unterrainer J, Schulze-Bonhage A. Cognitive functions in juvenile and adult patients with gelastic epilepsy due to hypothalamic hamartoma. *Epilepsia.* 2006;47(1):153–158.

53. Striano S, Striano P, Coppola A, Romanelli P. The syndrome gelastic seizures-hypothalamic hamartoma: severe, potentially reversible encephalopathy. *Epilepsia.* 2009;50(Suppl 5):62–65.

54. Arita K, Ikawa F, Kurisu K, et al. The relationship between magnetic resonance imaging findings and clinical manifestations of hypothalamic hamartoma. *J Neurosurg.* 1999;91 (2):212–220.

55. Chibbaro S, Cebula H, Scholly J, et al. Pure endoscopic management of epileptogenic hypothalamic hamartomas. *Neurosurg Rev.* 2017;40(4):647–653.

56. Leal AJ, Moreira A, Robalo C, Ribeiro C. Different electroclinical manifestations of the epilepsy associated with hamartomas connecting to the middle or posterior hypothalamus. *Epilepsia.* 2003;44 (9):1191–1195.

57. Kameyama S, Shirozu H, Masuda H, et al. MRI-guided stereotactic radiofrequency thermocoagulation for 100 hypothalamic hamartomas. *J Neurosurg.* 2016;124 (5):1503–1512.

58. Tellez-Zenteno JF, Serrano-Almeida C, Moien-Afshari F. Gelastic seizures associated with hypothalamic hamartomas. An update in the clinical presentation, diagnosis and treatment. *Neuropsychiatr Dis Treat.* 2008;4(6):1021–1031.

59. Delalande O, Fohlen M. Disconnecting surgical treatment of hypothalamic hamartoma in children and adults with refractory epilepsy and proposal of a new classification. *Neurol Med Chir (Tokyo).* 2003;43(2):61–68.

60. Valdueza JM, Cristante L, Dammann O, et al. Hypothalamic hamartomas: with special reference to gelastic epilepsy and surgery. *Neurosurgery.* 1994;34(6):949–958.

61. Berkovic SF, Andermann F, Melanson D, et al. Hypothalamic hamartomas and ictal laughter: evolution of a characteristic epileptic syndrome and diagnostic value of magnetic resonance imaging. *Ann Neurol.* 1988;23(5):429–439.

62. Troester M, Haine-Schlagel R, Ng YT, et al. EEG and video-EEG seizure monitoring has limited utility in patients with hypothalamic hamartoma and epilepsy. *Epilepsia.* 2011;52(6):1137–1143.

63. Wu J, Gao M, Shen JX, Qiu SF, Kerrigan JF. Mechanisms of intrinsic epileptogenesis in human gelastic seizures with hypothalamic hamartoma. *CNS Neurosci Ther.* 2015;21(2):104–111.

64. Fenoglio KA, Wu J, Kim DY, et al. Hypothalamic hamartoma: basic mechanisms of intrinsic epileptogenesis. *Semin Pediatr Neurol.* 2007;14(2):51–59.

65. Coons SW, Rekate HL, Prenger EC, et al. The histopathology of hypothalamic hamartomas: study of 57 cases. *J Neuropathol Exp Neurol.* 2007;66 (2):131–141.

66. Beggs J, Nakada S, Fenoglio K, et al. Hypothalamic hamartomas associated with epilepsy: ultrastructural features. *J Neuropathol Exp Neurol.* 2008;67 (7):657–668.

67. Maixner W. Hypothalamic hamartomas – clinical, neuropathological and surgical aspects. *Childs Nerv Syst.* 2006;22 (8):867–873.

68. Munari C, Kahane P, Francione S, et al. Role of the hypothalamic hamartoma in the genesis of gelastic fits (a video-stereo-EEG study). *Electroencephalogr Clin Neurophysiol.* 1995;95(3):154–160.

69. Rasmussen T, Olszewski J, Lloydsmith D. Focal seizures due to chronic localized encephalitis. *Neurology.* 1958;8(6):435–445.

70. Oguni H, Andermann F, Rasmussen TB. The syndrome of chronic encephalitis and epilepsy: a study based on the MNI series of 48 cases. *Adv Neurol.* 1992;57:419–433.

71. Pardo CA, Nabbout R, Galanopoulou AS. Mechanisms of epileptogenesis in pediatric epileptic syndromes: Rasmussen encephalitis, infantile spasms, and febrile infection-related epilepsy syndrome (FIRES). *Neurotherapeutics*. 2014;11 (2):297–310.

72. Varadkar S, Bien CG, Kruse CA, et al. Rasmussen's encephalitis: clinical features, pathobiology, and treatment advances. *Lancet Neurol*. 2014;13(2):195–205.

73. Bien CG, Granata T, Antozzi C, et al. Pathogenesis, diagnosis and treatment of Rasmussen encephalitis: a European consensus statement. *Brain*. 2005;128 (Pt 3):454–471.

74. Dubeau F, Andermann F, Wiendl H, Bar-Or A. Rasmussen's encephalitis (chronic focal encephalitis). In: Engel JJ, Pedley TA, eds., *Epilepsy: A Comprehensive Textbook*. 2nd edn. Philadelphia, PA: Lippincott Williams & Wilkins; 2008:2439–2453.

75. Bien CG, Urbach H, Deckert M, et al. Diagnosis and staging of Rasmussen's encephalitis by serial MRI and histopathology. *Neurology*. 2002;58 (2):250–257.

76. Granata T, Gobbi G, Spreafico R, et al. Rasmussen's encephalitis: early characteristics allow diagnosis. *Neurology*. 2003;60(3):422–425.

77. Ramesha KN, Rajesh B, Ashalatha R, et al. Rasmussen's encephalitis: experience from a developing country based on a group of medically and surgically treated patients. *Seizure*. 2009;18(8):567–572.

78. Avbersek A, Miserocchi A, McEvoy AW, et al. Multiphasic presentation of Rasmussen's encephalitis. *Epileptic Disord*. 2015;17(3):315–320.

79. Press C, Wallace A, Chapman KE. The Janus-faced nature of Rasmussen's encephalitis. *Semin Pediatr Neurol*. 2014;21 (2):129–136.

80. Muto A, Oguni H, Takahashi Y, et al. Nationwide survey (incidence, clinical course, prognosis) of Rasmussen's encephalitis. *Brain Dev*. 2010;32 (6):445–453.

81. Casciato S, Di Bonaventura C, Fattouch J, et al. Extrarolandic electroclinical findings in the evolution of adult-onset Rasmussen's encephalitis. *Epilepsy Behav*. 2013;28 (3):467–473.

82. Gambardella A, Andermann F, Shorvon S, Le Piane E, Aguglia U. Limited chronic focal encephalitis: another variant of Rasmussen syndrome? *Neurology*. 2008;70 (5):374–377.

83. Guan Y, Luan G, Zhou J, Liu X. Bilateral Rasmussen encephalitis. *Epilepsy Behav*. 2011;20(2):398–403.

84. Tobias SM, Robitaille Y, Hickey WF, et al. Bilateral Rasmussen encephalitis: postmortem documentation in a five-year-old. *Epilepsia*. 2003;44(1):127–130.

85. Frucht S. Dystonia, athetosis, and epilepsia partialis continua in a patient with late-onset Rasmussen's encephalitis. *Mov Disord*. 2002;17(3):609–612.

86. Takei H, Wilfong A, Malphrus A, et al. Dual pathology in Rasmussen's encephalitis: a study of seven cases and review of the literature. *Neuropathology*. 2010;30(4):381–391.

87. Longaretti F, Dunkley C, Varadkar S, et al. Evolution of the EEG in children with Rasmussen's syndrome. *Epilepsia*. 2012;53 (9):1539–1545.

88. So N, Gloor P. Electroencephalographic and electrocorticographic findings in chronic encephalitis of the Rasmussen type. In: Andermann F, ed., *Chronic Encephalitis and Epilepsy Rasmussen's Syndrome*. Stoneham, MA: Butterworth-Heinemann; 1991:37–45.

89. Pardo CA, Vining EP, Guo L, et al. The pathology of Rasmussen syndrome: stages of cortical involvement and neuropathological studies in 45 hemispherectomies. *Epilepsia*. 2004;45 (5):516–526.

90. Bauer J, Elger CE, Hans VH, et al. Astrocytes are a specific immunological target in Rasmussen's encephalitis. *Ann Neurol*. 2007;62(1):67–80.

91. Chiapparini L, Granata T, Farina L, et al. Diagnostic imaging in 13 cases of Rasmussen's encephalitis: can early MRI

suggest the diagnosis? *Neuroradiology.* 2003;45(3):171–183.

92. Yamazaki E, Takahashi Y, Akasaka N, Fujiwara T, Inoue Y. Temporal changes in brain MRI findings in Rasmussen syndrome. *Epileptic Disord.* 2011;13 (3):229–239.

93. Bhatjiwale MG, Polkey C, Cox TC, Dean A, Deasy N. Rasmussen's encephalitis: neuroimaging findings in 21 patients with a closer look at the basal ganglia. *Pediatr Neurosurg.* 1998;29(3):142–148.

94. Cauley KA, Burbank HN, Filippi CG. Diffusion tensor imaging and tractography of Rasmussen encephalitis. *Pediatr Radiol.* 2009;39(7):727–730.

95. Wagner J, Schoene-Bake JC, Bien CG, et al. Automated 3D MRI volumetry reveals regional atrophy differences in Rasmussen encephalitis. *Epilepsia.* 2012;53(4):613–621.

96. Fiorella DJ, Provenzale JM, Coleman RE, Crain BJ, Al-Sugair AA. (18)F-fluorodeoxyglucose positron emission tomography and MR imaging findings in Rasmussen encephalitis. *Am J Neuroradiol.* 2001;22(7):1291–1299.

97. Shetty-Alva N, Novotny EJ, Shetty T, Kuo PH. Positron emission tomography in Rasmussen's encephalitis. *Pediatr Neurol.* 2007;36(2):112–114.

98. Scheffer IE, Phillips HA, O'Brien CE, et al. Familial partial epilepsy with variable foci: a new partial epilepsy syndrome with suggestion of linkage to chromosome 2. *Ann Neurol.* 1998;44(6):890–899.

99. Berkovic SF, Serratosa JM, Phillips HA, et al. Familial partial epilepsy with variable foci: clinical features and linkage to chromosome 22q12. *Epilepsia.* 2004;45 (9):1054–1060.

100. Klein KM, O'Brien TJ, Praveen K, et al. Familial focal epilepsy with variable foci mapped to chromosome 22q12: expansion of the phenotypic spectrum. *Epilepsia.* 2012;53(8):e151–155.

101. Dibbens LM, de Vries B, Donatello S, et al. Mutations in DEPDC5 cause familial focal epilepsy with variable foci. *Nat Genet.* 2013;45(5):546–551.

102. Callenbach PM, van den Maagdenberg AM, Hottenga JJ, et al. Familial partial epilepsy with variable foci in a Dutch family: clinical characteristics and confirmation of linkage to chromosome 22q. *Epilepsia.* 2003;44 (10):1298–1305.

103. International League Against Epilepsy: Engel J, Jr. A proposed diagnostic scheme for people with epileptic seizures and with epilepsy: report of the ILAE Task Force on Classification and Terminology. *Epilepsia.* 2001;42(6):796–803.

104. Antebi D, Bird J. The facilitation and evocation of seizures. *Br J Psychiatry.* 1992;160:154–164.

105. Epilepsy Foundation of America Working Group: Fisher RS, Harding G, Erba G, Barkley GL, Wilkins A. Photic- and pattern-induced seizures: a review for the Epilepsy Foundation of America Working Group. *Epilepsia.* 2005;46(9):1426–1441.

106. Koepp MJ, Caciagli L, Pressler RM, Lehnertz K, Beniczky S. Reflex seizures, traits, and epilepsies: from physiology to pathology. *Lancet Neurol.* 2016;15 (1):92–105.

107. Italiano D, Ferlazzo E, Gasparini S, et al. Generalized versus partial reflex seizures: a review. *Seizure.* 2014;23(7):512–520.

108. Verrotti A, Beccaria F, Fiori F, Montagnini A, Capovilla G. Photosensitivity: epidemiology, genetics, clinical manifestations, assessment, and management. *Epileptic Disord.* 2012;14 (4):349–362.

109. Striano S, Coppola A, del Gaudio L, Striano P. Reflex seizures and reflex epilepsies: old models for understanding mechanisms of epileptogenesis. *Epilepsy Res.* 2012;100(1–2):1–11.

110. Harding G, Wilkins AJ, Erba G, Barkley GL, Fisher RS, Epilepsy Foundation of America Working Group. Photic- and pattern-induced seizures: expert consensus of the Epilepsy Foundation of America Working Group. *Epilepsia.* 2005;46 (9):1423–1425.

111. Hill RA, Chiappa KH, Huang-Hellinger F, Jenkins BG. Hemodynamic and metabolic aspects of photosensitive epilepsy revealed

by functional magnetic resonance imaging and magnetic resonance spectroscopy. *Epilepsia.* 1999;40(7):912–920.

112. Ricci GB, Chapman RM, Erne SN, et al. Neuromagnetic topography of photoconvulsive response in man. *Electroencephalogr Clin Neurophysiol.* 1990;75(2):1–12.

113. Kasteleijn-Nolst Trenite DG, Guerrini R, Binnie CD, Genton P. Visual sensitivity and epilepsy: a proposed terminology and classification for clinical and EEG phenomenology. *Epilepsia.* 2001;42 (5):692–701.

114. Ferlazzo E, Zifkin BG, Andermann E, Andermann F. Cortical triggers in generalized reflex seizures and epilepsies. *Brain.* 2005;128(Pt 4):700–710.

115. Guerrini R, Genton P. Epileptic syndromes and visually induced seizures. *Epilepsia.* 2004;45(Suppl 1):14–18.

116. Miller S, Razvi S, Russell A. Reading epilepsy. *Pract Neurol.* 2010;10(5):278–281.

117. Koutroumanidis M, Koepp MJ, Richardson MP, et al. The variants of reading epilepsy. A clinical and video-EEG study of 17 patients with reading-induced seizures. *Brain.* 1998;121(Pt 8):1409–1427.

118. Salek-Haddadi A, Mayer T, Hamandi K, et al. Imaging seizure activity: a combined EEG/EMG-fMRI study in reading epilepsy. *Epilepsia.* 2009;50(2):256–264.

119. Stern J. Musicogenic epilepsy. *Handb Clin Neurol.* 2015;129:469–477.

120. Kaplan PW. Musicogenic epilepsy and epileptic music: a seizure's song. *Epilepsy Behav.* 2003;4(5):464–473.

121. Wieser HG, Hungerbuhler H, Siegel AM, Buck A. Musicogenic epilepsy: review of the literature and case report with ictal single photon emission computed tomography. *Epilepsia.* 1997;38 (2):200–207.

122. Avanzini G. Musicogenic seizures. *Ann N Y Acad Sci.* 2003;999:95–102.

123. Pittau F, Tinuper P, Bisulli F, et al. Videopolygraphic and functional MRI study of musicogenic epilepsy. A case report and literature review. *Epilepsy Behav.* 2008;13(4):685–692.

124. Bebek N, Gurses C, Gokyigit A, et al. Hot water epilepsy: clinical and electrophysiologic findings based on 21 cases. *Epilepsia.* 2001;42(9):1180–1184.

125. Satishchandra P. Hot-water epilepsy. *Epilepsia.* 2003;44(Suppl 1):29–32.

126. Nagaraja D, Chand RP. Eating epilepsy. *Clin Neurol Neurosurg.* 1984;86(2):95–99.

127. Loreto V, Nocerino C, Striano P, et al. Eating epilepsy. Heterogeneity of ictal semiology: the role of video-EEG monitoring. *Epileptic Disord.* 2000;2 (2):93–98.

128. Aguglia U, Tinuper P, Gastaut H. Startle-induced epileptic seizures. *Epilepsia.* 1984;25(6):712–720.

129. Fernandez S, Donaire A, Maestro I, et al. Functional neuroimaging in startle epilepsy: involvement of a mesial frontoparietal network. *Epilepsia.* 2011;52 (9):1725–1732.

130. Nolan MA, Otsubo H, Iida K, Minassian BA. Startle-induced seizures associated with infantile hemiplegia: implication of the supplementary motor area. *Epileptic Disord.* 2005;7(1):49–52.

131. Ricci S, Cusmai R, Fusco L, Vigevano F. Reflex myoclonic epilepsy in infancy: a new age-dependent idiopathic epileptic syndrome related to startle reaction. *Epilepsia.* 1995;36(4):342–348.

132. Northrup H, Krueger DA, International Tuberous Sclerosis Complex Consensus Group. Tuberous sclerosis complex diagnostic criteria update: recommendations of the 2012 International Tuberous Sclerosis Complex Consensus Conference. *Pediatr Neurol.* 2013;49 (4):243–254.

133. El-Hattab AW, Adesina AM, Jones J, Scaglia F. MELAS syndrome: clinical manifestations, pathogenesis, and treatment options. *Mol Genet Metab.* 2015;116(1–2):4–12.

134. Middlebrooks EH, Ver Hoef L, Szaflarski JP. Neuroimaging in epilepsy. *Curr Neurol Neurosci Rep.* 2017;17(4):32.

135. Krumholz A, Shinnar S, French J, Gronseth G, Wiebe S. Evidence-based guideline: management of an unprovoked first seizure in adults. Report of the Guideline Development Subcommittee of the American Academy of Neurology and the American Epilepsy Society. *Neurology.* 2015;85(17):1526–1527.

136. Gupta L, Janssens R, Vlooswijk MC, et al. Towards prognostic biomarkers from BOLD fluctuations to differentiate a first epileptic seizure from new-onset epilepsy. *Epilepsia.* 2017;58(3):476–483.

137. Semah F, Picot MC, Adam C, et al. Is the underlying cause of epilepsy a major prognostic factor for recurrence? *Neurology.* 1998;51(5):1256–1262.

138. Annegers JF, Hauser WA, Lee JR, Rocca WA. Incidence of acute symptomatic seizures in Rochester, Minnesota, 1935–1984. *Epilepsia.* 1995;36(4):327–333.

139. Maschio M. Brain tumor-related epilepsy. *Curr Neuropharmacol.* 2012;10(2):124–133.

140. Cowie CJ, Cunningham MO. Peritumoral epilepsy: relating form and function for surgical success. *Epilepsy Behav.* 2014;38:53–61.

141. Kasper BS, Kasper EM. New classification of epilepsy-related neoplasms: the clinical perspective. *Epilepsy Behav.* 2017;67:91–97.

142. Lote K, Stenwig AE, Skullerud K, Hirschberg H. Prevalence and prognostic significance of epilepsy in patients with gliomas. *Eur J Cancer.* 1998;34(1):98–102.

143. Ruda R, Bello L, Duffau H, Soffietti R. Seizures in low-grade gliomas: natural history, pathogenesis, and outcome after treatments. *Neuro Oncol.* 2012;14(Suppl 4): iv55–64.

144. Jooma R, Yeh HS, Privitera MD, Gartner M. Lesionectomy versus electrophysiologically guided resection for temporal lobe tumors manifesting with complex partial seizures. *J Neurosurg.* 1995;83(2):231–236.

145. van Breemen MS, Vecht CJ. Optimal seizure management in brain tumor patients. *Curr Neurol Neurosci Rep.* 2005;5 (3):207–213.

146. van Breemen MS, Wilms EB, Vecht CJ. Epilepsy in patients with brain tumours: epidemiology, mechanisms, and management. *Lancet Neurol.* 2007;6 (5):421–430.

147. Aronica E, Gorter JA, Redeker S, et al. Distribution, characterization and clinical significance of microglia in glioneuronal tumours from patients with chronic intractable epilepsy. *Neuropathol Appl Neurobiol.* 2005;31(3):280–291.

148. Chernov MF, Kubo O, Hayashi M, et al. Proton MRS of the peritumoral brain. *J Neurol Sci.* 2005;228(2):137–142.

149. Ivens S, Kaufer D, Flores LP, et al. TGF-beta receptor-mediated albumin uptake into astrocytes is involved in neocortical epileptogenesis. *Brain.* 2007;130(Pt 2):535–547.

150. Chan CH, Bittar RG, Davis GA, Kalnins RM, Fabinyi GC. Long-term seizure outcome following surgery for dysembryoplastic neuroepithelial tumor. *J Neurosurg.* 2006;104(1):62–69.

151. Tandon V, Bansal S, Chandra PS, et al. Ganglioglioma: single-institutional experience of 24 cases with review of literature. *Asian J Neurosurg.* 2016;11 (4):407–411.

152. Song JY, Kim JH, Cho YH, Kim CJ, Lee EJ. Treatment and outcomes for gangliogliomas: a single-center review of 16 patients. *Brain Tumor Res Treat.* 2014;2 (2):49–55.

153. Odia Y. Gangliocytomas and gangliogliomas: review of clinical, pathologic and genetic features. *Clin Oncol (Belmont).* 2016;1:1017.

154. Xue H, Sveinsson O, Tomson T, Mathiesen T. Intracranial meningiomas and seizures: a review of the literature. *Acta Neurochir (Wien).* 2015;157(9):1541–1548.

155. Lynam LM, Lyons MK, Drazkowski JF, et al. Frequency of seizures in patients with newly diagnosed brain tumors: a retrospective review. *Clin Neurol Neurosurg.* 2007;109(7):634–638.

156. Glantz MJ, Cole BF, Forsyth PA, et al. Practice parameter: anticonvulsant prophylaxis in patients with newly

diagnosed brain tumors. Report of the Quality Standards Subcommittee of the American Academy of Neurology. *Neurology*. 2000;54(10):1886–1893.

157. Singh G, Rees JH, Sander JW. Seizures and epilepsy in oncological practice: causes, course, mechanisms and treatment. *J Neurol Neurosurg Psychiatry*. 2007;78 (4):342–349.

158. Patchell RA, Tibbs PA, Walsh JW, et al. A randomized trial of surgery in the treatment of single metastases to the brain. *N Engl J Med*. 1990;322(8):494–500.

159. Chadehumbe MA, Khatri P, Khoury JC, et al. Seizures are common in the acute setting of childhood stroke: a population-based study. *J Child Neurol*. 2009;24 (1):9–12.

160. Szaflarski JP, Rackley AY, Kleindorfer DO, et al. Incidence of seizures in the acute phase of stroke: a population-based study. *Epilepsia*. 2008;49(6):974–981.

161. Ferlazzo E, Gasparini S, Beghi E, et al. Epilepsy in cerebrovascular diseases: review of experimental and clinical data with meta-analysis of risk factors. *Epilepsia*. 2016;57(8):1205–1214.

162. Silverstein FS, Barks JD, Hagan P, et al. Cytokines and perinatal brain injury. *Neurochem Int*. 1997;30(4–5):375–383.

163. Fitzgerald KC, Williams LS, Garg BP, Golomb MR. Epilepsy in children with delayed presentation of perinatal stroke. *J Child Neurol*. 2007;22(11):1274–1280.

164. Rosenbaum P, Paneth N, Leviton A, et al. A report: the definition and classification of cerebral palsy April 2006. *Dev Med Child Neurol Suppl*. 2007;109:8–14.

165. Golomb MR, Garg BP, Carvalho KS, Johnson CS, Williams LS. Perinatal stroke and the risk of developing childhood epilepsy. *J Pediatr*. 2007;151(4):409–413.

166. Krageloh-Mann I, Cans C. Cerebral palsy update. *Brain Dev*. 2009;31(7):537–544.

167. Vannucci RC. Hypoxic-ischemic encephalopathy. *Am J Perinatol*. 2000;17 (3):113–120.

168. Laptook AR, Shankaran S, Ambalavanan N, et al. Outcome of term infants using apgar scores at 10 minutes following hypoxic-ischemic encephalopathy. *Pediatrics*. 2009;124(6):1619–1626.

169. Tagin MA, Woolcott CG, Vincer MJ, Whyte RK, Stinson DA. Hypothermia for neonatal hypoxic ischemic encephalopathy: an updated systematic review and meta-analysis. *Arch Pediatr Adolesc Med*. 2012;166(6):558–566.

170. Ekert P, Perlman M, Steinlin M, Hao Y. Predicting the outcome of postasphyxial hypoxic-ischemic encephalopathy within 4 hours of birth. *J Pediatr*. 1997;131 (4):613–617.

171. Spitzmiller RE, Phillips T, Meinzen-Derr J, Hoath SB. Amplitude-integrated EEG is useful in predicting neurodevelopmental outcome in full-term infants with hypoxic-ischemic encephalopathy: a meta-analysis. *J Child Neurol*. 2007;22(9):1069–1078.

172. Carlsson M, Hagberg G, Olsson I. Clinical and aetiological aspects of epilepsy in children with cerebral palsy. *Dev Med Child Neurol*. 2003;45(6):371–376.

173. Kilpatrick CJ, Davis SM, Hopper JL, Rossiter SC. Early seizures after acute stroke. Risk of late seizures. *Arch Neurol*. 1992;49(5):509–511.

174. So EL, Annegers JF, Hauser WA, O'Brien PC, Whisnant JP. Population-based study of seizure disorders after cerebral infarction. *Neurology*. 1996;46(2):350–355.

175. Silverman IE, Restrepo L, Mathews GC. Poststroke seizures. *Arch Neurol*. 2002;59 (2):195–201.

176. Koopman WJ, Willems PH, Smeitink JA. Monogenic mitochondrial disorders. *N Engl J Med*. 2012;366(12):1132–1141.

177. Chinnery PF. Mitochondrial disorders overview. In: Adam MP, Ardinger HH, Pagon RA, et al., eds., *GeneReviews(R)*. Seattle, WA: University of Washington; 2000.

178. Schon EA, Bonilla E, DiMauro S. Mitochondrial DNA mutations and pathogenesis. *J Bioenerg Biomembr*. 1997;29(2):131–149.

179. Taylor RW, Chinnery PF, Clark KM, Lightowlers RN, Turnbull DM. Treatment

of mitochondrial disease. *J Bioenerg Biomembr.* 1997;29(2):195–205.

180. Baertling F, Rodenburg RJ, Schaper J, et al. A guide to diagnosis and treatment of Leigh syndrome. *J Neurol Neurosurg Psychiatry.* 2014;85(3):257–265.

181. Leigh PN, Al-Sarraj S, DiMauro S. Impact commentaries. Subacute necrotising encephalomyelopathy (Leigh's disease; Leigh syndrome). *J Neurol Neurosurg Psychiatry.* 2015;86(4):363–365.

182. Milone M, Massie R. Polymerase gamma 1 mutations: clinical correlations. *Neurologist.* 2010;16(2):84–91.

183. Saneto RP, Cohen BH, Copeland WC, Naviaux RK. Alpers-Huttenlocher syndrome. *Pediatr Neurol.* 2013;48 (3):167–178.

184. Barkovich AJ, Kuzniecky RI, Jackson GD, Guerrini R, Dobyns WB. A developmental and genetic classification for malformations of cortical development. *Neurology.* 2005;65(12):1873–1887.

185. Barkovich AJ, Dobyns WB, Guerrini R. Malformations of cortical development and epilepsy. *Cold Spring Harb Perspect Med.* 2015;5(5):a022392.

186. Tinkle BT, Schorry EK, Franz DN, Crone KR, Saal HM. Epidemiology of hemimegalencephaly: a case series and review. *Am J Med Genet A.* 2005;139 (3):204–211.

187. Leventer RJ, Phelan EM, Coleman LT, et al. Clinical and imaging features of cortical malformations in childhood. *Neurology.* 1999;53(4):715–722.

188. Blumcke I, Thom M, Aronica E, et al. The clinicopathologic spectrum of focal cortical dysplasias: a consensus classification proposed by an ad hoc task force of the ILAE Diagnostic Methods Commission. *Epilepsia.* 2011;52 (1):158-174.

189. Hauptman JS, Mathern GW. Surgical treatment of epilepsy associated with cortical dysplasia: 2012 update. *Epilepsia.* 2012;53(Suppl 4):98–104.

190. Aghakhani Y, Kinay D, Gotman J, et al. The role of periventricular nodular heterotopia in epileptogenesis. *Brain.* 2005;128(Pt 3):641–651.

191. Sheen VL, Dixon PH, Fox JW, et al. Mutations in the X-linked filamin 1 gene cause periventricular nodular heterotopia in males as well as in females. *Hum Mol Genet.* 2001;10(17):1775–1783.

192. Eksioglu YZ, Scheffer IE, Cardenas P, et al. Periventricular heterotopia: an X-linked dominant epilepsy locus causing aberrant cerebral cortical development. *Neuron.* 1996;16(1):77–87.

193. Granata T, Freri E, Caccia C, et al. Schizencephaly: clinical spectrum, epilepsy, and pathogenesis. *J Child Neurol.* 2005;20 (4):313–318.

194. Dobyns WB, Reiner O, Carrozzo R, Ledbetter DH. Lissencephaly. A human brain malformation associated with deletion of the LIS1 gene located at chromosome 17p13. *JAMA.* 1993;270 (23):2838–2842.

195. Leventer RJ. Genotype-phenotype correlation in lissencephaly and subcortical band heterotopia: the key questions answered. *J Child Neurol.* 2005;20 (4):307–312.

196. Devisme L, Bouchet C, Gonzales M, et al. Cobblestone lissencephaly: neuropathological subtypes and correlations with genes of dystroglycanopathies. *Brain.* 2012;135(Pt 2):469–482.

197. D'Agostino MD, Bernasconi A, Das S, et al. Subcortical band heterotopia (SBH) in males: clinical, imaging and genetic findings in comparison with females. *Brain.* 2002;125(Pt 11):2507–2522.

198. Mai R, Tassi L, Cossu M, et al. A neuropathological, stereo-EEG, and MRI study of subcortical band heterotopia. *Neurology.* 2003;60(11):1834–1838.

199. Leventer RJ, Jansen A, Pilz DT, et al. Clinical and imaging heterogeneity of polymicrogyria: a study of 328 patients. *Brain.* 2010;133(Pt 5):1415–1427.

200. Napolioni V, Curatolo P. Genetics and molecular biology of tuberous sclerosis complex. *Curr Genomics.* 2008;9 (7):475–487.

201. Korf BR, Bebin EM. Neurocutaneous disorders in children. *Pediatr Rev*. 2017;38 (3):119–128.

202. Wu JY, Peters JM, Goyal M, et al. Clinical electroencephalographic biomarker for impending epilepsy in asymptomatic tuberous sclerosis complex infants. *Pediatr Neurol*. 2016;54:29–34.

203. Comi AM. Sturge-Weber syndrome and epilepsy: an argument for aggressive seizure management in these patients. *Expert Rev Neurother*. 2007;7(8):951–956.

204. Assogba K, Ferlazzo E, Striano P, et al. Heterogeneous seizure manifestations in Hypomelanosis of Ito: report of four new cases and review of the literature. *Neurol Sci*. 2010;31(1):9–16.

205. Hubert JN, Callen JP. Incontinentia pigmenti presenting as seizures. *Pediatr Dermatol*. 2002;19(6):550–552.

206. Ostendorf AP, Gutmann DH, Weisenberg JL. Epilepsy in individuals with neurofibromatosis type 1. *Epilepsia*. 2013;54(10):1810–1814.

207. Drouet A. [Seizures in neurofibromatosis. What is the risk?]. *Rev Neurol (Paris)*. 2011;167(12):886–896.

208. Temkin NR. Preventing and treating posttraumatic seizures: the human experience. *Epilepsia*. 2009;50(Suppl 2):10–13.

209. Szaflarski JP. Is there equipoise between phenytoin and levetiracetam for seizure prevention in traumatic brain injury? *Epilepsy Curr*. 2015;15(2):94–97.

210. Szaflarski JP, Nazzal Y, Dreer LE. Post-traumatic epilepsy: current and emerging treatment options. *Neuropsychiatr Dis Treat*. 2014;10:1469–1477.

211. Annegers JF, Hauser WA, Coan SP, Rocca WA. A population-based study of seizures after traumatic brain injuries. *N Engl J Med*. 1998;338(1):20–24.

212. Asikainen I, Kaste M, Sarna S. Early and late posttraumatic seizures in traumatic brain injury rehabilitation patients: brain injury factors causing late seizures and influence of seizures on long-term outcome. *Epilepsia*. 1999;40(5):584–589.

213. Annegers JF, Grabow JD, Groover RV, et al. Seizures after head trauma: a population study. *Neurology*. 1980;30(7 Pt 1):683–689.

214. Ritter AC, Wagner AK, Fabio A, et al. Incidence and risk factors of posttraumatic seizures following traumatic brain injury: a Traumatic Brain Injury Model Systems Study. *Epilepsia*. 2016;57(12):1968–1977.

215. Ritter AC, Wagner AK, Szaflarski JP, et al. Prognostic models for predicting posttraumatic seizures during acute hospitalization, and at 1 and 2 years following traumatic brain injury. *Epilepsia*. 2016;57(9):1503–1514.

216. Chang B, Lowenstein D. Practice parameter: antiepileptic drug prophylaxis in severe traumatic brain injury. *Neurology*. 2003;60(1):10–16.

217. Szaflarski JP, Sangha KS, Lindsell CJ, Shutter LA. Prospective, randomized, single-blinded comparative trial of intravenous levetiracetam versus phenytoin for seizure prophylaxis. *Neurocrit Care*. 2010;12(2):165–172.

218. Taylor S, Heinrichs RJ, Janzen JM, Ehtisham A. Levetiracetam is associated with improved cognitive outcome for patients with intracranial hemorrhage. *Neurocrit Care*. 2011;15(1):80–84.

219. Turjman F, Massoud TF, Sayre JW, et al. Epilepsy associated with cerebral arteriovenous malformations: a multivariate analysis of angioarchitectural characteristics. *Am J Neuroradiol*. 1995;16 (2):345–350.

220. Crawford PM, West CR, Chadwick DW, Shaw MD. Arteriovenous malformations of the brain: natural history in unoperated patients. *J Neurol Neurosurg Psychiatry*. 1986;49(1):1–10.

221. Rosenow F, Alonso-Vanegas MA, Baumgartner C, et al. Cavernoma-related epilepsy: review and recommendations for management – report of the Surgical Task Force of the ILAE Commission on Therapeutic Strategies. *Epilepsia*. 2013;54 (12):2025–2035.

222. Josephson CB, Leach JP, Duncan R, et al. Seizure risk from cavernous or

arteriovenous malformations: prospective population-based study. *Neurology.* 2011;76 (18):1548–1554.

223. Striano S, Nocerino C, Striano P, et al. Venous angiomas and epilepsy. *Neurol Sci.* 2000;21(3):151–155.

224. Mills PB, Footitt EJ, Mills KA, et al. Genotypic and phenotypic spectrum of pyridoxine-dependent epilepsy (ALDH7A1 deficiency). *Brain.* 2010;133(Pt 7):2148–2159.

225. Wang D, Pascual JM, De Vivo D. Glucose transporter type 1 deficiency syndrome. In: Adam MP, Ardinger HH, Pagon RA, et al., eds. *GeneReviews®,* Seattle, WA: University of Washington; 2002.

226. Annegers JF, Rocca WA, Hauser WA. Causes of epilepsy: contributions of the Rochester epidemiology project. *Mayo Clin Proc.* 1996;71(6):570–575.

227. Khan NA, Kazzi SN. Yield and costs of screening growth-retarded infants for torch infections. *Am J Perinatol.* 2000;17 (3):131–135.

228. Misra UK, Tan CT, Kalita J. Viral encephalitis and epilepsy. *Epilepsia.* 2008;49(Suppl 6):13–18.

229. Annegers JF, Hauser WA, Beghi E, Nicolosi A, Kurland LT. The risk of unprovoked seizures after encephalitis and meningitis. *Neurology.* 1988;38(9):1407–1410.

230. Chuang MJ, Chang WN, Chang HW, et al. Predictors and long-term outcome of seizures after bacterial brain abscess. *J Neurol Neurosurg Psychiatry.* 2010;81 (8):913–917.

231. Granerod J, Ambrose HE, Davies NW, et al. Causes of encephalitis and differences in their clinical presentations in England: a multicentre, population-based prospective study. *Lancet Infect Dis.* 2010;10(12):835–844.

232. Burneo JG, Cavazos JE. Neurocysticercosis and epilepsy. *Epilepsy Curr.* 2014;14(1 Suppl):23–28.

233. Baird RA, Wiebe S, Zunt JR, et al. Evidence-based guideline: treatment of parenchymal neurocysticercosis. Report of the Guideline Development Subcommittee of the American Academy of Neurology. *Neurology.* 2013;80(15):1424–1429.

234. Khawaja AM, DeWolfe JL, Miller DW, Szaflarski JP. New-onset refractory status epilepticus (NORSE) – the potential role for immunotherapy. *Epilepsy Behav.* 2015;47:17–23.

235. Vezzani A, French J, Bartfai T, Baram TZ. The role of inflammation in epilepsy. *Nat Rev Neurol.* 2011;7(1):31–40.

236. Vezzani A, Friedman A. Brain inflammation as a biomarker in epilepsy. *Biomark Med.* 2011;5(5):607–614.

237. Kivity S, Agmon-Levin N, Zandman-Goddard G, Chapman J, Shoenfeld Y. Neuropsychiatric lupus: a mosaic of clinical presentations. *BMC Med.* 2015;13:43.

238. Joseph FG, Scolding NJ. Cerebral vasculitis: a practical approach. *Practical Neurology.* 2002;2(2):80–93.

239. Krumholz A, Stern BJ, Stern EG. Clinical implications of seizures in neurosarcoidosis. *Arch Neurol.* 1991;48 (8):842–844.

Seizures Not Diagnosed as Epilepsy

Michael DiSano, Elia Pestana-Knight, and Ajay Gupta

8.1 Introduction

Despite recent changes in the key criteria required for the diagnosis of epilepsy,[1] there remains a population of patients who suffer from seizures that can recur, but do not fit the clinical definition of epilepsy. In 1993, the International League Against Epilepsy (ILAE) developed standard definitions for use in the epidemiological study of epilepsy, including definitions of epilepsy and epileptic seizures.[2] At that time, the ILAE created two categories of patients with epileptic seizures who did not necessarily meet the criteria of epilepsy: febrile seizures and benign neonatal seizures. Febrile seizures are acute symptomatic and electrographic seizures that occur in the context of a febrile illness. Benign neonatal seizures are acute symptomatic seizures occurring in the neonatal or infantile period, with a demonstrable electrographic correlate, but are thought to result in a benign outcome and normal development. Since that time, the definition of epilepsy has been revised, and both of these categories of patients have been the subject of further study.[3] This chapter will review the most up-to-date information about febrile seizures and benign neonatal seizures.

8.2 Febrile Seizures

Febrile seizures (FS) are one of the most commonly encountered acute neurologic conditions in children.[4] The first formal definition of FS was developed by the National Institutes of Health in 1980 as an event usually occurring between 3 months to 5 years of age and associated with a fever, but without evidence of intracranial infection or a "defined cause."[5] An additional definition was proposed in 1993 by the ILAE as a seizure occurring in childhood after 1 month of age associated with a febrile illness, but not caused by an infection of the central nervous system (CNS), without history of neonatal seizures or unprovoked seizures, and not meeting criteria for other acute symptomatic seizures such as toxic or metabolic derangements, trauma, or stroke.[2]

In an early attempt to stratify risk of patients with FS for future development of epilepsy, FS were classified into two main subtypes: simple and complex. Simple FS are considered as isolated events occurring in the context of an illness, do not exhibit focal features, are not prolonged, and have a total duration of less than 10 min[6] to 15 min.[7] Complex FS are those that do not meet the criteria for simple, or occur more than once in 24 hours or the same illness, have focal symptomatology, or have a prolonged duration of greater than 10 to 15 min.[4,6] It is estimated that 20–30% of all FS may be complex.[6–8] In a study of population modeling of patients presenting with first time febrile seizure, a best fit was made when patients were assumed to represent two subpopulations based on seizure duration. The first population was those patients with shorter FS, lasting on average 3.8 min. The second population comprised patients with more prolonged FS, lasting an average of 39.8 min. Interestingly, the cutoff of seizure duration between the two models occurred at approximately 10 min, further substantiating this duration as the lower limit for classification of complex febrile seizure.[9]

Additionally, the classification of febrile status epilepticus is reserved for patients presenting with very prolonged FS lasting >30 min. This subgroup of patients is the subject of an ongoing multicenter prospective study known as the "Consequences of Prolonged FS in Childhood" (FEBSTAT) study.[8,10] The overall goal of FEBSTAT has been to prospectively study the associations of febrile status epilepticus and subsequent risk of developing epilepsy, as well as other long-term developmental issues.

8.2.1 Epidemiology

The incidence of FS in the white population is currently reported to be 2–5%,[7] and slightly higher in Asian populations, with a reported incidence of 8–10%.[11] The age range is 1 month up to 8 years, (typical 6 months to 6 years), with 90% of FS occurring prior to age 3 years, and a peak age of 18 to 24 months.[4,7] Only about 6% of FS occur before 6 months of age, and 4% after 3 years of age.[4] FS in general do not seem to demonstrate a sex predominance.[4] A more recent study suggested a male predominance for brief FS (<10 minutes), but suggested a female predominance for longer FS, although this difference was not statistically significant.[9] Prolonged FS are also associated with younger median age and developmental delay, suggesting that patients with very prolonged FS may represent a different subpopulation with different risks of developing epilepsy.[9] First time febrile status epilepticus is also associated with lower temperatures, longer duration of recognized elevated temperature, first-degree family history of febrile seizure, and structural temporal lobe abnormalities.[12] The overall incidence of febrile status epilepticus remains low, likely 5–10%.[6,8] However, febrile status epilepticus remains the most common cause of status epilepticus in the pediatric population.[13,14]

8.2.2 Pathophysiology

Most FS occur with the onset of fever.[4] Previously, it had been proposed that the time of occurrence is most likely to coincide with the period of highest rate of rise of the temperature and/or peak body temperature during the illness.[15]

Most often FS are attributed to relatively common and self-limited infectious processes experienced in the pediatric population, including viral or bacterial infections of the ear, nose, and throat, as well as respiratory and gastrointestinal infections,[4,16] although Berg et al. found that gastrointestinal infection appeared to be protective for development of FS.[15] Recently published data from the FEBSTAT study demonstrated acute viremia with human herpesvirus (HHV)-6B and to a lesser extent HHV-7 at the time of presentation in over one-third of patients presenting with febrile status epilepticus. This suggests these viruses as a potential etiology for prolonged FS.[17]

Cytokines are also believed to play a role in the development or predisposition toward FS. A number of biomarkers have been investigated, including the anti-inflammatory interleukin (IL)-1 receptor antagonist (IL-1RA), proinflammatory and epileptogenic IL-1β, and proinflammatory IL-6 and IL-8 concentrations.[18,19] In an earlier study, Virta et al. demonstrated a positive association between the IL-1RA:IL-1β ratio and IL-6 concentration, and FS. However, it was not clear in this study if the levels were causative of the seizure or a result of ictal activity.[18] A similar study of cytokines in patients presenting with febrile status epilepticus compared to febrile controls was performed as part of the FEB-STAT study for investigation of a potential biomarker of hippocampal injury. This study also suggested involvement of IL-1RA, IL-6, and IL-8 with febrile status epilepticus, although specific levels of individual cytokines were not associated with febrile status epilepticus or MRI abnormalities. Lower ratios of IL-1RA:IL-8 and IL-1RA:IL-6 were associated with febrile status epilepticus and MRI abnormalities. Lower ratios of IL-1RA: IL-6 were also strongly predictive of abnormal hippocampal T2 hyperintensity, suggesting a potential biomarker for predicting future risk of mesial temporal sclerosis in patients presenting with febrile status epilepticus.[19]

Genetics also clearly play a role in the pathophysiology of FS. Between 25 and 40% of patients with FS have a positive family history of FS.[4,10] Recent advances have demonstrated robust relationships between familial FS and genetically determined epilepsies. The best defined of these is the generalized epilepsy with FS plus (GEFS+). The GEFS+ phenotype is heterogeneous and includes patients with recurrent FS, FS lasting beyond early childhood, and afebrile seizures with atypical semiology, including absence, myoclonic, or atonic seizures.[20] Mutations of several genes affecting the subunits of the voltage-gated sodium channel, including SCN1A, SCN2A, and SCN1B,[21-23] and the GABA$_A$ receptor subunit (GABRG2) have also been implicated with FS.[23,24] Dravet syndrome is a severe form of inherited sodium channelopathy caused by a mutation involving the SCN1A subunit that often presents with FS and normal prior development. Over time, these patients typically go on to have recurrent and prolonged FS, and eventually develop unprovoked seizures of varying semiology including myoclonic, atypical absence, and generalized intractable epilepsy. They also suffer from profound developmental delays and severe cognitive impairment. Sodium channel blocking agents should be avoided in these patients, as they will often make seizures worse.[4,25]

8.2.3 Acute Management and Initial Diagnostic Workup

Given the above understanding of pathogenesis of most FS, emphasis on management involves accurate history and prompt assessment (Table 8.1).[4] While febrile status epilepticus remains a rare complication, in a review of the FEBSTAT population, approximately one-third of cases of febrile status epilepticus went unrecognized in the emergency department and almost 90% of cases of febrile status epilepticus were not expected to stop spontaneously and required administration of an antiseizure medication for cessation.[8,26] Therefore prompt attention should be given to basic resuscitative measures and intravenous (IV) antiseizure medication should be given when appropriate.[4] Similar to population-based studies for patients presenting with status epilepticus and the demonstrable benefits of prompt recognition and administration of therapeutic interventions,[27,28] rapid initiation of antiseizure medications, usually in the form of a benzodiazepine,[13] to patients presenting in febrile status epilepticus reduces total seizure duration and is associated with lower rates of respiratory failure requiring intervention.[26] Use of intermittent benzodiazepines or prophylactic use of antiseizure medications may reduce the risk of subsequent FS; however, this may also be associated with increased risk of adverse effects, and has not been shown to impact the long-term outcomes.[29]

Gradually reducing the fever with antipyretics is generally recommended as a means of comfort to the child and management of other symptomatology.[4] However, these measures

Table 8.1 Clinical practice guidelines for the diagnostic evaluation of a child who presents with simple FS

Diagnostic test	Recommendation	Level of evidence/ policy level	Rationale
Routine lab work	Measurement of serum electrolytes, calcium, phosphorus, magnesium, blood glucose, or complete blood cell count should not be performed routinely for the sole purpose of identifying the cause of a simple FS	B (overwhelming evidence from observational studies)/Strong recommendation	When a fever is present the decision regarding the need for laboratory testing should be directed toward identifying the source of the fever
Lumbar puncture (LP)	1a: LP should be performed if a child has meningeal signs or symptoms, or history or examination raises concerns for meningitis or intracranial infection	B (overwhelming evidence from observational studies)/Strong recommendation	Data no longer support the routine lumbar puncture in well-appearing, fully immunized children who present with a simple FS. Data for unimmunized or partially immunized children are lacking. There are also no definitive data on the outcome of children already on antibiotics. While 25% of young children have seizures at the presenting sign, some are obtunded or comatose, and the remainder most often have obvious clinical signs of meningitis
	1b: LP is an option in children 6–12 months of age and considered deficient in *Haemophilus influenza* Type b (Hib) or *Streptococcus pneumoniae* immunizations or immunization status cannot be determined	D (expert opinion, case reports)/Option	
	1c: LP is an option in a child pretreated with antibiotics, because such treatment can mask the signs and symptoms of meningitis	D (reasoning from clinical experience, case series)/Option	
Neuroimaging	Neuroimaging should not be performed in the routine evaluation of a child with simple FS	B (overwhelming evidence from observational studies)/Strong recommendation	No data have been published that either support or negate the need for CT or MRI in the evaluation of children with simple FS. CT scanning is associated with radiation exposure

Table 8.1 (*cont.*)

Diagnostic test	Recommendation	Level of evidence/ policy level	Rationale
			that may escalate future cancer risk. MRI is associated with risks from required sedation and high cost
Electroencephalogram (EEG)	EEG should not be performed in the otherwise neurologically healthy with simple FS	B (overwhelming evidence from observational studies)/Strong recommendation	No evidence that EEGs performed at the time of presentation or within the following month are predictive of either recurrence of FS or development of epilepsy

Data from reference 31.

have not been shown to reduce the duration of fever or risk of recurrence of another febrile seizure.[30]

Since the infections leading to FS are most often self-limiting viral illnesses, the current recommendations regarding routine diagnostic studies performed should be done with the goal of finding the source of the fever. Routine labs for seizure alone are discouraged.[31] According to the practice parameter recommendations on the assessment of the child presenting with status epilepticus, routine analysis of electrolyte abnormalities yielded abnormal results in approximately 6% of patients. While these results were often considered causative for the seizure, according to the authors, it was unclear if these abnormalities were truly responsible or whether seizures improved following their correction. Blood cultures revealed an abnormality in 2.5% of children with status epilepticus.[32]

Risk of CNS infection is very low and lumbar puncture is typically not recommended as part of the initial diagnostic work up unless there are other aspects of the history or presence of clinical signs or symptoms of concern for meningitis.[31,32] Study of cerebral spinal fluid (CSF) in patients presenting with febrile status epilepticus demonstrated relatively benign values, further confirming the presence of leukocytosis in the CSF is unlikely to be a purely ictal phenomenon and should raise concern for an underlying CNS infectious process.[33]

Neuroimaging, either with computed tomography (CT) or magnetic resonance imaging (MRI), is generally not indicated in the acute period following febrile seizure unless there is concern for a structural neurological abnormality.[4,31] However, for patients presenting with febrile status epilepticus, acute MRI findings have been considered as a potential biomarker for long-term implications such as hippocampal sclerosis and temporal lobe epilepsy. In the FEBSTAT study cohort, 11.5% demonstrated T2 signal hyperintensity involving either unilateral or bilateral hippocampi, which is considered a biomarker for hippocampal injury following the acute period. This finding was not demonstrated in control subjects presenting with simple FS or complex FS not considered status epilepticus.[34] In a follow-up study of neuroimaging of the patients with acute signal changes in the hippocampi 1 year later, 85.7% had decreased hippocampal volume, and 71.4% met visual criteria for hippocampal sclerosis.[35] Patients with febrile status epilepticus were also more likely to have developmental anomalies of the temporal lobe, particularly hippocampal malrotation,[34,36] and more subtle medial temporal lobe abnormalities on quantitative morphometric analysis.[37]

Electroencephalography (EEG) is of limited use in the acute setting and generally not recommended for otherwise neurologically healthy children presenting with simple FS.[31] EEG may show transient abnormalities in the immediate postacute phase, but usually does not change management.[4,31,38] For the minority of patients presenting for febrile status epilepticus, the FEBSTAT study demonstrated findings of focal slowing or attenuation most commonly on EEG performed within 72 hours of presentation, and these findings seem to be associated with abnormal imaging consistent with hippocampal injury.[39] However, in a retrospective study done of neurologically normal or mild developmentally delayed children presenting with first complex febrile seizure who underwent EEG, the presence of epileptiform abnormalities had a poor positive predictive value for patients who subsequently went on to develop epilepsy.[40]

8.2.4 Postacute Management and Counseling

Caregivers of children with FS often express a sense of anxiety after witnessing a seizure at home.[4] In a study of the immediate- and long-term parental perceptions following febrile status epilepticus compared to parents of patients presenting with simple FS, the FEBSTAT study team demonstrated, at baseline, parents of children presenting with simple FS had higher scores corresponding to elevated stress demonstrated on the Parenting Stress Index, Short Form, compared to parents of patients presenting with febrile status epilepticus. However, this finding normalized within 1 year. At 1 year follow-up, parents of patients that presented with febrile status epilepticus and developmental delay, reported higher parental stress and lower scores on the Pediatric Quality of Life Inventory compared to patients with febrile status epilepticus and normal development.[41]

Caregivers often confuse FS and epilepsy[4] and it is important to educate families not only on the difference between FS and epilepsy, but also in regards to seizure first aid and home administration of seizure rescue medications (Table 8.2).

8.2.5 Risk of Recurrence

A second FS will occur in about one-third of patients following FS of any type and a third FS will occur in up to half of those patients. Greater than three FS is rare and is seen in less than 5% of patients presenting following an FS.[4,7,42,43] Age at the first FS seems to be one of the most important factors in risk of recurrence, and younger patients are more likely for recurrence.[42–44] Younger patients at the time of their first FS spend more time during the critical age for developing FS, and therefore are at a higher cumulative risk for recurrence. In addition, a first-degree relative with FS is associated with higher risk of recurrence for FS; however, family history of afebrile seizure may not convey the same increased risk of recurrence.[42,44]

Duration of the fever prior to the onset of the seizure is also associated with recurrence. Berg et al. demonstrated that patients with first FS occurring at fever durations of <1 hour

Table 8.2 Seizure rescue medications for emergent home administration

Medication	Route of Administration	Dose
Diazepam	Rectal	Aged 2–5 years – 0.5 mg/kg/dose Aged 6–11 years – 0.3 mg/kg/dose Aged >12 years – 0.2 mg/kg/dose Maximum dose – 20 mg
	Oral/buccal	0.33 mg/kg/dose every 8 hours during febrile illness from onset of fever to 24 hours post fever
Midazolam	Intramuscular	13–40 kg – 5 mg >40 kg – 10 mg
	Intranasal	0.2 mg/kg/dose, divided per each nostril Maximum total dose – 10 mg
	Oral/buccal	0.5 mg/kg/dose Maximum total dose – 10 mg

were more than twice as likely to have recurrent FS when compared to patients with seizures following more than 24 hours of fever. Peak temperature also plays a role, where patients presenting with lower temperatures triggering FS were also more likely to have recurrent FS.[42]

As part of their analysis, the FEBSTAT study determined that patients presenting with first febrile status epilepticus were at a significantly increased risk for further episodes of febrile status epilepticus when compared to first simple FS. MRI abnormalities further increased this risk for recurrence of febrile status epilepticus.[45]

8.2.6 Risk of Epilepsy

Determining risk factors for patients with first time FS that are predictive of subsequent development of epilepsy has been a topic of debate for years. This was part of the differentiation of FS into simple and complex.[4,46,47] Early studies suggested epilepsy development at an overall rate of 2–6% following FS. This rate was higher for patients who had neurodevelopmental abnormalities, presentation with all three aspects of complex FS or family history of unprovoked seizures.[46–48] One consideration for eventual development of epilepsy following FS is the "second hit hypothesis" where children initially predisposed to seizure undergo a "second hit" during the febrile illness that leads to damage that can occasionally be appreciated on neuroimaging.[34,35]

8.2.7 Risk of Cognitive Impairment

Older longitudinal studies of the long-term neurodevelopmental outcomes of FS failed to demonstrate an increased risk of intellectual or cognitive disability or of behavioral or attention issues later in life, even in cases of prolonged febrile status epilepticus.[49–51]

In the more recent study of cognitive impacts following febrile status epilepticus, the FEBSTAT study group demonstrated that patients presenting with febrile status epilepticus did not differ when compared to the control cohort of patients presenting with simple febrile status on tasks of cognition, receptive language, and memory at close follow-up of

1 month. However, at 1 year follow-up, the febrile status group demonstrated slightly weaker motor development and receptive language and patients with acute T2 signal hyperintensity on MRI signifying hippocampal damage at presentation were also associated with weaker receptive language skills.[9,52] In a population-based study from Denmark, they found slightly increased risk of subsequent development of ADHD in patients with FS, but much lower risk when compared to patients with childhood onset epilepsy or both FS and epilepsy.[53]

8.3 Benign Neonatal and Infantile Seizures

Benign neonatal and infantile seizures typically occur in otherwise normally developing infants, are relatively easy to control, and usually follow a relatively benign neurodevelopmental course. One of the first descriptions of infantile seizures resulting in a normal developmental outcome was in 1963 by Fukuyama. Our knowledge of such entities was expanded upon in the 1980s and 1990s to include both familial and nonfamilial occurrences.[25,54]

In benign nonfamilial infantile seizures, patients typically present with seizure onset in infancy, with a peak age of 4–6 months. Patients usually present with clusters of seizures which may be subtle and comprised of focal movements with or without secondary generalization, behavioral arrest with decreased responsiveness, and simple automatisms. Interictal EEG is usually normal, however ictal EEG may demonstrate focal epileptiform discharges. Neuroimaging is also usually unremarkable; however, focal cortical dysplasia may be subtle and missed on imaging in this age group and close neurodevelopmental follow-up is essential. Seizures typically resolve with antiseizure medications including carbamazepine and phenobarbital.[25,54]

Generally, inherited benign seizures occurring in the neonatal or infant periods are rare, and demonstrate an autosomal dominant inheritance pattern often with clear familial inheritance. Multiple genes have been implicated, with similar phenotypic presentations, differing primarily based on age of onset of seizures. In benign familial neonatal epilepsy (BFNE), patients typically present with seizures between the 2nd and 8th days of life, and have multiple brief seizures of varying semiology, including tonic and focal clonic, with or without secondary generalization, with apneic or autonomic symptoms. Seizures typically resolve between the 1st and 6th to 12th months of life. This entity is most commonly associated with a mutation of the potassium channel KCNQ2. KCNQ2-related disorders also represent a spectrum of disease, with KCNQ2-BFNE at the mild end and KCNQ2-related neonatal encephalopathy (NEE) at the severe end, where patients typically present with multiple daily seizures in the neonatal period, an EEG representing interictal burst suppression pattern or multifocal epileptiform activity, and poor overall course with moderate to severe developmental delays.[55] An additional potassium channel gene mutation, *KCNQ3*, has also been implicated in presentation with clusters of seizures in the neonatal or infantile periods, resulting in benign neurodevelopmental outcomes, but some patients have been described with long-term developmental disability with this mutation.[56]

Patients with benign familial infantile seizures (BFIS) typically present after the neonatal period, with a peak age similar to benign nonfamilial infantile seizures (~6 months), with similar semiology, including focal seizures that can occur in clusters, are again preceded by normal neurodevelopment, and result in a benign outcome. Mutations of *KCNQ2* and *KCNQ3* have been implicated in such patients, as have mutations of *PRRT2* (proline-rich transmembrane protein 2), a membrane protein that interacts with the presynaptic protein SNAP-25. Interestingly, these genetic mutations have also been implicated in several other inherited neurologic symptoms such as myokymia, paroxysmal choreoathetosis or myoclonus-like dystonia, and familial hemiplegic migraine.[23,25,54–56]

Lastly, there has been an additional subset of patients reported presenting with a similar phenotype and seizure semiology, but at an intermediate age between the neonatal and infantile periods, termed benign familial neonatal-infantile seizures (BFNIS), which has been associated with sodium channel mutations of the SCN2A subunit. It is unclear how this may related to other sodium channelopathies, as it does not seem to share similar phenotypic characteristics.[23,54]

References

1. Fisher RS, Acevedo C, Arzimanoglou A, et al. ILAE official report: a practical clinical definition of epilepsy. *Epilepsia*. 2014;55(4):475–482.

2. Commission on Epidemiology and Prognosis, International League Against Epilepsy. Guidelines for epidemiologic studies on epilepsy. *Epilepsia*. 1993;34 (4):592–596.

3. Berg AT, Berkovic SF, Brodie MJ, et al. Revised terminology and concepts for organization of seizures and epilepsies: report of the ILAE Commission on Classification and Terminology, 2005–2009. *Epilepsia*. 2010;51(4):676–685.

4. Gupta A. Febrile seizures. *Continuum (Minneap Minn)*. 2016;22(1 Epilepsy):51–59.

5. Freeman JM. Febrile seizures: a consensus of their significance, evaluation, and treatment. *Pediatrics*. 1980;66(6):1009.

6. Berg AT, Shinnar S. Complex febrile seizures. *Epilepsia*. 1996;37(2):126–133.

7. Verity CM, Butler NR, Golding J. Febrile convulsions in a national cohort followed up from birth. I – Prevalence and recurrence in the first five years of life. *Br Med J (Clin Res Ed)*. 1985;290 (6478):1307–1310.

8. Hesdorffer DC, Shinnar S, Lewis DV, et al. Design and phenomenology of the FEBSTAT study. *Epilepsia*. 2012;53 (9):1471–1480.

9. Hesdorffer DC, Benn EK, Bagiella E, et al. Distribution of febrile seizure duration and associations with development. *Ann Neurol*. 2011;70(1):93–100.

10. Shinnar S, Hesdorffer DC, Nordli DR, Jr., et al. Phenomenology of prolonged febrile seizures: results of the FEBSTAT study. *Neurology*. 2008;71(3):170–176.

11. Tsuboi T. Epidemiology of febrile and afebrile convulsions in children in Japan. *Neurology*. 1984;34(2):175–181.

12. Hesdorffer DC, Shinnar S, Lewis DV, et al. Risk factors for febrile status epilepticus: a case-control study. *J Pediatr*. 2013;163 (4):1147–1151.

13. Abend NS, Loddenkemper T. Pediatric status epilepticus management. *Curr Opin Pediatr*. 2014;26(6):668–674.

14. Brophy GM, Bell R, Claassen J, et al. Guidelines for the evaluation and management of status epilepticus. *Neurocrit Care*. 2012;17(1):3–23.

15. Berg AT, Shinnar S, Shapiro ED, et al. Risk factors for a first febrile seizure: a matched case-control study. *Epilepsia*. 1995;36 (4):334–341.

16. Francis JR, Richmond P, Robins C, et al. An observational study of febrile seizures: the importance of viral infection and immunization. *BMC Pediatr*. 2016;16 (1):202.

17. Epstein LG, Shinnar S, Hesdorffer DC, et al. Human herpesvirus 6 and 7 in febrile status epilepticus: the FEBSTAT study. *Epilepsia*. 2012;53 (9):1481–1488.

18. Virta M, Hurme M, Helminen M. Increased plasma levels of pro- and anti-inflammatory cytokines in patients with

febrile seizures. *Epilepsia.* 2002;43
(8):920–923.

19. Gallentine WB, Shinnar S, Hesdorffer DC,
    et al. Plasma cytokines associated with
    febrile status epilepticus in children: a
    potential biomarker for acute hippocampal
    injury. *Epilepsia.* 2017;58(6):1102–1111.

20. Scheffer IE, Berkovic SF. Generalized
    epilepsy with febrile seizures plus: a genetic
    disorder with heterogeneous clinical
    phenotypes. *Brain.* 1997;120 (Pt 3)
    (3):479–490.

21. Wallace RH, Wang DW, Singh R, et al.
    Febrile seizures and generalized epilepsy
    associated with a mutation in the Na+-
    channel beta1 subunit gene SCN1B.
    Nat Genet. 1998;19(4):366–370.

22. Escayg A, MacDonald BT, Meisler MH,
    et al. Mutations of SCN1A, encoding a
    neuronal sodium channel, in two families
    with GEFS+2. *Nat Genet.* 2000;24
    (4):343–345.

23. Mulley JC, Scheffer IE, Petrou S, Berkovic
    SF. Channelopathies as a genetic cause of
    epilepsy. *Curr Opin Neurol.* 2003;16
    (2):171–176.

24. Wallace RH, Marini C, Petrou S, et al.
    Mutant GABAA receptor γ2-subunit in
    childhood absence epilepsy and
    febrile seizures. *Nat Genet.* 2001;28
    (1):49–52.

25. Wirrell E. Infantile childhood, and
    adolescent epilepsies. *Continuum (Minneap
    Minn).* 2016;22(1 Epilepsy):60–93.

26. Seinfeld S, Shinnar S, Sun S, et al.
    Emergency management of febrile status
    epilepticus: results of the FEBSTAT study.
    Epilepsia. 2014;55(3):388–395.

27. Lowenstein DH, Alldredge BK, Allen F,
    et al. The prehospital treatment of status
    epilepticus (PHTSE) study: design and
    methodology. *Control Clin Trials.* 2001;22
    (3):290–309.

28. Silbergleit R, Durkalski V, Lowenstein D,
    et al. Intramuscular versus intravenous
    therapy for prehospital status epilepticus.
    N Engl J Med. 2012;366(7):591–600.

29. Offringa M, Newton R, Cozijnsen MA,
    Nevitt SJ. Prophylactic drug management

for febrile seizures in children. *Cochrane
Database Syst Rev.* 2017;2:CD003031.

30. Steering Committee on Quality
    Improvement and Management,
    Subcommittee on Febrile Seizures
    American Academy of Pediatrics. Febrile
    seizures: clinical practice guideline for the
    long-term management of the child with
    simple febrile seizures. *Pediatrics.* 2008;121
    (6):1281–1286.

31. Subcommittee on Febrile Seizures,
    American Academy of Pediatrics.
    Neurodiagnostic evaluation of the child
    with a simple febrile seizure. *Pediatrics.*
    2011;127(2):389–394.

32. Riviello JJ, Jr., Ashwal S, Hirtz D, et al.
    Practice parameter: diagnostic assessment
    of the child with status epilepticus (an
    evidence-based review). Report of the
    Quality Standards Subcommittee of the
    American Academy of Neurology and the
    Practice Committee of the Child Neurology
    Society. *Neurology.* 2006;67(9):1542–1550.

33. Frank LM, Shinnar S, Hesdorffer DC, et al.
    Cerebrospinal fluid findings in children
    with fever-associated status epilepticus:
    results of the consequences of prolonged
    febrile seizures (FEBSTAT) study. *J Pediatr.*
    2012;161(6):1169–1171.

34. Shinnar S, Bello JA, Chan S, et al. MRI
    abnormalities following febrile status
    epilepticus in children: the FEBSTAT
    study. *Neurology.* 2012;79(9):871–877.

35. Lewis DV, Shinnar S, Hesdorffer DC, et al.
    Hippocampal sclerosis after febrile status
    epilepticus: the FEBSTAT study. *Ann
    Neurol.* 2014;75(2):178–185.

36. Chan S, Bello JA, Shinnar S, et al.
    Hippocampal malrotation is associated
    with prolonged febrile seizures: results of
    the FEBSTAT study. *Am J Roentgenol.*
    2015;205(5):1068–1074.

37. McClelland AC, Gomes WA, Shinnar S,
    et al. Quantitative evaluation of medial
    temporal lobe morphology in children with
    febrile status epilepticus: results of the
    FEBSTAT study. *Am J Neuroradiol.*
    2016;37(12):2356–2362.

38. Maytal J, Steele R, Eviatar L, Novak G. The
    value of early postictal EEG in children

with complex febrile seizures. *Epilepsia.* 2000;41(2):219–221.

39. Nordli DR, Jr., Moshe SL, Shinnar S, et al. Acute EEG findings in children with febrile status epilepticus: results of the FEBSTAT study. *Neurology.* 2012;79(22):2180–2186.

40. Harini C, Nagarajan E, Kimia AA, et al. Utility of initial EEG in first complex febrile seizure. *Epilepsy Behav.* 2015;52(Pt A):200–204.

41. Shinnar RC, Shinnar S, Hesdorffer DC, et al. Parental stress, pediatric quality of life, and behavior at baseline and one-year follow-up: Results from the FEBSTAT study. *Epilepsy Behav.* 2017;69:95–99.

42. Berg AT, Shinnar S, Hauser WA, et al. A prospective study of recurrent febrile seizures. *N Engl J Med.* 1992;327(16):1122–1127.

43. Berg AT, Shinnar S, Darefsky AS, et al. Predictors of recurrent febrile seizures: a prospective cohort study. *Arch Pediatr Adolesc Med.* 1997;151(4):371–378.

44. Berg AT, Shinnar S, Hauser WA, Leventhal JM. Predictors of recurrent febrile seizures: a metaanalytic review. *J Pediatr.* 1990;116(3):329–337.

45. Hesdorffer DC, Shinnar S, Lax DN, et al. Risk factors for subsequent febrile seizures in the FEBSTAT study. *Epilepsia.* 2016;57(7):1042–1047.

46. Annegers JF, Hauser WA, Elveback LR, Kurland LT. The risk of epilepsy following febrile convulsions. *Neurology.* 1979;29(3):297–303.

47. Nelson KB, Ellenberg JH. Predictors of epilepsy in children who have experienced febrile seizures. *N Engl J Med.* 1976;295(19):1029–1033.

48. Annegers JF, Hauser WA, Shirts SB, Kurland LT. Factors prognostic of unprovoked seizures after febrile convulsions. *N Engl J Med.* 1987;316(9):493–498.

49. Chang YC, Guo NW, Huang CC, Wang ST, Tsai JJ. Neurocognitive attention and behavior outcome of school-age children with a history of febrile convulsions: a population study. *Epilepsia.* 2000;41(4):412–420.

50. Ellenberg JH, Nelson KB. Febrile seizures and later intellectual performance. *Arch Neurol.* 1978;35(1):17–21.

51. Verity CM, Greenwood R, Golding J. Long-term intellectual and behavioral outcomes of children with febrile convulsions. *N Engl J Med.* 1998;338(24):1723–1728.

52. Weiss EF, Masur D, Shinnar S, et al. Cognitive functioning one month and one year following febrile status epilepticus. *Epilepsy Behav.* 2016;64(Pt A):283–288.

53. Bertelsen EN, Larsen JT, Petersen L, Christensen J, Dalsgaard S. Childhood epilepsy, febrile seizures, and subsequent risk of ADHD. *Pediatrics.* 2016;138(2):e20154654.

54. Specchio N, Vigevano F. The spectrum of benign infantile seizures. *Epilepsy Res.* 2006;70 Suppl 1:S156–167.

55. Miceli F, Soldovieri MV, Joshi N, et al. KCNQ2-related disorders. In: Adam MP, Ardinger HH, Pagon RA, et al., eds., *GeneReviews®*. Seattle, WA: University of Washington; 2010.

56. Miceli F, Soldovieri MV, Joshi N, et al. KCNQ3-related disorders. In: Adam MP, Ardinger HH, Pagon RA, et al., eds. *GeneReviews®*. Seattle, WA: University of Washington; 2014.

Nonepileptic Spells

Tasleema Khan and Selim Benbadis

9.1 Introduction

Seizures and epilepsy are frequently misdiagnosed. Only about 50% of patients transferred to ICUs in tertiary hospitals after presumed status epilepticus are found to have status epilepticus.[1] About 90% of those misdiagnosed with epilepsy actually have psychogenic nonepileptic event (PNEE).[2] There are many other disorders misdiagnosed as epilepsy, organic and nonorganic, seen in adults and children. This chapter discusses the common differential diagnoses for epilepsy in hopes of making recognition of epilepsy imitators easier. As with any disorder, misdiagnosis delays the appropriate treatment needed to provide relief to the patient. In PNEE, a completely different therapeutic approach is needed (versus epileptic seizures), including psychotherapy and psychotropic medications. Anti-seizure drugs (ASDs) used in those who do not need them place an unnecessary risk of common and rare side effects.

9.2 Psychogenic Nonepileptic Events

PNEE is the most common misdiagnosis of epileptic seizures. It is considered a somatic symptom (DSM-IV or DSM-V) and is not associated with any abnormal electrographic changes or any abnormal neuronal discharges.[3] PNEE is typically not considered a factitious disorder or malingering, which both imply intentional feigning, but it is instead thought to be an unconscious production of physical symptoms.[4] In the DSM-V criteria, symptoms described as "attacks or seizures" are specifically listed under "conversion disorder" also known as "functional neurological symptom disorder."[5] As such, patients with PNEE are not considered to be "faking" or purposefully trying to obtain a secondary gain, though that distinction is difficult to make in individual cases, even for mental health professionals.

Of the patients referred to epilepsy centers, at least 20–30% are found to have PNEE.[4] While it is difficult to estimate, the overall prevalence is about 2–33/100,000.[6] Annual incidence of PNEE has been estimated to be 1.4/100,000,[7] and a more recent study shows incidence of PNEE is 4.9/100,000 a year.[8] The incidence may be even higher now, which may partly be due to increased recognition of the diagnosis. About 75% of PNEE patients are women[9] and 80% of patients with PNEE are initially diagnosed with epilepsy and treated with ASDs.[10] On average, there is a 7-year delay in diagnosing PNEE, and one correlation with the delay is the number of ASDs that were tried. This suggests trials were continued despite no response and supports the notion that patients with presumed seizures should be referred to an epilepsy center after two failed ASDs.[11]

PNEE is not limited to just adults and can also be seen in children as young as the age of 5.[17] Of 32 children with paroxysmal events suspected to have PNEE, 29 were confirmed in one study; 90% of them were adolescents, 76% were girls, and 72% were Caucasian.[13]

9.2.1 What causes PNEE?

Simply stated it is a manifestation of psychological distress. One thought is that patients with PNEE, or conversion disorder in general, have the inability to rationalize and understand their "feelings" and emotions, which is also known as alexithymia. This lack of emotional identification can cause misplacement or "misattribution" of "autonomic symptoms" of anxiety to a true organic disease.[14] It is as if to provide oneself an explanation and reconcile the inexplicable anxiety one experiences. PNEE has been considered a defense mechanism, and there is discussion of the importance of dissecting the underlying defense mechanism, as the different types may require unique therapies.[15]

9.2.2 Suspecting a Diagnosis

9.2.2.1 History

Initial suspicion for PNEE should arise from clinical presentation with thorough history and examination.[16] The past medical history, including social and sexual history, can be particularly useful in raising suspicion for PNEE when certain psychiatric comorbidities are present. Greater than 40–80% of patients with PNEE can have other psychiatric conditions, such as somatoform disorders, affective disorders, personality disorders, post-traumatic stress disorder, and anxiety-related disorders. In the same study, 87% of patients had a history of trauma with more than 60% having a traumatic history of sexual or physical abuse.[9] These become the "pertinent positives" in the history taking. Other risk factors include concurrent diagnoses of what are considered "functional somatic syndromes" such as "fibromyalgia, chronic fatigue syndrome, chronic pain syndrome, tension headaches, IBS, asthma, migraines, and GERD."[17]

9.2.2.2 Clinical Presentation

Details of the semiology of the attacks can aid in PNEE diagnosis. Persistent stress-related triggers such as pain, getting angry, and certain sounds/movement resulting in an attack should also raise suspicion.[16] One study attempted to classify PNEE by semiology and describes common clinical presentation during the event, including auras prior to the event. Classifications included abnormal motor phenomena such as asynchronous "violent thrashing, grabbing, and kicking movements" and other examples included pelvic thrusting and whole body jerking/flaccidity. An example of partial motor phenomena is head shaking. Affective/emotional behavior phenomena included "grimacing, gasping, choking feeling, and coughing."[18]

Another type was characterized as "dialeptic," and patients were unresponsive and "flaccid" throughout the entire event. There was even description of nonepileptic auras with "dizziness" as one example. Other symptoms noted were a stop-and-go pattern with "cessation or decrease in intensity during the events" as well as "stereotypy" and "variability." "Vocalizations" prior to or during the event were described as "moaning, grunting, screaming/shouting, gasping, and snorting." Fifty patients in the study had "forceful eye closure," and some had staring with lateral movements of the eyeballs. Hyperventilation and abnormal breathing pattern were also noted in some patients.[18] Even if the classification is not implemented in clinical practices, this study provides a very thorough and descriptive portrayal of the common red flags that can help identify PNEE.

The duration of the ictal period can further provide a hint to help differentiate an epileptic from a nonepileptic event. Generally, PNEE activity lasts significantly longer than epileptic seizures. Events lasting more than 5 minutes are 24 more times likely to be PNEE.[19] As also stated in the study, this is a problem, since status epilepticus is also defined as seizure activity >5 minutes. This can result in intubation, sedation, and treatment with intravenous ASDs for PNEE patients, exposing yet another reason why PNEE can be easily misdiagnosed as epilepsy.

9.2.2.3 Examination

Examination and observation can also help in the diagnosis. Give-way weakness, over-dramatization, and histrionic demeanor can all be clues.[16] Many patients will have events in the office, and in one study, 10 of 13 patients with spells during the office visit turned out to have PNEE.[20]

9.2.3 Confirming a Diagnosis

By definition, PNEE does not have epileptic electrographic correlation on electroencephalogram (EEG). During movements of PNEE, as is expected with any movement, including epileptic activity, muscle artifacts can be seen in varying frequencies and amplitudes. Interestingly, "hypermotor" and "partial motor" PNEE can be differentiated on EEG by the characteristics of muscle artifacts.[18] Muscle artifacts may also obscure epileptic activity; however, in PNEE, after cessation of abnormal motor activity, no postictal changes are seen on EEG,[18] as would be expected in epileptic seizures.

The question becomes which type of EEG should be used. Typically, long-term video monitoring EEG is recommended and not ambulatory or routine EEG. The issue with ambulatory EEG is that often it is without video. Video of the actual event allows interpreting physicians to review the entire event and correlate it with the EEG to ensure no electrographic changes concerning for a seizure occurred. Additionally, reviewing the semiology of the event on video allows clinical confirmation that the patient is not having frontal lobe seizures and other small epileptic seizures that are not always detected on EEG.[12]

9.2.4 Management

9.2.4.1 Role of the Neurologist

Diagnosis of PNEE is the initial role of a neurologist, but there is continued obligation in management. The first step in management and often the most difficult part, is presenting the diagnosis of PNEE to patients and their families. It can be challenging to reverse the epilepsy diagnosis and provide an alternative disorder, especially one associated with mental health. The diagnosis should be clearly stated with compassion, but without ambiguity, in terms that the patient can clearly understand. For example, patients should be told using words such as "psychological" or "stress-induced."[12] Patients should leave the conversation without feeling accused of "faking" it or trying to obtain secondary gain.

Terminology and semantics are important. For example, throughout this chapter we have referred to these nonepileptic episodes as PNEE or psychogenic nonepileptic "events" rather than PNES, that is, psychogenic nonepileptic "seizures." Referring to the attacks or events as seizures can be misleading to patients and they may associate it with epileptic seizures, regardless of the "nonepileptic" adjective. Avoiding the term seizure is one way to prevent room for ambiguity,[21] and stating it as an uncontrollable symptom or manifestation of anxiety, depression, or stress, as can be seen with palpitations or gastrointestinal distress, can be relatable to patients, and can alleviate the stigma associated with mental health.

9.2.4.2 Role of Mental Health Professionals

Psychologists, psychiatrists, and other mental health professions should play a long-term role after a patient has been diagnosed with PNEE.

The psychiatrist's role to prescribe medicinal therapies as treatment for PNEE is not limited to psychotropic drugs and is inclusive of psychotherapy. One study took 37 patients with PNEE confirmed on video-EEG, who were all initially treated for refractory epilepsy with aggressive ASDs. They underwent individualized psychoanalytic therapy after correct diagnosis of PNEE. Eleven of these patients had complete resolution of their events and the remainder showed a decrease in frequency.[22]

It is imperative to recognize other concurrent psychiatric disorders that are playing a role and manifesting as PNEE. Specific psychiatric conditions or underlying defense mechanisms, as mentioned above, will have unique therapies.[15] For example, in another case study,[23] prolonged exposure was used to treat patients specifically with concurrent post-traumatic stress disorder (PTSD) and PNEE. Prolonged exposure therapy generally is a method used to treat patients with PTSD. The modifications made in this study for concurrent PNEE included psychoeducation including breathing and other "grounding" techniques exercised even during the actual nonepileptic attack. Additionally, other "in-vivo" exercises included exposures to scenarios, situations, locations, and events that were intentionally and at times, irrationally avoided by patients with PTSD as they presented a reminder of their traumatic events. Of the 16 patients to complete the study, 13 had complete resolution of PNEE with these techniques and the remainder had decreased seizure frequency.

9.2.4.3 Roadblocks to Management

There are roadblocks to successful management from both a patient and a physician perspective. There is fear of losing the patient's trust/loyalty or being unable to communicate the diagnosis to the patient. One complication from a patient perspective affects veterans who are 100% service connected due to their disabilities from PNEE.[24]

Another roadblock is that at times, psychiatrists question the neurologist's diagnosis, even after video-EEG has confirmed it, and this can obviously hinder treatment. To prevent such discrepancies, a multidisciplinary approach is recommended during diagnosis.[24,25]

There is an inherent discomfort with approaching psychiatric illness with patients, as discussed above, as well as specific concern that the patient may be "faking it" or malingering when somatoform disorders are discussed, given that many mimic organic conditions.[26] Additionally, there may be a lack of interest on the part of the American Psychiatric Association and American Psychological Association.[27] The omission does not appear accidental given the comprehensive nature of these organizations in covering rarer conditions. Additionally, a search of a large psychiatric journal in 2011 showed no articles under "somatoform or conversion," but many on depression and anxiety.[27] This raises concern about ignorance of the topic in the mental health profession whether it be a lack of interest, ignorance, or discomfort. Perhaps the issue is a lack of ownership given that, for somatoform disorders, organic disorders must be excluded, which requires nonpsychiatric work up. For example, for diagnosis of PNEE, epileptic seizures must be excluded. While the neurologists are responsible for ruling out epileptic seizures, they are not equipped to manage psychiatric illness and it is imperative that psychiatrists and psychologists recognize, accept, and manage PNEE.

9.2.5 Prognosis

Adequate treatment allows complete resolution of seizure-like activity in 60–70% of patients diagnosed with PNEE, and an even higher percentage in children and teens.[10] One study specifically aimed at the early outcome of PNEE noted employment was related to a better prognosis. Interestingly, in the same study, 24 of the 27 patients in the study became spell-free and this occurred almost immediately after they were informed of the diagnosis, suggesting that an early diagnosis and appropriate discussion may lead to a better prognosis.[8] In the study of 32 children described above, with appropriate psychological therapy, 59% had complete remission and emergency room visits were reduced sevenfold.[13]

9.3 Syncope

Syncope is another condition commonly misdiagnosed as seizure, and the distinction is important as the treatment course is very different. Syncope is the transient loss of consciousness from diffuse lack of cerebral blood flow and oxygenation. Spontaneous return of consciousness and baseline is expected. Simplistically, the etiology for syncope can broadly be divided into cardiac, noncardiac, and unknown origin. Misdiagnosing syncope can cause serious, fatal cardiac conditions to go undetected. Atonic seizures can resemble syncope, but they are usually seen only in children and have a very short duration. Prolonged loss of consciousness is not associated with atonic seizures.[16]

9.3.1 Convulsive Syncope

Syncope can present with convulsions. In one study, 15% of syncopal patients had convulsions.[28] In a study aimed to study the characteristics of syncope, complete syncopal events with loss of consciousness and fall were successfully induced in 42 of 59 volunteers with hyperventilation and squatting followed by the Valsalva maneuver. It was observed that 90% of those 42 patients had myoclonus during their event. In most cases, it was bilateral, asynchronous myoclonic jerks.[29] A retrospective study of blood donors revealed about 12% of syncopes were convulsive, and a prospective study revealed 41% with blood-donation-related syncopal reactions were convulsive. The majority of these convulsions were described as starting with paleness, diaphoresis, and a "glassy" stare, followed by eyes rolling back, head extension, nuchal rigidity, and arm flexion (tonic spasms). After the event, patients remained pale and were flaccid.[30]

9.3.1.1 Clinical Features

Sheldon et al. created a point-scoring system to diagnose seizure versus syncope. A yes/no questionnaire was designed and definitive answers were given a positive or negative point score based on distinguishable findings in seizure versus syncope. For example, tongue biting, postictal confusion, and de ja vu were positive points suggestive of seizure, whereas positional triggers, diaphoresis, and lightheadedness were given negative points for syncope. A score of

1 or greater was diagnostic of seizure and less than 1 diagnostic of syncope. In their study of greater than 500 subjects, 94% were diagnosed correctly using this points system.[28]

Chest pain, dyspnea, palpitations, nausea prior to the event are also suggestive of syncope rather than seizures.[28]

9.3.2 Cardiac Etiologies and Diagnostic Studies

Studies have shown that 20–30% of patients with convulsive syncope are of cardiac origin.[31] Approximately 42% of 74 in a study who were initially diagnosed with epilepsy were found to have another diagnosis. About 63% of the patients had convulsive activity described similarly to the tonic spasms discussed above.[32] Implantable loop recorders (ILR) should be considered if extensive neurologic work-up (including negative magnetic resonance imaging (MRI) and EEG) and cardiac work-up has been unrevealing, and there is no known etiology for the syncopal episodes. ILRs have revealed cardiac asystole as the cause of recurrent syncope when other cardiac monitoring including electrocardiogram (EKG), external event monitoring, cardiac catheterization, tilt table testing, and exercise stress testing were negative.[31]

9.3.3 Psychogenic Pseudosyncope

It is imperative to give some attention to psychogenic pseudosyncope when discussing imitators of epilepsy and syncope as a differential diagnosis. Psychiatric conditions were seen more commonly in participants with syncope of unknown cause in a study. The conditions that were evaluated were somatization, panic disorder, generalized anxiety, major depression disorders, and drug/alcohol dependence and abuse disorders. Of the study participants with syncope, 20% had one of the above disorders. Patients with one of the four psychiatric disorders, excluding drug and alcohol abuse reported more than four syncopal episodes with prodome a year. The recurrence rate of syncope in patients with any psychiatric illness was 35%, about 20% higher than the population without mental illness.[33]

Can one definitively diagnose pseudosyncope? Yes, in the same way we diagnose PNEE, using video-EEG with activation. The criteria are as follows: activation induced the typical event, loss of tone and unresponsiveness was noted during the event with eyes closed, and lastly, the EEG was normal, before, during and after the event, and did not exhibit background suppression or "slowing," as is expected with syncope.[34]

A negative EEG alone should not be the extent of work-up in syncope, and a cardiologic source should also be ruled out. Many times, basic, noninvasive cardiovascular work-up, including a tilt test can provide the correct diagnosis. If not, further minimally invasive work-up should be considered, especially in cases where recurring syncopal episodes have no other etiology. Once a full neurologic and cardiologic work-up has been done for syncope and there is no known etiology, it is important to consider nonorganic etiologies of habitual episodes.

9.4 Neurological Disorders

9.4.1 Myoclonus

Myoclonus is defined as a sudden, brief, involuntary jerk of a muscle or muscle groups lasting no more than 200 milliseconds. Myoclonic jerks can be of various etiologies including medication-related and toxic/metabolic causes, as well as epileptic. Hiccups and hypnic jerks (described below) are examples of benign, nonepileptic myoclonus all people have experienced.[16] At times, it can be difficult to distinguish nonepileptic myoclonus from epileptic myoclonus, even with an EEG.

For instance, Ritzenthaler et al. described a case of an ICU patient with osmotic demyelination syndrome, who was seen to have right-sided myoclonus thought to be seizures. The patient was given IV clonazepam without any improvement and then tried on IV phenytoin, IV levetiracetam, and eventually propofol and phenobarbital with no clinical improvement of myoclonus. A continuous EEG revealed lateralized periodic discharges (LPDs) from the left hemisphere, but no improvement was seen with additional ASDs, including IV clonazepam. There was no evolution of the LPDs to suggest seizure, and when some of the ASDs were weaned off, there was no worsening of the EEG. Levetiracetam and clonazepam were continued to aid with myoclonus. Eventually, the LPDs resolved, and the neurologic examination was normal except for the myoclonus, which continued. This eventually resolved after 4 months. Repeat MRI of the brain at that time also showed improvement of myelinolysis. Given that clinically there were no electrical changes with ASD adjustment or electrical evolution, it was suspected that the LPDs and myoclonus were related to the myelinolyis.[35] This is just one example that portrays how nonepileptic myoclonus can be difficult to recognize, since both myoclonus and LPDs can be seen in status epilepticus.

9.4.2 Hypnic Jerks

Hypnic jerks are physiologic, benign myoclonic jerks occurring during wake–sleep transitioning seen in stage 1 and especially in rapid eye movement (REM) sleep.[36] It was seen to be evoked by acoustic stimulus in one study, and that the hypnic jerks were intensified in a patient with chronic insomnia. It started in stage 2, non-REM sleep with cranial muscles, and spread caudally and rostrally, which had not been described before, suggesting sleep disorders can intensify hypnic jerks.[37]

9.4.3 Hemifacial Spasm

Another movement disorder that can be mistaken for seizures is hemifacial spasm. It is characterized by involuntary, brief, intermittent or persistent twitching, or tonic or clonic contractions of facial muscles.[38] It usually first affects periorbital muscles, most commonly and first the eyelids (blepharopasm), then later the cheek and then perioral, usually unilaterally, but can progress to other facial muscles. Benzodiazepines, gabapentin, baclofen, botulinum toxin, and cranial nerve 7 decompressive surgery can all be part of management.[38,39] Botulinum toxin has shown 95% improvement in patients.[39] Hemifacial spasms are commonly misdiagnosed as focal seizures, tics, tardive dyskinesias, and psychogenic movement disorders, among others.[40] Interestingly, psychogenic movement disorder is the most common differential diagnosis, and more frequently tonic muscle contractions, bilateral asynchronous hemifacial involvement, isolated lower facial involvement, and downward deviation of the mouth angle are some red flags that point towards a psychogenic diagnosis.[41]

In one case, a young patient initially misdiagnosed with new onset hemifacial spasms later presented with a generalized tonic–clonic seizure. The concurrent seizure, as well as successful treatment with antiepileptic drugs confirmed epileptic myoclonus as the etiology of facial twitching.[42] While an EEG may show epileptic activity for facial twitching related to seizure, it may still be normal as a small focal, motor seizure may not clearly show epileptiform discharges. One other way to differentiate hemifacial spasms is that they are more chronic than paroxysmal, as one would expect with seizures.[16]

9.4.4 Acute Dystonic Reactions

Acute dystonic reactions usually occur within the first few days of starting an antipsychotic, though they can also occur from other causes. Anticholinergics can be used as treatment and can show significant improvement. One way to lower the risk of such a reaction and prevent a more long-term effect such as tardive dystonia, is by using the lowest dose and using newer, atypical antipsychotics, which have a lower risk of extrapyramidal signs as compared to older, typical antipsychotics. Acute dystonic reactions are described as "prolonged muscle contractions provoking slow, repetitive, involuntary, often twisting, movements that result in sustained abnormal, at times bizarre, posture" and can last seconds to hours.[43] It is understandable that the sudden, abnormal movements described above, can be mistaken for seizure; however, it is imperative to be able to clinically distinguish the two based on the unique presentation, which differs from rhythmic, tonic–clonic seizure activity, and from a patient's history of recent antipsychotic agent use.

9.4.5 Migraine

The episodic, recurrent, paroxysmal nature of migraines place them as a differential diagnosis of epilepsy, especially complicated migraine. A migraine aura can involve all the senses, similar to that of an epileptic aura, and at times, can cause loss of consciousness. One way to differentiate them is the time course, as migraines evolve over minutes, whereas seizures evolve over seconds.[16] The situation is further muddied by the rare condition of migralepsy, or visual migraine auras that evolve into epileptic seizures, typically arising from the occipital lobe. This can be confirmed on an EEG.[44] Migraines associated with confusion will be discussed in Section 9.5.1.

9.4.6 Narcolepsy

Narcolepsy is defined by international classification as excessive sleepiness associated with cataplexy, hypnagogic hallucinations, automatic behavior, and sleep paralysis. Cataplexy is defined as loss of muscle tone triggered by emotions lasting seconds to minutes with immediate and full recovery.[45] There is an association with HLA (HLA-DQB1*0602 seen in over 90%) and low levels of hypocretin (orexin) levels in patients with narcolepsy and cataplexy.[46] Given the loss of tone, cataplexy is often confused with epileptic events, as evidenced by two case series; one involving three adult patients[47] and the other, a 6-year-old child.[48] All subjects were initially misdiagnosed with epilepsy and polysomnography and a Multiple Sleep Latency Test (MSLT) confirmed narcolepsy. The MSLT revealed decreased sleep latency and occurrence of sleep onset REM in all the patients. Polysomnography was not indicative of narcolepsy in the adult cases, but helped rule out other sleep disorders such as obstructive sleep apnea. Polysomnography in the child showed reduced sleep latency, increased awakenings, abnormal sleep–wake cycles, and immediate and prolonged REM sleep. Interestingly, in the adult patients, witnesses described attacks as seizures, for example, "muscle twitching," "tonic–clonic seizures which occur during sleep." The child was diagnosed with atypical seizures not seen on EEG. It is important to obtain polysomnography and MSLT testing in patients with excessive sleep and epilepsy is in the differential.

9.5 Common Pediatric Epilepsy Imitators

Many of the organic and nonorganic imitators of epilepsy seen in adults described above can be seen in the pediatric population. Syncope, migraine, nonepileptic myoclonus, among others, are also diagnoses that can be seen in children and misdiagnosed as epilepsy. However, the remainder of this section is mainly dedicated to those syndromes that are typically if not exclusively seen in a pediatric population.

9.5.1 Acute Confusional Migraine

In children, migraines can be rarely linked to changes in mentation, including confusion, disorientation, agitation, incoherence, and somnolence, which come on suddenly and are associated with typical migraine features. There is some retrograde amnesia of the events. The event lasts minutes to hours. EEG will show slow-wave activity, but no reported epileptiform activity. Given events are fleeting and self-limiting, no specific treatment is indicated during the event.[49,50] In a retrospective study of 2509 files of pediatric patients treated for migraine and migraine variants, 111 patients met the criteria for migraine. Only 2.7% of those patients had acute confusional migraine symptoms[50] and it is still only rarely seen. It is a differential diagnosis for epilepsy in childhood since there is a sudden change in sensorium, but it is important to distinguish and not mistreat.

9.5.2 Sandifer Syndrome

Sandifer syndrome is a paroxysmal, dystonic movement associated with gastroesophageal reflux disease (GERD), which may sometimes be related to hiatal hernias. Dystonic movements have been described as torticollis, generalized shaking, whole-body stiffening, back arching, and hyperextension of extremities and spine.[51] There are also gastrointestinal symptoms in addition to reflux, such as vomiting. Typically, episodes start in childhood, but few adult cases have been reported.[52] Due to paroxysmal, abnormal movements, it is often misdiagnosed as infantile spasms. An EEG is useful and Sandifer syndrome should be considered if movements have no electrographic correlations. Improvement in movements can be seen when GERD is treated and the overall prognosis is very good.[53]

9.5.3 Gratification Phenomena

Infantile gratification behavior is also known as infantile masturbation. The age range is anywhere from 3 months to 8 years. There are various features that can be seen with infantile masturbation, including facial flushing, sweating, and grunting. The types of movements that have been described are as follows: pressure to the perineum, contraction and extension of extremities, scissoring or rubbing of legs and rocking of the body. Movements were distractible and there is no associated loss of consciousness.[54]

9.5.4 Shuddering Attacks

Shuddering attacks are another uncommon childhood disorder. Typically, they are described as shivering episodes seen with sitting and standing.[55] Stiffening and shaking can also occur, involving the head and shoulders and less commonly the trunk. Episodes are brief, and neurologic exam is normal. There is no associated loss of consciousness, falls, or developmental abnormality with these attacks.[55] Greater than 50% of the referred participants in this study were initially misdiagnosed with epilepsy, and the remainder were misdiagnosed as a movement disorder.[55] It is a benign condition with a good prognosis.

9.5.5 Breath-Holding Spells

Breath-holding spells are another nonepileptic, involuntary, paroxysmal event. It usually occurs in the first year of life, but ranges to 4 years of age, rarely later.[56] It is divided into two types: cyanotic and pallid, categorized depending on skin color. There is loss of consciousness and convulsions from cerebral anoxia/hypoxia can be seen, described as generalized clonic jerking, limb stiffening, and eyes rolling back. Many times, it is provoked by emotional stress or minor trauma. There can be a positive family history of breath-holding spells. It is self-remitting and usually no therapy is indicated.[56] In a prospective study of 95 patients with breath-holding spells, who were followed over a 9-year period, episodes resolved by the age of 4 years; 29 had cyanotic spells, 27 had pallid spells, and 19 had both. In 15% of the patients, there was no notable color change. There was a positive family history in 34%.

9.5.6 Benign Neonatal Myoclonus of Sleep

Benign neonatal myoclonus of sleep is a movement disorder that occurs in sleep, and as the name suggests consists of benign, self-resolving myoclonic jerks seen in the first month of life. Developmental and neurologic exams, and EEGs before, during, and after the events, both awake and asleep are normal, and treatment is not indicated.[57] In a study of 12 neonates, all presented by day 1 to day 15 of life. The events were described as rapid (4–5 jerks per second), synchronous, sometimes bilateral jerks that only occurred during sleep and were generalized, usually involving arms more than legs but eventually spreading to other areas, and very rarely, the face. Myoclonus was daily and "bouts" would not last for any longer than a second, but would irregularly reoccur over the next 30 minutes. If the newborn was awakened, the jerking would immediately stop. At times the myoclonus was very violent resulting in the appearance of the whole body shaking. Long-term EEGs were normal, and complete resolution was seen in less than a year.[58] Myoclonic jerks and generalized shaking are often misconstrued as convulsive, epileptic activity. Once again, EEG is useful in distinguishing this benign, nonepileptic condition and can prevent unnecessary pharmacotherapy.

9.6 Conclusion

Recurring events that occur periodically, episodically, and intermittently are commonly mistaken for seizures, especially those associated with abnormal movements, loss of awareness, and confusion. The differential diagnosis includes a wide variety of disorders, both organic and nonorganic, in adults and children. This chapter focused on the more common imitators, but there are likely more beyond the scope of this chapter. It is important to suspect other differentials based on history, examination, and clinical presentation to pursue appropriate diagnostic studies. This allows for cardiac, metabolic, psychogenic, and other etiologies to be appropriately managed and treated.

References

1. Walker MC, Howard RS, Smith SJ, et al. Diagnosis and treatment of status epilepticus on a neurological intensive care unit. *QJM.* 1996;89(12):913–920.

2. Benbadis SR. Psychogenic nonepileptic seizures. In: Wyllie E, Gupta A, Lachhwani DK, eds., *The Treatment of Epilepsy: Principles and Practice.* 4th edn. Philadelphia, PA: Lippincott, Williams & Wilkins; 2006:623–630.

3. LaFrance WC, Jr., Bjjornaes H. Designing treatment plans based on etiology of psychogenic nonepileptic seizures. In: Schachter SC, LaFrance WC, Jr., eds., *Gates and Rowan's Nonepileptic Seizures.* 3rd edn. New York, NY: Cambridge University Press; 2010:266–280.

4. Benbadis SR. Psychogenic nonepileptic seizures. Available at: http://emedicine.medscape.com/article/1184694-overview. Accessed March, 2019.

5. American Psychiatric Association. *Diagnostic and statistical manual of mental disorders.* 5th edn. Arlington, VA: American Psychiatric Association; 2013.

6. Benbadis SR, Allen Hauser W. An estimate of the prevalence of psychogenic non-epileptic seizures. *Seizure.* 2000;9 (4):280–281.

7. Sigurdardottir KR, Olafsson E. Incidence of psychogenic seizures in adults: a population-based study in Iceland. *Epilepsia.* 1998;39(7):749–752.

8. Duncan R, Razvi S, Mulhern S. Newly presenting psychogenic nonepileptic seizures: incidence, population characteristics, and early outcome from a prospective audit of a first seizure clinic. *Epilepsy Behav.* 2011;20(2):308–311.

9. Bowman ES, Markand ON. Psychodynamics and psychiatric diagnoses of pseudoseizure subjects. *Am J Psychiatry.* 1996;153(1):57–63.

10. Benbadis SR, Stagno SJ, Kosalko J, Friedman AL. Psychogenic seizures: a guide for patients and families. *J Neurosci Nurs.* 1994;26(5):306–308.

11. Kerr WT, Janio EA, Le JM, et al. Diagnostic delay in psychogenic seizures and the association with anti-seizure medication trials. *Seizure.* 2016;40:123–126.

12. Benbadis SR. Nonepileptic behavioral disorders: diagnosis and treatment. *Continuum (Minneap Minn).* 2013;19(3 Epilepsy):715–729.

13. Sawchuk T, Buchhalter J. Psychogenic nonepileptic seizures in children - psychological presentation, treatment, and short-term outcomes. *Epilepsy Behav.* 2015;52(Pt A):49–56.

14. Demartini B, Petrochilos P, Ricciardi L, et al. The role of alexithymia in the development of functional motor symptoms (conversion disorder). *J Neurol Neurosurg Psychiatry.* 2014;85 (10):1132–1137.

15. Beghi M, Negrini PB, Perin C, et al. Psychogenic non-epileptic seizures: so-called psychiatric comorbidity and underlying defense mechanisms. *Neuropsychiatr Dis Treat.* 2015;11:2519–2527.

16. Benbadis SR. Differential diagnosis of epilepsy. *Continuum (Minneap Minn).* 2007;13(4):48–70.

17. Dixit R, Popescu A, Bagic A, Ghearing G, Hendrickson R. Medical comorbidities in patients with psychogenic nonepileptic spells (PNES) referred for video-EEG monitoring. *Epilepsy Behav.* 2013;28 (2):137–140.

18. Dhiman V, Sinha S, Rawat VS, et al. Semiological characteristics of adults with psychogenic nonepileptic seizures (PNESs): an attempt towards a new classification. *Epilepsy Behav.* 2013;27(3):427–432.

19. Seneviratne U, Minato E, Paul E. How reliable is ictal duration to differentiate psychogenic nonepileptic seizures from epileptic seizures? *Epilepsy Behav.* 2017;66:127–131.

20. Benbadis SR. A spell in the epilepsy clinic and a history of "chronic pain" or

"fibromyalgia" independently predict a diagnosis of psychogenic seizures. *Epilepsy Behav.* 2005;6(2):264–265.

21. Benbadis SR. Psychogenic nonepileptic "seizures" or "attacks"? It's not just semantics: attacks. *Neurology.* 2010;75(1):84–86.

22. Santos Nde O, Benute GR, Santiago A, Marchiori PE, Lucia MC. Psychogenic non-epileptic seizures and psychoanalytical treatment: results. *Rev Assoc Med Bras (1992).* 2014;60(6):577–584.

23. Myers L, Vaidya-Mathur U, Lancman M. Prolonged exposure therapy for the treatment of patients diagnosed with psychogenic non-epileptic seizures (PNES) and post-traumatic stress disorder (PTSD). *Epilepsy Behav.* 2017;66:86–92.

24. McMillan KK, Pugh MJ, Hamid H, et al. Providers' perspectives on treating psychogenic nonepileptic seizures: frustration and hope. *Epilepsy Behav.* 2014;37:276–281.

25. Harden CL, Burgut FT, Kanner AM. The diagnostic significance of video-EEG monitoring findings on pseudoseizure patients differs between neurologists and psychiatrists. *Epilepsia.* 2003;44(3):453–456.

26. Benbadis SR. The problem of psychogenic symptoms: is the psychiatric community in denial? *Epilepsy Behav.* 2005;6(1):9–14.

27. Benbadis SR. Mental health organizations and the ostrich policy. *Neuropsychiatry.* 2013;3(1):5–7.

28. Sheldon R, Rose S, Ritchie D, et al. Historical criteria that distinguish syncope from seizures. *J Am Coll Cardiol.* 2002;40(1):142–148.

29. Lempert T, Bauer M, Schmidt D. Syncope: a videometric analysis of 56 episodes of transient cerebral hypoxia. *Ann Neurol.* 1994;36(2):233–237.

30. Lin JT, Ziegler DK, Lai CW, Bayer W. Convulsive syncope in blood donors. *Ann Neurol.* 1982;11(5):525–528.

31. Kanjwal K, Karabin B, Kanjwal Y, Grubb BP. Differentiation of convulsive syncope

from epilepsy with an implantable loop recorder. *Int J Med Sci.* 2009;6(6):296 300.

32. Zaidi A, Clough P, Cooper P, Scheepers B, Fitzpatrick AP. Misdiagnosis of epilepsy: many seizure-like attacks have a cardiovascular cause. *J Am Coll Cardiol.* 2000;36(1):181–184.

33. Kapoor WN, Fortunato M, Hanusa BH, Schulberg HC. Psychiatric illnesses in patients with syncope. *Am J Med.* 1995;99(5):505–512.

34. Benbadis SR, Chichkova R. Psychogenic pseudosyncope: an underestimated and provable diagnosis. *Epilepsy Behav.* 2006;9(1):106–110.

35. Ritzenthaler T, Laurencin C, Andre Obadia N, Bodonian C, Dailler F. Not everything that shakes is a seizure... role of continuous EEG in the intensive care unit. *Neurophysiol Clin.* 2017;47(1):13–18.

36. Montagna P, Liguori R, Zucconi M, et al. Physiological hypnic myoclonus. *Electroencephalogr Clin Neurophysiol.* 1988;70(2):172–176.

37. Calandra-Buonaura G, Alessandria M, Liguori R, Lugaresi E, Provini F. Hypnic jerks: neurophysiological characterization of a new motor pattern. *Sleep Med.* 2014;15(6):725–727.

38. Chaudhry N, Srivastava A, Joshi L. Hemifacial spasm: the past, present and future. *J Neurol Sci.* 2015;356(1–2):27–31.

39. Wang A, Jankovic J. Hemifacial spasm: clinical findings and treatment. *Muscle Nerve.* 1998;21(12):1740–1747.

40. Martinez AR, Nunes MB, Immich ND, et al. Misdiagnosis of hemifacial spasm is a frequent event in the primary care setting. *Arq Neuropsiquiatr.* 2014;72(2):119–122.

41. Baizabal-Carvallo JF, Jankovic J. Distinguishing features of psychogenic (functional) versus organic hemifacial spasm. *J Neurol.* 2017;264(2):359–363.

42. Deluca C, Tommasi G, Moretto G, Fiaschi A, Tinazzi M. Focal motor seizures mimicking hemifacial spasm. *Parkinsonism Relat Disord.* 2008;14(8):649–651.

43. Raja M. Managing antipsychotic-induced acute and tardive dystonia. *Drug Saf.* 1998;19(1):57–72.

44. Hartl E, Remi J, Noachtar S. Two patients with visual aura - migraine, epilepsy, or migralepsy? *Headache.* 2015;55 (8):1148–1151.

45. American Academy of Sleep Medicine. Narcolepsy. *International Classification of Sleep Disorders: Diagnostic and Coding Manual.* Westchester, IL: American Academy of Sleep Medicine; 2005:298–299.

46. Mignot E, Lammers GJ, Ripley B, et al. The role of cerebrospinal fluid hypocretin measurement in the diagnosis of narcolepsy and other hypersomnias. *Arch Neurol.* 2002;59(10):1553–1562.

47. Zeman A, Douglas N, Aylward R. Lesson of the week: narcolepsy mistaken for epilepsy. *BMJ.* 2001;322(7280):216–218.

48. Zhou J, Zhang X, Dong Z. Case report of narcolepsy in a six-year-old child initially misdiagnosed as atypical epilepsy. *Shanghai Arch Psychiatry.* 2014;26 (4):232–235.

49. Bechtel K. Acute mental status change due to acute confusional migraine. *Pediatr Emerg Care.* 2004;20(4):238–241.

50. Pacheva I, Ivanov I. Acute confusional migraine: is it a distinct form of migraine? *Int J Clin Pract.* 2013;67(3):250–256.

51. Werlin SL, D'Souza BJ, Hogan WJ, Dodds WJ, Arndorfer RC. Sandifer syndrome: an unappreciated clinical entity. *Dev Med Child Neurol.* 1980;22(3):374–378.

52. Bonnet C, Roubertie A, Doummar D, et al. Developmental and benign movement disorders in childhood. *Mov Disord.* 2010;25(10):1317–1334.

53. Wirth M, Bonnemains C, Auger J, Raffo E, Leheup B. [Sandifer's syndrome in a 5-month-old child with suspicion of infantile spasms]. *Arch Pediatr.* 2016;23(2):159–162.

54. Yang ML, Fullwood E, Goldstein J, Mink JW. Masturbation in infancy and early childhood presenting as a movement disorder: 12 cases and a review of the literature. *Pediatrics.* 2005;116 (6):1427–1432.

55. Jan MM. Shuddering attacks are not related to essential tremor. *J Child Neurol.* 2010;25 (7):881–883.

56. Lombroso CT, Lerman P. Breathholding spells (cyanotic and pallid infantile syncope). *Pediatrics.* 1967;39(4):563–581.

57. Coulter DL, Allen RJ. Benign neonatal sleep myoclonus. *Arch Neurol.* 1982;39 (3):191–192.

58. Di Capua M, Fusco L, Ricci S, Vigevano F. Benign neonatal sleep myoclonus: clinical features and video-polygraphic recordings. *Mov Disord.* 1993;8(2):191–194.

Status Epilepticus

Chandan B. Mehta, Paul Brady, and Shailaja Gaddam

10.1 Introduction

Status epilepticus (SE) is a relatively common medical and neurologic emergency that requires prompt evaluation and treatment. It accounts for up to 5% of all emergency department (ED) visits.[1]

A widely accepted practical definition of SE in adults and children (>5 years old) is: (a) at least 5 min of continuous seizure or (b) two or more seizures between which there is incomplete recovery of consciousness.[2] The diagnosis is usually not difficult, other than for patients with prolonged seizures, who often develop increasingly subtle features.[2] More recently, a report of the International League Against Epilepsy (ILAE) Task Force on the Classification of Status Epilepticus has proposed a new definition of SE which states the following:

> Status epilepticus is a condition resulting either from the failure of the mechanisms responsible for seizure termination or from the initiation of mechanisms, which lead to abnormally, prolonged seizures (after time point t_1). It is a condition, which can have long-term consequences (after time point t_2), including neuronal death, neuronal injury, and alteration of neuronal networks, depending on the type and duration of seizures.[3]

In the case of convulsive SE, both time points (t_1 at 5 min and t_2 at 30 min) have been based on animal experiments and clinical research; however, with incomplete evidence, these time points should be considered as the best estimate currently available.[3]

The reported yearly incidence of SE ranges from 7 to 41 cases per 100,000. Typically, the incidence of SE follows a U-shaped distribution, with relatively high incidence rates in children less than 1 year of age and then rising again in older adults over the age of 60 years.[1,4] There are a number of SE syndromes, which may be defined by clinical features and EEG findings. The most widely accepted classification of SE is a pragmatic and operational scheme distinguishing between convulsive SE, which is usually easy to recognize on clinical grounds, and nonconvulsive SE, in which the behavioral and/or cognitive changes persist as compared to baseline and where electroencephalogram (EEG) confirmation is mandatory.[5] SE was included in the classification of seizures by the ILAE of 1970 and 1981.[3] At that time, SE was divided into partial, generalized, or unilateral types, and basically mirrored the seizure classification.[3] A recent report of the ILAE Task Force in 2016 on Classification of Status Epilepticus has categorized SE in various subgroups, as seen in Figure 10.1.[5]

Most cases of SE in adults are symptomatic of an underlying structural brain lesion or a toxic metabolic derangement.[6] Other factors include acute and remote symptomatic causes and previous episodes of SE. If the underlying medical or structural cause is of recent

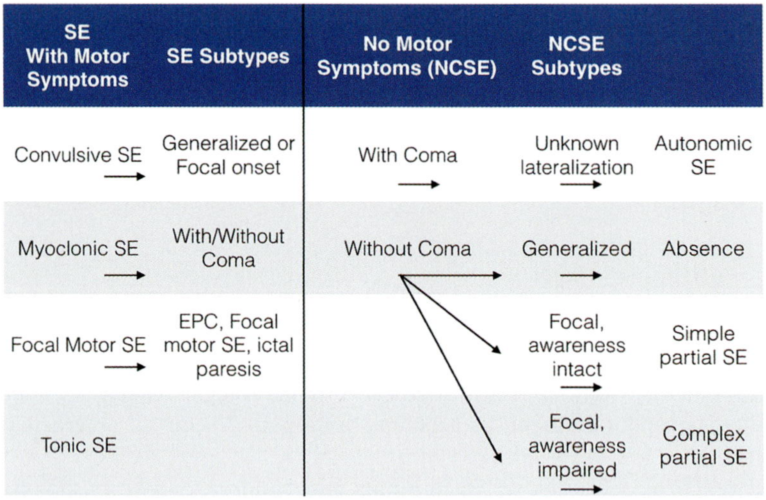

SE With Motor Symptoms	SE Subtypes	No Motor Symptoms (NCSE)	NCSE Subtypes	
Convulsive SE →	Generalized or Focal onset	With Coma →	Unknown lateralization →	Autonomic SE
Myoclonic SE →	With/Without Coma	Without Coma	Generalized →	Absence
Focal Motor SE →	EPC, Focal motor SE, ictal paresis		Focal, awareness intact →	Simple partial SE
Tonic SE			Focal, awareness impaired →	Complex partial SE

Figure 10.1 Classification of SE, adapted from the report of the ILAE Task Force on Classification of SE. (Adapted from Legriel S., Brophy GM. Managing Status Epilepticus in the Older Adult. *J Clin Med* 2016; 5(5):53.)

origin, SE is referred to as acute symptomatic. Episodes generated by a combination of an earlier lesion and a superimposed new metabolic, infectious, or pharmacologic stressor are referred to as remote symptomatic. In adults, the most common etiologies are acute symptomatic (50% of all cases), followed by remote symptomatic, and low antiseizure drug (ASD) levels in patients with known epilepsy.[7,8] Common causes of SE include stroke (hemorrhagic and ischemic), low ASD levels (due to altered metabolism or noncompliance), alcohol and substance withdrawal (benzodiazepines, barbiturates, baclofen), drug intoxication (ex-cocaine, isoniazid, imipenem, bupropion), anoxic or hypoxic brain injury, metabolic disturbance, brain or spinal cord infection, traumatic brain injury, malignancy, febrile seizures, congenital brain malformations, or idiopathic.[7] SE is also more commonly found in patients with secondary generalized epilepsy than in those with primary (genetic) generalized epilepsy.[9]

10.2 Status Epilepticus

10.2.1 Generalized Convulsive Status Epilepticus

Generalized convulsive status epilepticus (GCSE) is the most dramatic form of SE, with the potential for serious complications, morbidity, or even mortality. It consists of a self-perpetuating generalized tonic–clonic seizure or of a series of generalized tonic–clonic seizures without return to consciousness in between seizures. A study that included GCSE only, reported an incidence rate of 7 per 100,000.[10] In addition to GCSE, there are additional SE subtypes which present with prominent motor symptoms, including focal onset SE evolving into bilateral convulsive SE, myoclonic SE, tonic status, and hyperkinetic SE.[3]

Generally, the diagnosis of GCSE is fairly straightforward and based on clinical seizure activity. When an EEG is obtained for a patient with GCSE, it may be over shadowed by movement and myogenic artifact and thus, of limited diagnostic value.[3] However, in many cases, the EEG may show continuous spike-and-wave activity indicative of generalized seizure activity. Indeed, five identifiable EEG patterns have been described that occur in a predictable sequence during the course of GCSE: discrete seizures with interictal slowing, merging seizures with waxing and waning amplitude and recurrent build-up and slowing of frequency of EEG rhythms, continuous ictal activity consisting of rhythmic sharp or spike-and-wave discharges, continuous ictal activity punctuated by low-voltage flat periods, and periodic epileptiform discharges on a flat background.[11] In some cases of GCSE, a focal onset may manifest itself on EEG, and this can help to focus the evaluation on an underlying focal cause.

10.2.2 Myoclonic Status Epilepticus

Myoclonic SE (MSE) is a condition in which generalized myoclonic jerks are repeated continuously or occur in clusters lasting for a sufficiently long period, usually greater than 30 minutes.[12] It consists of irregular, usually bilateral or generalized myoclonic jerking without interference with consciousness.

It is most often seen in patients with insufficiently controlled juvenile myoclonic epilepsy (JME), Dravet syndrome, and in nonprogressive myoclonic epilepsy in infancy, particularly Angelman syndrome.[13] Primary forms of epilepsy syndrome-related MSE are those in which myoclonus is a characteristic finding, such as in JME. Secondary epilepsy syndromes causing MSE are usually more severe and commonly occur in childhood, as seen in Lennox–Gastaut syndrome. In other cases, MSE is symptomatic of a more widespread neurologic dysfunction or an acute encephalopathy, the most ominous causes being hypoxic-ischemic encephalopathy, or anoxia (Figure 10.2).

The EEG of patients with MSE demonstrates generalized periodic complexes usually correlating with myoclonus, with marked attenuation of activity between the complexes.[14] Differentiation from subcortical myoclonus, which mimics MSE, must be made by administration of a paralytic agent to rid the EEG of myogenic artifact, to determine if there is presence of underlying SE.

10.2.3 Focal Status Epilepticus

Focal SE has many clinical manifestations and consists of repeated focal motor seizures, epilepsia partialis continua, adversive status, oculoclonic status, and ictal paresis.[3] The manifestations of focal SE are largely dependent on the location of the epileptogenic brain focus. Focal SE tends to be the most easily recognized amongst the SE classification spectrum, and can present with progression of focal jerking activity of a limb commonly referred to as "Jacksonian March." However, it can also evolve and proceed into bilateral convulsive SE.[15]

Compared to GCSE, focal SE is much less common. Indeed, except for series of patients with epilepsia partialis continua (EPC), discussed below, or simple partial seizures, most reports of focal SE are restricted to isolated cases or small series.[15] For other forms of focal SE, other than EPC, the relative frequency is difficult to determine, and causes and response to ASDs are even less well established.[15]

Frequent recurrent discrete electrographic seizures on EEG support a diagnosis of focal SE.[16] However, continuous epileptiform discharges are also a frequent finding and patients may alternate between these two patterns.[17]

10.2.3.1 Epilepsia Partialis Continua

EPC is the most readily recognized variant of simple focal motor SE in which frequent repetitive muscle jerks, usually arrhythmic, continue over prolonged periods of time.

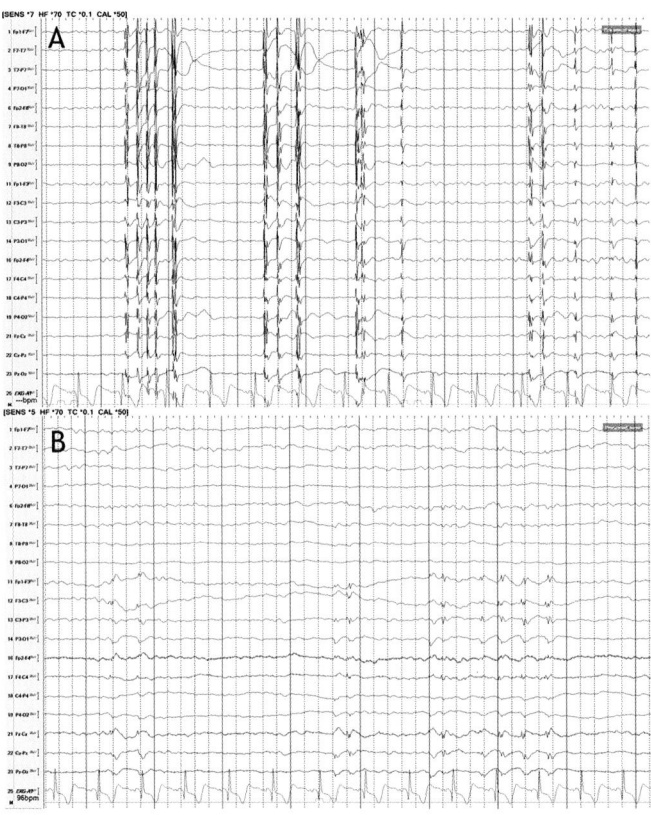

Figure 10.2 Patient s/p pulseless electrical activity (PEA) arrest, with continuous myoclonic jerks with time-locked generalized spike/polyspike wave discharges (A). Post administration of paralytic, bipolar montage demonstrates mid-line and bi-frontal spikes with resolution of myogenic artifact (B).

The jerks tend to be stereotyped, affecting single muscles, muscle groups, an entire limb, or larger parts of one hemibody.[18] EPC appears as a subclass of focal motor status in the recent report of the ILAE Task Force on Classification of SE.[3]

No formal epidemiological data appear to exist for EPC; however, several centers were able to collect a substantial series of patients in a limited time period.[19] There are a number of EPC etiologies, which can be local like stroke and Rasmussen syndrome,[20] or systemic, particularly mitochondrial diseases and nonketotic hyperglycemia.[18]

In some patients, the myoclonic jerks of EPC are not always accompanied by correlated discharges on surface EEG.[21] However, when captured electrographically, EPC is reported to present as irregularly occurring focal discharges of cortical origin that commonly consist of discrete spikes, sharp waves or slow-wave activity, and periodic lateralized epileptiform discharges.[18]

10.3 Nonconvulsive Status Epilepticus

Nonconvulsive status epilepticus (NCSE) can be defined as a condition of ongoing or intermittent seizure activity without convulsions, without recovery of consciousness between attacks, and lasting more than 10 minutes. Further, NCSE comprises a group of syndromes that display a great diversity regarding response to ASDs, ranging from virtually self-limiting variants to entirely refractory forms.[22] In the ILAE classification, NCSE is subdivided according to the level of consciousness and clinical EEG features seen in Figure 10.1.[5] Up to 34% of patients undergoing CEEG demonstrate nonconvulsive seizures (NCS), and 76% of these cases are NCSE. Comatose patients require CEEG for prolonged periods (greater than 24 hours), as they are more likely to have their first seizure detected after this point (20% versus 5% of noncomatose patients).[23]

The underlying causes of NCSE are varied and differ according to the patient population being studied. Approximately one-half to two-thirds of patients have a prior history of seizures or epilepsy. NCSE can be the presenting symptom of infectious or autoimmune encephalitis including anti-NMDA receptor encephalitis, Hashimoto's encephalopathy, lupus cerebritis, and neurosyphilis. In the critically ill patient, common causes of NCSE include subarachnoid hemorrhage, traumatic brain injury, malignancy, stroke, and hypoxic or anoxic injury.

A high index of suspicion is necessary to confirm NCSE, since clinical signs and symptoms are subtle and variable, and confirmation of the diagnosis is largely based on prolonged confirmatory EEG showing frequent or continuous nonconvulsive seizures. Patients however, may display subtle signs of jerking or twitching, and may have episodes of staring, speech arrest, or gaze deviations with focal seizures.[1] Approximately 10–19% of patients in an ICU setting demonstrate presence of subclinical seizures when monitored on continuous EEG.[23,24] Greater than 90% of patients with seizures in the ICU have nonconvulsive seizures.[24]

The EEG changes most importantly include, in traditional terminology, periodic lateralized epileptiform discharges, bilateral independent periodic lateralized epileptiform discharges, generalized periodic epileptiform discharges, and stimulus-induced rhythmic periodic ictal-like discharges.[22] When these periodic discharges are present, continuous EEG monitoring should be considered to rule out nonconvulsive seizures in patients who are lethargic or unresponsive.

10.4 Refractory and Super-Refractory Status Epilepticus

Status epilepticus is considered refractory (RSE) if the first- and second-line treatments with benzodiazepines and an antiepileptic drug fail to terminate seizure activity. Up to 40% of cases of SE become RSE.[25]

SE is defined as super-refractory (SRSE) if it continues for more than 24 hours after the first administration of general anesthesia.[26] Less than 50% of patients with SE have had previous seizures or epilepsy.[27] SRSE is hypothesized to occur due to failure of self-terminating mechanisms; changes in receptor configuration, reduction in GABA receptors in the cells affected by seizure discharges, and an increase in glutaminergic receptors, resulting in reduced GABA-ergic activity and resulted decreased effectiveness of GABA-ergic ASDs in controlling seizures.[28]

Population-based incidence data for RSE and SRSE are scarce.[26] A recent hospital-based 9-year cohort study of RSE and SRSE from Switzerland suggests that 33% of SE becomes RSE and 4% of SE becomes SRSE, resulting in incidence for RSE of 3.3–5.3/100,000 and for SRSE 0.4–0.6/100,000.[29] The etiology of RSE in developing countries is dominated by central nervous system infections and head injury compared to stroke and drug withdrawal in developed countries. New-onset refractory status epilepticus (NORSE) is a syndrome described in several reports of patients who present with severe generalized seizures and SE of unclear etiology, often in the setting of a prodromal febrile illness suggesting a viral encephalitis.[30,31]

The diagnostic approach to NORSE includes a computed tomography (CT) of the head, continuous EEG, lumbar puncture (LP), and microbe serologies that include herpes simplex virus (HSV), varicella zoster virus (VZV), and bacterial evaluation, within the initial 24 hours of patient presentation. Thereafter, a magnetic resonance image (MRI) of the brain followed by a repeat LP to evaluate for an autoimmune or neoplastic cause should be obtained.[32] The utility of the EEG for patients with RSE is to monitor for burst suppression after initiating intravenous anesthetic therapy (IVAT) for treatment. The goal of IVAT is to stop RSE, but the depth of anesthesia is unknown. Current guidelines state that IVAT may be titrated (using EEG) to seizure suppression or burst suppression, in which the patient's EEG becomes discontinuous, with bursts of activity separated by periods of suppression. Targeting an interburst interval of about 10 s for 24 hours (followed by tapering IVAT) is a standard recommendation.[25]

10.5 Management of Status Epilepticus

Management may be divided into multiple stages, dependent on how long seizure activity has occurred. The goals of therapy include cessation of seizure activity, identification of etiology/reversible causes, and prevention of further seizures and subsequent complications. Care must be taken to delineate etiology of SE; as this may be helpful in treatment and management of SE. Evaluation and treatment of SE should begin in the field. Appropriate medical history must be obtained, and evaluation of vital signs and blood glucose should be established. On arrival in the emergency department, basic laboratory workup, including a comprehensive metabolic profile, blood count, lactate, blood, urine, and sputum cultures should be drawn.[33] Intravenous access must be established, if not already done. Neurologic examination must be obtained.

Treatment for drug intoxication/withdrawal, hypo- or hyperglycemia, electrolyte disturbances, toxo-metabolic states, and/or infections must concurrently occur. Appropriate neuro-imaging, including CT of the brain and/or MRI of the brain, with and without contrast, should be considered to delineate causative intracranial pathology, which may necessitate prompt treatment.

Further consideration can be made for completion of LP, toxicology panel, serum ASD levels, and testing for inborn errors of metabolism on a case-by-case basis.[33] Airway management, including mechanical ventilation, must be considered if there is no return to consciousness after seizure activity, or if the patient is not protecting their airway. If the patient remains obtunded after repeated seizure activity, continuous EEG (cEEG) must be established, if available. The algorithm for medical management of SE includes first-, second- (urgent control), and third-line (refractory and super refractory control) agents, which are shown in Table 10.1. Intravenous (IV) administration of first-line agents must be used as abortive therapy. Second- and third-line agents may be instituted once a patient has reached established SE (greater than 5 minutes of seizure activity) or refractory SE (seizure activity occurring for more than 24 hours, despite first- and second-line therapies).[34]

10.5.1 Stage 1: First-Line Therapy

First-line agents are comprised of benzodiazepines (BZDs), which may be administered intravenously (IV), intramuscularly (IM), or rectally if no IV access is available. Administration of BZDs should be possibly prior to transfer to ED for seizure cessation. Typically lorazepam and midazolam are commonly used in the emergency setting. Diazepam IV or

Table 10.1 Mechanisms of action, dosing, and side effects of first-, second , and third-line agents

Drug	Loading/ maintenance and continuous infusion (CI) doses	Mechanism	Side effects	Key notes
Diazepam	10 mg/dose, up to 0.15 mg/kg IV q 5 min, max 30 mg	Binds BZD receptors, GABA-ergic	Respiratory depression, hypotension	IV has propylene glycol
Lorazepam	2–4 mg/dose, up to 0.1 mg/kg IV q 5 min	Binds BZD receptors, GABA-ergic	Respiratory depression, hypotension	IV has propylene glycol
Midazolam	0.2 mg/kg IM/IV, up to max dose 10 mg, 0.05–2 mg/mg/h IV CI	Binds BZD receptors, GABA-ergic	Respiratory depression, hypotension, tachyphylaxis	Short duration
Ketamine	1–2 mg/kg IV q 3–5 min load (max 4.5 mg/kg), 1–10 mg/kg/h IV CI	NMDA receptor antagonist	Respiratory depression	Neurotoxicity, memory impairment
Lacosamide	200–400 mg IV load, 25–200 mg PO q 12 h	Enhances slow inactivation of voltage sensitive Na channels	PR prolongation causing AV nodal blockade	Minimal drug interactions
Levetiracetam	1–3 g IV load, 500 mg–2 g IV/PO q 12 h	Binds synaptic vesicle glycoprotein SV2A, inhibits presynaptic calcium channels	Agitation, suicidality	Minimal drug interactions
Phenytoin	15–20 mg/kg IV, 100 mg IV/PO q 8 h	Modulated voltage-dependent Na and Ca channels	Hypotension, purple glove syndrome, arrhythmia, fever, thrombocytopenia	IV has propylene glycol
Phenobarbital	10–20 mg/kg IV (half or full load), max 400 mg/day (divided) PO	Blockade of glutamate signaling, increases flux of chloride ions into neurons decreasing excitability	Hypotension, respiratory depression	IV has propylene glycol
Pentobarbital	10–20 mg/kg IV (half or full load), 0.5–5 mg/kg/h IV CI	Potentiation of GABA-ergic tone, inhibition of excitatory AMPA-glutamate receptor	Hypotension, respiratory depression, ileus	Requires mechanical ventilation, IV has propylene glycol

Table 10.1 (*cont.*)

Drug	Loading/ maintenance and continuous infusion (CI) doses	Mechanism	Side effects	Key notes
Propofol	1–2 mg/kg IV load, 30–200 µg/kg/min IV CI	Positive modulation of GABA inhibitory effects through GABA$_A$ receptors	Hypotension, respiratory depression, propofol infusion syndrome	Requires mechanical ventilation, must adjust caloric needs/intake
Topiramate	200–400 mg PO load, 300–1600 mg/ day (divided) PO	Carbonic anhydrase inhibitor, antagonizes glutamate and voltage-dependent Na receptors, potentiates GABA inhibition	Metabolic acidosis, decreased hunger, weight loss	Metabolic acidosis
Valproate sodium	20–40 mg/kg IV, max 60 mg/kg/day (divided) PO	GABA-ergic, inhibits glutamate/NMDA receptor mediated excitation	Hepatotoxicity, thrombocytopenia, fever, hyper-ammonemia	Contraindicated in mitochondrial disease

mg, milligram; g, gram; kg, kilogram; min, minute; h, hour; IV, intravenous; IM, intramuscular; PO, per os (by mouth); max, maximum; BZD, benzodiazepine; GABA, gamma-aminobutyric acid; NMDA, N-methyl-d-aspartate; AMPA, α-amino-3-hydroxy-5-methyl-4-isoxazolepropionic acid; SV2A, synaptic vesicle glycoprotein 2A; Na, sodium; Ca, calcium.

rectally and clonazepam sublingually may additionally be used as breakthrough medications. Benzodiazepines bind to GABA$_A$ receptors, increasing the frequency of chloride channel opening, and heightening the inhibitory effects of the receptors.[35]

The RAMPART study was a double-blinded, randomized, noninferiority trial comparing administration of IM midazolam (10 mg) followed by IV placebo (n = 448), to administration of IM placebo followed by IV lorazepam (4 mg) (n = 445) in children and adults with SE (seizures lasting >5 min) in the prehospital setting by emergency medical services (EMS).[36,37] Seizures had stopped prior to arrival in the ED without administration of rescue therapy in 73.4% of subjects with active IM treatment and in 63.4% of subjects given active IV therapy. The study demonstrated that use of IM route of midazolam allowed for more reliable and rapid administration of therapy, leading to lower rates of hospital, as well as ICU admission.

Alldredge et al.[38,39] conducted a randomized, double-blinded study on 258 patients to evaluate the use of IV diazepam (5 mg), lorazepam (2 mg), or placebo on patients with repetitive generalized convulsive seizures, or seizures lasting greater than 5 min; in order to evaluate treatment with benzodiazepines in the prehospital setting. Patients could receive a second injection if seizures did not cease. SE terminated on arrival in the ED in 59.1% of patients receiving lorazepam, 42.6% of patients receiving diazepam, and 21.1% of patients receiving placebo.

If the physician is unable to abort seizure activity, or if the patient does not return to baseline mental status, then proceeding with urgent therapy is indicated.

10.5.2 Stage 2: Urgent Therapy

If SE does not abort with BZDs, the patient must be loaded with maintenance ASDs intravenously. Maintenance ASD therapy should be initiated in the ED or critical care setting unless a frank, reversible cause of seizure is established (i.e. hypoglycemia).[33] Renal and hepatic function should be investigated. Continuous EEG should be started in order to monitor response to therapy. Frequent neurologic checks and evaluation of airway protection should occur. Current mainstays of therapy include valproate, levetiracetam, phenytoin, fosphenytoin, lacosamide, and topamax[1,39], which may be used separately, or in conjunction with one another, with loading doses as noted in Table 10.1. Care must be taken to check for AV nodal blockade before lacosamide is administered.

In the acutely ill, IV administration of these medications is preferable, as delayed absorption or clearance may hinder resolution of SE.

On the basis of a number of studies, it can be concluded that phenytoin, valproate, phenobarbital, levetiracetam, and lacosamide are all suitable choices as second-line agents.[40–45] Consideration must be given at this point to imaging with a head CT or brain MRI if there is any focality in neurologic exam, and for lumbar puncture if routine laboratory testing and infectious workup is unrevealing.

10.5.3 Stages 3 and 4: Management of Refractory and Super-Refractory SE

Continuous infusions of anesthetic agents, barbiturates, or benzodiazepines may be considered as third-line agents for management of RSE and SRSE. These agents should be instituted in patients that are unresponsive to the IV antiepileptic therapy listed above after 24 hours. They are utilized in addition to the IV ASDs described above, and also in combination with enterally administered ASDs for the treatment of RSE and SRSE. Up to 10–15% of patients with RSE fail to respond to third-line therapies, and are considered to have SRSE.[28,46] The objective of IV anesthetic use is to ablate RSE. IV anesthetics should be titrated to seizure and burst suppression lasting 5–10 s in duration for 24 48 hours before weaning attempts take place.[25,28]

On a retrospective case survey of 553 cases in 44 countries, midazolam proved to be the most widely used first-line anesthetic (59%). Propofol was used first 32% of the time, followed by barbiturates 8% of the time.[47]

Midazolam may be utilized separately, or in conjunction with other third-line infusions.

Propofol is often utilized in ED or in patients who may require frequent neurologic re-examination due to the potential need for operative intervention due to trauma. It has a short half-life and rapid CNS penetration, and patients may be awakened within 10 to 15 min.[29,48] Prolonged usage at high doses (>4 mg/kg/h) places patients at risk of propofol infusion syndrome, which consists of rhabdomyolysis, renal failure, metabolic acidosis, and cardiac failure. Hyperkalemia, elevated triglycerides, and hepatomegaly may also be present.[29,48] Daily creatine phosphokinase (CPK) and triglycerides should be checked, along with intermittent liver function tests.

If midazolam or propofol are unsuccessful in breaking RSE, pentobarbital may be used. Pentobarbital 10 mg/kg IV may be loaded and repeated once, with maintenance dosing starting at 0.5 mg/kg/h up to 10 mg/kg/h, and titrated every 6 hours to burst suppression of

10–30 s. The main disadvantage of utilizing barbiturates includes the prolonged half-life, and the highly sedating effects, which may blunt the neurologic exam on the critically ill neurologic patient, even at modest doses. Additionally, patients are predisposed to developing a significant ileus due to slowed GI motility, and may require total parenteral nutrition (TPN).[28]

Ketamine may be used on nonintubated patients; but at higher doses, intubation must be considered.[28,49] Hofler et al. retrospectively reviewed data from 44 patients with RSE and SRSE who received two anesthetic drugs and three ASD drugs prior to ketamine administration in the neuro-ICU setting, with 3-day median latency from SE to treatment with ketamine. Median duration of SE was 10 days, ketamine administration was 4 days, mortality 45.2%, and SE control 64%. No adverse events were demonstrated.[50]

Anesthetic agents may not be used unless a patient is intubated (except ketamine). Continuous EEG must be established by this point. Hemodynamic monitoring and aggressive ICU care must be undertaken to prevent the risks of infection, deep vein thrombosis, ileus, and hypotension associated with medically induced coma. Patients should be placed in a therapeutic coma for at least 24–48 hours prior to re-emergence, if tolerated.[33] Weaning should occur in intervals such that the continuous infusions are tapered from the patient's system in a slow manner. Abrupt discontinuation of these agents may trigger withdrawal seizures.

In 2016, Alvarez et al. compared the use of a therapeutic coma with IV anesthetic agents for RSE of all etiologies except postanoxic across multiple hospital systems to evaluate the potential effects on mortality and length of stay.[51] They noted that therapeutic coma was not associated with mortality after controlling for SE severity, refractoriness, comorbidities, and demographics, but that it correlated to a 60% increase in length of stay in acute facilities.[51]

Combination of multiple IV anesthetics may be used; but after multiple weaning attempts, if unable to control SRSE, consideration should be given to family discussion for goals of care if all treatment options have been exhausted. If suspicion is for SRSE secondary to an autoimmune condition, high-dose steroids may be started (methylprednisolone 1g IV daily for 5 days followed by prednisone taper); IVIG 0.4 g IV daily × 5 doses, or plasmapheresis (PLEX) for five sessions.[28]

10.5.4 Other Considerations

In cases in which focal SE cannot be controlled; consideration should be made for placement of depth electrodes for mapping of epileptogenic foci for potential surgical resection. Interventions include callosotomy, hemispherectomy or lobectomy, focal cortical resection, or resection of mass lesion (including malignancy, tuber, etc.) or vascular malformation. Surgical treatment may be curative, or may at least lead to reduction in the need for multiple oral ASDs. A ketogenic diet, hypothermia and vagus nerve stimulation, and magnesium and pyridoxine therapy have also been reported as mechanisms for therapy.[28]

10.5.5 Outcomes

Outcomes for SE vary based on etiology and subtype classification. Mortality rates are low for SE cases in ambulatory patients from absence or complex partial seizures.[1] Patients with SE requiring inpatient therapy however, have very different outcomes. Old age (greater than

65–75 in variable studies[5]), severity of end organ dysfunction, super-refractoriness of SE, and premorbid clinical function are predictors of long-term mortality.[27] Thirty-day mortality rates are between 19 and 27% for SE.[46] Ferlisi et al. reported a 22% mortality rate out of 413 cases. Of the patients who survived, just 42.6% of them had a modified Rankin score less than 2 (slight disability or less).[47] The more prolonged the SE course is, and the longer the delay in recognition and treatment, the poorer the outcome may be. Etiology of SE is an important predictor of outcome. If SE is secondary to metabolic disturbance, alcohol withdrawal, or noncompliance with ASD regimen, mortality may be less than 10%.[46] A study in Finland has reported long-term mortality rates of 26–34% with poor functional outcome in 11–28% of patients at 1–12-month follow-ups.[26,27] Patients requiring use of IV anesthetics have a poorer outcome, specifically those requiring use of multiple IV anesthetics.[47] Those patients with "high risk" EEG characteristics of monomorphic bursts and maximum amplitude bursts may have difficulty in weaning attempts from burst suppression, and may suffer from recurrent SE.[25] Anoxia causing SE is a poor predictor of outcome.

Two scores have been developed to help predict outcome after SE.[52–54] The Status Epilepticus Severity Score (STESS) is based on the level of consciousness before treatment, worst seizure time, age, and history of previous seizures. Scores >3 predict a high risk of death after an SE episode; however, independent validations of the study demonstrate a cutoff value >4 may be best for predicting in-hospital death.[53]

The Epidemiology-based Mortality score in Status Epilepticus (EMSE) was introduced in 2015, and utilizes etiology, age, comorbidities, and EEG patterns – lateralized periodic discharges, generalized periodic discharges, after-SE ictal discharges, and spontaneous burst suppression. Points >64 predict a higher likelihood of death.[52] Giovannini et al. evaluated 162 patients, for a total of 175 SE episodes. Thirty-day mortality was 31.5%. In this review, 69% of patients demonstrated STESS scores ≥3, and 34% of patients had STESS scores ≥4; 49% of patients demonstrated EMSE scores >64. An EMSE score of 64 had the highest accuracy in predicting 30-day mortality after SE (88%), thus indicating that a patient with high score should be treated rapidly and aggressively. A score <64 suggested that a patient had a high probability of surviving (98%) without significant functional decline after SE.[52]

10.6 Conclusion

SE is a challenging diagnosis to treat. Outcomes are frequently dictated by etiology, and rapidity of treatment. Clinical outcomes have improved over time with use of continuous EEG recording and prompt recognition of SE, with aggressive treatment starting earlier on, due to changes in diagnostic criteria for SE. Improvements in outcome will continue to rise with education of practitioners in the prehospital and emergency settings. Future research should focus on therapy and management of RSE and SRSE.

References

1. Varelas PN, Spanaki MV, Mirski MA. Status epilepticus: an update. *Curr Neurol Neurosci Rep.* 2013;13(7):357.

2. Lowenstein DH, Bleck T, Macdonald RL. It's time to revise the definition of status epilepticus. *Epilepsia.* 1999;40 (1):120–122.

3. Trinka E, Cock H, Hesdorffer D, et al. A definition and classification of status epilepticus – report of the ILAE Task Force on Classification of Status Epilepticus. *Epilepsia.* 2015;56(10):1515–1523.

4. Chin RF, Neville BG, Scott RC. A systematic review of the epidemiology of status epilepticus. *Eur J Neurol.* 2004;11 (12):800–810.

5. Legriel S, Brophy GM. Managing status epilepticus in the older adult. *J Clin Med.* 2016;5(5):53.

6. Barry E, Hauser WA. Status epilepticus: the interaction of epilepsy and acute brain disease. *Neurology.* 1993;43(8):1473–1478.

7. DeLorenzo RJ, Hauser WA, Towne AR, et al. A prospective, population-based epidemiologic study of status epilepticus in Richmond, Virginia. *Neurology.* 1996;46(4):1029–1035.

8. Hesdorffer DC, Logroscino G, Cascino G, Annegers JF, Hauser WA. Incidence of status epilepticus in Rochester, Minnesota, 1965–1984. *Neurology.* 1998;50(3):735–741.

9. Jozwiak J, Kotulska K, Jozwiak S. Similarity of balloon cells in focal cortical dysplasia to giant cells in tuberous sclerosis. *Epilepsia.* 2006;47(4):805.

10. Wu YW, Shek DW, Garcia PA, Zhao S, Johnston SC. Incidence and mortality of generalized convulsive status epilepticus in California. *Neurology.* 2002;58(7):1070–1076.

11. Treiman DM, Walton NY, Kendrick C. A progressive sequence of electroencephalographic changes during generalized convulsive status epilepticus. *Epilepsy Res.* 1990;5(1):49–60.

12. Baysal Kirac L, Aydogdu I, Acarer A, et al. Myoclonic status epilepticus in six patients without epilepsy. *Epilepsy Behav Case Rep.* 2013;1:10–13.

13. Engel J, Jr. Report of the ILAE Classification Core Group. *Epilepsia.* 2006;47(9):1558–1568.

14. Jumao-as A, Brenner RP. Myoclonic status epilepticus: a clinical and electroencephalographic study. *Neurology.* 1990;40(8):1199–1202.

15. Drislane FW, Blum AS, Schomer DL. Focal status epilepticus: clinical features and significance of different EEG patterns. *Epilepsia.* 1999;40(9):1254–1260.

16. Scholtes FB, Renier WO, Meinardi H. Simple partial status epilepticus: causes, treatment, and outcome in 47 patients. *J Neurol Neurosurg Psychiatry.* 1996;61(1):90–92.

17. So EL, Ruggles KH, Ahmann PA, et al. Clinical significance and outcome of subclinical status epilepticus in adults. *J Epilepsy.* 1995;8(1):11–15.

18. Mameniskiene R, Wolf P. Epilepsia partialis continua: a review. *Seizure.* 2017;44:74–80.

19. Cockerell OC, Rothwell J, Thompson PD, Marsden CD, Shorvon SD. Clinical and physiological features of epilepsia partialis continua: cases ascertained in the UK. *Brain.* 1996;119(Pt 2):393–407.

20. Mameniskiene R, Bast T, Bentes C, et al. Clinical course and variability of non-Rasmussen, nonstroke motor and sensory epilepsia partialis continua: a European survey and analysis of 65 cases. *Epilepsia.* 2011;52(6):1168–1176.

21. Li H, Xue J, Qian P, et al. Electro-clinical-etiological associations of epilepsia partialis continua in 57 Chinese children. *Brain Dev.* 2017;39(6):506–514.

22. Holtkamp M, Meierkord H. Nonconvulsive status epilepticus: a diagnostic and therapeutic challenge in the intensive care setting. *Ther Adv Neurol Disord.* 2011;4(3):169–181.

23. Claassen J, Mayer SA, Kowalski RG, Emerson RG, Hirsch LJ. Detection of electrographic seizures with continuous EEG monitoring in critically ill patients. *Neurology.* 2004;62(10):1743–1748.

24. Fogang Y, Legros B, Depondt C, Mavroudakis N, Gaspard N. Yield of repeated intermittent EEG for seizure detection in critically ill adults. *Neurophysiol Clin.* 2017;47(1):5–12.

25. Johnson EL, Martinez NC, Ritzl EK. EEG characteristics of successful burst suppression for refractory status epilepticus. *Neurocrit Care.* 2016;25(3):407–414.

26. Kantanen AM, Reinikainen M, Parviainen I, Kalviainen R. Long-term outcome of refractory status epilepticus in adults: a retrospective population-based study. *Epilepsy Res.* 2017;133:13–21.

27. Kantanen AM, Kalviainen R, Parviainen I, et al. Predictors of hospital and one-year mortality in intensive care patients with

refractory status epilepticus: a population based study. *Crit Care.* 2017;21(1):71.

28. Cuero MR, Varelas PN. Super-refractory status epilepticus. *Curr Neurol Neurosci Rep.* 2015;15(11):74.

29. Delaj L, Novy J, Ryvlin P, Marchi NA, Rossetti AO. Refractory and super-refractory status epilepticus in adults: a 9-year cohort study. *Acta Neurol Scand.* 2017;135(1):92–99.

30. Costello DJ, Kilbride RD, Cole AJ. Cryptogenic new onset refractory status epilepticus (NORSE) in adults-infectious or not? *J Neurol Sci.* 2009;277(1–2):26–31.

31. Wilder-Smith EP, Lim EC, Teoh HL, et al. The NORSE (new-onset refractory status epilepticus) syndrome: defining a disease entity. *Ann Acad Med Singapore.* 2005;34 (7):417–420.

32. Cabrera Kang CM, Gaspard N, LaRoche SM, Foreman B. Survey of the diagnostic and therapeutic approach to new-onset refractory status epilepticus. *Seizure.* 2017;46:24–30.

33. Brophy GM, Bell R, Claassen J, et al. Guidelines for the evaluation and management of status epilepticus. *Neurocrit Care.* 2012;17(1):3–23.

34. Zaccara G, Giannasi G, Oggioni R, et al. Challenges in the treatment of convulsive status epilepticus. *Seizure.* 2017;47:17–24.

35. Patel SI, Birnbaum AK, Cloyd JC, Leppik IE. Intravenous and intramuscular formulations of antiseizure drugs in the treatment of epilepsy. *CNS Drugs.* 2015;29 (12):1009–1022.

36. Neurological Emergency Treatment Trials (NETT) Investigators: Silbergleit R, Lowenstein D, Durkalski V, Conwit R, RAMPART (Rapid Anticonvulsant Medication Prior to Arrival Trial): a double-blind randomized clinical trial of the efficacy of intramuscular midazolam versus intravenous lorazepam in the prehospital treatment of status epilepticus by paramedics. *Epilepsia.* 2011;52(Suppl 8):45–47.

37. Silbergleit R, Lowenstein D, Durkalski V, Conwit R, Investigators N. Lessons from the RAMPART study – and which is the best route of administration of benzodiazepines in status epilepticus. *Epilepsia.* 2013;54(Suppl 6):74–77.

38. Alldredge BK, Gelb AM, Isaacs SM, et al. A comparison of lorazepam, diazepam, and placebo for the treatment of out-of-hospital status epilepticus. *N Engl J Med.* 2001;345 (9):631–637.

39. Varelas PN, Spanaki MV, Mirski MA. Seizures and the neurosurgical intensive care unit. *Neurosurg Clin N Am.* 2013;24 (3):393–406.

40. Navarro V, Dagron C, Elie C, et al. Prehospital treatment with levetiracetam plus clonazepam or placebo plus clonazepam in status epilepticus (SAMUKeppra): a randomised, double-blind, phase 3 trial. *Lancet Neurol.* 2016;15 (1):47–55.

41. Treiman DM, Meyers PD, Walton NY, et al. A comparison of four treatments for generalized convulsive status epilepticus: Veterans Affairs Status Epilepticus Cooperative Study Group. *N Engl J Med.* 1998;339(12):792–798.

42. Agarwal P, Kumar N, Chandra R, et al. Randomized study of intravenous valproate and phenytoin in status epilepticus. *Seizure.* 2007;16(6):527–532.

43. Chakravarthi S, Goyal MK, Modi M, Bhalla A, Singh P. Levetiracetam versus phenytoin in management of status epilepticus. *J Clin Neurosci.* 2015;22(6):959–963.

44. Alvarez V, Januel JM, Burnand B, Rossetti AO. Second-line status epilepticus treatment: comparison of phenytoin, valproate, and levetiracetam. *Epilepsia.* 2011;52(7):1292–1296.

45. Garces M, Villanueva V, Mauri JA, et al. Factors influencing response to intravenous lacosamide in emergency situations: LACO-IV study. *Epilepsy Behav.* 2014;36:144–152.

46. Al-Mufti F, Claassen J. Neurocritical care: status epilepticus review. *Crit Care Clin.* 2014;30(4):751–764.

47. International Steering Committee of the StEp Audit: Ferlisi M, Hocker S, Grade M, Trinka E, Shorvon S. Preliminary results of the global audit of treatment of refractory

status epilepticus. *Epilepsy Behav.*
2015;49:318–324.

48. Grover EH, Nazzal Y, Hirsch LJ. Treatment
of convulsive status epilepticus. *Curr Treat
Options Neurol.* 2016;18(3):11.

49. Alvarez V, Lee JW, Drislane FW, et al.
Practice variability and efficacy of
clonazepam, lorazepam, and midazolam in
status epilepticus: a multicenter
comparison. *Epilepsia.* 2015;56
(8):1275–1285.

50. Hofler J, Rohracher A, Kalss G, et al. (S)-
ketamine in refractory and super-refractory
status epilepticus: a retrospective study.
CNS Drugs. 2016;30(9):869–876.

51. Alvarez V, Lee JW, Westover MB, et al.
Therapeutic coma for status epilepticus:

differing practices in a prospective
multicenter study. *Neurology.* 2016;87
(16):1650–1659.

52. Giovannini G, Monti G, Tondelli M, et al.
Mortality, morbidity and refractoriness
prediction in status epilepticus: comparison
of STESS and EMSE scores. *Seizure.*
2017;46:31–37.

53. Kang BS, Kim DW, Kim KK, et al.
Prediction of mortality and functional
outcome from status epilepticus and
independent external validation of STESS
and EMSE scores. *Crit Care.* 2016;20(1):25.

54. Pacha MS, Orellana L, Silva E, et al. Role of
EMSE and STESS scores in the outcome
evaluation of status epilepticus. *Epilepsy
Behav.* 2016;64(Pt A):140–142.

Chapter 11

EEG Instrumentation and Basics

Amit Ray and Naoum P. Issa

11.1 The Electroencephalogram Signal

The scalp electroencephalogram (EEG) signals detect the extracellular electrical field generated by the columns underneath the electrodes closer to the cortical surface and represent near-synchronous summated potentials (excitatory postsynaptic potential (EPSP) and inhibitory postsynaptic potential (IPSP)) generated by these columns of the cerebral cortex.[1–4]

Only a fraction of the activity generated by the cerebral cortex is seen on the scalp EEG. Due to the attenuating properties of the skull, most of the cortical EEG potentials do not produce a scalp EEG correlate.[5,6] Multiple factors determine whether a given potential produced at the cortex of the brain can be recorded by the scalp EEG (see box).

Major Determinants of Scalp EEG potential

- Cerebral Source Area
- Synchrony
- Dipole orientation
- Source depth
- Amplitude of individual cortical potentials
- Propagation and recruitment of potential.

11.1.1 Cerebral Source Area

The active area of cortex is among the most important determinants of whether a cortical electrical potential can be recorded on the scalp EEG. Early *in vitro* work by Cooper et al.[7] suggested that an area of 6 cm^2 of synchronously active cortex is needed to produce a recordable field on scalp electrodes. However, subsequent work[6,8,9] done using simultaneous scalp and intracranial EEG recordings demonstrated that this is probably the lower limit of area, i.e., while spikes involving an area of less than 6 cm^2 would never be seen, spikes are rarely seen unless a cortical area of the order of 10 cm^2 is activated. Additionally, prominent scalp EEG spikes require a much larger area of cortical activation, of the order of 20–30 cm^2 (Figure 11.1).

11.1.2 Synchrony

Aside from source area, synchrony is another important determinant of the scalp EEG potential. Again using simultaneous scalp and intracranial EEGs, it has been demonstrated

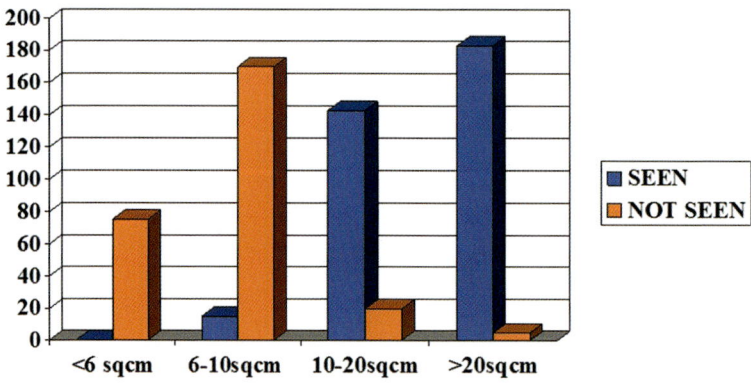

611 Spikes Analyzed

Figure 11.1 Scalp EEG spikes relative to intracranial source area. A total of 611 spikes were analyzed. No scalp spikes were seen if less than 6 cm² cortical source area was involved. Additionally, most cortical spikes with source area between 6 and 10 cm² were not seen on the scalp EEG. As the active cortical spike area increased, there was a greater chance for the spike to produce a visible scalp potential. Prominent scalp spikes were, however, seen only with activation of greater than 20 cm² of cortical surface. (Data summarized from reference 6).

that synchronously occurring cortical discharges will have a better chance of being visible on the scalp EEG than temporal distributed discharges.

11.1.3 Orientation

Source orientation is also a major determinant of the scalp EEG potential.[10] The electrical currents important to the EEG are oriented radially, along the pia-to-white-matter axis of the cerebral cortex. When electrical potentials are generated in gyri, which by definition run parallel to the skull, then the radially directed potentials can be detected by an overlying scalp EEG sensor.

The polarity of surface EEG depends on the location of synaptic activity within the cortical neurons. Synchronous excitation of numerous afferent inputs into the dendritic layer leads to entry of positive charges at the synapse, causing negative charges in the extracellular space near it and positive charges at a more distant site. This separation of charge along the vertical main dendrite creates a "vertical dipole." This dipole generates an electrical field projecting out, wherein the deflection of the pen appears opposite: negative (upward) deflection indicates superficial excitatory or deep inhibitory inputs, and positive (downward) deflection signifies deep excitatory or superficial inhibitory inputs.

If, however, the currents are generated in the walls of sulci, which are orthogonal to the skull, then the relevant potentials would not be detectable by the immediately overlying EEG sensor. These potentials can produce "horizontal dipoles," which might be detected in distant EEG sensors or could be detected by magnetoencephalography (MEG) because of the magnetic field induced by electrical currents.[11,12]

The orientation of adjacent sources (e.g., groups of pyramidal neurons) can modify the amplitude of the scalp EEG signal as well. If neighboring sources are similarly oriented, there will likely be a summation of the source voltages and a higher possibility of them generating a scalp EEG potential. However, if the sources are oriented in opposite

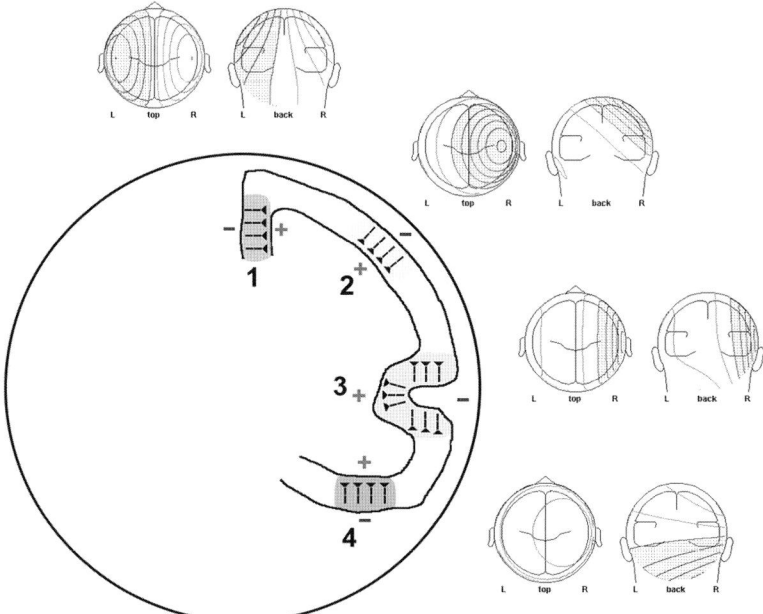

Figure 11.2 Effect of source orientation on scalp EEG potential. Four representative cortical EEG potentials are seen (Adapted with permission from Ebersole JS. Cortical generators and EEG voltage fields. In: Ebersole JS, Pedley TA, eds. *Current Practice of Clinical Electroencephalography*, 3rd edn. Philadelphia: Lippincott Williams & Wilkins; 2003:12–31).

directions, the individual potentials will likely cancel out, resulting in no potentials being seen on the scalp EEG electrode, just above it (Figure 11.2).

11.1.4 Additional Factors

The depth of the electric source, amplitude of the individual cortical potentials, and propagation and recruitment of sufficient cortex by electrical potentials are other factors that potentially determine if a given cortical potential will be seen on the scalp EEG.

The contribution of deep sources to the scalp EEG potential is being increasingly recognized. Electrical signals from deep sources travel through the brain in two general ways: volume conduction and propagation through neuronal transmission.[13–16] Volume conduction is simply the electrical field in a three-dimensional conductor induced by a voltage step (that is, a brain discharge). The voltage changes from volume conduction happen nearly instantaneously (at the speed of light), and fall off in intensity with the square of the distance from the source ($V \propto 1/r^2$). As a result, the amplitude of the volume-conducted voltage signal from a deep source is very small compared to the amplitude of a superficial source. This is despite the shielding effect of the skull, which is hypothesized to affect superficial discharges more than deep discharges.[1,17] Deep sources are influenced by similar factors to superficial sources, namely source area, synchrony, orientation, propagation, and amplitude.

An important deep source of abnormal EEG potentials is the hippocampus. Given its anatomy, with neurons and fields oriented opposite to each other, very little (if any) purely hippocampal electrical activity is seen on the scalp EEG. The primary mechanism by which discharges originating in deep sources reach the scalp is propagation through neuronal transmission, and this is how hippocampal discharges most commonly affect the scalp EEG. When hippocampal discharges propagate and subsequently recruit a sufficient number of neurons in the basal temporal cortex, activity can be seen on the scalp EEG.[1,18,19] Given the orientation of neurons in the basal temporal cortex, discharges are best seen over the subtemporal (as opposed to the standard temporal) electrodes with positive maxima over the vertex.[20] Orientation and determination of negative and positive scalp EEG maxima are important for pinpointing these actual source generators.[21] Because axonal propagation and neurotransmission are not instantaneous, these scalp discharges are delayed by many milliseconds compared to the original hippocampal discharges.

11.2 Scalp EEG Recording Techniques

Now that we have discussed some of the determinants of the scalp EEG potential we can proceed to a brief overview of EEG recordings, electrode placement, and localization.

11.2.1 10-20 Electrode Placement System

Initially proposed by Jasper in 1958,[22] the 10-20 electrode placement system is the most commonly used system for placement of scalp EEG electrodes (Figure 11.3). It is a standardized and reproducible system with consistent use across time and geography. This system is based on the relationship between the location of an electrode and the underlying area of the cerebral cortex. Typically using 21 electrodes, the electrode sites are thought to provide accurate voltage recordings of similar underlying anatomic structures regardless of skull size and shape. The "10" and "20" refer to the fact that the electrode positions are at either 10% or 20% of the total front–back or right–left distance at homologous points of the skull.[23] While ensuring a high level of standardization, the 10-20 system does have its drawbacks. The relatively large interelectrode distance is recognized as one of the main negatives of this system. While historically this electrode placement system has served us well, in this current era of high-resolution brain imaging when it has become imperative, especially from the standpoint of epilepsy surgery, to localize epileptogenic foci as accurately as possible, this may lead to imperfect localization. Additionally, the incomplete

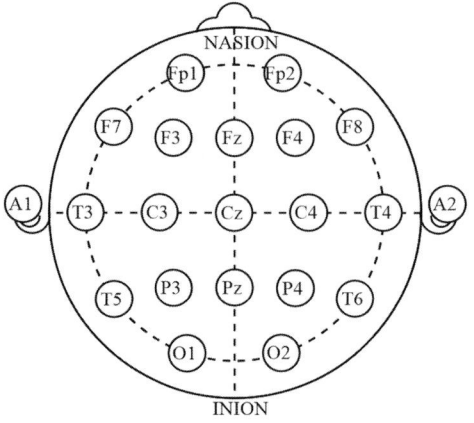

Figure 11.3 Electrodes in the commonly used 10-20 system of electrode placement.

coverage of important areas especially in the subtemporal region (which as we have seen before is responsible for recording scalp EEG abnormalities in cases with mesial temporal lobe epilepsy) may lead to incorrect diagnoses and localizations. The nonintuitive and relatively arbitrary nature of the numbering of the electrodes is also a known drawback of this system.

11.2.2 10-10 Electrode Placement

Proposed by Chatrian et al. in 1985,[24] this system attempts to overcome some of the drawbacks of the 10-20 system. Using 81 electrodes, the interelectrode distances are reduced to 10% of the distance between homologous points on the skull, leading to a higher electrode density,[25–28] which in turn may improve localization (Figure 11.4). Additionally, the nomenclature of electrodes is more intuitive, with electrode positions along the same sagittal line having the same number and electrodes along the same coronal line having the same letter (Fp1/Fp2, O1/O2 being exceptions). An additional row of subtemporal electrodes 10% below the standard temporal electrodes may also help better localize mesial temporal epileptogenic foci. The new "modified combinatorial system" substitutes the T3/T4 and T5/T6 terms with consistent T7/T8 and P7/P8 terms. In some centers, high-density electrode placement systems using as many as 300 electrode positions (e.g., 10-5 system) are also being used.[29–31]

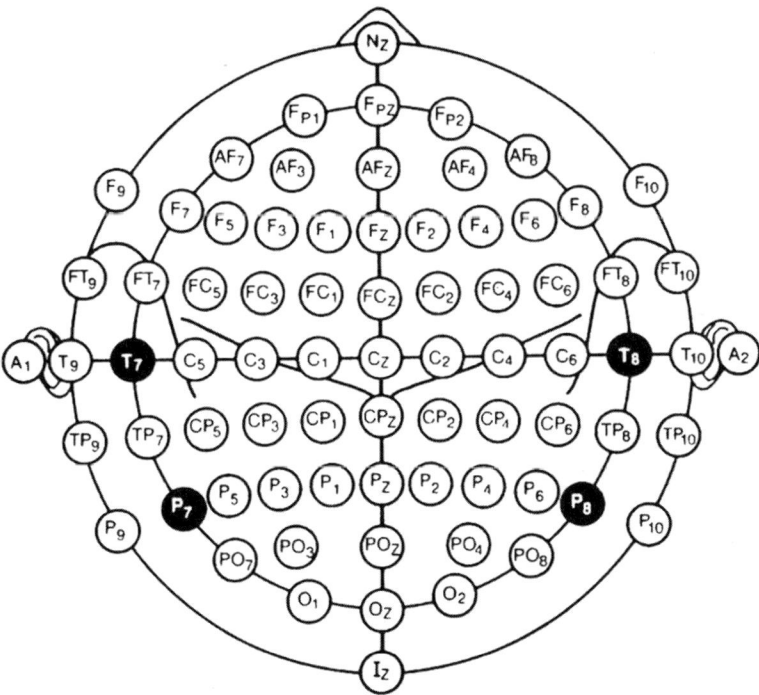

Figure 11.4 Electrodes in the 10-10 system of electrode placement. Note the much more densely placed electrodes with smaller interelectrode distances. Additionally T3 and T4 are changed to T7 and T8, and T5 and T6 to P7 and P8, respectively.

11.2.3 Polarity and Recording Conventions

EEG recordings are based on the principle of differential amplification with rejection of common mode noise. The scalp EEG potential that is seen is the difference between the two inputs at the amplifier. Convention designates that electrode symbols separated by a dash represent electrodes connected to the two amplifier inputs with the first electrode connected to input 1 and the second to input 2, e.g., Fp2-F8 designates Fp2 as input 1 and F8 as input 2. If input 1 is more negative than input 2, then by convention, an upward (negative) deflection is seen (Fp2 is more negative than F8 in the aforementioned example). On the other hand if input 2 is more negative than input 1, then downward (positive) deflection is seen (F8 is more negative than Fp2 in the aforementioned example, Figure 11.5).

11.3 Electrode Montages

Montages are specific combinations of EEG channels arranged to represent EEG activity simultaneously across the entire scalp in a logical way to represent three-dimensional source data with two-dimensional EEG traces. Montages can be classified as bipolar or referential. Bipolar montages have a different electrode connected to input 2 of the amplifier at each channel in a series. However, adjacent channels in a series have 1 electrode in common. The electrode connected to input 2 of the first channel will be serially connected to input 1 at the second channel, and so on. Bipolar montages can be arranged longitudinally (common double banana montage, Figure 11.6) or coronally (transverse montage, Figure 11.7). Bipolar montages emphasize the spatial gradient of a signal, meaning they are most useful for identifying the origin of highly focal discharges, at the expense of poor detection of signals with broad spatial fields.

A referential montage has different electrodes connecting to input 1 of the amplifiers but a common reference input connected to input 2 (Figure 11.8). This common reference can be a single electrode (e.g. Cz reference, as in Figure 11.8), or it can be the result of a combination of electrodes (e.g., linked ear reference A1-A2). The choice of reference electrode has been a source of considerable controversy among electroencephalographers. Given the fact that traditional EEG interpretation has focused on spikes only as a negative potential, the electrode chosen as the reference electrode was supposed to be an inactive electrode (typically as distant as possible from the potential of interest). However, with recognition that EEG spikes are dipolar, i.e., have positive and negative maxima, it is now accepted that in the head no given area can be truly inactive. The choice of a particular

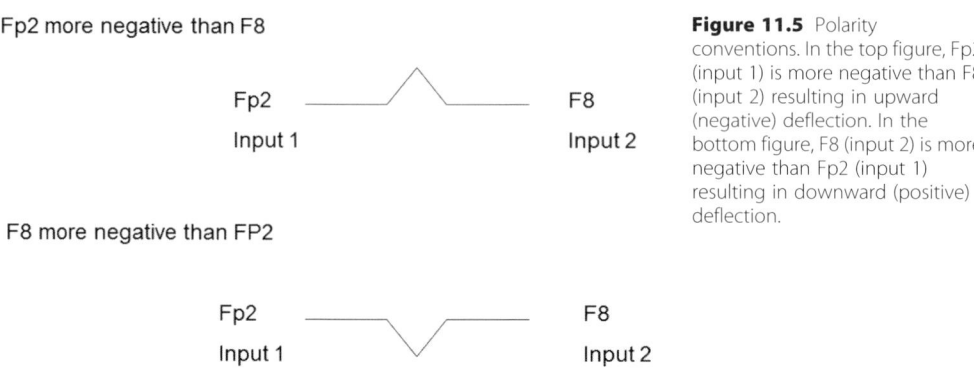

Fp2 more negative than F8

Fp2 ———⋀——— F8

Input 1　　　　　Input 2

F8 more negative than FP2

Fp2 ———⋁——— F8

Input 1　　　　　Input 2

Figure 11.5 Polarity conventions. In the top figure, Fp2 (input 1) is more negative than F8 (input 2) resulting in upward (negative) deflection. In the bottom figure, F8 (input 2) is more negative than Fp2 (input 1) resulting in downward (positive) deflection.

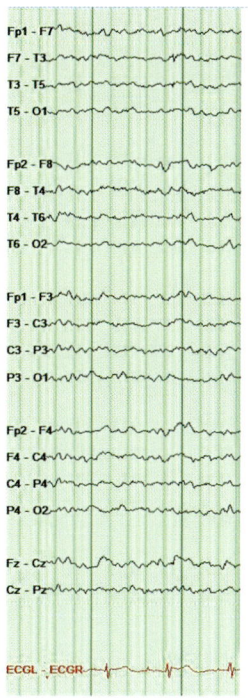

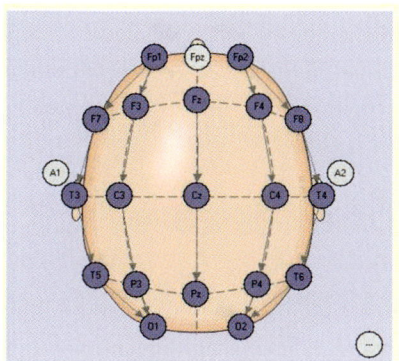

Figure 11.6 Longitudinal bipolar montage, commonly known as the double banana montage. Adjacent channels in a series have 1 electrode in common. Input 2 in the first channel becomes input 1 in the next channel and so on.

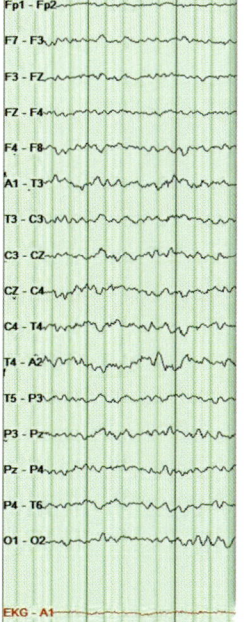

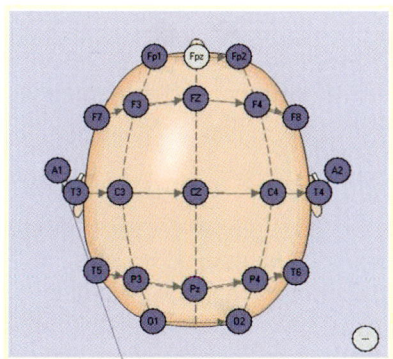

Figure 11.7 Transverse bipolar montage. Electrodes are connected coronally across the head in a left-to-right fashion.

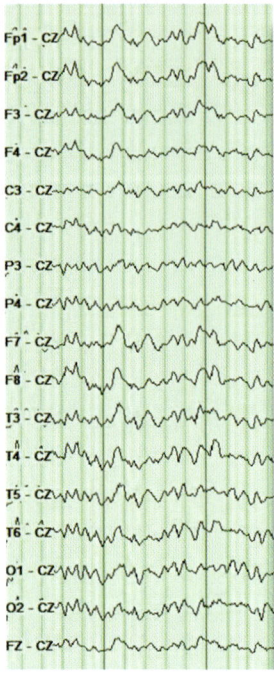

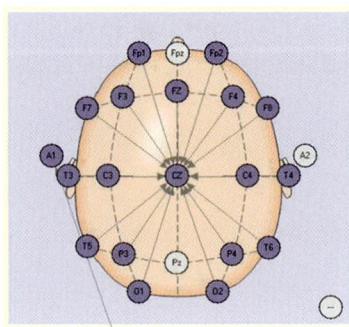

Figure 11.8 Referential montage. Different electrodes connect to input 1 of the amplifiers, but a common reference input is connected to input 2, in this case the Cz electrode – known as a Cz reference montage.

electrode as reference, thus, may only influence the appearance of the potential on the EEG, and if properly interpreted, any electrode can be chosen as the reference electrode. The Laplacian montage is a special type of reference montage in which input 2 is the result of a combination of the surrounding electrodes to the electrode connected to input 1. The common average reference is another referential montage in which input 2 is the average of all electrode potentials recorded from the head. If this resultant potential is now considered as the reference zero potential, then both the maximum negative and positive fields will be appropriately emphasized. As a result, the average referential montage is thought to give the best estimate of signal amplitude in any EEG channel.[32,33]

11.3.1 Localization in Bipolar and Referential Montages

While a detailed discussion of the principles of localization is outside the scope of this chapter, some general principles will be mentioned here.

In bipolar montages, localization of the area of maximum negativity (or positivity) is achieved using the principle of phase reversals. A phase reversal is defined as two channels within a chain of electrodes (each adjacent channel sharing one electrode) in which the EEG deflection is in the opposite direction. Channels in which the deflections point towards each other are defined as negative phase reversals, and those where the deflections point away from each other are described as positive phase reversals (Figure 11.9A and B). In the case of a negative phase reversal, the common electrode between the two channels is the area of maximal negative potential (or minimal positivity as compared to the noncommon electrodes). Similarly, with a positive phase reversal, the common electrode between the two channels is the area of maximal positive potential (or minimal negative potential, as

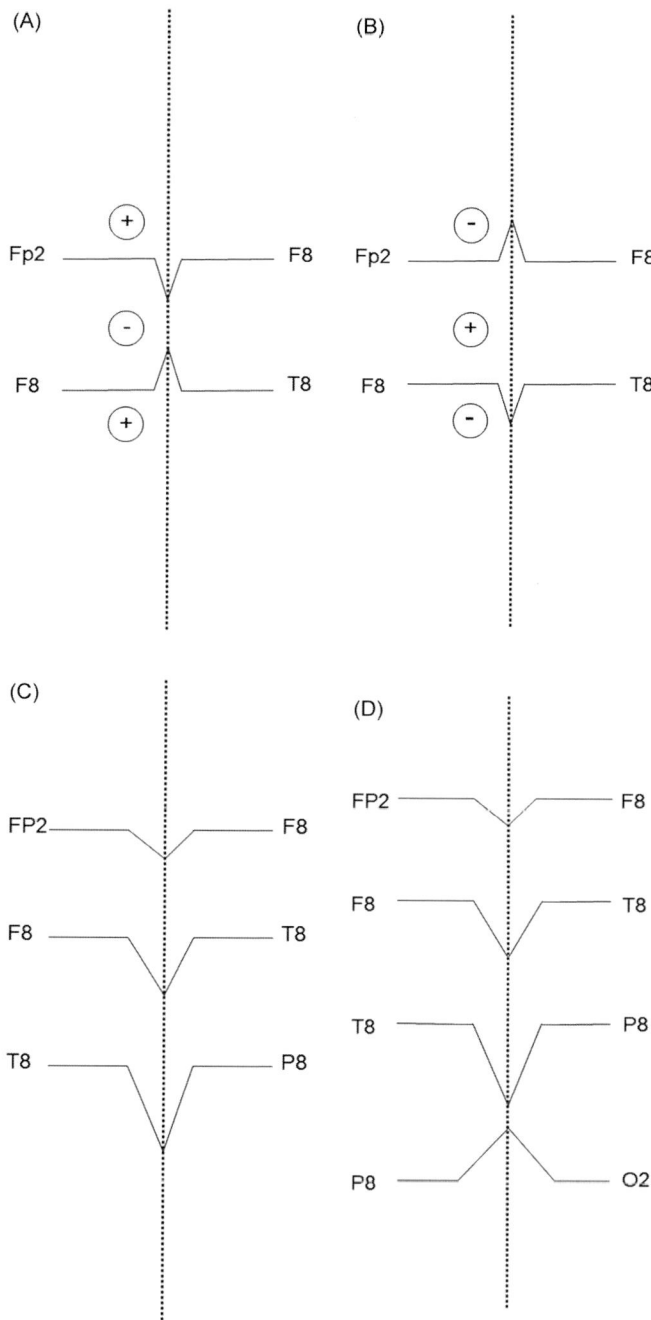

Figure 11.9 Localization in bipolar montage using phase reversals. Part (A) demonstrates a negative phase reversal. In this example, F8 is more negative than Fp2 and F8 is also more negative than T8. A negative phase reversal is seen at F8, which is the common electrode and also the electrode with maximal negative potential. Part (B) demonstrates a positive phase reversal. F8 is more positive than Fp2 and also more positive than T8. A positive phase reversal is seen at F8, which is the common electrode and also the electrode with maximal positive potential. Part (C) demonstrates a bipolar montage in which no phase reversal is seen, suggesting the maximal negative (or positive) potential is at the end of the chain, in this case it is at P8 or beyond. Part (D) shows the same potential as (C) with an additional channel P8-O2 showing a negative phase reversal at P8, suggesting that P8 is the electrode with the maximal negative potential.

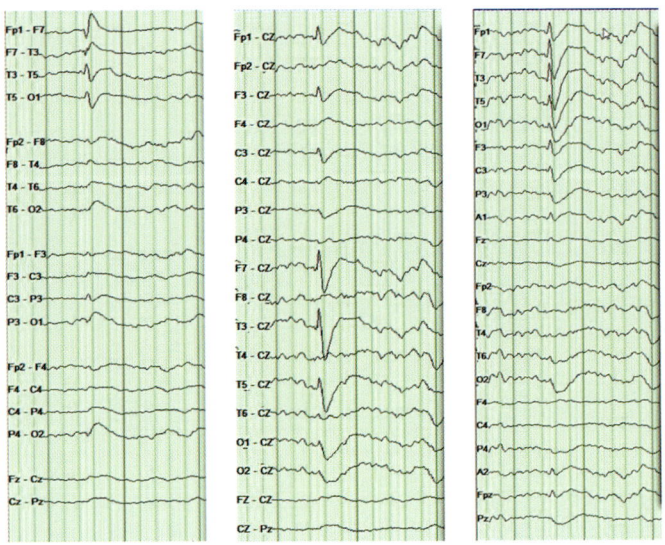

Figure 11.10 Left temporal spike seen on longitudinal bipolar (left panel), Cz reference (center panel) and common average reference (right panel) montages. Negative phase reversal is seen at the F7-T3 channel, suggesting that these are the electrodes with the maximal negative potential. The same is corroborated with the Cz referential montages, which show maximal negative potentials at the F7 and T3 electrodes.

compared to the noncommon electrodes). However, in cases in which there is no phase reversal seen, the area of maximal negativity (or positivity) is located at the end of a chain of electrodes (Figure 11.9C and D).[34]

In a referential montage on the other hand, the areas of maximal negativity and positivity are determined by the amplitude of the potential. The area of maximal negative potential is at the channel with the largest negative amplitude (upward deflection on EEG) and the area of maximal positive potential is at the channel with the largest positive amplitude (downward deflection on EEG), relative to the chosen reference potential (Figure 11.10). As discussed earlier, altering the reference may change the appearance of this potential[1] (but not the actual potential itself).

11.4 Digitization

In the modern age of electrophysiology, all signals are captured on a digital system, meaning a computer. In the predigital era, signal measurements were "analog," so the signals could vary smoothly and could be measured at an arbitrarily high precision depending on the physical properties of the measurement system (e.g., the mass of the pens used to mark the EEG paper). Digital signal acquisition differs from analog in many important ways, and if the analog-to-digital conversion (ADC) is not done properly, then electrophysiological signals will be degraded. Fortunately, EEG machine manufacturers take care of the ADC to avoid these problems, but it is important for clinicians to know what has been done to the signals in order to interpret the data correctly. Here are some typical questions that come up in practice: Our EEG machine samples at 250 Hz (samples per second), what is the highest frequency I can read on the EEG? The high frequency filter is set at 15 Hz, why can I count oscillations at 18 Hz? Our EEG software shows a time constant not a cut-off frequency, how are they related?

11.4.1 Analog-to-Digital Conversion

Analog electrical signals can have any amplitude and fluctuate at any frequency, but computers can store only limited ranges of voltage amplitude and frequency. The wider the range of amplitudes and frequencies needed and the more precisely signals are sampled, the more computer memory and processing power is needed. The first step in converting an analog electrical signal to a digital signal is, therefore, to rescale the incoming signal to match the range that a computer can easily capture and store.

11.4.2 Pre-sampling Amplification

Raw EEG signals are amplified before digital sampling by a preamplifier, or "preamp." Typical EEG signals have amplitudes in the range of 1–100 µV, small enough to be significantly affected by noise introduced by an analog-to-digital converter. When the signal is amplified by the preamp, it becomes large enough that the noise introduced at ADC is small compared to the signal.

In clinical EEG systems the electrodes on the scalp are passive (no circuitry in them) and the preamps (one for each scalp electrode) are in a box connected to the electrodes by wires. If the wires move, an artifact is introduced, and because the unamplified EEG signals are small, these artifacts can be large in comparison. In research EEG systems active electrodes are often used. Active electrodes have the preamp built into the electrode. As a result, the amplified EEG signal is much larger than any noise introduced by movement of wires after the electrode. At the time of this writing, active electrodes (and wireless signal transmission) are on the verge of being approved for use in the clinical setting.

11.4.3 Low-pass Filtering Based on the Nyquist Criterion

The second processing step before ADC is filtering out high frequencies (or "low-pass filtering"). The higher the frequency in a signal that is of interest, the more quickly the computer needs to sample and the more data it needs to store. Harry Nyquist of Bell Laboratories developed the theory that specifies how often a signal needs to be sampled (the sampling rate) to preserve information about high frequencies.[35,36] The Nyquist criterion requires sampling at more than twice the highest frequency in an analog signal.

Nyquist criterion: Sampling rate $> 2 \times$ highest frequency in the signal

For example, to capture a 1 Hz signal, the Nyquist criterion requires that the signal be sampled more than twice a second. The more densely a signal is sampled, the better it can be reconstructed. Sampling at 10 samples/s produces a much better representation of a 1 Hz signal than would sampling at 3 samples/s. It is because of the Nyquist criterion that EEG machines sample at 250 samples/s or more despite the clinical frequencies of interest in scalp EEG ranging from 1 to ~40 Hz.

So why do high frequencies need to be filtered out of the signal before ADC? If frequencies above the Nyquist cutoff are not removed before sampling, low frequencies that do not exist in the original signal will be erroneously inserted into the digitized data (Figure 11.11, bottom left and bottom right panels). This distortion is known as "aliasing" and aliasing cannot be reversed after sampling. There are many examples of aliasing in everyday life, and it is most easily observed in car commercials, where spinning wheels can look stationary or even appear to rotate backwards. In these commercials, TV images are taken at about 60 frames per second, but a hubcap spoke appears at the top of the wheel about 100 times a second. The video does not capture all the different phases of the wheel rotation, but catches just the ones that make it look like its rotating much more slowly than it actually is. The same thing can happen with EEG signals – a high frequency signal sampled too infrequently will look like a

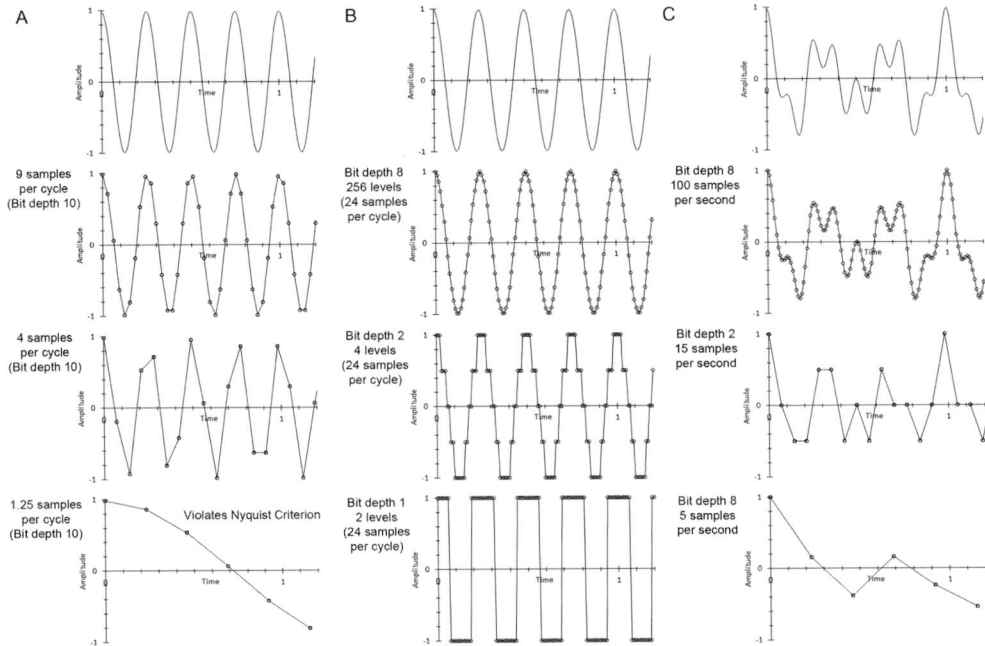

Figure 11.11 How ADC sampling parameters affect data quality. (A) The effect of sampling frequency on data quality. The top curve is the original signal to be sampled. The middle two traces show the sampled signal with sampling rates that are above the Nyquist frequency; the higher the sampling rate, the better the quality of the recording. The bottom trace shows the effect of sampling below the Nyquist frequency; the sampled signal looks like a low-frequency signal and bears no similarity to the original signal. (B) The effect of bit depth on signal quality is shown in the middle column. The smaller the bit depth, the fewer levels of the original signal are captured. The first iteration of ADCs had a bit depth of 8; modern systems have bit depths of 16. (C) The effect of sampling parameters on acquisition of unfiltered, complex waveforms. The original waveform is shown in the top panel. A well-sampled signal is shown in the second panel. A poorly sampled signal, with a low sampling rate and low bit depth, is shown in the third panel. A high bit depth cannot compensate for a low sampling rate, as shown in the bottom panel. Symbols show individual digital samples.

very low frequency signal. To avoid aliasing, it is necessary to remove any frequencies from the original signal that are too fast for the analog-to-digital converter. For example, if the computer samples at 1000 samples/s, any frequency at or above 500 Hz needs to be filtered out prior to the ADC. EEG machines typically filter signals above ~1/3 the sampling frequency (for 1000 samples/s the filter should attenuate frequencies greater than ~333 Hz). This filtering is usually fixed by the manufacturer and is not changed by the clinician.

11.4.4 High-Pass Frequency Filtering

Very low frequencies must also be removed from a signal before digitization. ADCs have a limited range of voltages they can digitize. If signals drift slowly over the course of the day, they will fall out of the range of voltages the ADC can handle. For example, if the voltage on an electrode fluctuates around 0 mV at the beginning of a recording session, it will be easily digitized by an ADC with an operating range of ± 5 mV, but if the average voltage decreases by 1 mV every minute, eventually it will be less than –5 mV and the ADC will only register –5 mV with no fluctuations. This kind of drift happens for a lot of reasons, like sweating or slow changes in the electrodes. To eliminate this, low-frequency changes in the signal need to be removed before digitization, because low frequencies are attenuated and high frequencies are preserved by this filtering, it is known as "high-pass filtering." EEG signals are typically high-pass filtered at ~0.1 Hz prior to digitization.

11.4.5 Bit Depth

The precision at which a signal is digitized is determined by the "bit depth" of the ADC (Figure 11.11B). If an ADC had a bit depth of 1, it would only be able to characterize the amplitude of a signal as High or Low. The greater the bit depth, the more levels can be used to describe the amplitude. In the early days of digital sampling, ADCs had a bit depth of 8, which would allow 256 levels (2^8 levels). Modern EEG ADCs usually have a bit depth of 16, allowing 65,536 levels (2^{16} levels). The "least significant bit" gives the exact precision of the sampling. For example, if a 16-bit ADC can convert signals between –5 mV and +5 mV, the "least significant bit" means that each level represents 0.15 µV (10 mV/65,536 samples).

11.4.6 Post-processing

One major benefit of digital systems is that after acquisition, signals can be processed without changing the stored data. In old analog EEG systems, in which traces were written directly on paper, the format of the EEG could not be changed. Remnants of this protocol can be found in modern digital EEGs. For example, classically trained EEG technicians still change montages at intervals while an EEG is being recorded, even though the montage can be easily changed at any point while reading a digital EEG. The most frequently used processing tools are temporal frequency filters, so these will be reviewed.

11.4.7 Temporal Filtering

Filters remove certain frequencies from a signal. This allows contaminants of a signal to be subtracted out if the frequency of the contaminant is known. For example, electrical energy is transmitted through the electrical grid with a current that alternates at 60 Hz in the United States (50 Hz in Europe), so filtering out 60 Hz (50 Hz) signals in an EEG removes most of the electrical noise from nearby electrical appliances.

The basic principle behind filtering comes from Fourier theory, which posits that any time-varying signal can be constructed from the sum of sine waves of different frequencies, amplitudes, and phases. When we talk about the frequencies in a signal, we are talking about the frequencies of the sine waves that are summed together to generate the overall signal. For example, in an EEG with an alpha-range posterior dominant rhythm (PDR), the signals in O1 or O2 are composed of sine waves with a wide range of frequencies (from 1 to 70 Hz in a typical EEG system), but the largest amplitude sine waves in the signal have a frequency around 10 Hz. If there is a large amount of electrical noise at 60 Hz in the signal, the PDR might be masked. Subtracting out the 60 Hz noise through filtering unmasks the underlying PDR (Figure 11.12).

In clinical practice we use three types of filtering. High-pass filters remove frequencies below the cutoff frequency, preserving higher frequencies. Standard high-pass cutoff frequencies in EEG range between 0.3 and 1.6 Hz. The cutoff frequency (F_{CO}) can be specified in one of two ways. In the simplest way, F_{CO} is specified in Hz such that sine waves with a frequency below the cutoff are attenuated strongly, and sine waves with a frequency above the cutoff are not attenuated much. The second way to specify a filter cutoff is by giving a time constant (t_{RC}). This is typically used for high-pass filters. The conversion from time

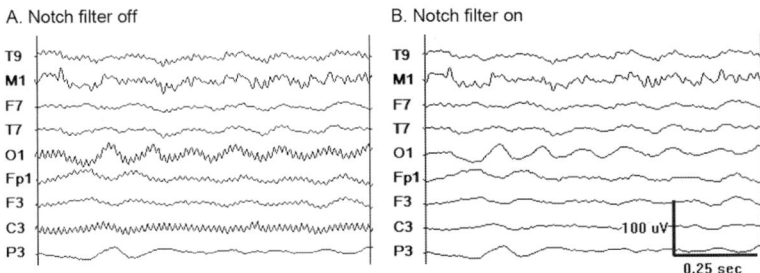

A. Notch filter off

B. Notch filter on

Figure 11.12 The effect of notch filtering on signals. (A) The unfiltered signal shows a weak alpha frequency in O1 with superimposed 60-Hz electrical line artifact. (B) Implementing the 60-Hz notch filter removes the line-associated noise and makes the background brain signal clearer.

constant to cutoff frequency comes from electrical engineering, where filters are constructed by putting resistors and capacitors together in a circuit (resistor-capacitor (RC) circuit) and measuring how long it takes for current to decay after a voltage step (characterized by the time constant). The conversion from t_{RC} to F_{CO} used in clinical practice is:

$$F_{CO} = 1/(2\pi t_{RC})$$

The second type of filtering is low-pass filtering, in which frequencies below the cutoff frequency are preserved, but higher frequencies are attenuated. This is useful for reducing quickly varying distortions, like electromyography (EMG) signals from muscle contraction. Clinically useful low-pass cutoff frequencies for scalp EEG are between 40 and 70 Hz. Although some clinicians use a low-pass cutoff of 15 Hz, such a low cutoff can lead to problems interpreting signals; for example, when low-pass filtered at 15 Hz, a chewing artifact can look like 3-Hz spike-and-wave discharges.

The third type of filtering used is a notch filter. The notch filter removes only a narrow range of frequencies, and is most useful when the exact frequency of a contaminant is known. A 60 Hz (50 Hz) notch filter can be used to attenuate electrical noise.

A filter is never perfect, so it cannot completely eliminate power at a frequency, and it often distorts the waveform of frequencies around the cutoff frequency. As a result, it is better to set filter cutoffs far from the frequencies of interest rather than to allow only the frequencies of interest through.

11.5 Sources of Noise

A variety of noncerebral electrical signals can contaminate EEG signals. The most prominent contaminants are usually line noise (60- or 50-Hz noise from electrical lines, discussed above), wire movement, and the signals of the electrocardiogram (EKG) and EMG. However, there are other common but more subtle contaminants that can affect EEG interpretation.

11.5.1 High-Impedance Electrodes

EEG voltages are detected as currents flowing into metal electrodes, and good electrical conductivity between an electrode and the scalp is needed for small signals to be detected. Resistance is the classic metric that describes how a medium conducts electricity; a good conductor has a low resistance and a poor conductor has a high resistance. Impedance is similar to resistance but is measured with an alternating voltage rather than a constant voltage. This is important because the interface between the electrode and the scalp is not a pure resistor; rather it has both resistive and capacitive components (a RC circuit). This means that with any change in voltage the resulting current decays with a time constant determined by the RC components, naturally acting to filter out frequencies from the signal. To account for this filtering, impedance rather than resistance is measured during EEG calibration procedures. To measure impedance, a small alternating voltage (usually at 1000 Hz) is applied across the electrode–scalp interface and the current generated is measured. A low-impedance interface would have a large current in response to the applied voltage, while a high-impedance interface would have a small current.

Impedance, like resistance, is measured in ohms. Good electrode–scalp connections have an impedance of less than 5 kohms. Because the capacitor in the circuit cannot easily be changed, high-impedance connections are fixed by resetting the electrode with a conducting gel between the electrode and the scalp to reduce the resistance. However, this needs to be done carefully, because if too much gel is used, it can bridge neighboring electrodes ("short-circuiting" the electrodes), putting them at the same voltage and making them redundant.

In summary, high-impedance electrode connections degrade signals, and when impedance is very high (that is when the electrode is not connected to the scalp), it can introduce arbitrary and large artifacts into a recording.

11.5.2 1/f Noise and Scalp Attenuation

The amplitude of brain activity tends to be larger at low frequencies than at high frequencies. Signal amplitudes decrease in proportion with the frequency, meaning, on average, amplitude $\propto$ 1/frequency.[37] This relationship is called "1/f noise" for short and is not unique to the brain. With an almost magical flavor, 1/f noise is found in all sorts of natural and artificial systems, from how people sway while standing on a platform, to the length of scenes in movies, to stock market fluctuations.[38] Change is larger at low frequencies than at high frequencies.

The practical implication of 1/f noise is that low frequencies are easier to detect on scalp EEG than high frequencies. This is compounded by the degradation of EEG signals as they cross from brain tissue through dura, skull, and skin. Estimates of this attenuation vary from 10–30-fold,[39,40] and the attenuation appears reasonably constant across all frequencies. Because brain activity at high frequencies is smaller in amplitude than at low frequencies, the attenuation at the scalp makes signals with a frequency above ~40 Hz small enough that they are easily buried in noise on a scalp EEG.

11.6 EEG and Electrical Safety

EEG in general is a very safe procedure; however, there are small but definite risks, with potentially serious consequences, associated with this procedure. Injuries due to EEG can range from skin burns at the site of the electrode to more devastating consequences like cardiac arrhythmias and, rarely, even death. Electric current intensity (amperes), and not voltage, is the major factor responsible for injuries during the EEG. For example, a shock of 10,000 volts which drives only 10 milliampere (mA) through the body is less severe than a shock of 100 volts that drives 1 A through the body. While any amount of current over

10 mA is capable of producing painful-to-severe shock with tetanic muscle contractions, currents above 100 mA are potentially lethal. Currents as low as 20 mA may cause labored breathing, with cessation of respirations at about 75 mA. Table 11.1[1,41] summarizes the effects of various current intensities on humans. However, these thresholds have been established for normal individuals. Sick patients may have higher susceptibility to ill effects of electrical injury, secondary to their current debility as well as other factors discussed below.

11.6.1 Macroshock versus Microshock

Macroshock is a perceptible sensation that occurs when there is direct contact between an individual and the power supply resulting in the individual receiving a high intensity current. This situation is rare, albeit possible, in patients undergoing an EEG, especially if the EEG machine is improperly grounded. In case of a spark or fault in the machine, the current can leak into the EEG chassis (if the patient touches the metal chassis) then conduct into the ground through the patient, on occasion via the heart, which may be potentially fatal (Figure 11.13 A and B). However, of even greater importance in the EEG patient is microshock, which is low-intensity electric current that may pass through a strategic organ like the heart through a low-resistance pathway like a central line or transvenous catheter and result in a fatal cardiac arrhythmia.[42-44]

Besides current intensity, additional factors that might influence the extent of injury include current frequency, duration, point of entry, and patient body weight.

11.6.2 Grounding

Improper grounding of EEG equipment can result in both macroshock and microschock to the patient. It is for this reason that it is key to connect EEG machines to hospital-grade ground receptacles labeled appropriately so, typically with a green dot.[45,46] Additionally, to avoid the problem of double grounding, all electrical devices need to be connected to a common ground connection. Given that no two grounds are at identical voltage, current may flow between the two grounds through the patient, also known as a ground loop.

Table 11.1 Effects at various current intensities at 60 Hz for 1 s

Current Intensity	Effect
0.1 mA	Ventricular fibrillation if applied directly to the heart
0.3 mA	Sensory threshold
1.0 mA	Pain threshold
5 mA	Maximal harmless level
15 mA	Tetany
50 mA	Tissue injury
100 mA	Ventricular fibrillation/death

Adapted with permission from Ebersole JS. Cortical generators and EEG voltage fields. In: Ebersole JS, Pedley TA, eds. Current Practice of Clinical Electroencephalography. 3rd ed. Philadelphia: Lippincott Williams & Wilkins; 2003:12-31[1] and Tyner FS, Knott JR, Mayer WB. Fundamentals of EEG technology: basic concepts and methods. Philadelphia: Raven Press; 1983.

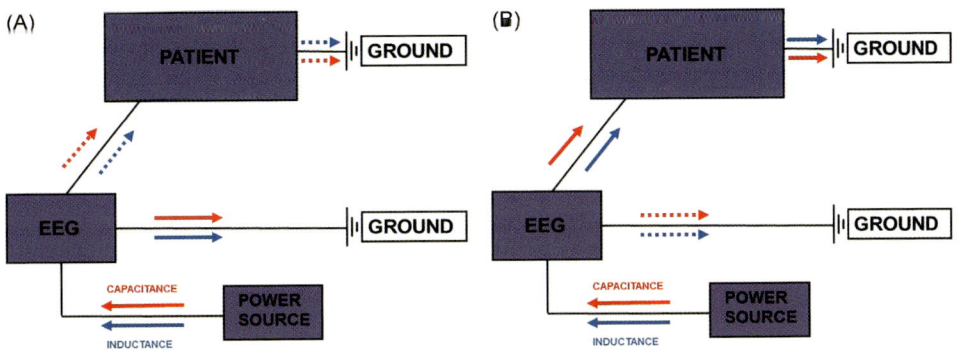

Figure 11.13 Role of a ground electrode in electrical safety during EEG recordings. Part (A) illustrates an EEG machine with an intact and well-functioning ground. Any leakage capacitance (red) or inductance (blue) currents or current that leaks into the chassis of the EEG machine as a result of sparking or faults in the EEG machine are conducted to the ground through the intact ground contact (solid arrows) and no current is conducted through the patient (dashed arrows). However, in case of malfunctioning of the ground contact attached to the EEG machine (B), currents may go through the path of least resistance to the ground via the patient (solid arrows), resulting in injury, while no electrode flows to the EEG ground contact (dashed arrows).

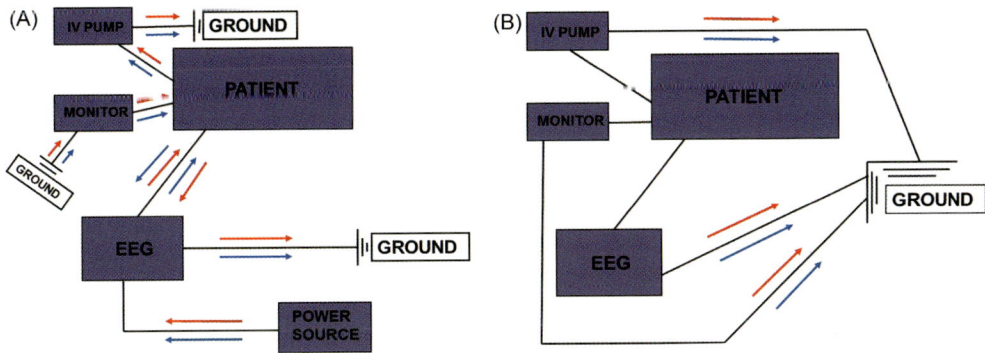

Figure 11.14 This schematic illustrates the importance of maintaining a common ground. In (A), the EEG machine, the intravenous pump, and the monitor are all attached to the patient as well as to different ground electrodes (double grounding), which do not have exactly identical voltage potentials. This potential difference between grounds creates ground loops that cause currents to flow between the individual ground electrodes (often through the patient). These currents may again be secondary to faults in the machine, or capacitance (red) or inductance (blue) currents. This problem of double grounding and resultant ground loops can be eliminated by ensuring that all electric equipment connected to the patient is connected to a common (B), functioning, hospital-grade ground electrode.

Avoiding ground loops is especially important in cases where multiple devices, often invasive, are connected to the patient, which is often the situation in intensive care units (Figure 11.14).

11.6.3 Leakage Currents

Leakage current is stray current that builds up on electrical equipment and is secondary to the inherent flow of current from the live electrical parts of an appliance or instrument to the accessible metal casing or parts. These can be mainly divided into capacitive and inductive currents. Capacitive currents are generated by multiple power sources, e.g., the EEG power cord, electrical mains wiring, etc. The alternating current running in the live wire of the power cord connecting the EEG machine generates capacitive currents in neutral and ground wires. Normally this leakage current is shunted directly to the ground contact and the patient is not harmed. However, in the absence of a well-functioning ground, such current may flow through the patient. While the magnitude of this current is small, if it finds mechanical conduits to strategic organs like the heart via invasive instruments, it can result in serious consequences. For the same reasons, extension cords should not be used in EEG machines as this can result in an increase in capacitance, which is a direct function of wire length.

Inductive currents are another type of leakage current, typically smaller in intensity than capacitive currents. As is known from the laws of physics, electric current induces a magnetic field, which in turn can generate electric currents that may travel through other wires, including ground and neutral wires. In well-functioning systems, the magnitude of this electric current is small and typically routed to the ground contact. As discussed earlier, in cases of poorly functioning ground, there is a possibility of the same current being routed through the patient via critical organs. Ground loops or double grounds may also produce similar inductive currents.

The maximum allowable leakage current for EEG recordings of patients with intact ground should be limited to 10 μA.

11.7 Safety Recommendations

1. Maintain a common ground for all electric equipment connected to the patient. Always use hospital grade three-pronged electric plugs and receptacles for medical electric equipment. In high-risk situations (for example where patients have transvenous catheters), isolated power supplies and electrically isolated jack boxes should be utilized to protect electrically sensitive patients from injury.
2. Avoid use of extension cords to minimize capacitive currents.
3. Visually inspect all equipment, wires, and plugs periodically and prior to using on patients. In addition, chassis leakage current should be periodically measured and be under 100 μA.
4. EEG equipment should be powered on prior to hooking up the patient and disconnected prior to powering off.
5. Minimize electrode leakage current to below 10 μA with connected ground.

References

1. Ebersole JS. Cortical generators and EEG voltage fields. In: Ebersole JS, Pedley TA, eds. *Current Practice of Clinical Electroencephalography.* 3rd edn. Philadelphia: Lippincott Williams & Wilkins; 2003:12–31.

2. Li CL, Jasper H. Microelectrode studies of the electrical activity of the cerebral cortex in the cat. *J Physiol.* 1953;121 (1):117–140.

3. Humphrey DR. Re-analysis of the antidromic cortical response. II. On the contribution of cell discharge and PSPs to the evoked potentials. *Electroencephalogr Clin Neurophysiol.* 1968;25(5):421–442.

4. Purpura DP, Grundfest H. Nature of dendritic potentials and synaptic mechanisms in cerebral cortex of cat. *J Neurophysiol.* 1956;19(6):573–595.

5. Abraham K, Marsan CA. Patterns of cortical discharges and their relation to

routine scalp electroencephalography. *Electroencephalogr Clin Neurophysiol.* 1958;10(3):447–461.

6. Tao JX, Ray A, Hawes-Ebersole S, Ebersole JS. Intracranial EEG substrates of scalp EEG interictal spikes. *Epilepsia.* 2005;46 (5):669–676.

7. Cooper R, Winter AL, Crow HJ, Walter WG. Comparison of subcortical, cortical and scalp activity using chronically indwelling electrodes in man. *Electroencephalogr Clin Neurophysiol.* 1965;18:217–228.

8. Tao JX, Baldwin M, Ray A, Hawes-Ebersole S, Ebersole JS. The impact of cerebral source area and synchrony on recording scalp electroencephalography ictal patterns. *Epilepsia.* 2007;48 (11):2167–2176.

9. Ray A, Tao JX, Hawes-Ebersole SM, Ebersole JS. Localizing value of scalp EEG spikes: a simultaneous scalp and intracranial study. *Clin Neurophysiol.* 2007;118(1):69–79.

10. Haueisen J, Funke M, Gullmar D, Eichardt R. Tangential and radial epileptic spike activity: different sensitivity in EEG and MEG. *J Clin Neurophysiol.* 2012;29 (4):327–332.

11. Hunold A, Funke ME, Eichardt R, Stenroos M, Haueisen J. EEG and MEG: sensitivity to epileptic spike activity as function of source orientation and depth. *Physiol Meas.* 2016;37(7):1146–1162.

12. Cohen D, Cuffin BN. EEG versus MEG localization accuracy: theory and experiment. *Brain Topogr.* 1991;4 (2):95–103.

13. van den Broek SP, Reinders F, Donderwinkel M, Peters MJ. Volume conduction effects in EEG and MEG. *Electroencephalogr Clin Neurophysiol.* 1998;106(6):522–534.

14. Holsheimer J, Feenstra BW. Volume conduction and EEG measurements within the brain: a quantitative approach to the influence of electrical spread on the linear relationship of activity measured at different locations. *Electroencephalogr Clin Neurophysiol.* 1977;43(1):52–58.

15. Gloor P. Neuronal generators and the problem of localization in electroencephalography: application of volume conductor theory to electroencephalography. *J Clin Neurophysiol.* 1985;2(4):327–354.

16. Alarcon G, Guy CN, Binnie CD, et al. Intracerebral propagation of interictal activity in partial epilepsy: implications for source localisation. *J Neurol Neurosurg Psychiatry.* 1994;57(4):435–449.

17. Delucchi MR, Garoutte B, Aird RB. The scalp as an electroencephalographic averager. *Electroencephalogr Clin Neurophysiol.* 1962;14:191–196.

18. Pacia SV, Ebersole JS. Intracranial EEG substrates of scalp ictal patterns from temporal lobe foci. *Epilepsia.* 1997;38 (6):642–654.

19. Pacia SV, Ebersole JS. Intracranial EEG in temporal lobe epilepsy. *J Clin Neurophysiol.* 1999;16(5):399–407.

20. Bach Justesen A, Eskelund Johansen AB, Martinussen NI, et al. Added clinical value of the inferior temporal EEG electrode chain. *Clin Neurophysiol.* 2018;129 (1):291–295.

21. Ebersole JS. EEG dipole modeling in complex partial epilepsy. *Brain Topogr.* 1991;4(2):113–123.

22. Jasper HH. Report of the committee on methods of clinical examination in electroencephalography. *Electroencephalogr Clin Neurophysiol.* 1958;10(2):370–375.

23. Acharya JN, Hani A, Cheek J, Thirumala P, Tsuchida TN. American Clinical Neurophysiology Society Guideline 2: Guidelines for standard electrode position nomenclature. *J Clin Neurophysiol.* 2016;33 (4):308–311.

24. Chatrian GE, Lettich E, Nelson PL. Modified nomenclature for the "10%" electrode system. *J Clin Neurophysiol.* 1988;5(2):183–186.

25. Spitzer AR, Cohen LG, Fabrikant J, Hallett M. A method for determining optimal interelectrode spacing for cerebral topographic mapping. *Electroencephalogr Clin Neurophysiol.* 1989;72(4):355–361.

26. Sohrabpour A, Lu Y, Kankirawatana P, et al. Effect of EEG electrode number on epileptic source localization in pediatric patients. *Clin Neurophysiol.* 2015;126 (3):472–480.

27. Lascano AM, Perneger T, Vulliemoz S, et al. Yield of MRI, high-density electric source imaging (HD-ESI), SPECT and PET in epilepsy surgery candidates. *Clin Neurophysiol.* 2016;127(1):150–155.

28. Lantz G, Grave de Peralta R, Spinelli L, Seeck M, Michel CM. Epileptic source localization with high density EEG: how many electrodes are needed? *Clin Neurophysiol.* 2003;114(1):63–69.

29. Seeck M, Koessler L, Bast T, et al. The standardized EEG electrode array of the IFCN. *Clin Neurophysiol.* 2017;128 (10):2070–2077.

30. Laarne PH, Tenhunen-Eskelinen ML, Hyttinen JK, Eskola HJ. Effect of EEG electrode density on dipole localization accuracy using two realistically shaped skull resistivity models. *Brain Topogr.* 2000;12 (4):249–254.

31. Jurcak V, Tsuzuki D, Dan I. 10/20, 10/10, and 10/5 systems revisited: their validity as relative head-surface-based positioning systems. *Neuroimage.* 2007;34 (4):1600–1611.

32. Rosenzweig I, Fogarasi A, Johnsen B, et al. Beyond the double banana: improved recognition of temporal lobe seizures in long-term EEG. *J Clin Neurophysiol.* 2014;31(1):1–9.

33. Knott JR. Further thoughts on polarity, montages, and localization. *J Clin Neurophysiol.* 1985;2(1):63–75.

34. Jayakar P, Duchowny M, Resnick TJ, Alvarez LA. Localization of seizure foci: pitfalls and caveats. *J Clin Neurophysiol.* 1991;8(4):414–431.

35. Nyquist H. Certain factors affecting telegraph speed. *Bell System Technical Journal.* 1924;3(2):324–346.

36. Nyquist H. Certain topics in telegraph transmission theory. *Transactions of the American Institute of Electrical Engineers.* 1928;47(2):617–644.

37. Linkenkaer-Hansen K, Nikouline VV, Palva JM, Ilmoniemi RJ. Long-range temporal correlations and scaling behavior in human brain oscillations. *J Neurosci.* 2001;21(4):1370–1377.

38. Greenwood P, Ward L. 1/f noise. *Scholarpedia.* 2007;2(12):1537.

39. Zhang Y, van Drongelen W, He B. Estimation of in vivo brain-to-skull conductivity ratio in humans. *Appl Phys Lett.* 2006;89(22):223903–2239033.

40. Lai Y, van Drongelen W, Ding L, et al. Estimation of in vivo human brain-to-skull conductivity ratio from simultaneous extra- and intra-cranial electrical potential recordings. *Clin Neurophysiol.* 2005;116 (2):456–465.

41. Tyner FS, Knott JR, Mayer WB. *Fundamentals of EEG Technology: Basic Concepts and Methods.* Philadelphia: Raven Press; 1983.

42. Electrical safety Q&A: a reference guide for the clinical engineer. *Health Devices.* 2005;34(2):57–75.

43. Walczak TS, Chokroverty S. Electroencephalography, electromyography, and electro-oculography. In: *Sleep Disorders Medicine:* Elsevier; 2009:157–181.

44. Schwartz JJ. Electrical safety. In: Atlee JL, ed. *Complications in Anesthesia.* 2nd edn. Philadelphia: Elsevier; 2007:560–561.

45. Grimnes S, Martinsen OG. Selected applications. In: *Bioimpedance and Bioelectricity Basics.* 3rd edn. London: Elsevier; 2015:405–494.

46. Backes J. Safety testing of medical devices: IEC 62353 explained. *Med Device Technol.* 2007;18(7):46–47.

Interpreting the Normal Electroencephalogram of an Adult

Vibhangini S. Wasade

12.1 Introduction

Interpreting an electroencephalogram (EEG) record requires correlating the observed waveforms to the specific scalp location and to the patient's state and age. EEG waveforms are described in terms of frequency, amplitude, morphology, synchrony and symmetry, rhythmicity, and reactivity.

12.2 Features of EEG Waveforms

12.2.1 Frequency

Frequency refers to the number of waves recorded in 1 s (unit – hertz (Hz)). Four standard frequency ranges are divided in the ranges alpha (8–13 Hz), beta (13–25 Hz), theta (4–8 Hz), and delta (<4 Hz) (see Table 12.1). The designation of Greek letter names to the frequency bands is not sequential, and can be understood from historical perspective as the waveforms were described.[1] In 1929, Berger announced the term "alpha" and "beta" as he labelled the particular frequencies. In 1936, Walter introduced the term "delta" to designate all frequencies below alpha. However, he himself found a need to designate a range for 4–7.5 per second, with a presumed thalamic origin for these waves, hence he skipped the Greek letters epsilon, zeta, and eta, and chose "theta."

12.2.2 Amplitude

Amplitude refers to the voltage of the EEG signal and is measured in microvolts (μV), often as the highest to lowest point of the wave. It is reported as low (<25 μV), medium or moderate (25 to 75 μV), or high (>75 μV). The normal amplitude of alpha rhythm usually ranges from 15 to 50 μV.

12.2.3 Morphology

Morphology refers to the appearance of the waveform, with regards to its shape and phases. The shapes could be of different types, including sinusoidal as usually seen with alpha, spindle-shaped as with sleep spindles, saw-toothed as with lambda waves or slow waves, or epileptiform, noted as sharp or spike waves. The waves may be monomorphic, which appear more regular, or irregular or polymorphic, which change in duration and shape. The phases describe the number of deflections in a wave from the baseline and are seen as mono-, bi-, tri-, or polyphasic waveforms.[2]

Table 12.1 Features of identified frequencies/rhythms in Greek alphabetical order from a historical perspective

Band (frequency)/ rhythm	Historical perspective (year, described by)	Usual location, state	Features
Alpha (8–13 Hz)	1929, Hans Berger	Posterior, rounded, sinusoidal waveforms, in relaxed wakefulness, with eyes closed	Blocked by influx of light (eye opening), either afferent stimuli and mental activity
Beta (13–25 Hz)	1929, Hans Berger	Frontal, fairly common, very fast, can be seen in light sleep and REM sleep Central, partly the basis of Rolandic mu often intermixed	Normal amplitude typically low, usually less than 25 μV Anxiety can enhance normal beta activity Induced by centrally acting medications – benzodiazepines, phenobarbital, stimulants, alcohol
Gamma (>30 Hz)	1938, Jasper and Andrews (eventually abandoned, made a comeback during the 1990s)	Superimposed on occipital alpha	Also known as "fast" beta or "very fast" gamma range activity
Delta (<4 Hz)	1936, Walter	Diffuse, slow-wave sleep	Initially designated for all frequencies below alpha, later defined as <4 Hz after theta frequencies were described
Theta (4–7 Hz)	1944, Walter and Dovey	Usually frontal midline region with mental activity, seen in drowsiness	Initially presumed thalamic origin
Kappa rhythm	1937, Laugier and Liberson	Initially anterior temporal rhythm in alpha frequency, later thought to be possibly, an ocular artifact caused by eye oscillations	Later thought to be unlikely cerebral rhythm
Lambda rhythm	1951, Gastaut	Occipital regions of awake subject during reading/ scanning/visual searching	Triangular/saw tooth shaped, 100–300 ms duration, biphasic/ triphasic, mainly positive, time-locked to saccadic eye movements, varying amplitude – generally 50 μV Often seen in those who also show POSTS and photic driving response

Table 12.1 (*cont.*)

Band (frequency)/ rhythm	Historical perspective (year, described by)	Usual location, state	Features
Mu rhythm (7–11 Hz)	1952, Gaustaut	Rolandic (central) region, strongly related to motor cortex	Known as en arceau, arch-like morphology, central alpha rhythm, somatosensory alpha rhythm, comb rhythm Blocked by active, passive or reflexive movements
Pi rhythm (3–4 Hz)	1977, Dutertre (hardly used since the 1990s)	Posterior region	Designated for posterior slow rhythm
Rho rhythm	1973, Kugler and Laub	Posterior	Known as POSTS
Sigma rhythm (11–14 Hz)	1981, Kugler	Frontal/central/midline	Was also known as "sigma activity", instead of "sleep spindles"
Tau rhythm	1990s, Niedermeyer	Temporal region	Known as "third rhythm," "independent temporal alphoid rhythm," rhythmical alpha and upper theta range, not detected by scalp electrodes unless bone defect in the mid-temporal region Can be picked up from epidural electrodes
Phi rhythm	Daly 1983, Belsh	Posterior region	Monorhythmic posterior delta waves (<4 Hz), different from background, occur within 2 s of eye closure Described by Belsh as "posterior rhythmic slow activity after eye closure"

POSTS, posterior occipital sharp transients of sleep; REM, rapid eye movement
Collated from Neidermeyer[1]

12.2.4 Synchrony and Symmetry

Interhemispheric coherence of waveforms is noted by assessing synchrony and symmetry. Synchrony refers to the coincidence of waveforms occurring simultaneously. The waves can be bisynchronous, when they appear concurrently over bilateral hemispheres, or asynchronous, when they occur independently at different times.[2] Synchrony is commonly appreciated in normal sleep architecture, generally seen in stage 2 sleep.

Symmetry is described with regards to amplitude and frequency. Sometimes, the normal asymmetry of alpha rhythm can be noted with 50% higher amplitude on the right. Some of this may be related to the thickness asymmetry of the occipital bone.[2]

12.2.5 Rhythmicity

Rhythmicity implies repetition of waveforms, in a manner described as rhythmic or semi-rhythmic. Sleep spindles are usually seen to exhibit this rhythmic feature in normal sleep architecture. Depending on the regularity of occurrence, the waves can be periodic or quasi-periodic (nearly periodic).

12.2.6 Reactivity

Reactivity is one of the important features of waveforms that helps in overall EEG interpretation. Reactivity denotes a change in waveforms with different maneuvers, including those of activation procedures described later in this chapter. Reactivity is routinely assessed by eye closure and opening in a normal relaxed state, when the posterior alpha rhythm appears and abates. In an encephalopathic patient, somatosensory stimulation is used to assess reactivity, and noted changes in EEG background help in grading the level of encephalopathy.

12.3 EEG Patterns in Wakefulness

Wakefulness in a normal adult EEG record is characterized by alpha rhythm (usually 8.5–12 Hz) over the posterior derivations, of low to moderate amplitude (15–65 μV), seen in a relaxed state with eyes closed. In about a third of people, it may be noted over parietal or posterior temporal aspects. This is reactive and may disappear with eye opening due to an influx of light, with any mental activation, or with transition to sleep stages. A frequency of 8 Hz or below is usually considered abnormal, even in elderly people. Posterior dominant rhythm changes with age, and maturation of EEG rhythms from infancy to childhood is described in detail in Chapter 14.

The phenomenon of "alpha squeak" is often observed and refers to an increase in frequency by 1 Hz, soon after eye closure (Figure 12.1). Physiologic variations with ongoing alpha activity in the EEG record have been described as alpha variants. When the frequency appears to slow to half of the noted alpha frequency, it is referred to as a "slow alpha variant" and with higher frequency, it is referred to as a "fast alpha variant," which is also described as a beta rhythm. Failure of alpha blocking on one side after eye opening is sometimes noted in those with ipsilateral parietal and temporal lesions and is described as Bancaud's phenomenon.[3]

12.4 EEG Patterns in Drowsiness and Sleep

Different sleep stages are characterized by different waveforms. Common waveforms are discussed below, followed by overall patterns seen in different stages of sleep.

12.4.1 Vertex Waves

Vertex waves are bilaterally synchronous waves with prominent amplitude of up to 250 μV at the vertex, and maximal at the Cz electrode and adjacent C3 and C4 electrodes. They may

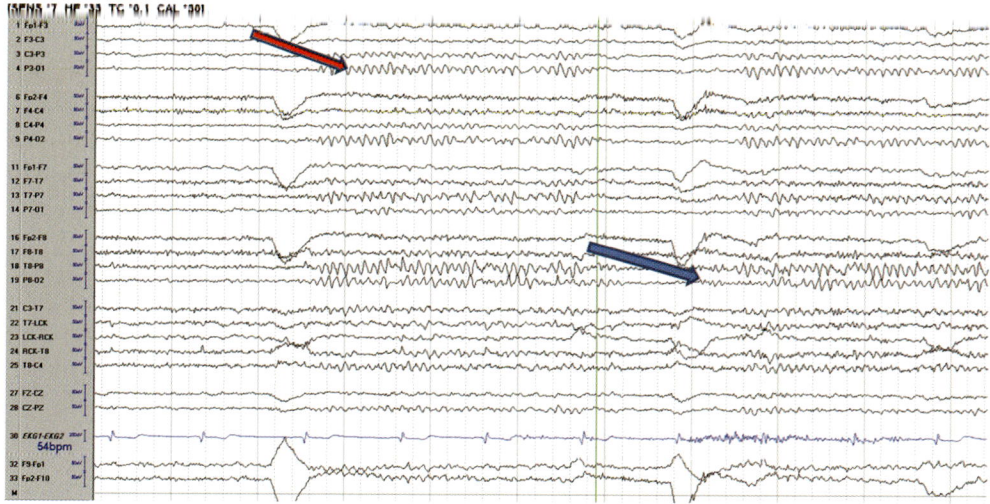

Figure 12.1 Note a posterior dominant rhythm of 11 Hz (red arrow), and alpha squeak of 12 Hz (blue arrow).

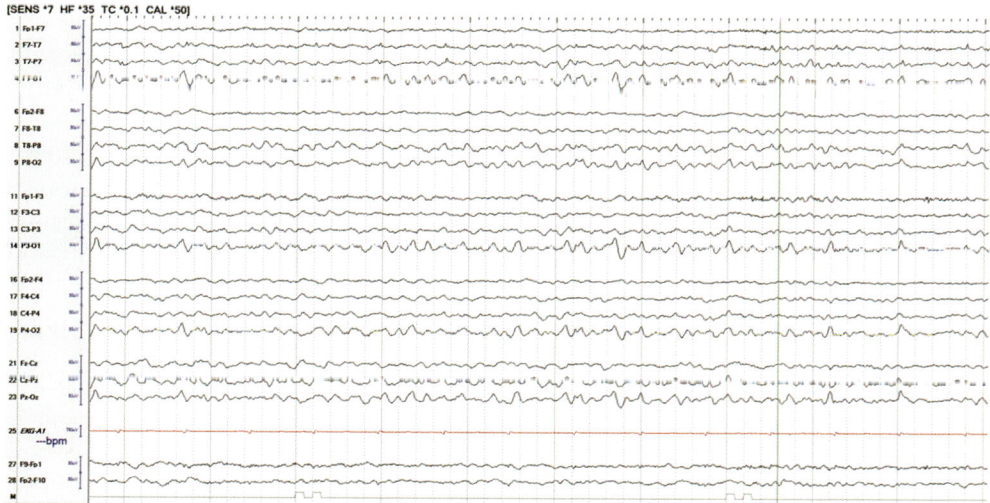

Figure 12.2 Posterior occipital sharp transients of sleep are seen synchronously in the occipital regions in drowsiness.

appear in isolation, or more often appear repetitively in runs, at irregular intervals. They can be mistaken for abnormal epileptiform activity, given their morphology.

12.4.2 Positive Occipital Sharp Transients of Sleep

Positive occipital sharp transients of sleep (POSTS) emerge in the later stage of drowsiness in a normal adult, and show monophasic or biphasic, triangular-shaped morphology with a positive polarity over the occipital derivations (Figure 12.2). They occur synchronously or independently over both sides. They can occur in trains or at an irregular frequency.

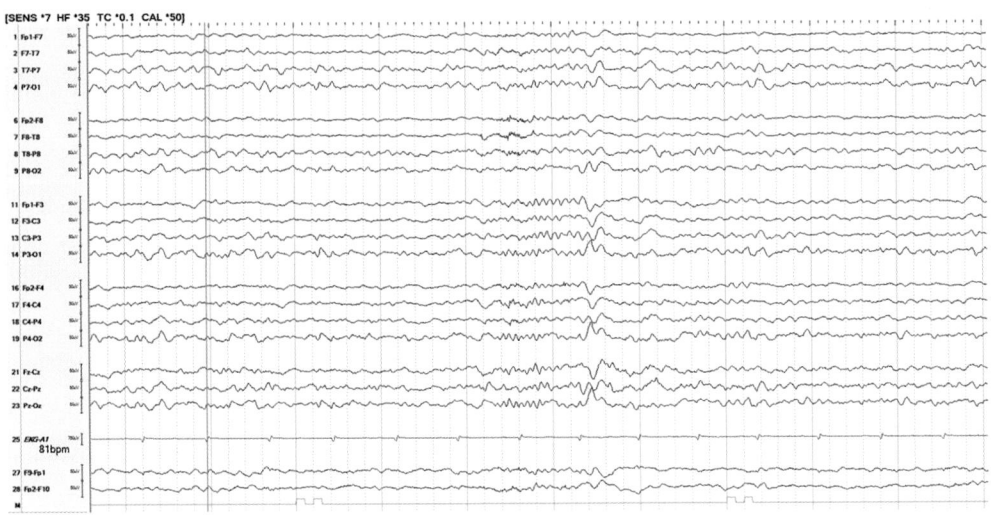

Figure 12.3 Sleep spindles in stage 2 sleep, noted over the fronto-central and midline derivations in a bipolar montage.

These have also been referred to as "lambdoid waves" in the past, given their similarity with lambda waves in wakefulness; however, the mechanism for generating these waves remains unspecified, and the term is not currently used.

12.4.3 Sleep Spindles

Sleep spindles are spindle-shaped trains, usually synchronous in adults, with frequencies around 12–14 Hz (range of 11–15 Hz), and are maximal over the central/vertex regions (Figure 12.3). The thalamic reticular nucleus is considered to be involved in generation of spindle activity in sleep.[4]

12.4.4 K-Complexes

K-complexes are of biphasic morphology, initially negative high-amplitude ($>$200 µV) sharp waves, followed by a longer, positive, slow wave (duration 500 ms to 1 s) component, superimposed by the fast component of sleep spindles. They are thought to be elicited during sleep by sensory/auditory stimulation. The generators of K-complexes are not definitively known; however, highly synchronized cortical frontal and prefrontal gray matter is assumed to be involved.[5] K-complexes have been related to information processing and memory consolidation.

12.4.5 Sleep Stages and Patterns

In adults, early stages of drowsiness are characterized by the dropout of alpha and appearance of theta-range slow waves with brief alpha waves. Slow lateral eye movements ($>$0.5 Hz) are often the earliest sign of drowsiness. "Paradoxical alpha rhythm," instead of eye closure and relaxation, may appear with slight alertness. Vertex waves and POSTS occur in the later stages of drowsiness.

Stage 2 sleep, which is considered a light sleep, is demonstrated by sleep spindles and K-complexes, as well as ongoing vertex waves and POSTS.

Stages 3 or 4, together referred to as deep or slow-wave sleep, is noted as very slow delta (<2 Hz) with high amplitude (>75μV). In sleep scoring, deep sleep is differentiated as stage 3 sleep when 20–50% of the 30-second epoch is dominated by these slow delta waves with ongoing K-complexes and some spindles, and as stage 4 sleep when >50% of the epoch exhibits slowing, with some K-complexes.[6]

Rapid eye movement (REM) sleep is noted normally about 60 to 90 min after sleep onset and is characterized by low-voltage activity with saw-tooth waves with 2–6 Hz frequency, occurring in bursts in conjunction with the rapid eye movements. REM sleep occurring soon after sleep onset (termed sleep-onset REM period or SOREMP) can be observed in those with narcolepsy or other sleep disorders, or even with sleep deprivation.

12.5 Activation Procedures

Activation procedures are performed to provoke abnormal EEG patterns and may also elicit normal physiologic patterns that are not routinely seen on EEG.

12.5.1 Photic Stimulation

Photic stimulation is a routine technique used during EEG, with intermittent strobe flash frequencies from 1 to 30 Hz.[7] This can produce different responses that include photic driving response, photomyogenic (photomyoclonic) response, photoparoxysmal (photoconvulsive) response, and photoelectric (photovoltaic) response.

Photic driving response is the activity recorded at occipital derivations, occurring about 70 to 150 ms from the onset of flash stimulus, time-locked to the stimulus, and appearing at the same, subharmonic, or supraharmonic to the stimulus frequency (Figure 12.4).

Photomyogenic (photomyoclonic) response refers to a muscle artifact, especially of the periocular frontalis muscles, time-locked to the flash frequency, and stopping with stimulus.

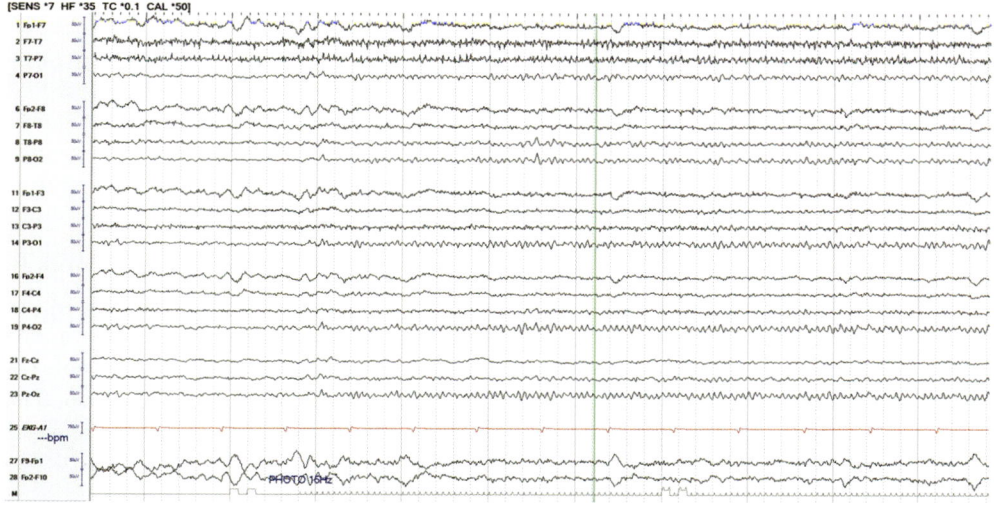

Figure 12.4 Photic driving response at 16 Hz flash frequency.

Photoparoxysmal (photoepileptiform or photoconvulsive) response refers to generalized or anterior-dominant spike/polyspike-and-wave discharges that often outlasts the stimulus and can be reproduced. It is often provoked by flash frequencies of 10–20 Hz and can lead to a clinical seizure.

Photoelectric (photovoltaic) response refers to an artifact caused by a high-impedance electrode due to a photochemical reaction of the adhesive used to place the electrode on the scalp. It is noted as a brief spike-like transient that disappears on covering the involved electrode.

12.5.2 Hyperventilation

Hyperventilation is one of the oldest known provocative techniques, when over breathing is carried out for 3 to 5 min to activate any EEG changes. Hyperventilation leads to increased loss of CO_2, resulting in a decrease in P_aCO_2, and hypocapnia. This can cause cerebral vasoconstriction, mild cerebral hypoperfusion, and hypoxia, leading to EEG background changes to diffuse theta and delta activity.[6] Hypoglycemia may accentuate such slowing. As per the American Clinical Neurophysiology Society, hyperventilation is avoided in those with medically justifiable reasons, including severe cardiopulmonary disease, sickle cell disease or trait, a recent intracranial hemorrhage, acute stroke, large vessel stenosis, documented Moyamoya disease, or a patient's inability to cooperate.[8] Hyperventilation can provoke generalized spike-and-slow-wave discharges, as well as focal sharps/spikes and can accentuate any focal slowing.

12.6 Benign Variants

Benign variants are variations in normal rhythm or waveforms that often appear similar to epileptiform discharges and can lead to over interpretation of the EEG record. Some have related these to various symptoms/conditions; however, these are now considered to be a nonspecific finding of uncertain significance.

12.6.1 Wicket Rhythm, Wicket Spikes

These waves occur with a frequency of 6–11 Hz and an amplitude of 60–200 μV, over the temporal derivations, either in isolation (wicket spikes) or in trains (wicket rhythm) (Figure 12.5). They are present in drowsiness, light sleep, and, at times, wakefulness and are noted predominantly in adults older than 30 years, occurring bilaterally or independently over either hemisphere. They are not blocked by eye opening and become obvious when the alpha activity disappears. They can be mistaken for a temporal epileptiform discharge and can be differentiated by the absence of a subsequent slow wave, without disruption of the background, and absence in deep sleep.

12.6.2 Rhythmic Temporal Theta Bursts of Drowsiness (RTTB), Rhythmic Mid-temporal Discharges (RMTD), or Psychomotor Variants

These waveforms are trains of rhythmic theta (5–7 Hz) activity with a monomorphic flat-topped, notched, or sharp appearance in the temporal regions, noted in relaxed wakefulness or drowsiness. These can occur bilaterally or independently over either hemisphere. They may last for up to 10 seconds, and should be differentiated from ictal discharge by a monomorphic pattern without clear evolution in frequency.

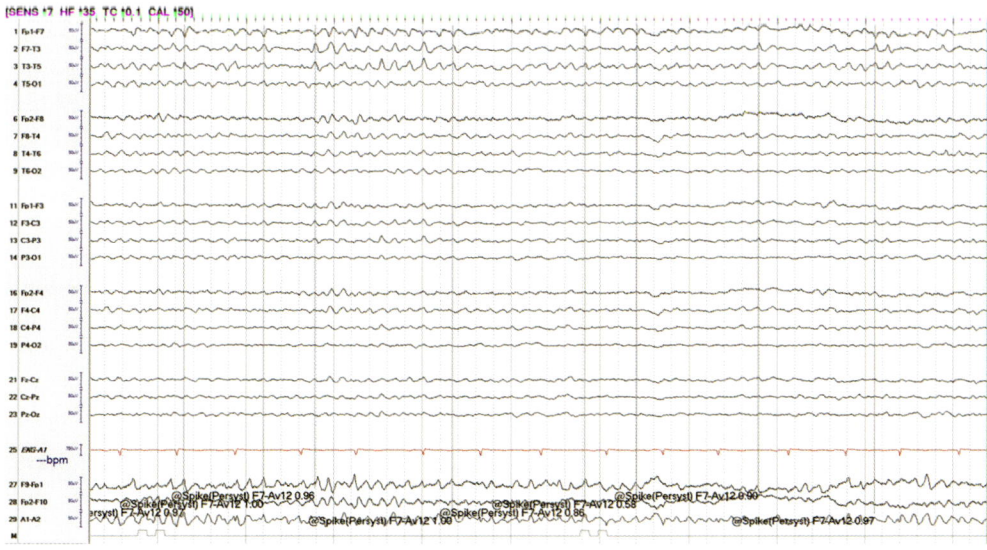

Figure 12.5 Burst of wicket rhythm noted in the left temporal derivations.

12.6.3 Midline Theta Rhythm or Ciganek Rhythm

These are trains of rhythmic theta (4–7 Hz) activity with a sinusoidal, smooth, spiky, mu-like, or arci-form morphology in the central/midline derivations, noted in wakefulness and drowsiness. These can last for 4 to 20 s. They have inconsistent reactivity to eye opening, alerting, and movement.

12.6.4 Small Sharp Spikes (SSS), Benign Epileptiform Transients of Sleep (BETS), or Benign Sporadic Sleep Spikes (BSSS)

These are low voltage (<50 μV), short duration (50 ms), single mono- or diphasic spikes, with abrupt ascending and steep descending slopes, noted in drowsiness and light sleep. They are not stereotypical in appearance and exhibit a broad field, appreciated more over the temporal derivations. These are generally unilateral, but on longer EEG sampling, they are seen bilaterally, and occur independently with a field conforming to an oblique transverse dipole across both hemispheres. They can be differentiated from an epileptiform spike by their distinctive morphology and disappearance in slow-wave sleep.

12.6.5 Subclinical Rhythmic Electrographic Discharges in Adults (SREDA)

Subclinical rhythmic electrographic discharges in adults is a rare pattern seen in people older than 50 years, occurring at rest, or drowsiness. This pattern can be provoked by hyperventilation. The pattern occurs in rhythmic runs lasting from 20 s to a few minutes, with mixed frequencies exhibiting evolution from delta- to theta- (5–7 Hz)-range frequencies (Figure 12.6). The activity is maximal over the parietal-posterior temporal head derivations. These have a tendency to be present in subsequent EEGs. This can be differentiated from ictal discharge by evolution to faster frequencies and absence of postictal slowing.

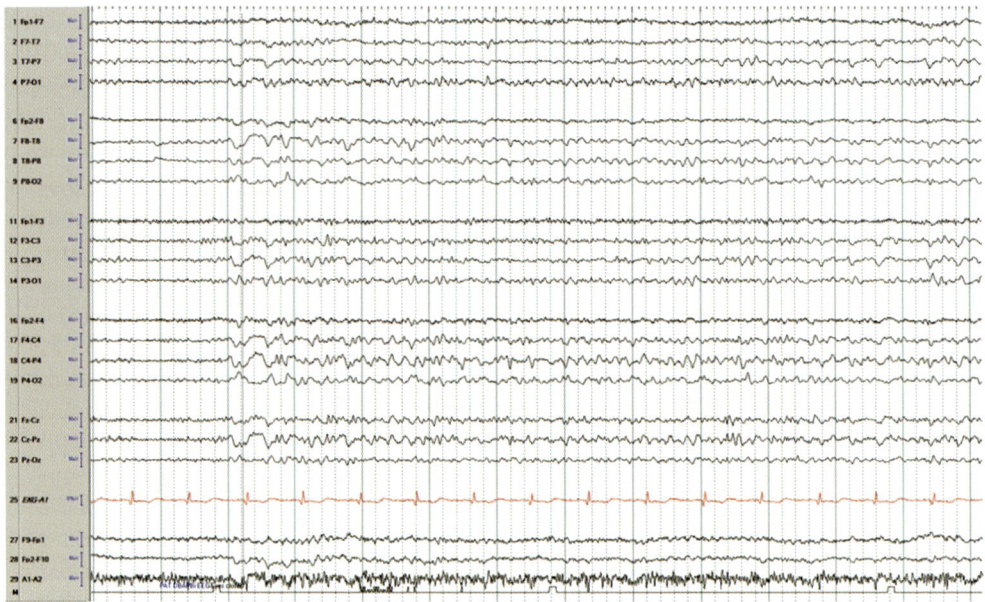

Figure 12.6 A subclinical rhythmic electrographic discharge in adults starting with a burst of delta waves evolving to theta-range activity predominantly over the right parietal derivations.

12.6.6 Fourteen and Six Positive Bursts or Ctenoids

These waves are rhythmic bursts that appear in short runs (<1 s) of an arch-shaped positive spiky component, alternating with a rounded negative component, at a rate of 13–17 Hz (14 Hz) or 5–7 Hz (6 Hz), and medium amplitude (20–60 μV, usually <75 μV). The 14-Hz component is more common and often resembles a sleep spindle. These are predominantly noted during drowsiness and light sleep, and are located mostly posterior-temporal or parietal, unilaterally or bilaterally, independent or synchronous. They are best seen in referential montage. They can be observed at any age, but are expressed maximally in adolescents (aged 13–14 years). The 6-Hz component predominates in children younger than 1 year, and the 14-Hz component predominates or combines with 6-Hz spikes in other age groups. They have been described in advanced stages of metabolic (hepatic) coma and in children with Reye's syndrome.

12.6.7 Six-Hertz Spike and Wave Bursts or Phantom Spike and Wave

These are usually 6 Hz (range 5–7 Hz) spike-and-wave discharges, lasting 1 to 2 s, noted in relaxed wakefulness or drowsiness. The spikes are typically small, very brief (<30 μV and <30 ms), with a diphasic spike followed by a larger (50–100 μV) slow-wave component, and the bursts are bilaterally synchronous. Two types have been noted: the WHAM (wake, high-amplitude, anterior, male), more likely to be associated with epilepsy, and the FOLD (female, occipital, low-amplitude, drowsy), considered to be a more benign variant.[9]

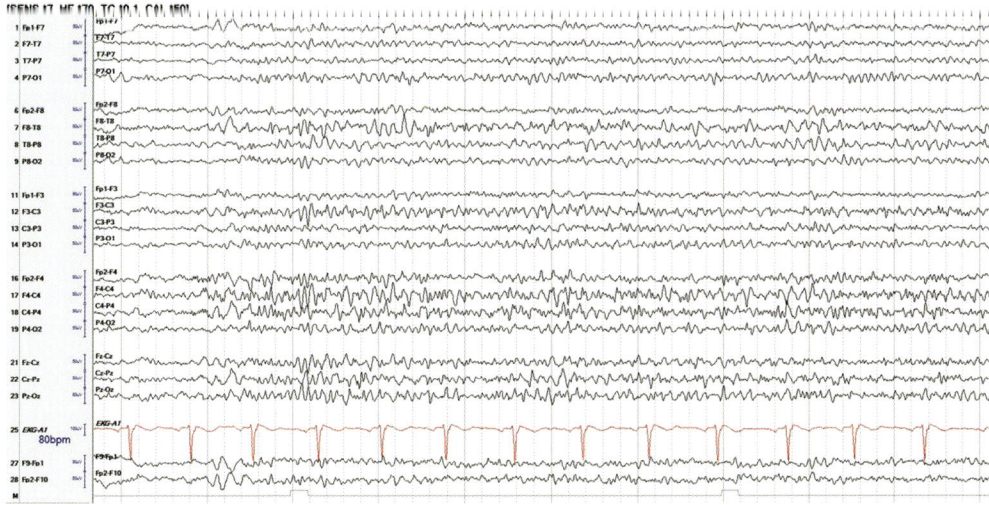

Figure 12.7 Breach rhythm seen over the right fronto-central region noted as higher-voltage, higher-frequency activity in a patient after craniotomy for meningioma resection in that region.

12.6.8 Breach Rhythm

Breach rhythm is noted as a relatively higher-voltage activity in comparison to the other hemisphere that is sharply contoured or spiky in appearance and occasionally intermixed with higher-frequency activity in the area of a skull defect (Figure 12.7). Accentuation of underlying cerebral activity occurs due to the absence of skull bone, which acts as a high-frequency filter. Often the sharp/spiky appearance can be misinterpreted as epileptogenic; however, absence of a subsequent slow wave with a lack of spread and a believable field could help in differentiating the two. Focal slowing or epileptiform discharges can be noted embedded in the breach rhythm, implying the presence of underlying focal cerebral dysfunction or cortical irritability.

12.6.9 Texting Rhythm

Texting rhythm was described in 2016 in patients using personal electronic devices during EEG and seen as a time-locked, task-specific, generalized fronto-central-predominant 5–6 Hz theta activity that occurred with active texting.[10] It is reproducible and unique, present with eyes open, and not seen as a result of any other forms of physical, mental, or emotional activation. This could be mistaken for an ictal pattern and can be differentiated by paroxysmal onset and offset, and absence of evolution.

12.7 Artifacts

Artifacts noted in EEG are waveforms recorded that have a non-cerebral source of origin. It is important to recognize such patterns to avoid any misinterpretations. Some of these occur spontaneously, and comments from the observing technologist could help in their identification, and for others, following strict technical requirement guidelines in performing EEG could aid in minimizing them. Artifacts in EEG can have physiological or nonphysiological sources,[11] and the common ones are described below.

12.7.1 Physiologic Artifacts

12.7.1.1 Eye Movements

These are noted with movements at Fp1, Fp2, F7, and F8 electrodes, which are located close to the eyeball. Vertical eye movements, like blinks or eye flutter, or horizontal slow lateral and saccadic eye movements can be recognized by observing deflections on these electrodes. The corneo-retinal dipole potential, with the cornea as positive and retina as negative is considered a generator for this artifact. Basic concepts of G1 and G2 electrodes suggest that when G1 is more positive than G2, the signal deflects downwards; and when G1 is more negative than G2, then the signal deflects upwards. During eye blink, with eyelid closure, eyeballs move upwards (Bell's phenomenon) leading to increased momentary positivity over Fp1 and Fp2, causing a downward deflection in the frontal electrodes (Figure 12.8). Eye flutter in comparison to eye blinks are lower amplitude, more rhythmic, and more rapid. Application of an additional electrode below the eye can help distinguish frontal delta activity from eye movement in the ipsi-ear referential montage. An out-of-phase deflection with positivity in frontal and negativity in eye electrodes is noted with eye movements, whereas an in-phase deflection is noted with frontal delta activity.

For the horizontal eye movements, F7 and F8 electrodes exhibit out-of-phase deflections. For example, during slow lateral eye movements noted in drowsiness, if eyes deviate to the right, the right eyeball approaches the right temporal electrode (F8), while the left eyeball turns away from the left temporal electrode (F7). This leads to a positive potential at F8 and a negative potential at the F7, producing simultaneous corresponding deflections in the right temporal electrode (appearance of "positive phase reversal" at F8) and the left temporal electrode (appearance of "negative phase reversal" at F7) (Figure 12.9). With saccadic eye movements, sharper waveforms are noted (Figure 12.8).

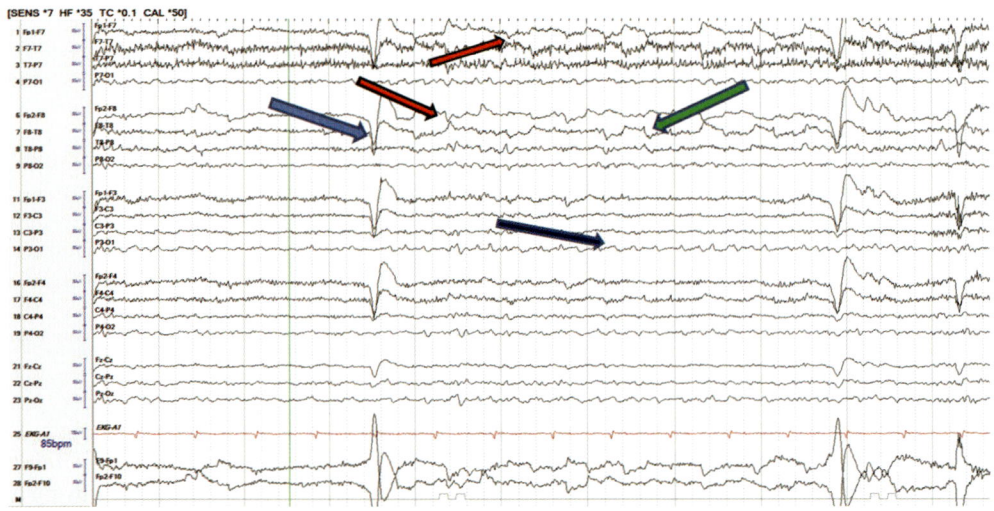

Figure 12.8 Eye blink artifact (blue arrow), in a patient who was reading, as noted with a saccadic eye movement artifact (red arrows), lateral rectus spike artifact (green arrow), and triangular shaped lambda waves in occipital derivations (navy blue arrow).

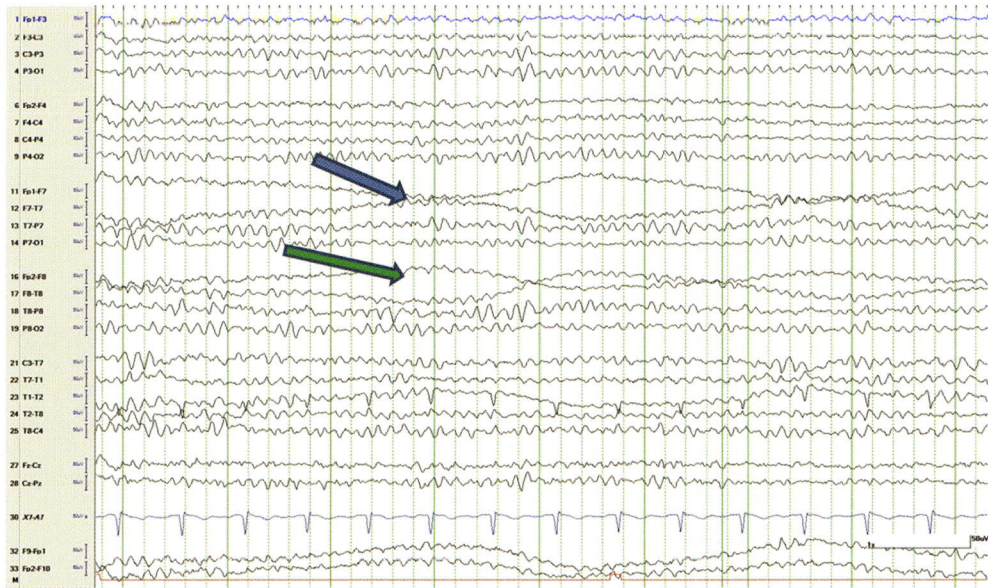

Figure 12.9 Horizontal slow lateral eye movements in drowsiness, with negative phase reversal appearance seen at the F7 electrode (blue arrow) and positive phase reversal appearance seen at the F8 electrode (green arrow).

12.7.1.2 Lateral Rectus Spike Artifact

These are low-amplitude, short-duration spikes noted over the frontal/temporal electrodes (Figure 12.8), which just precede lateral eye movement (usually saccadic) and are caused by contraction of the lateral rectus muscle.

12.7.1.3 Glossokinetic and Chewing Artifacts

The tongue tip is considered negatively charged compared to its base, and so movement of the tongue generates an electrical field that is recorded as a muscle artifact predominantly over the temporal or frontal (Figure 12.10) electrodes, or entire face. In addition, if there are chewing movements, the muscle artifact is noted to be repetitive, intermittent, time-locked, and involving all electrodes (Figure 12.11).

12.7.1.4 Sweat Artifact

Sweat artifact is noted in patients with excessive perspiration, as a high-amplitude, slow potential (<1 Hz), with EEG baseline swaying due to sodium chloride reacting with contact electrodes (salt bridge). This could be reduced by using a low-frequency filter. Cooling the patient and drying the scalp can help resolve this artifact.

12.7.1.5 Electrocardiogram and Pulse Artifacts

An electrocardiogram (ECG) artifact refers to one generated by potential changes in heart beat recorded at the scalp, representing a "far-field potential." It implies involvement of mainly the R wave of the QRS complex or may involve other ECG components with a larger artifact. It is easily seen when there is simultaneous heart monitoring on a separate ECG channel in the EEG record (Figure 12.12). It is usually noted in a referential montage with

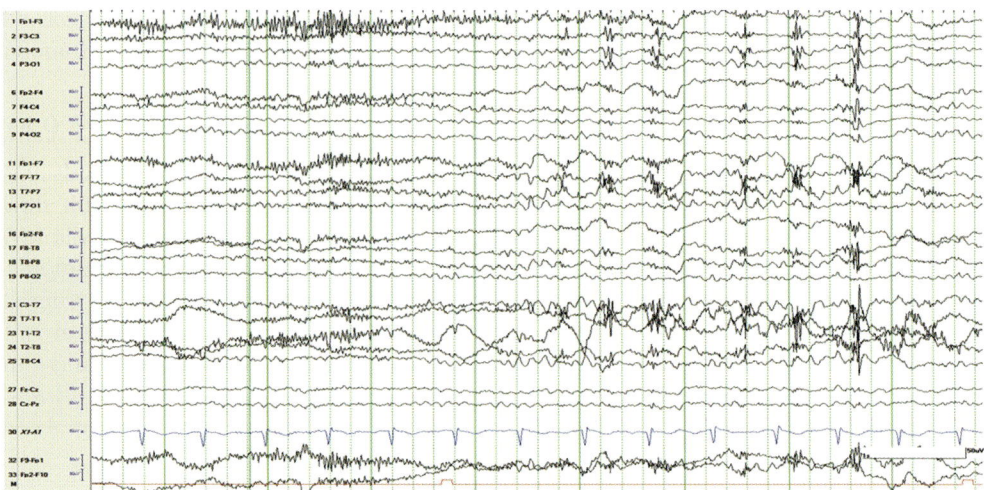

Figure 12.10 Glossokinetic artifact noted with slurping juice.

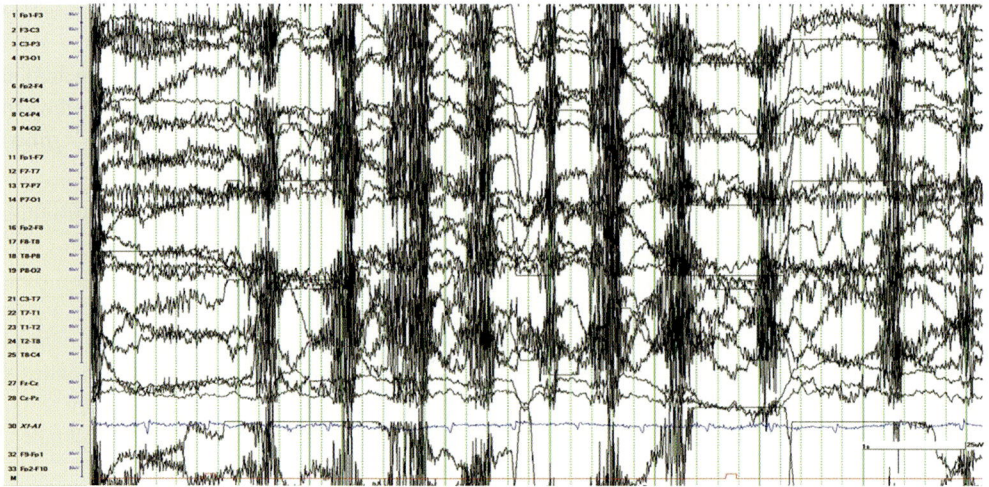

Figure 12.11 Chewing movements causing repetitive, brief, diffuse muscle artifact.

wide interelectrode distances, especially ear references, and detects a negative polarity artifact from one side (A1 or A2) and a positive polarity artifact from the other side (A2 or A1). This is often seen in those with a short neck, those whose head is close to the thorax, or obese people. This artifact can be minimized by neck extension, by using a Cz reference, or by combining both ears as references.

A pulse artifact refers to a smooth, rhythmic, slow-wave potential over a single electrode, most obvious when an electrode is loosely applied over or near an artery. It is caused by a pulse wave generating slight electrical changes between the electrode and scalp. It is time-locked to heart beats noted on the ECG channel and can be resolved by replacing the electrode at some distance from the artery.

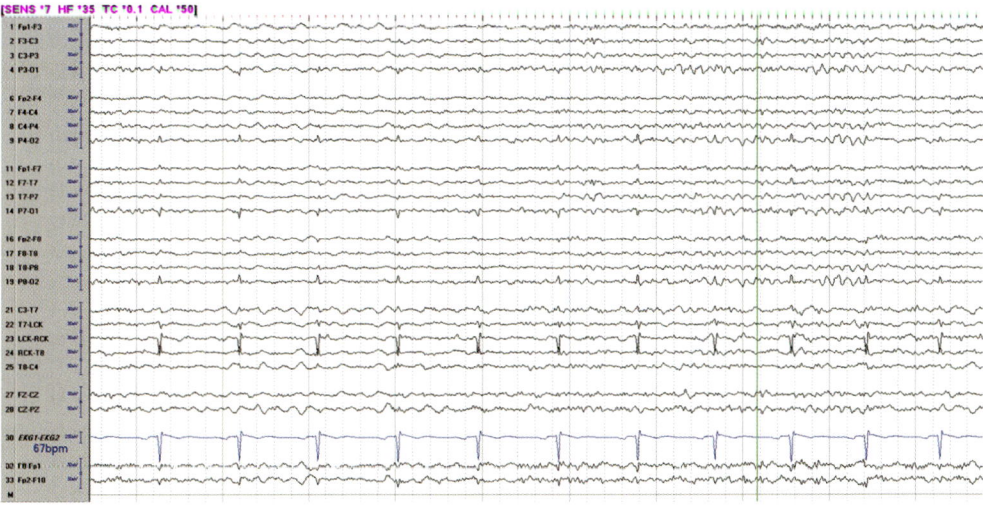

Figure 12.12 Note ECG artifact in multiple channels in relation to the QRS complex in the ECG channel.

12.7.1.6 Muscle or Electromyographic Artifacts

This artifact is frequently noted in EEG due to contraction or movement of respective muscles. It appears due to repetitive negative or positive deflections of motor units, in the form of short duration (<50 ms) spike discharges on EEG. This artifact can be lessened by relaxation maneuvers, and technically to some extent by decreasing the high-frequency filter to up to 35 Hz, bearing in mind that over filtering may falsely alter the waveforms.

12.7.2 Nonphysiologic Artifacts

12.7.2.1 Interference and Equipment Artifacts

Common sources of electrical interference artifacts can originate from electrical power lines and equipment near or on the patient. This has a 60-Hz frequency in North America and 50 Hz in other countries. It can appear on one, a few, or all channels, and can be eliminated during the recording by adequate grounding, shielding, and proper wiring. A 60-Hz filter setting can be used during EEG review to lessen the artifact. In addition, other equipment surrounding the patient, including mechanical ventilators, electronic pumps, devices, and the bed can cause artifacts and these are often noted in patients in intensive care units.

12.7.2.2 Electrode or Electrode Pop Artifacts

A poorly applied electrode can cause an electrode pop artifact due to buildup and then sudden release of charge in that particular electrode. This is noted as a brief, odd-looking discharge on EEG, appearing out of phase in adjacent channels, with no plausible field, limited to a single electrode, and differing significantly from the background (Figure 12.13). These features make it relatively easy to distinguish from epileptiform discharges.

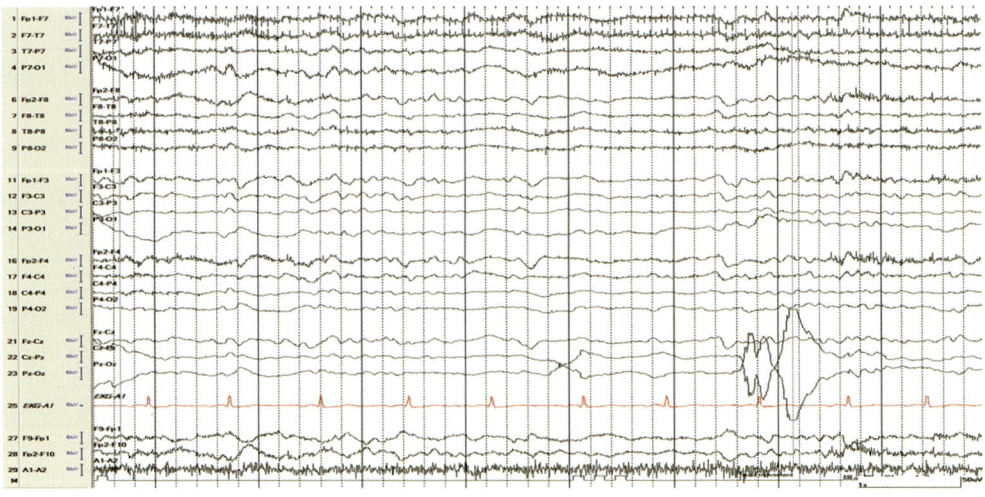

Figure 12.13 Note sudden, bizarre, electrode pop artifact at Pz electrode.

References

1. Niedermeyer E. The normal EEG of the waking adult. In: Niedermeyer E, Lopes Da Silva F, eds., *Electroencephalography: Basic Principles, Clinical Applications and Related Fields*, 5th edn. Philadelphia: Lippincott Williams & Wilkins; 2005:167–192.

2. Fisch BJ. Descriptors of EEG activity. In: Fisch BJ, ed., *Fisch & Spehlmann's EEG primer: Basic Principles of Digital and Analog EEG*, 3rd edn. San Diego, CA: Elsevier; 1999:145–154.

3. Fisch BJ. Deviations from normal patterns. In: *Fisch & Spehlmann's EEG primer: Basic Principles of Digital and Analog EEG*, 3rd edn. San Diego, CA: Elsevier; 1999:419–432.

4. Lüthi A. Sleep spindles: where they come from, what they do. *Neuroscientist*. 2014;20 (3):243–256.

5. Crowley K, Trinder J, Colrain IM. An examination of evoked K-complex amplitude and frequency of occurrence in the elderly. *J Sleep Res*. 2002;11 (2):129–140.

6. Dement W, Kleitman N. Cyclic variation in EEG during sleep and their relation to eye movements, body motility and dreaming. *Electrenephalogr Clin Neurophysiol*. 1957;9:673–690.

7. Fisch BJ, So EL. Activation methods. In: Ebersole JS, Pedley TA, eds., *Current Practice of Clinical Electroencephalography*, 3rd edn. Philadelphia: Lippincott Williams & Wilkins; 2003:246–270.

8. Sinha SR, Sullivan L, Sabau D, et al. American Clinical Neurophysiology Society guideline 1: minimum technical requirements for performing clinical electroencephalography. *J Clin Neurophysiol*. 2016;33(4):303–307.

9. Hughes JR. Two forms of the 6/sec spike and wave complex. *Electroencephalogr Clin Neurophysiol*. 1980;48(5):535–550.

10. Tatum WO, DiCiaccio B, Kipta JA, Yelvington KH, Stein MA. The texting rhythm: a novel EEG waveform using smartphones. *J Clin Neurophysiol*. 2016;33 (4):359–366.

11. Klem GH. Artifacts. In: Ebersole JS, Pedley TA, eds., *Current Practice of Clinical Electroencephalography*, 3rd edn. Philadelphia: Lippincott Williams; 2003:271–287.

Ictal and Interictal Epileptiform Electroencephalogram Patterns

Alma Yum and Vladimir Shvarts

13.1 Introduction

According to the International Federation of Societies for Electroencephalography and Clinical Neurophysiology (IFSECN), epileptiform activity is defined as distinctive waveforms or complexes resembling those recorded in a proportion of human subjects suffering from epileptic disorders and in animals rendered epileptic experimentally.[1] The suggestibility of epileptiform findings should not be considered absolute, and the patient's clinical history should be taken into account when considering a diagnosis of epilepsy. Though the diagnosis of epilepsy can be entirely based on clinical history without evidence of epileptiform activity on the patient's electroencephalogram (EEG), the presence of interictal discharges without an appropriate clinical history does not qualify the patient for a diagnosis of epilepsy. About 10% of patients who do not have epilepsy have been known to have nonspecific abnormalities on their EEG, and about 1% can have epileptiform interictal discharges without seizures. The incidence of such interictal activity is increased in children. Eeg-Olofsson et al. reported that 1.9% of 743 normal children had epileptiform discharges on their EEGs.[2] Others report even more frequent occurrence of epileptiform abnormalities, up to 2–3%, in the pediatric population. In addition, several factors – including medications, skull defects, certain medical conditions, and artifacts from multiple sources – can modify recorded activity and ultimately render EEG interpretation abnormal.

13.2 Interictal EEG Patterns

13.2.1 Focal Spikes and Sharp Waves

Whether a waveform appears epileptiform or not is judged by its morphology, amplitude, effect on the concurrent background activity, and topology. The waveforms are classified as "sharp waves" or "spikes" depending on their duration: sharp waves last 70–200 ms, while spikes are briefer than 70 ms. Sharp waves are transient waveforms that are biphasic or polyphasic, with an upward peak that usually has surface-negative voltage maxima. Surface-positive epileptiform discharges with true cortical generators have been described in the setting of benign Rolandic epilepsy, periventricular hemorrhage in neonates, red fiber myoclonus, and disturbance of the anatomic structures due to prior injury or resection. The morphology of the spikes usually features a much sharper-appearing peak. If multiple smaller irregular discharges are seen in the initial component of a spike–wave complex, they are referred to as "polyspikes." Typically, an epileptiform discharge is of higher amplitude, usually by a factor of two, and is immediately followed by a slow wave. These elements should be sufficient enough for the discharge to stand out from the surrounding background activity. The discharges should be seen with an adequate associated voltage field spread, which is evidenced by its appearance in one or more adjacent electrodes. This field is a representation of the extent of influence that a charge has on its surrounding area and associated leads. The field of an abnormal discharge is not always symmetric. It tends to fade away due to the decrease in the source strength over distance from the maximal focus of the discharge recorded on the scalp EEG. A discharge that is so focal and can only be detected in one electrode without affecting the other leads is highly unusual with spontaneous cerebral activity. Such a discharge is likely an artifact, most commonly caused by lead movement, or conduction of static or extraneous electric activity through the recording wire.

When a sharp wave or spike is determined to be epileptiform, this suggests a higher risk or susceptibility for developing seizures in the region it originates from. EEG recording during sleep increases the yield of demonstrating interictal epileptiform discharges to about 80–85%. The interictal discharges captured during non-rapid eye movement (REM) sleep have been known to carry high localizing value, demonstrating more accuracy than the same discharges captured during wakefulness.[3]

13.2.2 Temporal Lobe Discharges

Often, focal epileptiform spikes can be seen in combination with focal slowing in the same region. A region of maximal surface-voltage negativity can carry distinct clinical implications and sometimes be associated with a correlating structural lesion. Anterior temporal spikes have been shown to have a high association with mesial temporal lobe epilepsy. In patients with hippocampal sclerosis, interictal discharges can be found in the anterior temporal lobe region 90% of the time.[4] Independently, the likelihood of hippocampal sclerosis is less when frequent sharp waves were seen in the posterior or extratemporal regions.[5] Posterior temporal epileptiform discharges must also be distinguished from similar-appearing nonepileptiform wicket spikes (Figure 13.1).

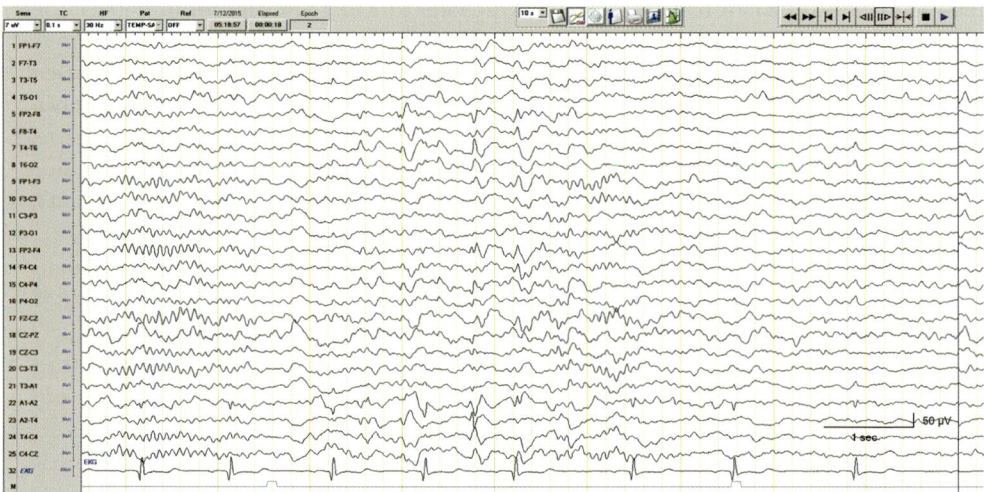

Figure 13.1 Temporal spike–wave discharges. Interictal scalp EEG, bipolar montage. A 23-year-old woman, with right temporal spike–wave discharges seen maximally over F8/T4, captured during non-REM stage II sleep.

13.2.3 Frontal Lobe Discharges

While interpreting frontal discharges indicative of frontal lobe epilepsy, special consideration should be given to discharges emanating from the deep midline regions, such as the cortex on the banks of the interhemispheric fissure or deep sulci. The synchronous activity of the pyramidal cells summates to produce a dipole, the negative maxima of which is detected by the recording surface electrode. Whether the epileptiform activity is seen by a given electrode depends on the dipole source location, its strength, and the solid angle of its vector in relation to the plane of the scalp electrode. If the dipole is horizontal or largely tangential to the scalp surface, the epileptiform discharge will remain invisible to the recording electrode. Alternatively, the propagation of the dipole angle may result in a maximal voltage surface negativity in the electrode over the contralateral hemisphere. Another scenario involves propagation of an epileptiform discharge bidirectionally from its deep source, resulting in the appearance of bisynchronous spikes or sharp waves in the adjacent electrodes over both hemispheres. The presence of these discharges may lead to the erroneous interpretation of the activity in question as representing generalized epileptiform waveforms. A differentiating clue might be provided by the presence of a consistent time lead of the epileptiform discharge over one hemisphere, as compared to the other.

Triphasic waves that are commonly seen with hepatic, renal, or toxic-metabolic encephalopathies, as well as with deep focal lesions, are typically frontally dominant and state-dependent, occurring in awake or stimulated states. Triphasic waves are usually slow waves in the 2–3 Hz frequency range, with a classically described "upward-downward-upward" deflection pattern that earned them their name. In cases where these waveforms are frontally dominant, they usually have a broad associated field that shows an anterior-to-posterior lag of the second downward phase that might help to distinguish them from generalized epileptiform discharges. Less commonly, these discharges might have a posterior predominance – in these instances, a posterior-to-anterior phase lag is more likely to be seen.

13.2.4 Occipital Lobe Discharges

Occipital spikes can be seen in early- or late-onset childhood occipital epilepsies, known as Panayiotopoulos syndrome and Gastaut-type occipital epilepsy, respectively. These discharges are seen in two-thirds of recordings obtained in patients with a suggestive clinical history. They can be unilateral or bilateral, and classically attenuate with eye opening ("fixation-off effect") or become more prominent when the lights are turned off. Less commonly, interictal epileptiform waveforms in these patients have also been described originating from extraoccipital areas. Additionally, sharp morphology waveforms with occipital predominance have also been mentioned in patients with migraines,[6] celiac disease,[7] and Lafora body disease.[8] Benign occipital waveforms that should not be mistaken for epileptiform discharges include positive occipital sharp transients of sleep (POSTS), lambda waves, or a normal driving response evoked by photic stimulation during the study.

13.2.5 Focal Slowing

Spontaneous activity in the theta–delta range in an awake state can be abnormal. When these waveforms appear asymmetrically over just one hemisphere or over a smaller region it is referred to as focal slowing. Focal slowing should be described in terms of its duration, abundance, rhythmicity, amplitude, and localization. Focal slowing typically suggests cerebral dysfunction associated with underlying subcortical white matter. When the slow waves are focal and seen in a rhythmic manner (usually in the delta frequency), it can carry epileptiform significance, depending on their location, and is termed lateralized rhythmic delta activity (LRDA). In the temporal lobe, this finding is called temporal intermittent rhythmic delta activity (TIRDA), and has a high association with temporal lobe epilepsy (TLE). Several publications have confirmed that TIRDA strongly correlates with the diagnosis of temporal lobe epilepsy,[9–11] and particularly with mesial temporal lobe epilepsy.[12]

Generalized rhythmic delta activity (GRDA) or former frontally dominant intermittent rhythmic delta activity (FIRDA) is not considered a focal or epileptiform finding. Instead, it is a marker of diffuse encephalopathy of toxic or metabolic etiology, and can be an indication of an expanding deep midline lesion, such as a midline tumor, hemorrhage, edema, or hydrocephalus.

Occipital intermittent rhythmic delta activity (OIRDA) is most commonly found in pediatric patients; its posterior predominance is largely explained by incomplete myelination of the frontal lobes at this stage of neuronal development. It can be a sign of toxic or metabolic encephalopathy; nevertheless, a form of OIRDA appearing as prolonged runs of 3-Hz delta activity has been associated with childhood absence epilepsy.

13.2.6 Periodic Discharges

When waveforms with relatively uniform morphology and duration recur at regular intervals and are separated by definable intervening background activity, they are termed periodic (or quasiperiodic when they occur at nearly regular intervals) discharges. In contrast, rhythmic waveforms do not have an interval of baseline activity between consecutive waveforms[1]. Periodic discharges demonstrate spike, sharp wave, or polyspike morphology at the usual amplitudes of 50–150 µV, occasionally reaching up to 300 µV. The repetition rate varies from 0.2 to 3 per second. When waveforms appear faster than three times per second, the intervening background activity disappears, causing periodic discharges to appear rhythmic and making the distinction between ictal and interictal activity subjective. Based on their distribution, periodic discharges are designated lateralized periodic discharges (LPDs), bilateral periodic lateralized epileptiform discharges (bi-PLEDs), or generalized periodic discharges (GPDs). Bi-PLEDs are characterized by asynchronous discharges over each hemisphere that frequently have different amplitudes, fields, and repetition rates. GPDs are generalized and synchronous with low amplitude (<10 µV) intervening background activity. Periodic discharges tend to resolve within days to weeks; rarely can they persist for months or years. Their morphological frequency and complexity decreases over time, without a clear relationship with specific antiseizure therapies.

The incidence of LPDs in most EEG series is approximately 0.4% to 1.0%.[13–15] In the pediatric patient population, central nervous system infections are the dominant causes of quasiperiodic activity on EEG.[16] In adult patients, the potential causes are quite diverse, and include acute cerebral infarction (with watershed-type stroke being the most common), hemorrhagic stroke, neoplasms, post-traumatic coma, status epilepticus, herpes simplex encephalitis, postanoxic insults, metabolic imbalances, drug or alcohol withdrawal, multiple sclerosis, inflammatory disorders, hemiplegic migraines, sickle cell disease, cerebral amyloidosis, hyperperfusion after endarterectomy, acquired immune deficiency syndrome, neuro-Behçet's, tuberous sclerosis, aminophylline intoxication, infectious mononucleosis encephalitis, posterior reversible encephalopathy syndrome, and neurosyphilis. Bi-PLEDs have most commonly been reported with anoxic brain injuries, infections of the central nervous system, chronic seizure disorders, and vascular causes.[17] GPDs are seen in the setting of extensive anoxic cortical injury, dementia, intracerebral hemorrhage, severe toxic-metabolic encephalopathies, head injuries with seizures, early Creutzfeldt–Jakob disease, and subacute sclerosing panencephalitis. The interval between the periodic discharges is shorter in Cruetzfeldt–Jakob disease compared to subacute sclerosing panencephalitis.

Chatrian et al. demonstrated that functional isolation of the cortex is sufficient as a generator of periodic epileptiform discharges.[18] Early observations concluded that either direct cortical injury or subcortical dysfunction resulting in denervation of the cortical neurons and, in turn, disturbance of the balance between synaptic inhibition and excitation is a key pathophysiologic feature responsible for the generation of periodic discharges on the EEG. An abnormal cortical response to reticular thalamic nuclear rhythmic burst firing, evoked as a possible mechanism for origin of quasiperiodic discharges was initially introduced by Gloor et al.[19] and later revisited by Gross et al.[20] Other specific etiologies may shine additional light on the pathophysiologic mechanisms responsible for generation of periodic discharges. Focal hyperexcitabilty in the penumbra zone of ischemic stroke was given significance by Pohlmann Eden et al.[21] In patients with herpes simplex encephalitis, virus-induced fusion of neuronal processes leading to electrotonic coupling between cells and, in turn, to large cellular aggregates firing in synchrony has been proposed as a mechanism of cortical periodicity.[22,23] It has been commonly observed that in patients with quasiperiodic discharges on EEG, seizures can evolve from these epileptiform waveforms, starting in the same region, but preceded by attenuation of periodic discharges, or appear independently from persistent and simultaneous periodic discharges. This observation led to the notion that the trigger site for the discharges is poorly defined and could be minimally involved or not involved in the specific pathophysiologic process affecting the patient. Clinically, this uncertainty generated a controversy of whether periodic discharges are consistent with ongoing epileptic activity or if they are an electrographic epiphenomenon and more likely to represent an abnormal response of the cortex to a recent injury.[24,25] Studies utilizing functional modalities, such as PET, SPECT, and MEG, have been used to argue both views.[26–30] LPDs are most commonly associated with focal or secondarily-generalized seizures while bi-PLEDS and GPDs are accompanied by generalized seizures. Overall, a given patient's clinical outcome is largely dictated by the associated etiology and extent of cortical injury; hence, outcome prognostication of bi-PLEDs and GPDs is less favorable than LPDs.

13.2.7 Generalized Discharges

In generalized epilepsy, epileptiform activity involves large areas of the cortex. By the time the activity propagates to the surface electrodes, EEG findings are bilateral and synchronized. However, in many instances the generalized epileptiform discharges may appear fragmented and with greater prominence in one specific region. In addition, secondary bilateral synchrony of an epileptiform discharge that can be seen in focal epilepsies, may be difficult to distinguish from a fragment of generalized epilepsy, as it spreads bilaterally rapidly and appears generalized at first glance if not examined closely for asynchrony. There may be a brief but consistent lead-in marking a subtle focal onset (Figure 13.2).

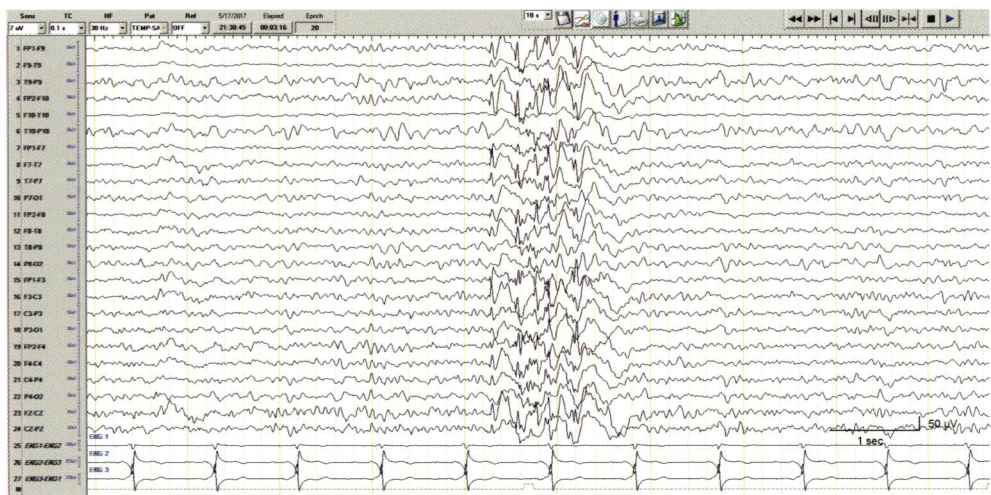

Figure 13.2 Generalized discharges. Interictal scalp EEG, bipolar montage. A 66-year-old woman with genetic generalized epilepsy (juvenile myoclonic epilepsy). EEG shows brief 1–2 s bursts of fast polyspike-and-slow-wave discharges, captured during sleep.

13.2.7.1 Generalized 3-Hz Spike-and-Wave Pattern

An EEG pattern of high-amplitude, generalized spike-and-slow-wave discharges with an average frequency of 3 Hz, occurring in abrupt bursts amid an otherwise normal background is characteristic of genetic (idiopathic) generalized epilepsy. The frequency of 3 Hz is typically seen in young patients with absence epilepsy. The spike–wave discharges can be seen with higher amplitude in the fronto-central leads, and may become more prominent with eye closure, hyperventilation (which often triggers an actual seizure with clinical signs), drowsiness, and hypoglycemia. At times, the spike–wave frequency can be initially faster, around 4 Hz, and slows slightly towards the end. Occurrence of generalized epileptiform discharges in some cases can have genetic predisposition that may or may not progress to the clinical seizures.

13.2.7.2 Fast Spike-and-Wave Pattern

A faster frequency spike–wave pattern, ranging from 3.5 to 6.0 Hz is seen in juvenile myoclonic epilepsy (JME). The generalized spike-and-slow-wave morphology can appear more fragmented, and often has an initial polyspike component demonstrating up to eight subsequent waveforms. The discharges may be more prominent with sleep deprivation. A number of pharmacological agents causing excessive GABA activation have been known to exacerbate epileptiform activity, sometimes causing spike–wave stupor when severe. Similar to typical absence epilepsy, the underlying background EEG pattern should be normal. A photoparoxysmal response characterized by bilateral and synchronous polyspike or polyspike-and-slow-wave discharges can be seen in these patients with photic stimulation, frequently with higher flash frequencies in the 12–20 Hz range. The discharges may not be time locked to the flash frequency, and can also occur after the flash stimulus has been terminated. The incidence of photic sensitivity is increased in JME, reported in up to 31% in comparison to 18% seen in childhood absence epilepsy patients.[31] This fast spike–wave pattern can also be seen in progressive myoclonic epilepsies of varied etiologies, though the concomitant background in these cases will likely show varying degrees of slowing and clinically the patient would exhibit cognitive dysfunction.

13.2.7.3 Slow Spike-and-Wave Pattern

A slow spike-and-wave pattern occurring around 1–2.5 Hz is typically seen in association with symptomatic generalized epilepsies. The spike component in particular can appear broader with a longer duration, consistent with a sharp wave rather than a spike. The EEG background is slow, frequently exhibiting independent multifocal sharp waves and spikes. These patients are often cognitively delayed due to perinatal brain insult or de novo genetic mutation, and may have structural abnormalities on imaging studies. They often carry a diagnosis of Lennox–Gastaut syndrome, although, this is only one of many potential clinical syndromes in which this pattern occurs.

13.2.7.4 Hypsarrhythmia

Hypsarrhythmia refers to a distinct EEG pattern consisting of high-voltage irregular activity that is often sharply contoured and contains multifocal spikes, which ultimately give the overall background pattern a very disorganized and chaotic appearance. This was first defined by Gibbs and Gibbs in 1952, and was described as "random high-voltage waves and spikes."[32] They stated that these spikes vary from moment to moment, both in time and in location. At times they appear to be focal, and a few seconds later they seem to originate from multiple foci. Occasionally the spike discharge becomes generalized, but it never appears as a rhythmically repetitive and highly organized pattern that could be confused with a discharge of a petit mal or petit mal variant type. This pattern is classic for infantile spasms, which are seen in very young patients (aged 4 months to 4 years old), who usually exhibit significant cognitive delay. Tuberous sclerosis is a common etiology, but hypsarrhythmia can also have other infectious, metabolic, or genetic causes. The hypsarrhythmia pattern evolves over time as the patient ages due to progressive myelination and synaptogenesis.

13.3 Ictal EEG Patterns

13.3.1 Generalized-Onset Seizure

In generalized epilepsy, ictal activity typically manifests as high-amplitude bursts of epileptiform discharges with abrupt onset and offset that is prominent and distinct relative to the background. The ictal EEG pattern may appear similar to the interictal pattern, but with prolonged runs of increased duration with evolution of discharges. These EEG findings are expected to coincide with objectively apparent clinical signs, confirming the diagnosis of a seizure (Figure 13.3).

Generalized paroxysmal fast activity (GPFA) is a pattern consisting of diffuse repetitive spikes and blunted waves appearing at frequencies from 8–20 Hz. Its duration is typically measured in seconds. This pattern can be seen in generalized epilepsies with prominent tonic seizures, and can occur in combination with a diffuse electrodecrement of the background activity.

Electrodecrement is an ictal pattern seen with the tonic and atonic seizures in symptomatic generalized epilepsies. It is commonly preceded by a high-amplitude slow wave and over-riding GPFA. The EEG exhibits abrupt diffuse background attenuation, occurring within 1–2 s and lasting less than 4–5 s. Since the baseline background activity is commonly

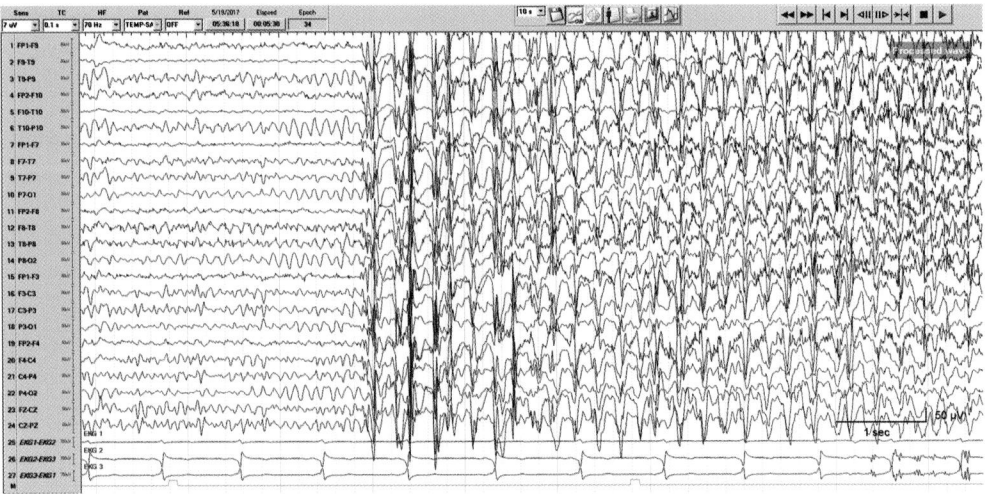

Figure 13.3 Generalized-onset seizure. Ictal scalp EEG, bipolar montage. A 56-year-old woman with genetic generalized epilepsy (juvenile myoclonic epilepsy). EEG shows abrupt seizure onset in the form of generalized fast frequency polyspike-and-slow-wave discharges.

abnormal due to the presence of slowing and multifocal sharp discharges, the brief attenuation period that transiently resolves these abnormalities may give the EEG a "normal" appearance. Hence it is also referred to as "pseudonormalization."

13.3.2 Focal-Onset Seizure

For focal-onset ictal patterns, the key to distinguishing seizures from interictal discharges or abnormal background activity is identifying the evolution of a waveform's characteristic features. The EEG terminology guidelines set forth by the American Clinical Neurophysiology Society in 2012 define evolution as an unequivocal sequential change in frequency, location, and morphology, lasting at least three cycles each, consisting of two consecutive time periods, showing sequential spread to two or more channels in the 10-20 international electrode placement system, or exhibiting two or more consecutive changes to a novel morphology.[1] An evolving ictal pattern typically begins with low-amplitude, faster activity that becomes gradually more prominent in its amplitude and morphology, then it slows to rhythmic lower-frequency activity, at times incorporating spike-and-slow-wave discharges spreading over a broader area. With movements during the seizure, the EEG becomes obscured by lead and myogenic artifacts. Ictal offset may be abrupt or gradual, and is often followed by diffuse background attenuation and diffuse high-amplitude delta-range slowing. Asymmetry of the postictal slowing is an indication of increased cerebral dysfunction in the involved hemisphere, and may be helpful in lateralizing the seizure onset.[33–35] Particularly in temporal lobe epilepsy, postictal delta slowing has been reported to lateralize the ictal onset correctly in up to 96% of seizures.[36]

The region of seizure onset is an important feature that suggests an epileptogenic focus in a patient with intractable epilepsy who is being considered for resective surgery. Electrographically, the ictal pattern can take on various forms: rhythmic slow-wave activity,

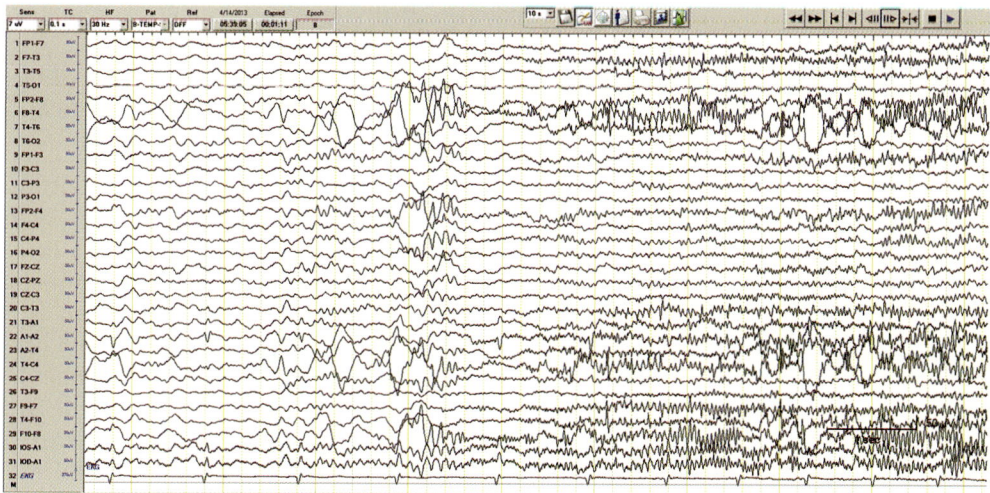

Figure 13.4 Focal-onset seizure. Ictal scalp EEG, bipolar montage. A 51-year-old woman with focal neocortical epilepsy. EEG shows heralding polyspikes in the right frontotemporal region, followed by low amplitude rhythmic fast activity in the right hemisphere.

a "heralding spike" in the form of a high-amplitude epileptiform discharge, irregular fast spike activity, or abrupt background attenuation (Figure 13.4). The onset pattern of partial seizures in scalp recordings could be seen as sinusoidal waves, repetitive discharges such as spikes and sharp waves, or an electrodecremental response. Rhythmic 5–9 Hz activity is a common pattern seen within the first 30 s of a seizure This has been reported with higher frequency in mesial temporal lobe seizures – up to 65–90% when localized to the temporal leads,[37–40] – and even more frequently in patients with advanced hippocampal atrophy – up to 79%.[41] This onset pattern is only rarely reported in extratemporal lobe epilepsy. Neocortical temporal lobe epilepsy may exhibit slower 2–5 Hz, rhythmic or polymorphic, and irregular activity at the onset of seizures.[42] Initial ictal changes from midline frontal or orbito-frontal lobe seizures may be difficult to capture, especially with scalp recordings. This difficulty is also explained by the overall brief duration of the seizures, rapid spread, and significant artifacts that tend to obscure the EEG due to hyperkinetic movements. The aforementioned bilateral synchrony can be seen frequently due to deep epileptogenic focus and rapid generalization. There may just be subtle findings such as rhythmic slowing or background attenuation preceding or following the seizure.

Electrical decrement or attenuation seen at the onset of seizures can be a very subtle finding that marks the beginning of a seizure. This is seen as an abrupt suppression that disrupts the background activity briefly prior to more obvious ictal activity, which can be seen focally, involving just a few electrodes. Otherwise, the background attenuation may be diffuse and, though helpful in identifying seizure onset, has no localizing or lateralizing value. For seizures with a midline or deep epileptogenic source, as seen in many frontal lobe epilepsies, the ictal EEG may appear normal overall, with only this subtle background change as a clue to the presence of a seizure. Sudden cessation of previously recurring interictal discharges can also mark the onset of a seizure. Other seizure-onset patterns that can be seen in extratemporal lobe epilepsies include paroxysmal fast activity or repetitive spiking. When the fast activity appears in a restricted region on the EEG, it has high localizing value, reflective of close proximity between the overlying electrode and seizure onset zone. Repetitive paroxysms of spikes, also known as "trains of spikes," are characterized by higher-amplitude spikes that may precede the paroxysmal fast activity as a component of the overall evolving ictal pattern.

References

1. Hirsch LJ, LaRoche SM, Gaspard N, et al. American Clinical Neurophysiology Society's standardized critical care EEG terminology: 2012 version. *J Clin Neurophysiol.* 2013;30(1):1–27.

2. Eeg-Olofsson O, Petersen I, Sellden U. The development of the electroencephalogram in normal children from the age of 1 through 15 years. Paroxysmal activity. *Neuropadiatrie.* 1971;2(4):375–404.

3. Adachi N, Alarcon G, Binnie CD, et al. Predictive value of interictal epileptiform discharges during non-REM sleep on scalp EEG recordings for the lateralization of epileptogenesis. *Epilepsia.* 1998;39(6):628–632.

4. Ebersole JS, Wade PB. Spike voltage topography identifies two types of frontotemporal epileptic foci. *Neurology.* 1991;41(9):1425–1433.

5. Hamer HM, Najm I, Mohamed A, Wyllie E. Interictal epileptiform discharges in temporal lobe epilepsy due to hippocampal sclerosis versus medial temporal lobe tumors. *Epilepsia.* 1999;40(9):1261–1268.

6. Beaumanoir A, Grandjean E. Occipital spikes, migraine and epilepsy. In: Andermann F, Lugaresi E, eds. *Migraine and Epilepsy.* Boston: Butterworths; 1987:97–110.

7. Gobbi G, Sorrenti G, Santucci M, et al. Epilepsy with bilateral occipital calcifications: a benign onset with progressive severity. *Neurology.* 1988;38(6):913–920.

8. Tassinari CA, Bureau-Paillas M, Dalla Bernardina B, et al. [Lafora disease (author's transl)]. *Rev Electroencephalogr Neurophysiol Clin.* 1978;8(1):107–122.

9. Reiher J, Beaudry M, Leduc CP. Temporal intermittent rhythmic delta activity (TIRDA) in the diagnosis of complex partial epilepsy: sensitivity, specificity and predictive value. *Can J Neurol Sci.* 1989;16(4):398–401.

10. Blume WT, Borghesi JL, Lemieux JF. Interictal indices of temporal seizure origin. *Ann Neurol.* 1993;34(5):703–709.

11. Gambardella A, Gotman J, Cendes F, Andermann F. Focal intermittent delta activity in patients with mesiotemporal atrophy: a reliable marker of the epileptogenic focus. *Epilepsia.* 1995;36(2):122–129.

12. Di Gennaro G, Quarato PP, Onorati P, et al. Localizing significance of temporal intermittent rhythmic delta activity (TIRDA) in drug-resistant focal epilepsy. *Clin Neurophysiol.* 2003;114(1):70–78.

13. Kuroiwa Y, Celesia GG. Clinical significance of periodic EEG patterns. *Arch Neurol.* 1980;37(1):15–20.

14. Snodgrass SM, Tsuburaya K, Ajmone-Marsan C. Clinical significance of periodic lateralized epileptiform discharges: relationship with status epilepticus. *J Clin Neurophysiol.* 1989;6(2):159–172.

15. Walsh JM, Brenner RP. Periodic lateralized epileptiform discharges – long-term outcome in adults. *Epilepsia.* 1987;28(5):533–536.

16. Fitzpatrick W, Lowry N. PLEDs: clinical correlates. *Can J Neurol Sci.* 2007;34(4):443–450.

17. de la Paz D, Brenner RP. Bilateral independent periodic lateralized epileptiform discharges. Clinical significance. *Arch Neurol.* 1981;38(11):713–715.

18. Chatrian GE, Shaw CM, Leffman H. The significance of periodic lateralized epileptiform discharges in EEG: an electrographic, clinical and pathological

study, *Electroencephalogr Clin Neurophysiol.* 1964;17(2):177–193.

19. Gloor P, Kalabay O, Giard N. The electroencephalogram in diffuse encephalopathies: electroencephalographic correlates of grey and white matter lesions. *Brain.* 1968;91(4):779–802.

20. Gross DW, Quesney LF, Sadikot AF. Chronic periodic lateralized epileptiform discharges during sleep in a patient with caudate nucleus atrophy: insights into the anatomical circuitry of PLEDs. *Electroencephalogr Clin Neurophysiol.* 1998;107(6):434–438.

21. Pohlmann-Eden B, Hoch DB, Cochius JI, Chiappa KH. Periodic lateralized epileptiform discharges – a critical review. *J Clin Neurophysiol.* 1996;13(6):519–530.

22. Cobb WA. Evidence on the periodic mechanism in herpes simplex encephalitis. *Electroencephalogr Clin Neurophysiol.* 1979;46(3):345–350.

23. Traub RD, Pedley TA. Virus-induced electrotonic coupling: hypothesis on the mechanism of periodic EEG discharges in Creutzfeldt-Jakob disease. *Ann Neurol.* 1981;10(5):405–410.

24. Treiman DM, Walton NY, DeGiorgio C. Predictable sequence of EEG changes during generalized convulsive status epilepticus in man and three experimental models of status epilepticus in the rat [abstract]. *Neurology.* 1987;37(3 Suppl 1):244–245.

25. Walton NY, Treiman DM. Response of status epilepticus induced by lithium and pilocarpine to treatment with diazepam. *Exp Neurol.* 1988;101(2):267–275.

26. Ali II, Pirzada NA, Vaughn BV. Periodic lateralized epileptiform discharges after complex partial status epilepticus associated with increased focal cerebral blood flow. *J Clin Neurophysiol.* 2001;18(6):565–569.

27. Assal F, Papazyan JP, Slosman DO, Jallon P, Goerres GW. SPECT in periodic lateralized epileptiform discharges (PLEDs): a form of partial status epilepticus? *Seizure.* 2001;10(4):260–265.

28. Handforth A, Finch DM, Peters R, Tan AM, Treiman DM. Interictal spiking increases 2-deoxy[14C]glucose uptake and c-fos-like reactivity. *Ann Neurol.* 1994;35 (6):724–731.

29. Handforth A, Treiman DM. Functional mapping of the late stages of status epilepticus in the lithium-pilocarpine model in rat: a 14C-2-deoxyglucose study. *Neuroscience.* 1995;64(4):1075–1089.

30. Shvarts V, Zoltay G, Bowyer SM, et al. Periodic discharges: insight from magnetoencephalography. *J Clin Neurophysiol.* 2017;34(3):196–206.

31. Wolf P, Goosses R. Relation of photosensitivity to epileptic syndromes. *J Neurol Neurosurg Psychiatry.* 1986;49 (12):1386–1391.

32. Gibbs FA, Gibbs EL. *Atlas of electroencephalography: Epilepsy.* Vol 2. Reading, MA: Addison-Wesley Publishing Company; 1952.

33. Kaibara M, Blume WT. The postictal electroencephalogram. *Electroencephalogr Clin Neurophysiol.* 1988;70(2):99–104.

34. Walczak TS, Radtke RA, Lewis DV. Accuracy and interobserver reliability of scalp ictal EEG. *Neurology.* 1992;42 (12):2279–2285.

35. Hufnagel A, Elger CE, Pels H, et al. Prognostic significance of ictal and interictal epileptiform activity in temporal lobe epilepsy. *Epilepsia.* 1994;35 (6):1146–1153.

36. Jan MM, Sadler M, Rahey SR. Lateralized postictal EEG delta predicts the side of seizure surgery in temporal lobe epilepsy. *Epilepsia.* 2001;42(3):402–405.

37. Risinger MW, Engel J, Jr., Van Ness PC, Henry TR, Crandall PH. Ictal localization of temporal lobe seizures with scalp/ sphenoidal recordings. *Neurology.* 1989;39 (10):1288–1293.

38. Ebersole JS, Pacia SV. Localization of temporal lobe foci by ictal EEG patterns. *Epilepsia.* 1996;37(4):386–399.

39. Caboclo LO, Garzon E, Oliveira PA, et al. Correlation between temporal pole MRI abnormalities and surface ictal EEG

patterns in patients with unilateral mesial temporal lobe epilepsy. *Seizure*. 2007;16 (1):8–16.

40. Foldvary N, Klem G, Hammel J, et al. The localizing value of ictal EEG in focal epilepsy. *Neurology*. 2001;57 (11):2022–2028.

41. Vossler DG, Kraemer DL, Knowlton RC, et al. Temporal ictal

electroencephalographic frequency correlates with hippocampal atrophy and sclerosis. *Ann Neurol*. 1998;43 (6):756–762.

42. Foldvary N, Lee N, Thwaites G, et al. Clinical and electrographic manifestations of lesional neocortical temporal lobe epilepsy. *Neurology*. 1997;49 (3):757–763.

Chapter 14

Neonatal and Pediatric Electroencephalogram

Basanagoud Mudigoudar, Stephen Fulton, Sarah Weatherspoon, and James W. Wheless

14.1 Introduction

Interpretation of the pediatric electroencephalogram (EEG) is challenging due to the dramatic changes in EEG patterns that occur in neonates, infants, and children secondary to rapid anatomic and physiological development of the brain. Knowledge of orderly maturational changes in the EEG is an essential skill for proper interpretation in this age group.

14.2 Neonatal EEG

Precise information about the conceptual age (CA) of the child is needed for accurate analysis of EEG in neonates and young infants. CA is calculated by adding legal age (age since birth) to the estimated gestational age. For the purpose of interpretation of EEG, rate of brain development is considered to be the same whether in utero or after birth.

The international 10-20 system of electrode placement is modified in neonates below 32 weeks CA in view of the small head size and immature frontal lobes.[1] A minimum of nine electrodes (F1, F2, C3, C4, CZ, T7, T8, O1, and O2) is required in addition to the referential electrodes placed on ear lobes (A1 and A2). Polygraphic measures (eye movement, electromyography, electrocardiogram, and respiration) are crucial in providing information about the behavioral state (awake or asleep) of the child and identifying artifacts. Simultaneous video-EEG monitoring and technician notes are essential for interpreting neonatal EEG.

14.3 Principles of Interpreting Neonatal EEG Background

Initial visual analysis of EEG is based on assessing the behavioral state of the child and the continuity of EEG background. Further evaluation should include analyzing the symmetry and interhemispheric synchrony of waveforms. In addition, identification of specific waveforms and patterns that occur during the neonatal period is required to correctly evaluate the developmental maturation of EEG.

14.3.1 Continuity and State Changes

Except during the neonatal period, all pediatric EEGs should have a continuous background in all states (awake, drowsy, and asleep). The earliest evidence of brain electric activity is seen after 8 weeks of CA, characterized by long periods of quiescence interrupted by bursts of activity. This pattern in premature neonates is termed tracé discontinu (Figure 14.1) and the periods of quiescence are termed interburst intervals (IBI). As the CA increases, the

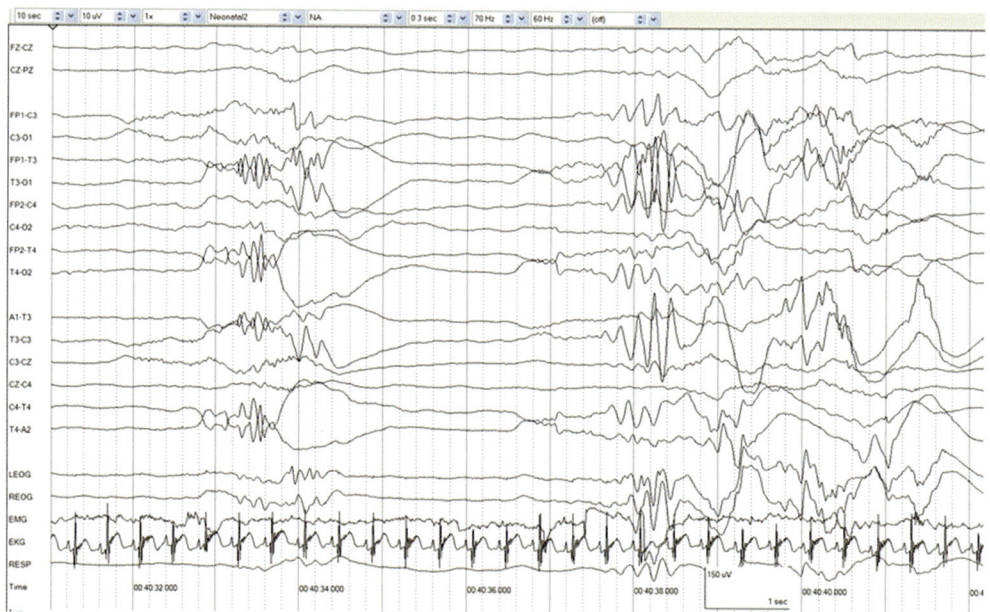

Figure 14.1 Tracé discontinu pattern at 26 weeks CA.

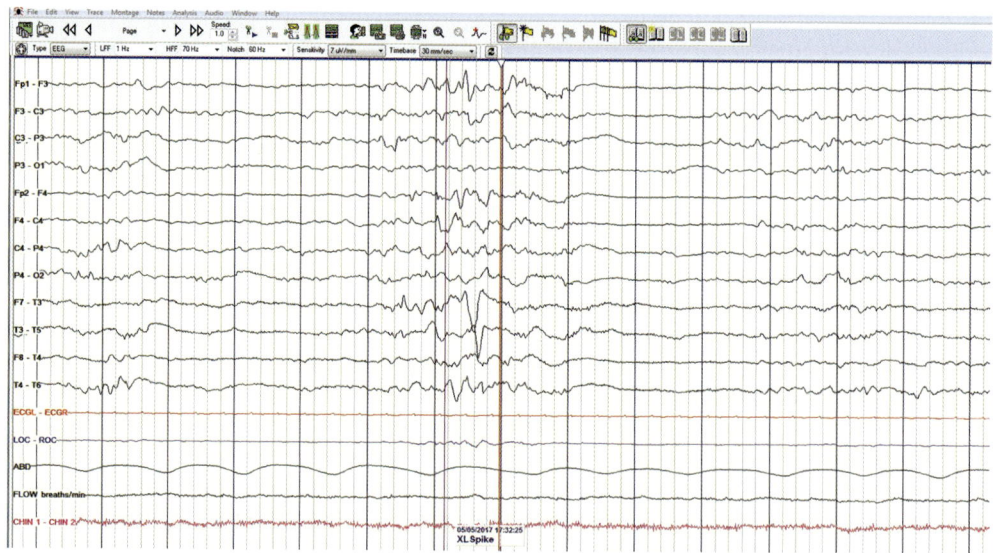

Figure 14.2 Tracé alternant pattern at 37 weeks CA.

duration of the IBI shortens and the EEG becomes more continuous. The maximum amplitude of IBI during tracé discontinu is less than 25 μV.[2] In neonates older than 37–38 weeks CA, the background in quiet sleep (what will later become non-rapid-eye-movement (NREM) sleep) changes to periods of relative generalized voltage attenuation (amplitude > 25 μV) instead of complete quiescence and is now termed tracé alternant (Figure 14.2).

The EEG background changes, depending on the behavioral state of the child, as the infant gets older. Prior to 36–37 weeks of CA the state of the child is mainly determined by changes in behavior and polygraphic recordings. Eye opening indicates the awake state and eye closure, sleep. Irregular respiration, rapid eye movements, and decreased muscle tone are associated with active sleep (later what will become REM (rapid eye movement) sleep). Quiet sleep (what will later become NREM sleep) is associated with regular respiration, variable muscle tone, and random eye movements. In a neonate, even after careful analysis of the behavioral signs, polygraphic recordings, and EEG, sometimes it is difficult to distinguish the different sleep cycles. When this occurs it is termed indeterminate or transitional sleep. The newborn sleep–wake cycle has a periodicity of 50–60 minutes, and lengthens with increasing age.

14.3.2 Synchrony and Symmetry

EEG activity between the two hemispheres should be symmetric at any age. If the difference in amplitude of the EEG activity arising from homologous regions of the two hemispheres exceeds a 2:1 ratio then it is considered to be abnormal (typically on the side with the lower voltage).[3] The degree of synchrony in EEG activity between the two hemispheres increases with increasing central nervous system (CNS) maturity. Bursts of activity from two homologous regions separated by more than 1.5–2 s are considered to be asynchronous. Around 70% of bursts are synchronous during quiet sleep at 31–32 weeks CA, increasing to 100% by 37 weeks.[4] In infants, sleep spindles and vertex sharp waves are usually synchronous by 18 to 24 months of age.

14.3.3 Specific Normal Neonatal Background Patterns and Waveforms

14.3.3.1 Delta Brushes

These waveforms are considered to be a marker of prematurity. They consist of high-amplitude delta waves with over-riding bursts of 8–22 Hz fast activity (Figure 14.3). These can be seen over any head region, but are less frequent over frontal head regions. They are predominantly present over temporal, occipital, and central head regions. They are seen frequently between 26 and 38 weeks of gestation. In neonates less than 33 weeks CA, they are more commonly seen during active sleep, but appear to be more frequent during quiet sleep in older neonates. At 37 weeks CA, they are seen only during quiet sleep and then disappear by 44 weeks CA.

14.3.3.2 Rhythmic Temporal Theta Activity

These are brief (<2 s) bursts of sharply contoured theta waveforms seen over both temporal head regions, either synchronously or independently (Figure 14.4). They are exclusively seen between 31 and 33 weeks of CA. Sometimes they are confused with temporal sharp transients.

14.3.3.3 Anterior Dysrhythmia

This pattern consists of intermittent runs of quasirhythmic high-amplitude delta activity over the bifrontal regions. Sometimes the waveforms are very sharply contoured and are seen admixed with frontal sharp transients (encoches frontales). This activity is usually symmetric and synchronous over both frontal regions. It is a normal feature in term and near-term neonates. Though this can be seen in any behavioral state, it is more common

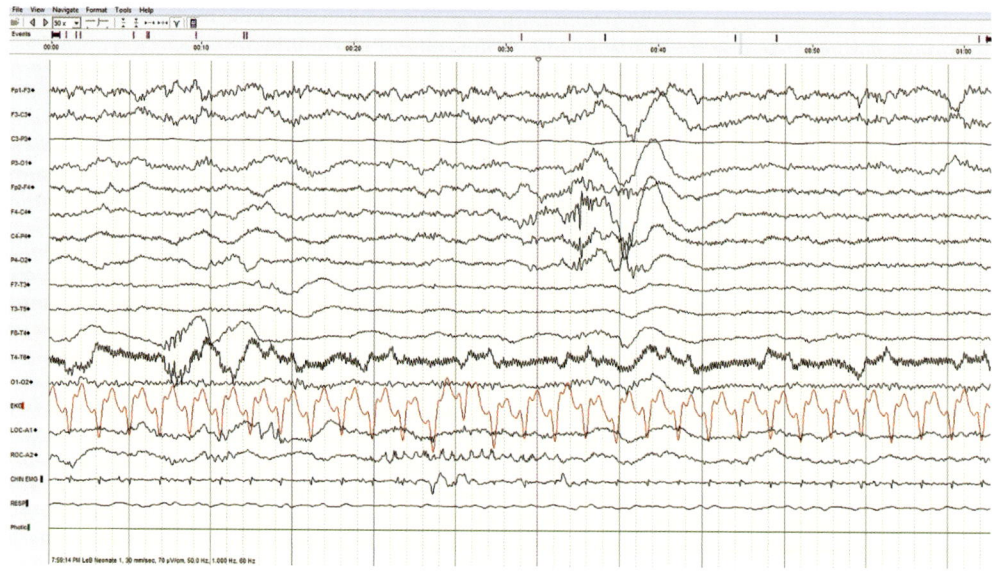

Figure 14.3 Beta range fast-frequency activity over-riding high-amplitude delta activity in a delta brush pattern at 27 weeks CA.

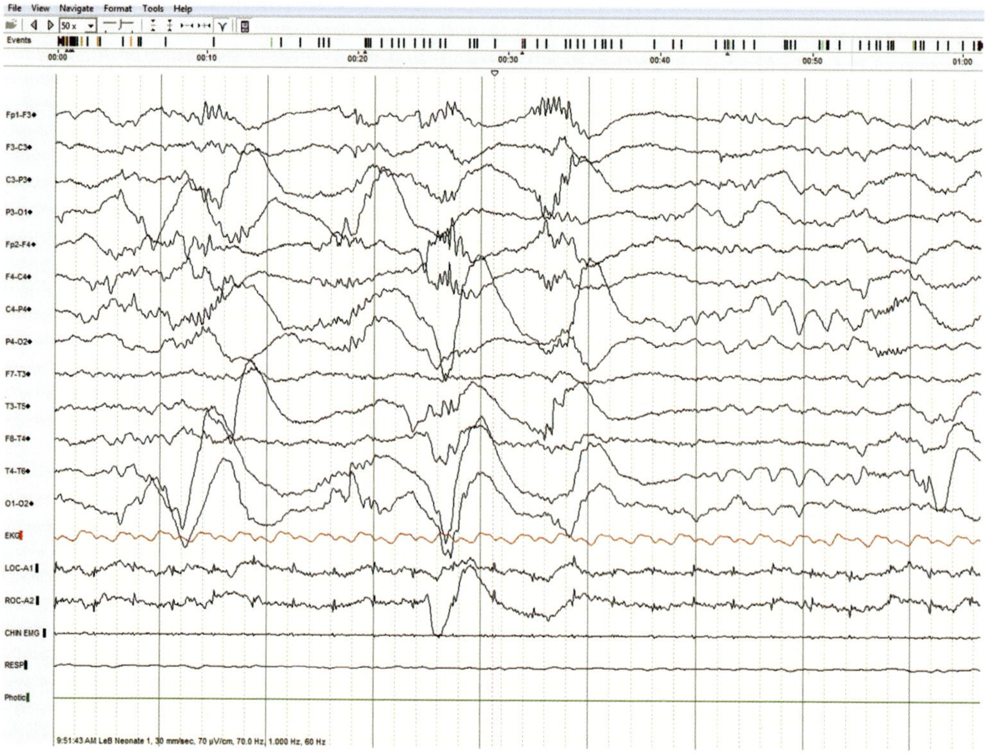

Figure 14.4 Rhythmic temporal theta activity at 31 weeks CA.

during transitional sleep. Excessive amounts of this pattern are sometimes seen in diffuse encephalopathies and are considered to be a nonspecific abnormal finding.[5]

14.3.3.4 Encoche Frontales (Frontal Sharp Waves)

Presence of high-amplitude biphasic sharp waves over the frontal regions is considered to be a normal finding in neonates. They usually appear symmetrically and synchronously over the frontal regions, and frequently are seen admixed with the anterior dysrhythmia pattern. They appear at 34 weeks of CA and disappear by 44 weeks of CA. They can be distinguished from spikes, which have a typical morphology and are usually seen in an asymmetric fashion.[3]

14.4 Normal Maturation of the Neonatal EEG

Orderly changes in EEG background are seen with advancement of age paralleling brain development in a predictable manner. Knowledge of EEG ontogeny is critical in distinguishing normal findings from abnormal features in different age groups.

14.4.1 Less than 29 Weeks CA

EEG background at this age is discontinuous with bursts of activity separated by periods of very low voltage (<25 μV, tracé discontinu). Typically IBI are 8–12 s in duration, but longer intervals up to 30 s can be seen. The EEG background does not change with state changes. Bursts consist of high-amplitude delta waves seen maximally over the occipital regions, along with delta brushes. Almost all bursts at this age are synchronous.

14.4.2 30 to 34 Weeks CA

At this age differences in EEG background start to show up between the awake state/active sleep (these can have similar EEG findings, knowledge of eye opening or closure and the other polygraphic variables helps distinguish the two) and quiet sleep. EEG activity also begins to show reactivity to stimuli. Awake and active sleep consist of longer periods of bursts of activity separated by briefer inactive IBI. Occurrence of paroxysms of rhythmic theta activity over the temporal regions is a characteristic finding between 31 and 33 weeks CA. Quiet sleep is characterized by tracé discontinu with shorter IBI, lasting 5–8 s.

14.4.3 35 to 36 Weeks CA

At this CA, the EEG background is continuous during the awake and active sleep states and consists of polyfrequency activity with fewer delta brushes over the temporal, central, and occipital head regions. During quiet sleep, IBIs of 4–6 s duration with amplitude of >25 μV are seen, separated by bursts of activity suggesting tracé alternant pattern for the first time.

14.4.4 37 to 40 Weeks CA

At this age, awake and active sleep are easily distinguishable from quiet sleep. Awake state EEG (Figure 14.5) shows an admixture of theta activity with lower amplitude delta activity, which is continuous. Quiet sleep is characterized by tracé alternant pattern with IBIs lasting for 2–4 s. Brief periods of continuous delta activity, a marker of continuous slow-wave sleep (NREM), are noticed during quiet sleep for the first time at this age (Figure 14.6).

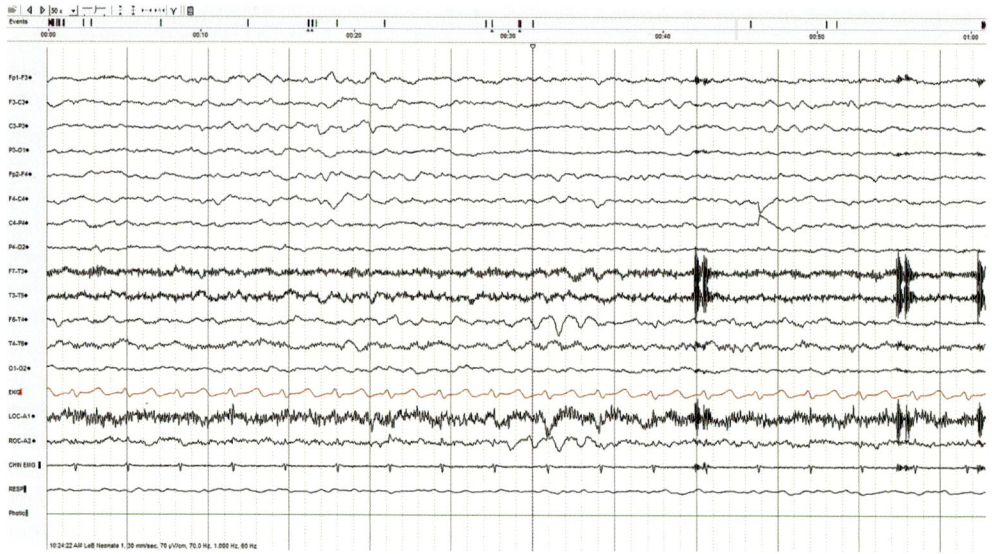

Figure 14.5 Awake EEG with theta and lower-amplitude delta activity at 40 weeks CA.

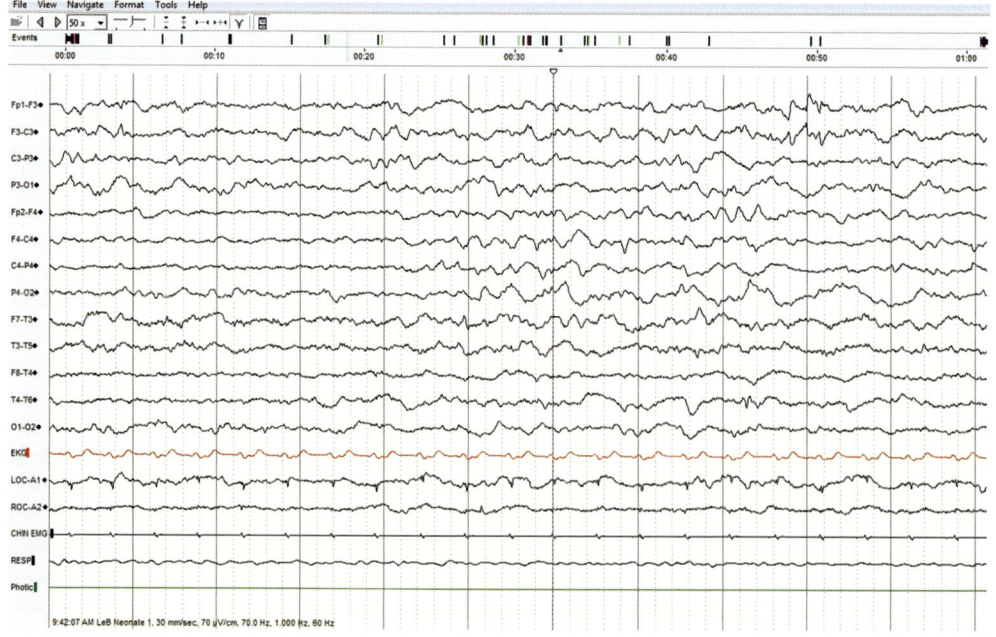

Figure 14.6 Quiet sleep pattern at 41 weeks CA.

14.4.5 40 to 46 Weeks CA

Around this age the trace alternant pattern gradually disappears and is replaced by continuous slow-wave sleep. Delta brushes are also seen sparingly during quiet sleep and tend to disappear by 44 weeks. Sleep spindles (12–14 Hz) start appearing around 46 weeks of CA over the central regions.

14.4.6 46 Weeks CA to 3 Months of Age

Wakefulness (Figure 14.7) is characterized by an admixture of delta and theta activity without a definite anterior to posterior gradient. The majority of the time sleep onset starts with quiet sleep (Figure 14.8) consisting of high-amplitude delta activity (active sleep or REM sleep occurs after wakfulness until the age of 6 weeks, when quiet sleep or NREM sleep occurs at sleep onset, the sequence that is seen throughout childhood and into adulthood). Symmetric asynchronous long duration sleep spindles (lasting 2.5-4 seconds) are seen in this age. Absence of sleep spindles over one hemisphere or an amplitude asymmetry of >50% should be considered abnormal.

14.4.7 3 Months to 2 Years of Age

Around 3 months of age, the awake background begins to show an anterior to posterior frequency and voltage gradient with appearance of poorly regulated 3–4 Hz delta activity over the occipital regions that is reactive to eye opening and closure. A prominent central theta rhythm begins to appear at 6 months of age. The posterior dominant rhythm increases in frequency to 6 Hz by 1 year of age and then to 7–8 Hz around 2 years of age. During the transition from awake to drowsiness and immediately after arousal from sleep, high-amplitude semirhythmic delta activity is seen, lasting for several seconds, and is referred to as hypnogogic and hypnopompic hypersynchrony (Figure 14.9), respectively.

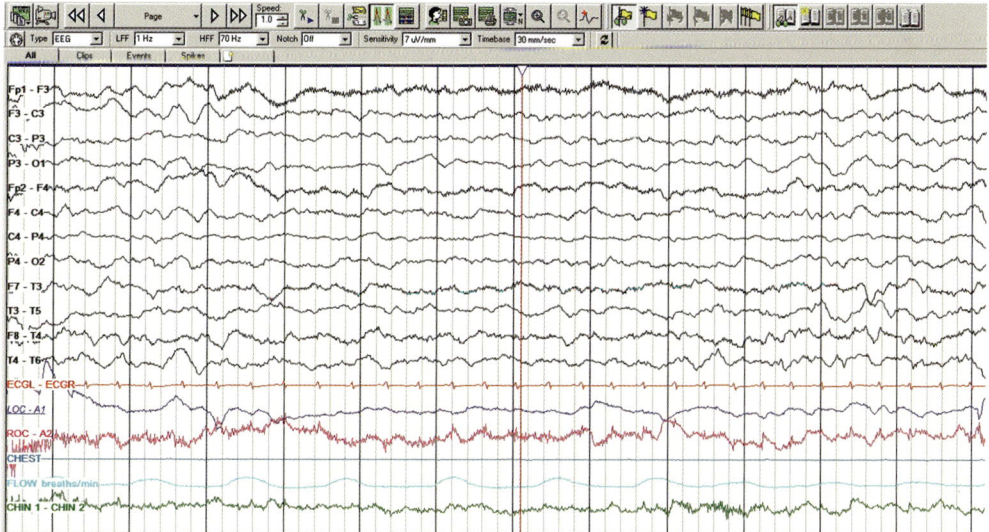

Figure 14.7 Admixture of delta–theta activity without definite anterior–posterior gradient in wakefulness at 48 weeks CA.

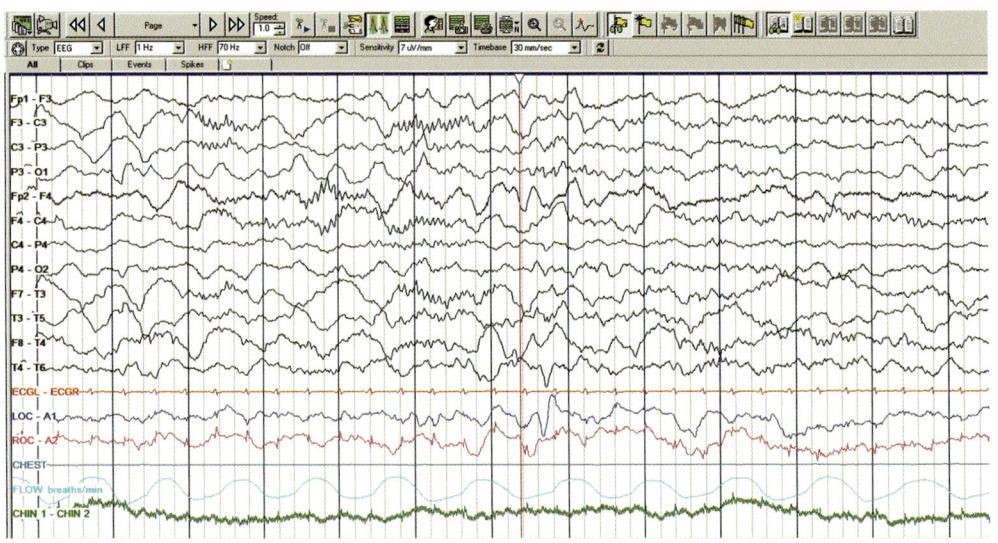

Figure 14.8 Quiet sleep consisting of high-amplitude delta activity at 48 weeks CA.

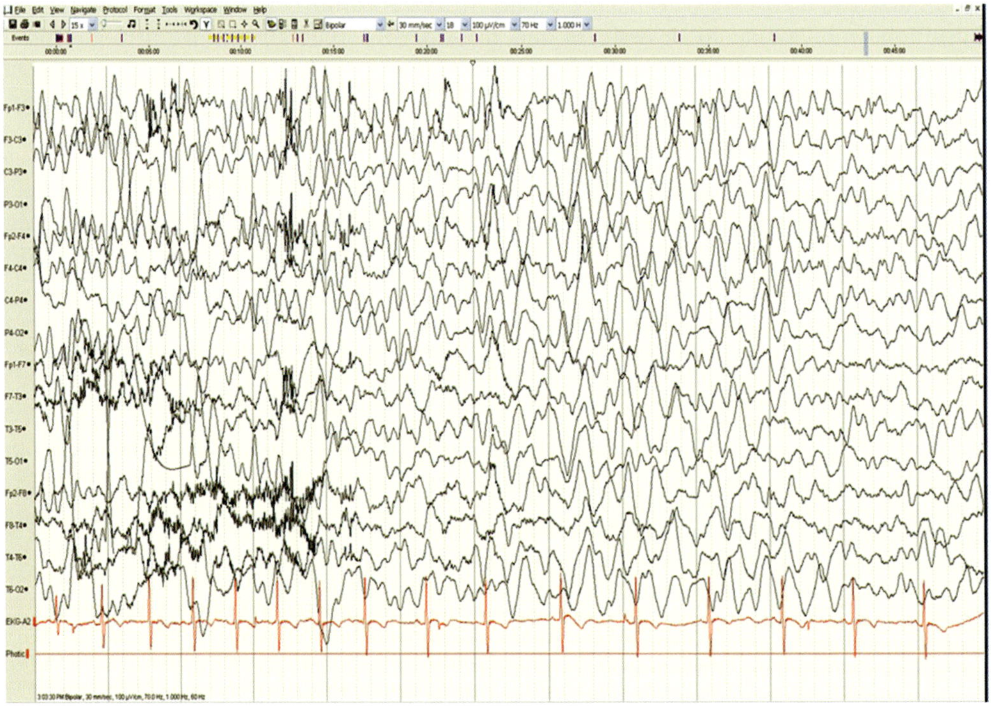

Figure 14.9 High-amplitude semirhythmic delta during transition to drowsiness in hypnogogic hypersynchrony at 38 months.

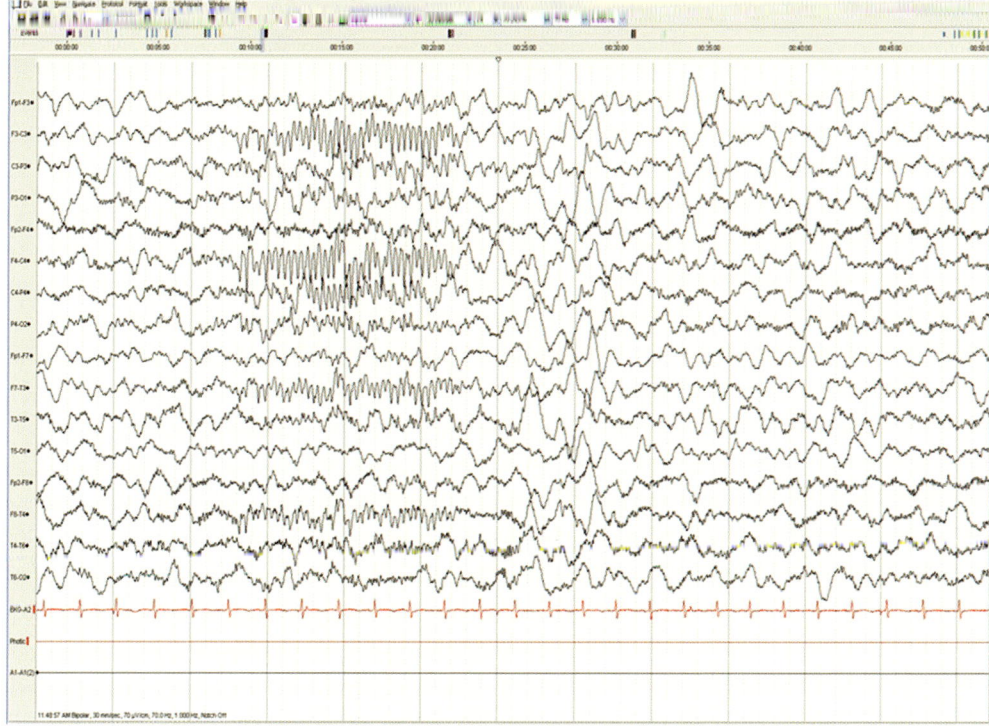

Figure 14.10 Symmetric sleep spindles noted to be synchronous by 24 months.

Sleep shows symmetric sleep spindles and vertex sharp waves (Figure 14.10). Sleep architecture should be synchronous by 24 months of age. Vertex sharp waves appear between 3 and 6 months of age. K-complexes start appearing during sleep at this age. High-amplitude delta waves, termed "cone waves," are seen over the occipital regions during sleep.

14.4.8 Childhood and Adolescence

As the infant enters childhood and adolescence, there is progressive maturation of the anterior–posterior gradient seen during wakefulness. The posterior dominant rhythm increases in frequency to 8 Hz at 3 years of age and up to 11 Hz by early adolescence. Well-defined 7–11 Hz activity is seen over the central regions suggestive of mu rhythm. Older children and adolescents tend to show a dramatic build-up of high-amplitude, synchronous and symmetric delta activity with hyperventilation (Figure 14.11).

14.5 Abnormal Neonatal EEG Backgrounds

14.5.1 Excessive Discontinuity

Any discontinuity in EEG after 46 weeks CA is always abnormal. Though the presence of discontinuity is normal in preterm neonates, excessively prolonged IBI for the CA is considered abnormal. When the EEG shows excessive discontinuity, it is important to

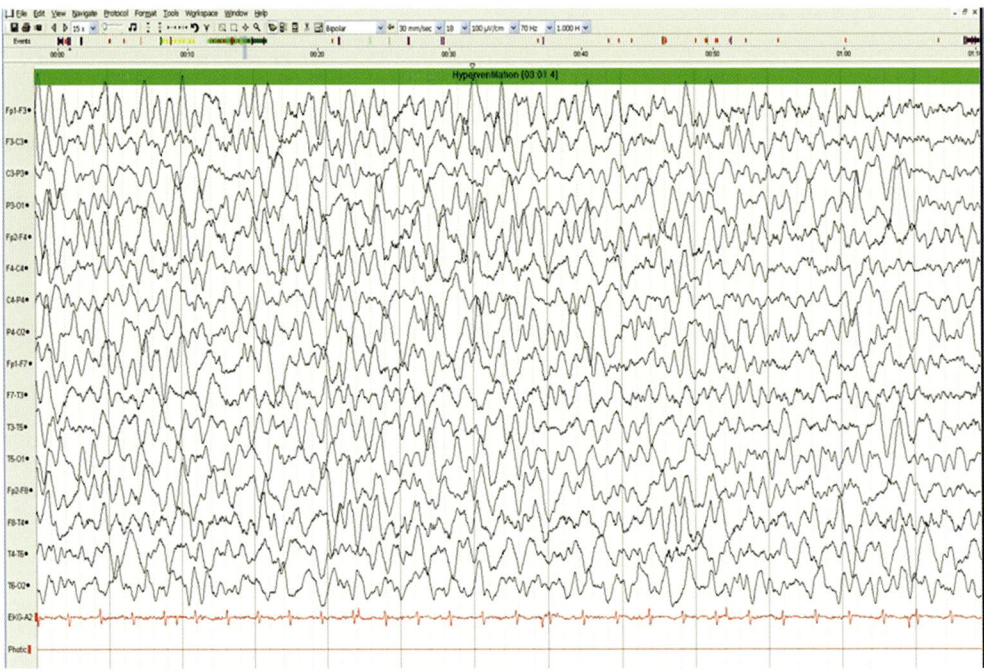

Figure 14.11 Build-up of high-amplitude synchronous and symmetric delta activity with hyperventilation in a 14 year old.

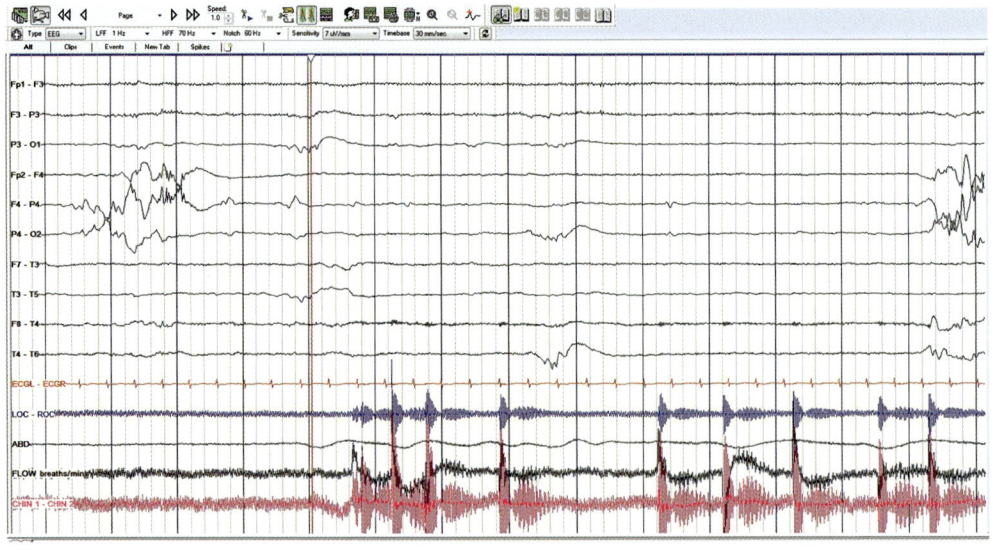

Figure 14.12 Excessive discontinuity with long IBI, worse on the left, at 29 weeks CA.

make sure that bursts of activity contain normal patterns expected for the age. The longest accepted IBI for <30 weeks of gestational age (GA) is 30 s (Figure 14.12), for 31–33 weeks, 20 s, for 34–36 weeks, 10 s, and for 37–40 weeks, 6 s.[6] This abnormality is etiologically nonspecific and indicates a diffuse encephalopathy.

14.5.2 Burst Suppression

This pattern consists of periods of extremely low-voltage activity (<5 µV) separated by brief bursts of synchronous or asynchronous delta and theta activity (Figure 14.13). This pattern does not vary with state and shows no reactivity to stimuli. The bursts themselves lack the age-appropriate normal patterns and waveforms.[7] A burst suppression pattern indicates an underlying severe encephalopathy with poor prognosis. It is seen in many conditions including hypoxic ischemic encephalopathy, nonketotic hyperglycinemia, Ohtaharra syndrome, and early myoclonic epileptic encephalopathy.

14.5.3 Depressed and Undifferentiated Background

In this neonatal EEG abnormality, the background consists of very low-amplitude (<10 µV) monotonous activity with lack of different frequencies (Figure 14.14). The EEG background does not change with state or stimulation. This is another nonspecific abnormality seen in many encephalopathic processes.

14.5.4 Isoelectric (Electrocerebral Inactivity)

Absence of any discernible cerebral activity of greater than 2 µV is defined as electrocerebral inactivity when the EEG is performed according the American Clinical Neurophysiology Society (ACNS) criteria. (It should be noted that these criteria do not apply to preterm

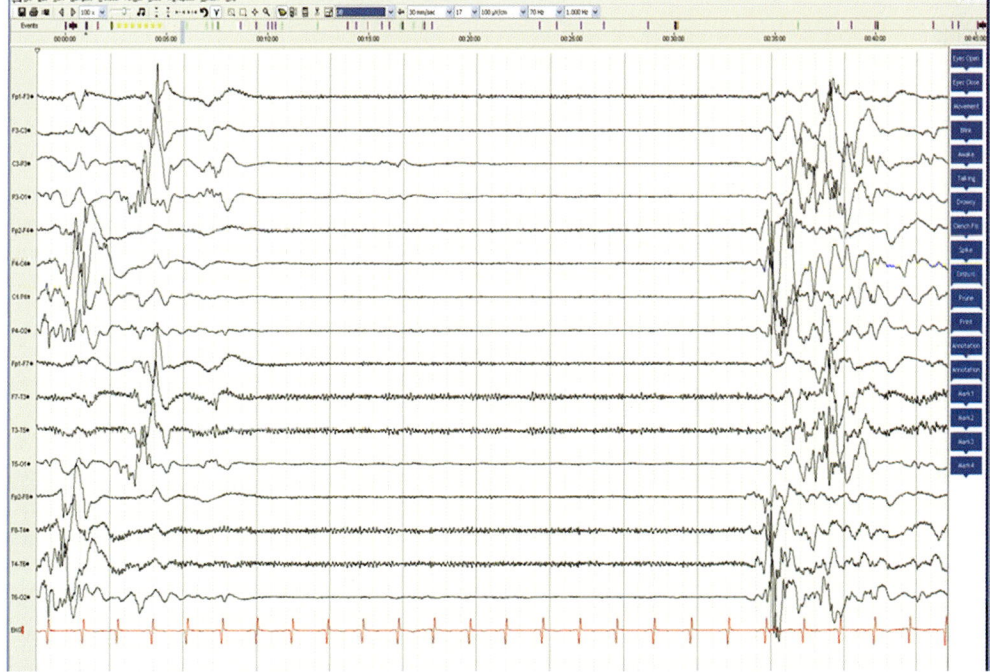

Figure 14.13 Burst suppression pattern at 3 months with periods of extremely low-voltage activity separated by brief bursts of synchronous or asynchronous delta and theta activity.

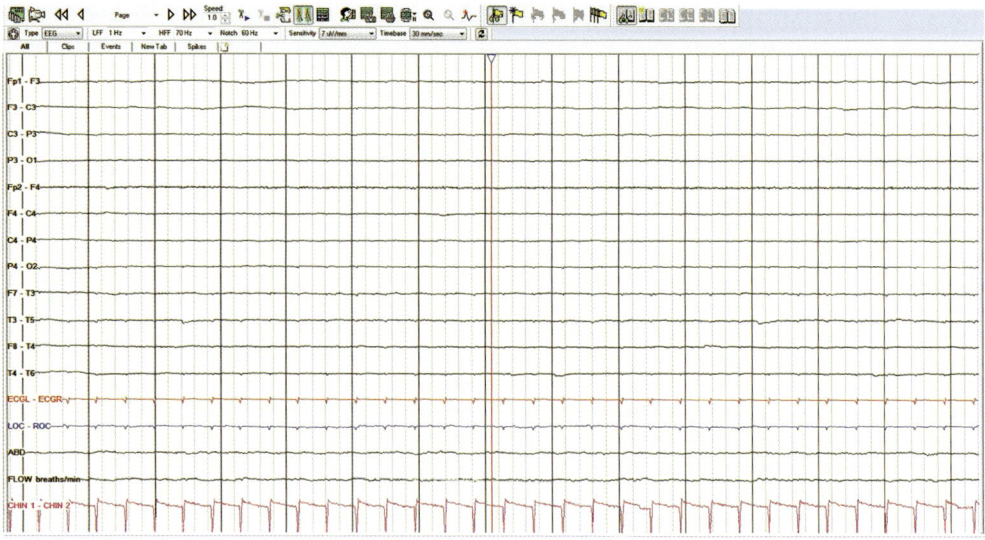

Figure 14.14 Background of very low-amplitude monotonous activity with lack of different frequencies at 40 weeks CA.

infants or neonates.)[8] In sick neonates it is challenging to be certain about the absence of cerebral activity (Figure 14.15). As such, this EEG finding is not interpreted as electrocerebral inactivity in this age group, but rather as a marked low-voltage tracing.

14.5.5 Dysmaturity

If the neonatal EEG background shows features that are normal for an infant 2 or more weeks younger than the current CA, then it is considered to be dysmature. To assess dysmaturity one has to consider degree of asynchrony, frequency and location of delta brushes, presence of frontal sharp transients and temporal theta bursts, and duration of IBI. A dysmature EEG correlates with CNS immaturity and indicates diffuse cerebral dysfunction.[9]

14.6 Sharp EEG Transients and Neonatal Seizures

14.6.1 Negative Sharp Transients

A finding of negative sharp waves in the neonatal EEG may not predict a risk of seizures, as in older children and adults.[10] Infrequent sharp transients can be seen in normal neonates over any scalp region, but are typically seen more often over the temporal (Figure 14.16), central, and frontal regions. Normal sharp transients are seen during the bursts of activity in quiet sleep. An excessive number of multifocal sharp waves are considered a nonspecific abnormality, indicating cortical irritability. This is a subjective finding and there are no objective criteria to define it. Most neonates with confirmed seizures have excessive sharp waves and spikes, and an abnormal background. In these patients with seizures, spikes and sharp waves are typically seen in a repetitive fashion over one region or hemisphere, and also occur during IBI.

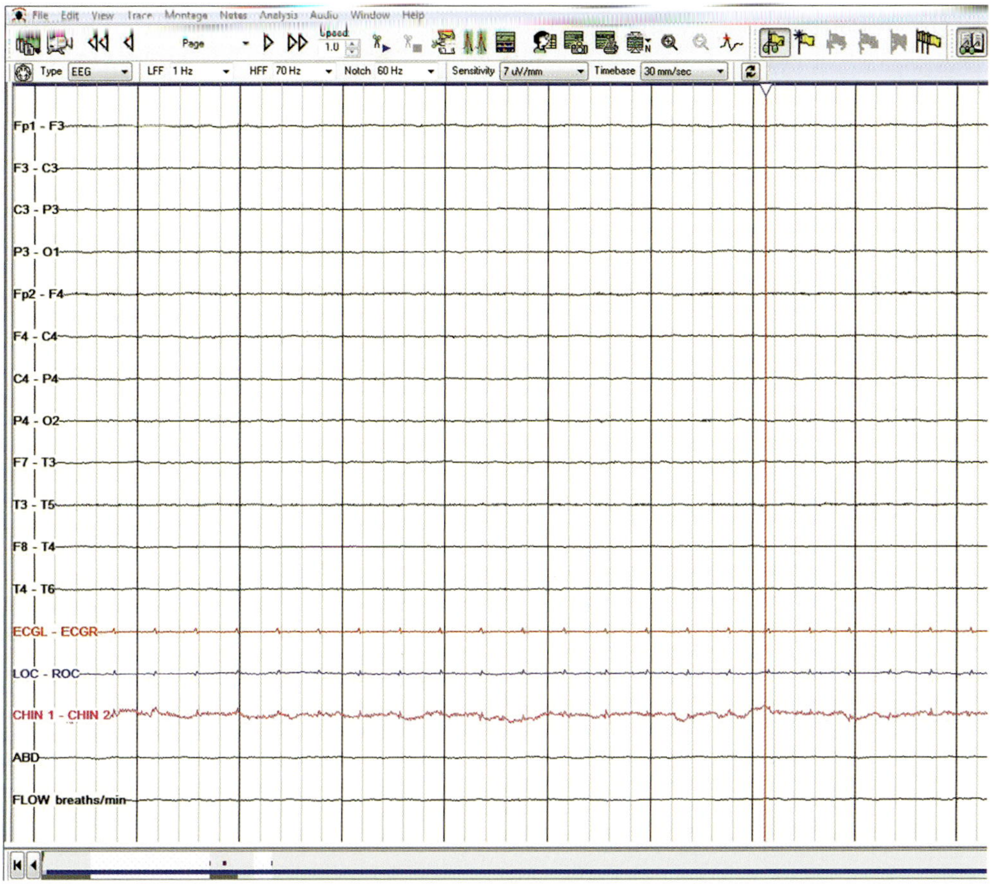

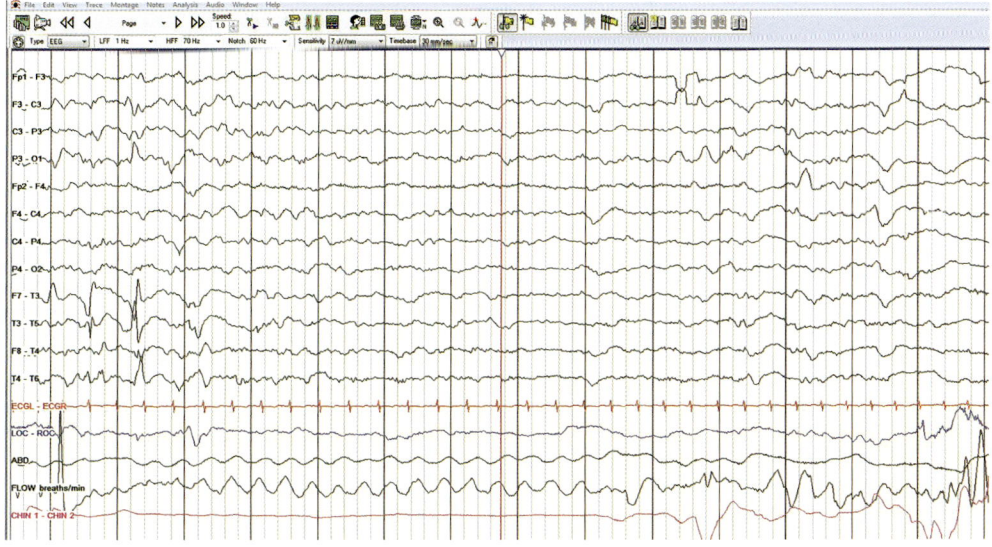

Figure 14.15 Absence of any discernible cerebral activity at 42 weeks CA.

Figure 14.16 Note sharp transients over the temporal derivations (T7 spikes) in a normal neonate.

14.6.2 Positive Sharp Waves

These are sharp transients with surface-positive polarity. They are usually seen over the rolandic, vertex, and temporal regions (Figure 14.17). They are more likely to be seen in premature neonates. Their presence may indicate underlying structural brain damage, common examples including periventricular leukomalacia and intraventricular hemorrhage.[11] Studies have shown that they are not associated with an increased risk of seizures.

14.6.3 Neonatal Seizures

The neonatal period is the most vulnerable time for hypoxic and metabolic derangements, and the majority of seizures are acute symptomatic seizures. Only a minority are manifestations of neonatal-onset epilepsy syndromes. It is important to distinguish epileptic seizures from nonepileptic paroxysmal behaviors, and video-EEG plays an important role.[12] The EEG characteristic of an epileptic seizure is the sudden occurrence of repetitive discharge that evolves in amplitude and frequency, with a changing field, and a definitive beginning and end.[13] The discharge during a neonatal seizure may be represented by any frequency waveform. Seizures could be electroclinical or electrographic only. Electrographic seizures can be seen in neonates with severe encephalopathy or in those treated with antiseizure drugs (ASDs) (ASD treatment can lead to decoupling of electrical from clinical activity).[12] A minimum duration of 10 s is required to define a repetitive waveform as an electrographic seizure.[13] Discharges showing typical ictal evolution but lasting less than 10 s are termed brief rhythmic discharges (BRDs).[14] BRDs indicate a lower seizure threshold.

The majority of neonatal seizures are focal in onset. Central and temporal regions are the most common sites of origin, although they may arise over any head region.

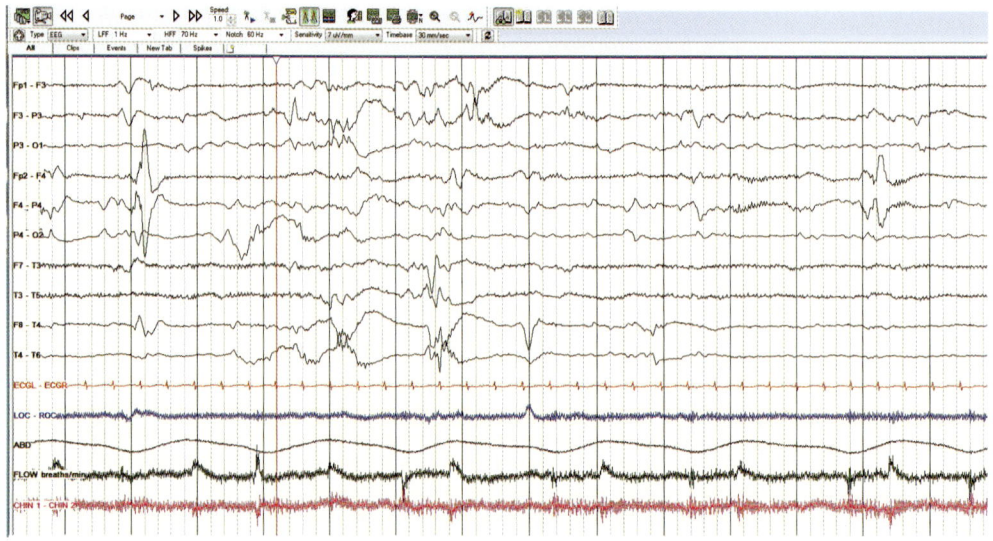

Figure 14.17 Positive sharp waves in a premature neonate at 34 weeks CA.

They can be unifocal or multifocal in origin. Recurrent seizures from a single focus should raise suspicion of an underlying focal structural lesion.[15] Sometimes simultaneously occurring focal seizures may be seen from independent foci. Generalized seizures are rare and only a few specific seizure types are seen in neonates. Generalized myoclonic seizures are associated with generalized sharp transients and spasms with generalized voltage attenuation or diffuse slow waves. The impact of neonatal seizures on subsequent development is hard to determine, but, in general, neonates with seizures superimposed on a normal background have better outcome compared to those with an abnormal background.[16] Much of the prognosis depends on the etiology of the acute seizure.

14.7 Neonatal Epilepsy Syndromes

Four epilepsy syndromes have been described in neonates; two are benign and two are catastrophic. The benign syndromes are benign neonatal convulsions and benign familial neonatal epilepsy. Benign neonatal convulsions, also termed "fifth day fits," consist of brief clonic seizures in full-term neonates between the 4th and 6th days of life. The majority of these neonates have a specific interictal EEG background named "theta pointu alternant," in which bursts of sharply contoured theta waves are seen over the central regions in the discontinuous parts of the record.[17] Benign familial neonatal epilepsy is an genetic epilepsy syndrome caused by mutations leading to a defective KCNQ2 channel.[18] These patients have a broad clinical spectrum ranging from a benign course to severe encephalopathy. Their interictal EEG may be normal or may contain excessive sharp transients.[19]

The two catastrophic neonatal epilepsies are early myoclonic encephalopathy (EME) and early infantile epileptic encephalopathy (EIEE or Ohtahara syndrome). Neonates with EME have fragmentary myoclonus in the beginning and later develop focal seizures and tonic spasms. Their EEG background is markedly abnormal, showing a burst-suppression pattern and the myoclonus is usually seen during the bursts.[20] This is a multifactorial disease, with inborn errors of metabolism being the most common cause (nonketotic hyperglycinemia, etc.). Neonates with EIEE (Ohtahara syndrome) have early-onset tonic seizures and severe encephalopathy. Their EEG background also shows a burst-suppression pattern (Figure 14.18), which may later evolve into hypsarrhythmia.[21] Etiologies for EIEE include structural brain abnormalities and metabolic disorders or genetic mutations (i.e., *ARX*, *CDKL5*, and *STXBP1*, among others). Seizures in both of these conditions are usually resistant to antiepileptic drugs.

14.8 Pediatric EEG

Interpretation of the EEG during childhood requires a foundational knowledge of the normal variants that may be encountered in the pediatric age group. Care must be taken in recognizing that some waveforms may appear unusual or epileptiform in morphology but may in fact be normal for age. Features such as the behavioral state of the patient (awake, drowsy, and asleep), location (central, temporal, etc.), frequency (alpha, theta, and delta), and rhythmicity (6 Hz, for example) aid in distinguishing these findings as normal versus abnormal.

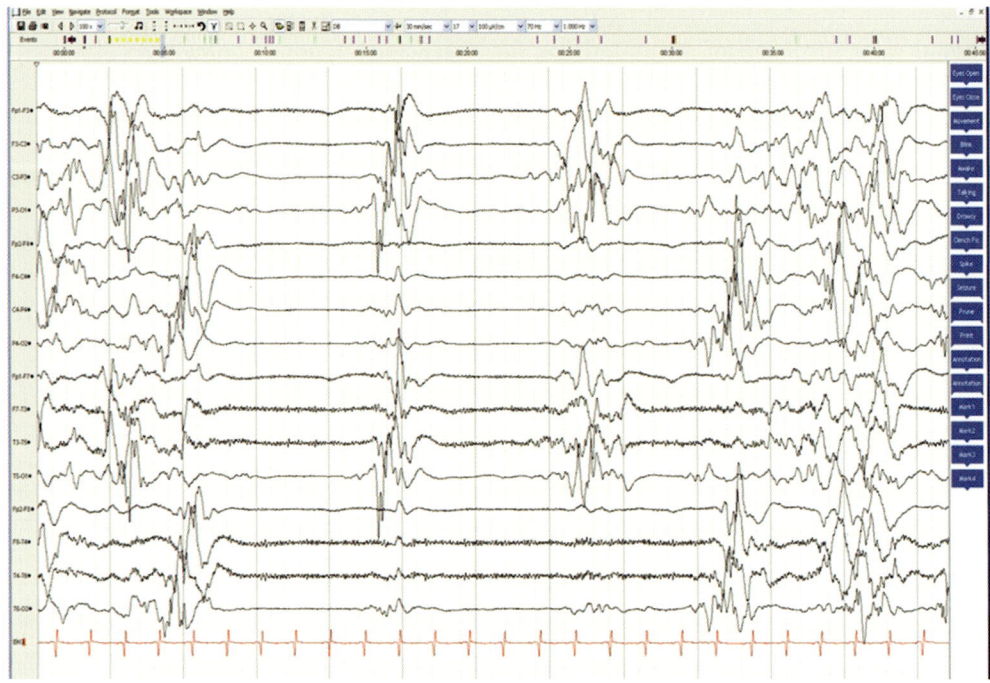

Figure 14.18 Burst suppression pattern in Ohtahara syndrome in a 2 month old.

14.9 Normal Pediatric EEG Variants

14.9.1 Slow and Fast Alpha Variants

The posterior dominant rhythm reaches alpha frequency (8–12 Hz) by the third year of life (Figure 14.19). Slow and fast alpha variants occur in both children and adults and are apparent in the awake state with eye closure. They may be brief or last several seconds. An unusual morphology such as a notched or archiform appearance may be noted. They may be unilaterally or bilaterally synchronous. Slow alpha variant is a subharmonic of the posterior dominant rhythm, and is usually half of the person's typical rhythm. Fast alpha variant is a supraharmonic of the posterior dominant rhythm and is usually double that of the person's typical rhythm.[22]

14.9.2 Alpha Squeak

When eye closure occurs, there is a brief increase in the alpha frequency of the posterior dominant rhythm, which may also appear slightly lower in voltage. This phenomenon dissipates quickly, within 0.5–2 s. It is facilitated by visual attention prior to eye closure. This is a normal finding.[22]

14.9.3 Posterior Slow Waves of Youth

Posterior slow waves of youth (Figure 14.20) are arrhythmic moderate voltage slow waves visualized over the posterior EEG leads, either occipital, parieto-occipital, or

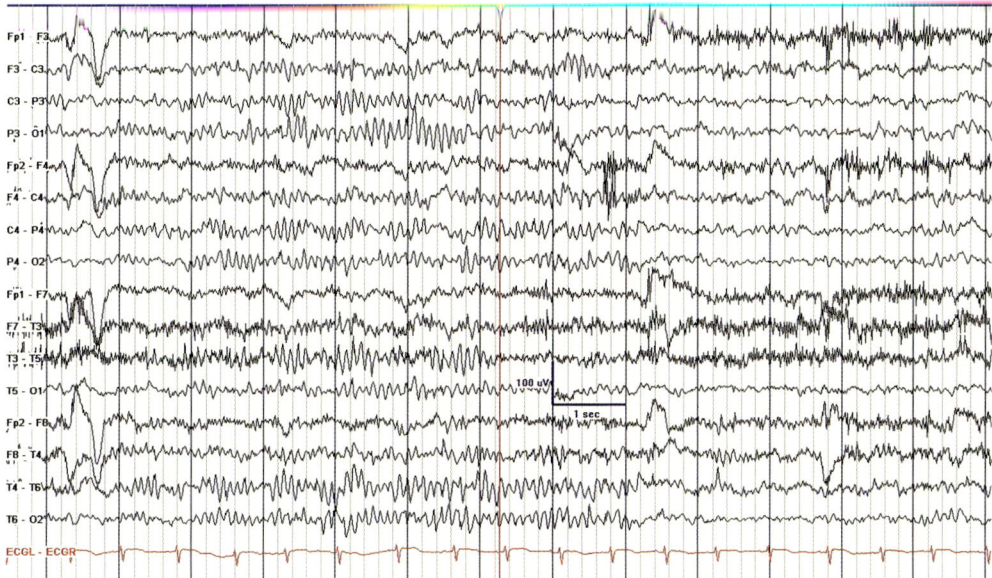

Figure 14.19 Posterior dominant rhythm in a 4 year old.

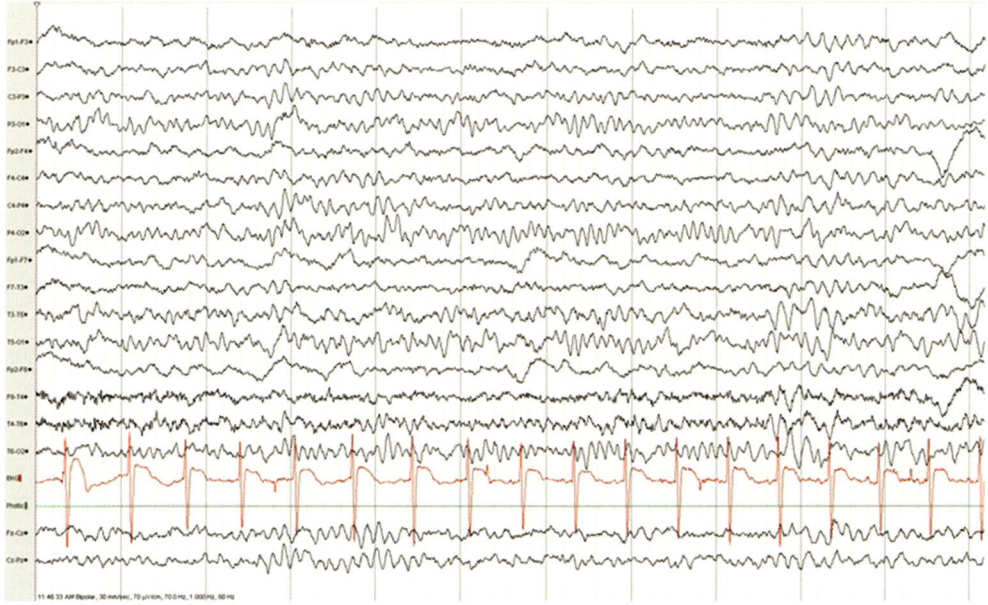

Figure 14.20 Posterior slow waves of youth noted as arrhythmic moderate voltage slow waves visualized over the posterior EEG leads.

occipito-temporal. They may appear after 2 years of age and are most prominent from 8–14 years of age.[23] The morphology of a posterior slow wave of youth is that of a delta wave with overlying or intermixed alpha activity and may be preceded by a sharply contoured wave. This waveform is more prominent when the eyes are closed and is blocked with eye opening, just like the posterior dominant rhythm. Posterior slow waves of youth are either unilaterally or bilaterally synchronous.

14.9.4 Mu Rhythm

Mu, also known as Rolandic mu due to its location in the central head regions, is designated with this particular Greek character due to its relationship to motor phenomena.[24] It typically appears during the second year of life and peaks at 11–15 years of age.[23] The morphology is archiform with a negative spike phase and a positive curved phase (Figure 14.21). It is often an alpha frequency and occurs in trains lasting several seconds. Mu is typically bilateral but asynchronous. Mu can be blocked by passive or active movement of the contralateral upper extremity, however it does not disappear with eye opening. Even the mere thought of moving the contralateral upper extremity is sufficient to block mu.

14.9.5 Lambda Wave

Lambda waves are seen most commonly at 3–12 years of age, but persist through adulthood (Figure 14.22). They are maximal over the occipital head regions and are seen during wakefulness with eyes open.[25] These should disappear with eye closure, which helps differentiate this normal variant from abnormal posterior sharp waves. The morphology is that of a sharp wave with a prominent positive phase. Amplitude is less than 50 µV. They may be triggered by voluntary scanning movements of the eyes in a well-illuminated room.[26]

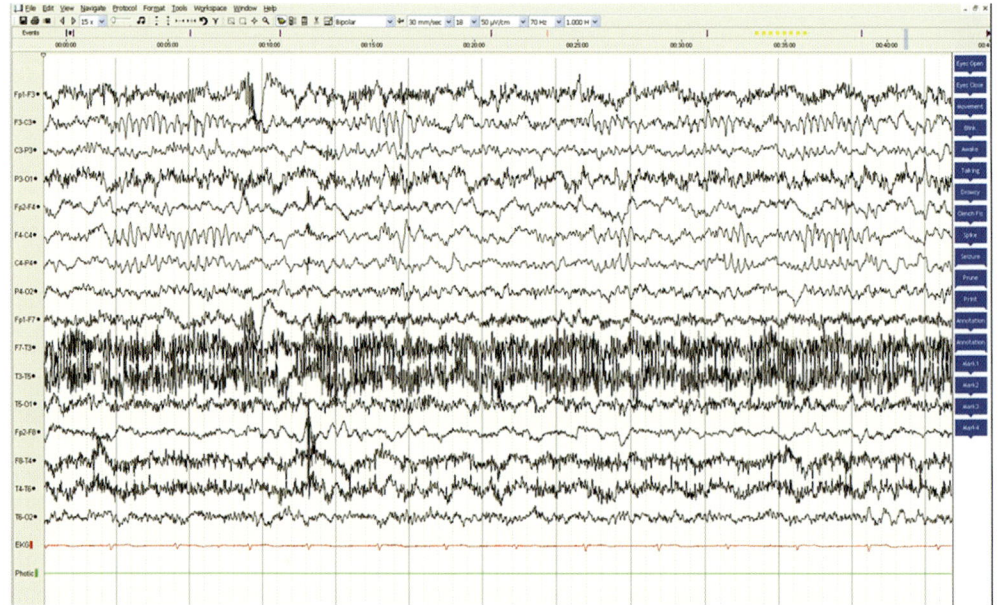

Figure 14.21 Rolandic mu rhythm noted with archiform morphology with a negative spike phase and a positive curved phase.

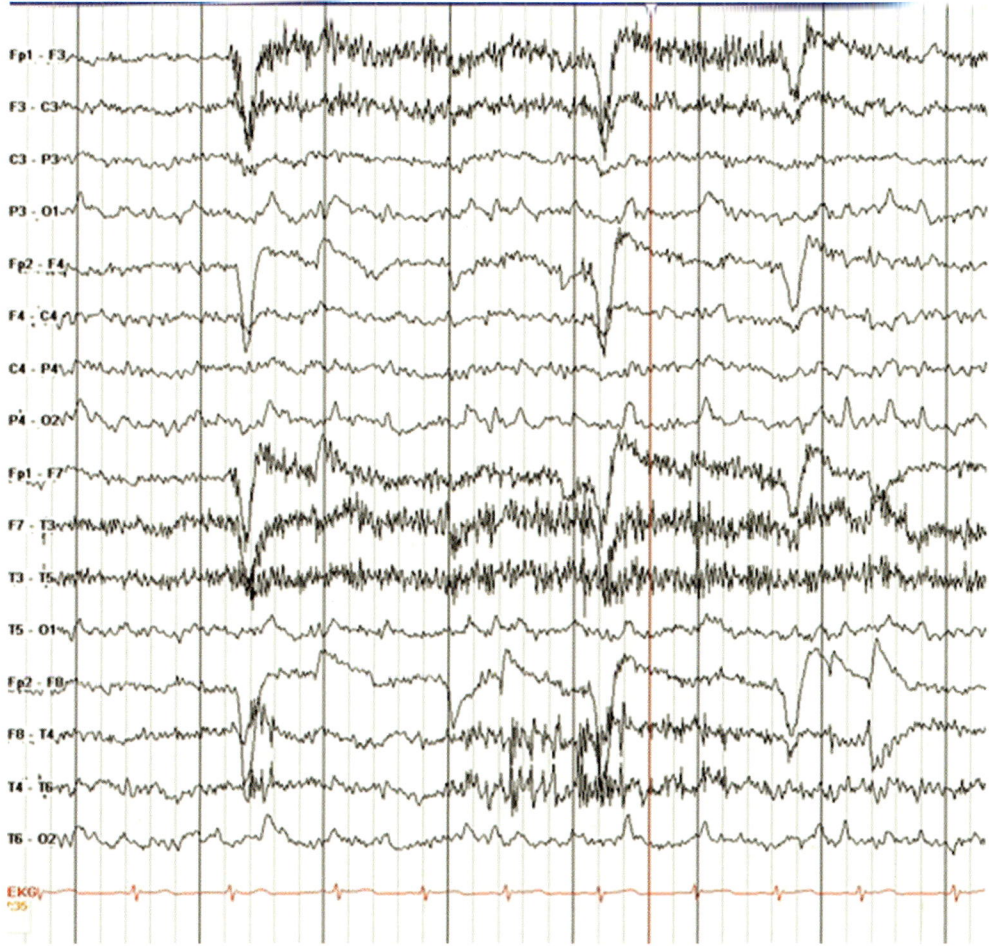

Figure 14.22 Lambda waves over the occipital head regions seen during wakefulness with eyes open.

14.9.6 Positive Occipital Sharp Transients of Sleep

Positive occipital sharp transients of sleep (POSTS), also known as lambdoid waves ("lambda-like"), bear a resemblance to lambda waves, but are instead seen during drowsiness and may persist in light and deep sleep (Figure 14.23).[27] They, too, are maximal in the occipital head region and have a sharp wave morphology with a prominent positive phase. They can occur in trains of 4–5 Hz. POSTS are seen in adolescence and continue through adulthood. It is hypothesized that they represent a playback of images obtained by the visual cortex during the day. Of note, they are absent in the blind.[28]

14.9.7 Arousal Patterns

Frontal arousal rhythm (FAR) is a pattern of childhood described as an arousal, usually from Stage II sleep, where rhythmic slow waves in the alpha or theta range are seen in the bifrontal head regions, usually maximal at F3/F4.[22] It was originally described in children

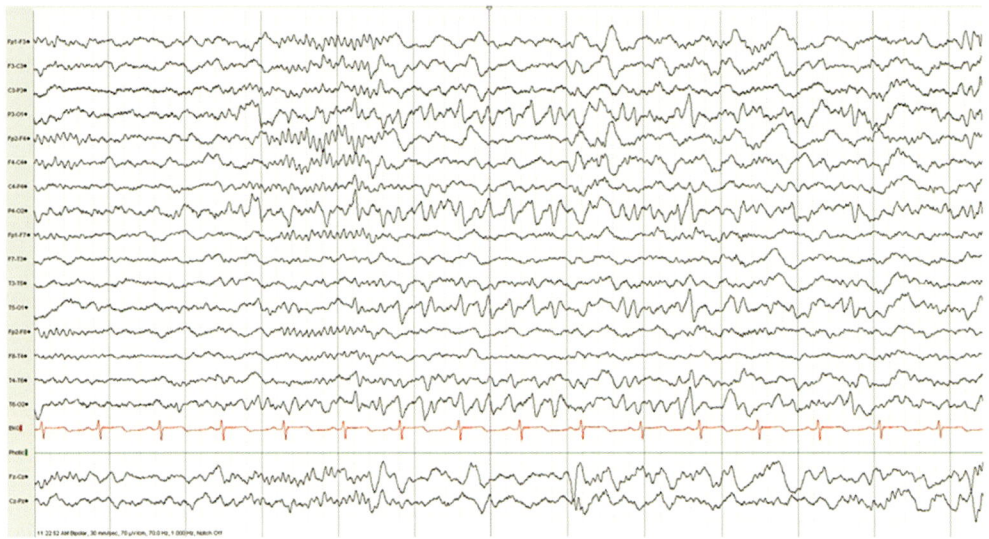

Figure 14.23 Positive occipital sharp transients of sleep (POSTS), or lambdoid waves ("lambda-like"), during sleep.

with seizures and/or mild cerebral dysfunction and thought to be definitively abnormal.[29] However, it is now considered a pattern of uncertain significance.

Hypnagogic hypersynchrony refers to diffuse rhythmic delta activity seen in children during the transition from wakefulness to sleep.[23] *Hypnopompic hypersynchrony* refers to the same pattern, but upon transition from sleep to wakefulness.

14.9.8 Psychomotor Variant (Rhythmic Midtemporal Theta Bursts of Drowsiness or RMTD)

RMTD is a finding mainly seen in adults, but also may be present in adolescents and rarely in children, that occurs during light drowsiness and/or wakefulness (Figure 14.24). Runs of repetitive waves of a theta frequency (5–7 Hz usually) occur in the midtemporal head regions, although spread to adjacent regions is possible.[30] These waves may have a sharp, archiform, notched, or flat appearance with a prominent negative phase and occur in bursts lasting from 10–60 s. RMTD may be bilaterally synchronous, asynchronous, or asymmetric.

14.9.9 Midline Theta Rhythm (Ciganek Rhythm)

Ciganek rhythm bears a resemblance to RMTD yet differs primarily in terms of location and timing. Ciganek rhythm consists of repetitive 4–7 Hz theta activity lasting 3–20 s in duration that may have a sinusoidal, archiform, notched, or flat appearance.[31] It is maximal in the midline leads, typically at Cz, and may spread parasagittally. It is seen most commonly during wakefulness, but can also persist during drowsiness. Performance of mental tasks is associated with this rhythm.

14.9.10 14 and 6 Hz Positive Burst

14- and 6-Hz positive bursts, also known as ctenoids after the Greek term for "comb" to describe their appearance, are common in young children and adolescents (Figure 14.25).[32]

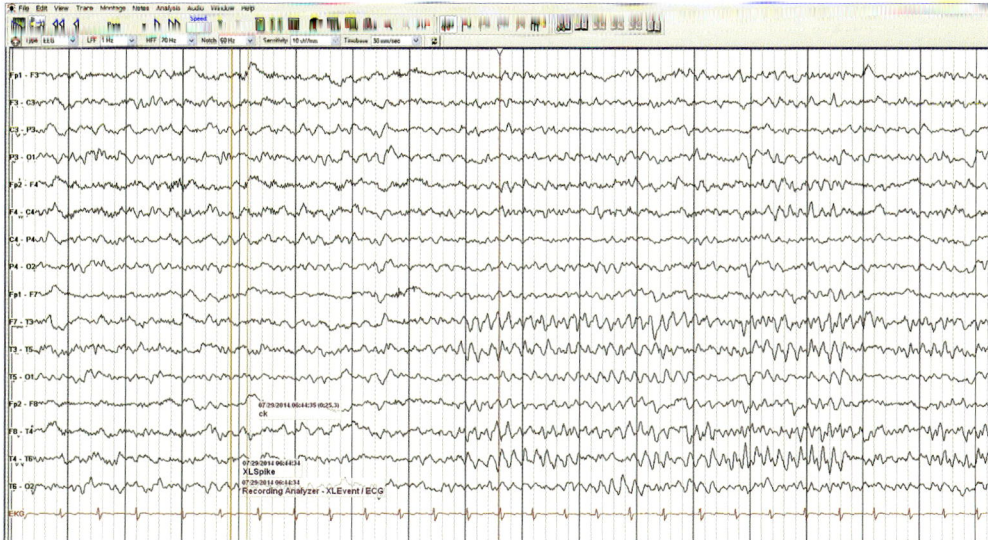

Figure 14.24 Rhythmic mid temporal theta of drowsiness (RMTD) during light drowsiness.

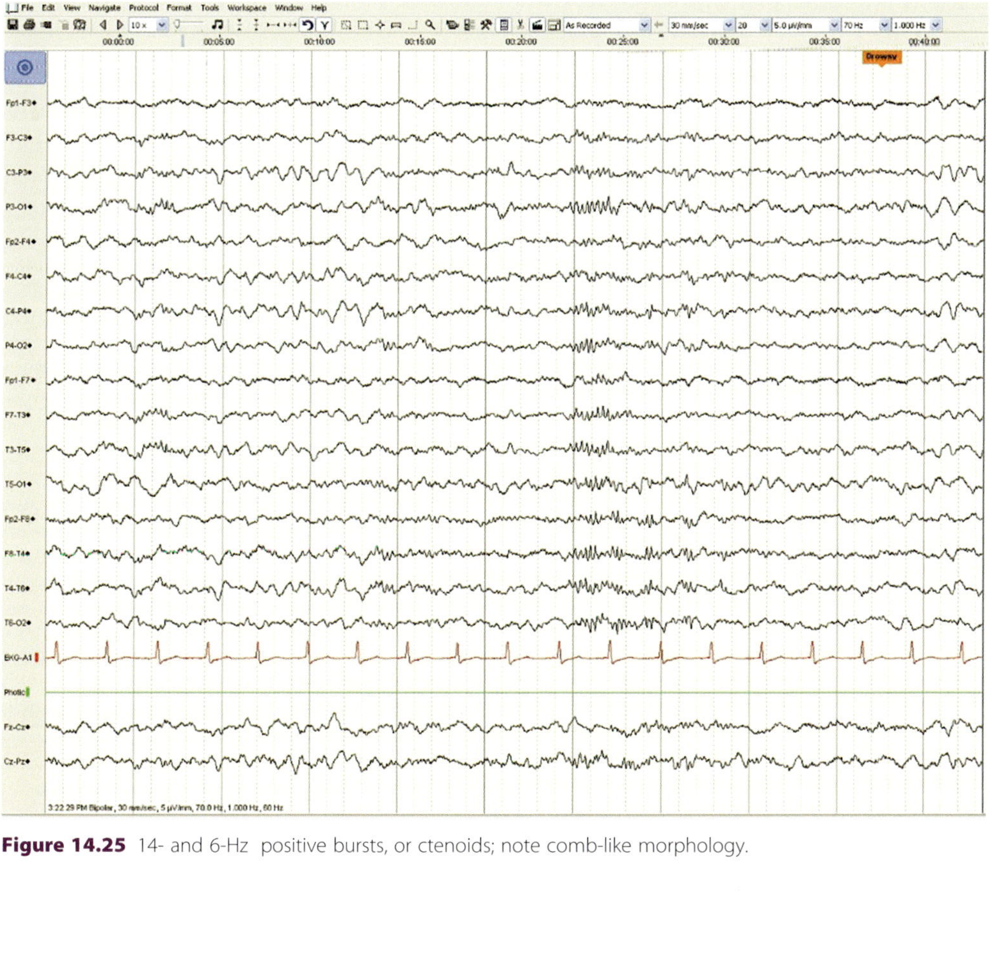

Figure 14.25 14- and 6-Hz positive bursts, or ctenoids; note comb-like morphology.

They occur during drowsiness and light sleep, and are located in the posterior temporal and occipital leads.[23] They may be unilateral or bilateral. 14- and 6-Hz positive bursts are rather lower in voltage, typically less than 75 μV, and have a dominant positive phase. They are a benign finding. However, a similar-appearing finding can be present in advanced hepatic coma, Reye's syndrome, or encephalopathy of a variety of causes.[33,34]

14.9.11 6-Hz Spike and Wave

The 6-Hz spike and wave, also known as phantom spike and wave, is seen during drowsiness and can occur in children up through adulthood. The term "phantom" refers to their resemblance to spike-and-wave complexes seen in absence epilepsy, although the former are lower in amplitude.[35] It is a 6-Hz generalized spike-and-slow-wave complex that lasts about 1 s. The wave component is dominant and higher in amplitude than the spike component, the latter often having a positive phase. Its disappearance rather than activation with sleep can help distinguish it from true epileptiform discharges.[36] The 6-Hz spike and wave is divided into two subtypes using the acronyms WHAM and FOLD. WHAM stands for waking, high amplitude, anterior in location, and male gender predominance. FOLD stands for female gender predominance, occipital in location, low amplitude, drowsiness (Figure 14.26). WHAM, or frontally located 6-Hz spike and wave, has a greater association with epilepsy. In contrast, FOLD, or occipitally located spike and wave, is not associated with epilepsy.

14.9.12 Breach Rhythm

Breach rhythm refers to focal changes in brain activity seen in the region of a craniotomy or skull fracture, particularly in the central and temporal head regions.[22] Normal physiologic patterns may appear sharper and higher in amplitude due to surgical or traumatic defects in

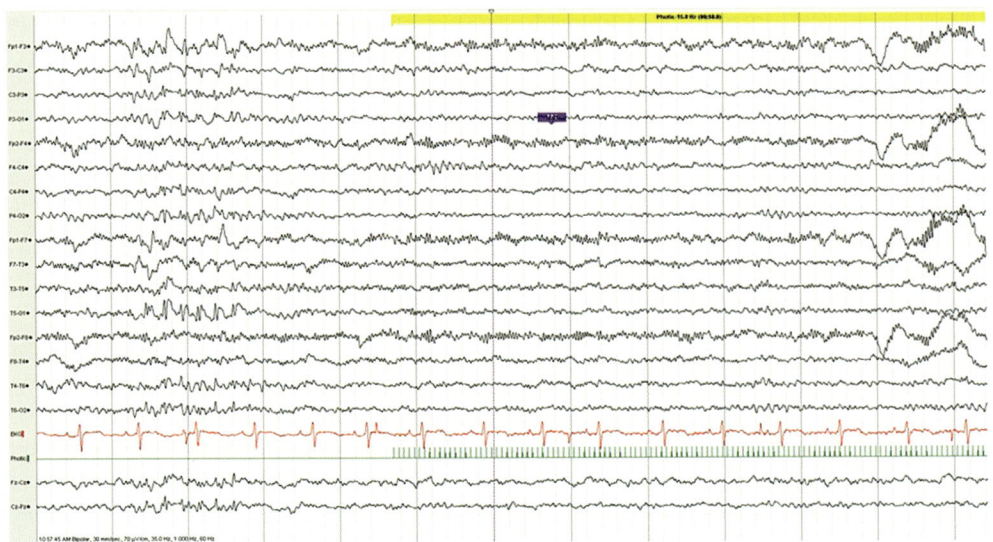

Figure 14.26 Note 6-Hz spike and wave pattern in a female as low-amplitude, occipital dominant spike in drowsiness (FOLD).

a region of the skull that would, in a normal state act as a high frequency filter.[37] It is important to distinguish these accentuated normal patterns from pathologic epileptiform discharges or focal slowing. Consideration should be paid to whether the location of the waveform(s) and state of the patient correlate with a known normal finding so as to distinguish it from truly abnormal activity. For example, in the case of mu rhythm, contralateral hand movement can be performed during the EEG recording to look for expected attenuation. Attention should be paid to known normal temporal region variants as well such as RMTD and wicket spikes. Sharp-appearing waveforms in breach rhythm should not have a subsequent slow wave, which can help distinguish these temporal and other location variants from abnormal findings.

14.10 Activation Procedures

The outpatient routine EEG provides a representative window into the baseline cerebral activity for a given patient. During that 30–60 min recording, epileptiform activity may or may not be present, depending on the state of the patient and their particular spike frequency. The initial routine EEG may be normal in 50–80% of patients who are ultimately diagnosed with epilepsy. Therefore, activation procedures should be used to enhance the yield during a recording.[38] These procedures include intermittent photic stimulation (IPS), hyperventilation (HV), and sleep deprivation (or an appropriate strategy to increase the yield of capturing sleep during the routine EEG). In addition, some abnormalities, such as 3-Hz spike-and-slow-wave complexes with HV or photoparoxysmal response with IPS, can provide specific information that allows the physician to further classify the patient's seizure, and in some cases, enable the diagnosis of a specific epilepsy syndrome in the appropriate clinical context.

14.10.1 Intermittent Photic Stimulation

IPS is applied using a strobe lamp placed 20–30 cm in front of the patient, whose eyes are closed. A range of flash frequencies is used from 1–30 Hz given in trains of 5–10 s.[38]

The photic driving response refers to the rhythmic activity seen over the posterior EEG leads that is time-locked to the flash rate (Figure 14.27). It should be the same frequency as the flash rate (e.g., a posterior driving rate of 10 Hz for a 10 Hz stimulus flash rate) or may be subharmonic (e.g,. a posterior driving rate of 5 Hz for a 10 Hz stimulus flash rate) or supraharmonic (e.g. a posterior driving rate of 20 Hz for a 10 Hz stimulus flash rate). Although it can be seen in infancy, it is more commonly seen starting in young childhood. Although amplitude asymmetries between the two hemispheres are of unlikely significance if this is the only abnormality seen during the EEG recording, unilaterally absent posterior driving response may represent a cortical lesion. Normal subjects may lack a posterior driving response. Those with prominent lambda waves are more likely to have a photic driving response.[25] Of note, at flash frequencies less than 5 Hz, a visually evoked response (rather than true photic driving) may be seen in the posterior leads.[38]

The photomyogenic (also known as photomyoclonic) response seen with IPS is not produced by cerebral activity, but rather is a myogenic artifact with muscle-generated spikes over the frontal head regions.[23] It is often associated with eyelid flutter or facial twitching in response to photic stimulation. It is most commonly seen at flash frequencies of 12–18 Hz. Although a normal finding, it can be seen in the setting of alcohol or barbiturate withdrawal or secondary to hypocalcemia.[39]

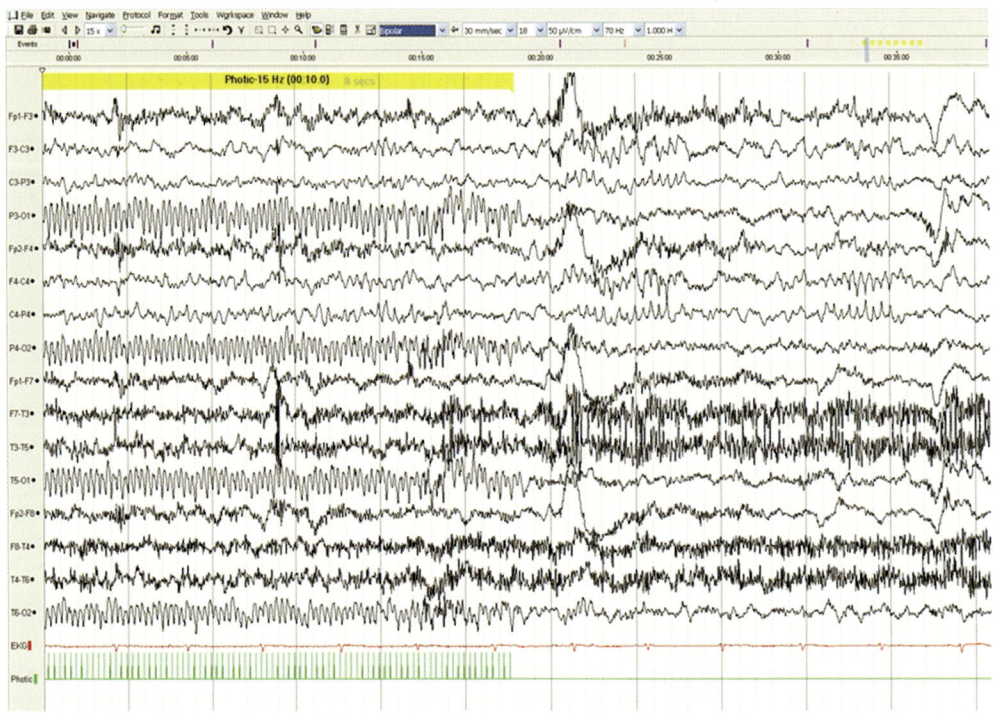

Figure 14.27 Note the photic driving response over the posterior EEG leads that is time-locked to the flash rate.

A photoelectric response is an EEG artifact created by high-impedance electrodes. The light causes a photochemical reaction in the electrode which appears on the EEG as narrow spikes similar to a myogenic artifact at the same frequency as the flash. It can be blocked by covering the electrode with a cloth.

A photoparoxysmal response (PPR) refers to epileptiform discharges triggered by IPS, usually of the spike-and-wave or polyspike patterns.[38] Stimulation at 15–18 Hz more commonly produces this response compared to other frequencies (Figure 14.28). PPR may be induced by eye closure during IPS. It is most commonly associated with genetic generalized epilepsies, such as juvenile myoclonic epilepsy. It is more common in females and in children and adolescents. PPRs that have a stronger association with a risk of seizures include those that are generalized rather than posterior predominant, those that persist at multiple flash frequencies, and those where the epileptiform discharges continue despite cessation of the photic stimulus. A posterior predominant PPR has a lower association with epilepsy and may be seen as an EEG "genetic trait." In terms of therapy, valproic acid has been demonstrated to be effective in abolishing the PPR response in 61% of patients.[40] Levetiracetam has also demonstrated efficacy.[41] Blue lenses can be very effective in blocking this response.

A photoconvulsive response is when IPS triggers an electroclinical seizure. Common seizure types that may occur include absence, myoclonic, and generalized tonic–clonic.

14.10.2 Hyperventilation

A patient is asked to hyperventilate for 3–5 min during the EEG recording. Hypocapnia develops as carbon dioxide is repetitively exhaled, subsequently leading to cerebral

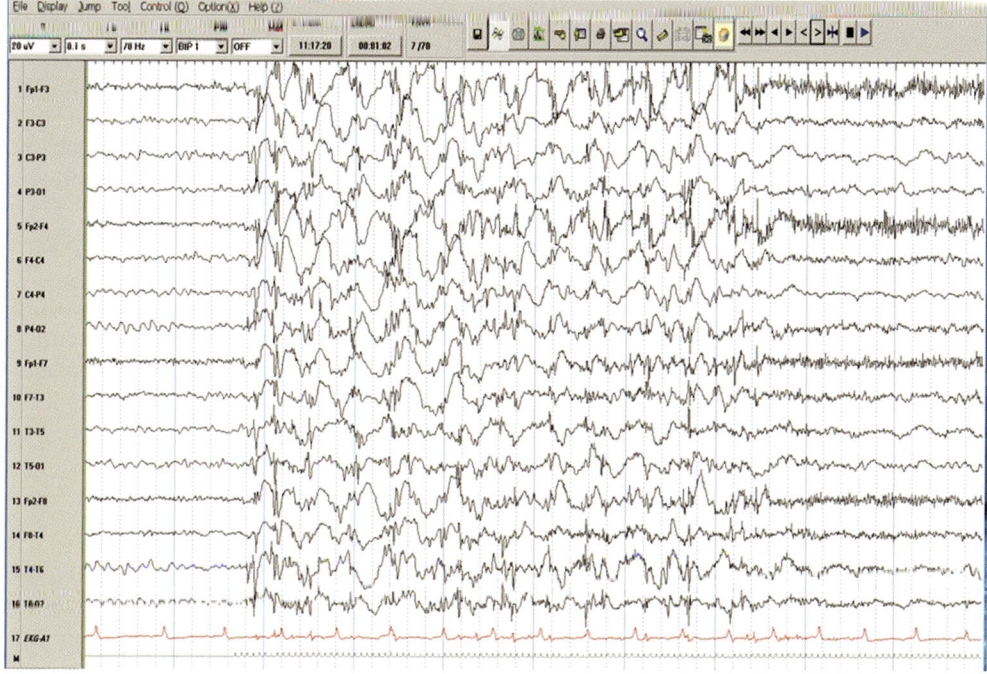

Figure 14.28 Note the photoparoxysmal response occurring as epileptiform discharges triggered by IPS.

vasoconstriction and thus reduced cerebral blood flow.[38] In response, the EEG demonstrates high-voltage diffuse polymorphic or sinusoidal slowing in the delta to theta range which can outlast the duration of the hyperventilation activity. The diffuse slow waves can have a notched appearance, which should not be mistaken for epileptiform discharges. This EEG response is more pronounced in the setting of fasting/hypoglycemia and when performed in the upright rather than the reclined position. This response of diffuse slowing is most pronounced in children and may not be seen in adults. Abnormalities unmasked by HV include interictal epileptiform discharges (particularly in genetic generalized epilepsies with generalized spike-and-wave complexes, but also focal epileptiform discharges), seizures (typically absence, but rarely focal seizures), and focal slowing (suggestive of a focal cerebral lesion). Hyperventilation should be avoided in patients with known cerebrovascular disease, Moyamoya syndrome, sickle cell anemia, recent stroke, intracerebral hemorrhage, and severe cardiopulmonary disease.

Although the duration of the HV response can be quite variable, from 30 s up to several minutes, the presence of a "rebuildup" where the response wanes but then waxes once again despite cessation of the HV process is concerning and associated with Moyamoya syndrome.

14.10.3 Sleep Deprivation

Sleep deprivation, which in the strictest terms means no sleep for the preceding 24 hours, may activate epileptiform abnormalities in 10–52% of patients.[42] The effect is greater in children. The patient should strive to stay awake for the initial portion of the recording as it is the fatigue not the sleep itself that is activating.[38] Sleep deprivation is more likely to trigger a seizure in those with generalized epilepsy as compared to focal epilepsy.

14.11 Abnormal Pediatric EEG Patterns

Particular EEG abnormalities in the pediatric population must be interpreted within the clinical context for a given patient. Findings such as occipital or frontal intermittent rhythmic delta activity do not necessarily represent focal dysfunction, but rather are indicators of some neurologic abnormality, whether an association with an epilepsy syndrome or encephalopathy. However, they do not necessarily predict seizure propensity. Generalized epileptiform discharges must also be interpreted with caution. Distinguishing between generalized versus focal with rapid secondary bilateral synchrony is important in choosing antiseizure medication, determining whether a patient is a resective epilepsy surgery candidate, and/or accurately diagnosing whether a patient has a specific epilepsy syndrome.

14.11.1 Occipital Intermittent Rhythmic Delta Activity

Occipital intermittent rhythmic delta activity (OIRDA or "phi rhythm") is a 3–4 Hz monomorphic delta activity seen over the occipital head regions that can have a notched appearance (Figure 14.29). It may be bilaterally synchronous or unilateral. It is most commonly seen in children from 6 to 10 years of age.[22] OIRDA is most commonly associated with childhood absence epilepsy. Its presence on EEG in children with typical absence seizures may confer a better prognosis and response to medication.[43] It also can be seen in association with other generalized seizure types such as atonic, myoclonic, and tonic–clonic, and has even been described in children with focal seizures.[44] However, it can be seen in children without seizures. It is activated by hyperventilation and eye closure.

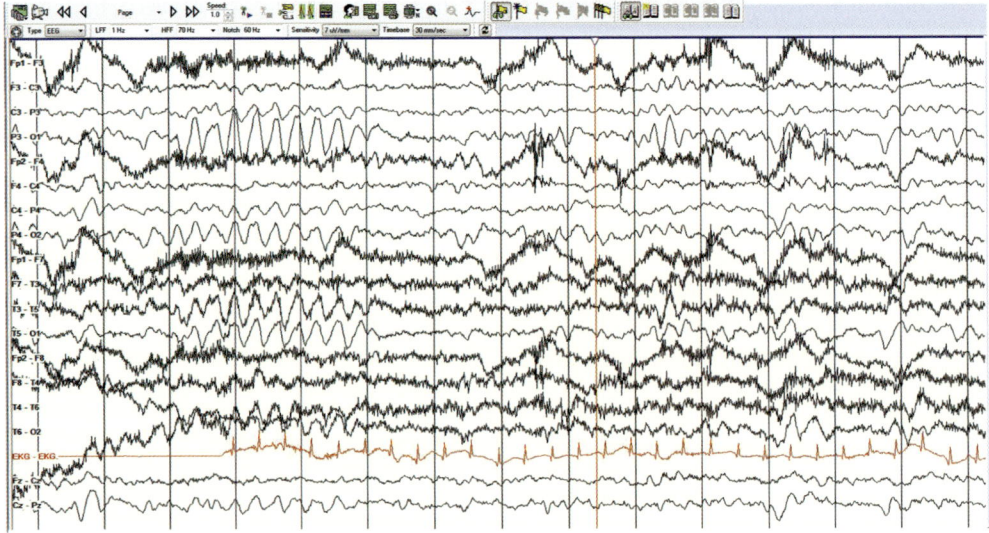

Figure 14.29 Occipital intermittent rhythmic delta activity (OIRDA), or "phi rhythm," as a 3–4 Hz monomorphic delta activity over the occipital head regions.

14.11.2 Frontal Intermittent Rhythmic Delta Activity

Frontal intermittent rhythmic delta activity (FIRDA) is bifrontally synchronous slow-wave activity that can be in the delta or theta frequency range. It is associated with encephalopathies of any cause, but most commonly metabolic derangements. It is also associated with deep midline lesions, subcortical abnormalities, and increased intracranial pressure. It is a relatively uncommon pattern in children. When present, it is typically nonspecific and may be seen in a variety of encephalopathies of metabolic or structural etiologies.[45] It is thought to be nonepileptiform and therefore unrelated to risk of seizures.

14.11.3 Secondary Bilateral Synchrony versus Generalized Epileptiform Discharges

Secondary bilateral synchrony (SBS) refers to epileptiform discharges (EDs) with a diffuse or generalized appearance, but from a focal cortical epileptogenic source. There are several theories as to why or how a focal source may appear to have such widespread activity on scalp EEG. The discharge may be rapidly spread via interhemispheric connections to the contralateral hemisphere. Widespread excitatory networks may facilitate the spread of focal activity. The limited scalp EEG coverage may not allow for precise localization (as opposed to intracranial EEG). Low-voltage fast activity may not penetrate the skull. Historically, the Wada test has been used to determine if EDs are truly generalized or lateralized.[46] When amobarbital is injected ipsilateral to the known side of abnormality, the bilaterally synchronous EDs are ameliorated. When amobarbital is injected contralateral to the side of abnormality, the discharges are reduced but not obliterated.[47] The source of SBS is most commonly frontal, but can originate in any cortical head region. In the modern era this distinction can be aided by mangnetoencephalography or computer-assisted EEG interpretation. Patients with SBS and intractable epilepsy tend to have poor resective surgery outcomes, as opposed to those without SBS.[46]

14.12 Pediatric Epilepsy Syndromes

Epilepsy syndromes are constituted by distinct EEG patterns and clinical features.[48] Identifying a specific syndrome in a particular patient allows for optimal antiseizure treatment choices, prognostication, and early identification of comorbidities. With recent pharmacologic and genetic advances, syndrome identification allows for research trial designs for new pharmacologic and nonpharmacologic interventions. The common pediatric epilepsy syndromes are presented here.

14.12.1 Childhood and Juvenile Absence Epilepsy

Childhood absence epilepsy (CAE) onset usually occurs at 5–7 years of age, but can range from 4–10 years of age and is one of the genetic generalized epilepsies. Childhood absence epilepsy is characterized by typical absence seizures. Typical absence seizures involve a behavioral arrest with staring, often with automatisms or subtle myoclonic jerks of the face and/or head. They are relatively brief, lasting about 10 s and have no aura or postictal phase. Consciousness is typically impaired. The absence seizures may occur tens to hundreds of times a day. In association with the clinical event, the EEG demonstrates generalized 3-Hz spike-and-slow-wave complexes (Figure 14.30). Interictally, shorter bursts of generalized

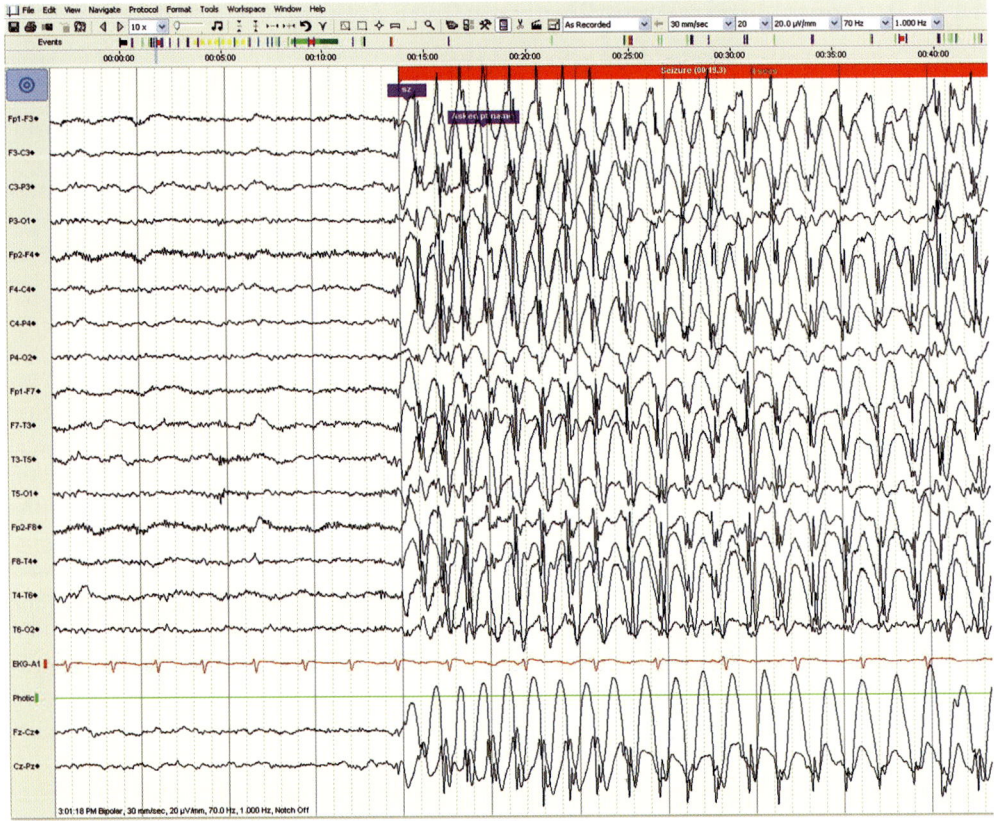

Figure 14.30 Generalized 3-Hz spike-and-slow-wave complexes noted during absence seizure.

spike and slow waves, as well as fragments of the epileptiform discharges may be seen. OIRDA may be present. OIRDA is high-amplitude rhythmic delta activity in the posterior leads triggered by hyperventilation and eye closure. Rarely, other generalized seizure types may be seen, such as tonic–clonic or myoclonic. IPS typically does not elicit an abnormal response. Absence seizures can be provoked with hyperventilation. Most patients have normal neurologic function although there is an association with attention deficit hyperactivity disorder and behavioral problems.[49] The treatments of choice are valproic acid or ethosuximide followed by lamotrigine.[50] Seizure resolution, if it occurs, typically is by 10–14 years of age. Family members without seizures may demonstrate generalized spike and slow waves suggesting this is an EEG "genetic trait." Genes associated with CAE include *CACNA1H* (encoding for Cav3.2 T-type channel) and $GABA_A$ receptor genes.[51]

Juvenile absence epilepsy (JAE) typically presents around puberty. The primary seizure types are typical absence, generalized tonic–clonic, and myoclonic. Unlike CAE where the absence seizures may occur hundreds of times a day, in JAE the absence seizures are less frequent, and more sporadic.[52] However, they may last longer and have a more prominent motor component. The EEG varies from CAE with slightly faster generalized spike-and-slow-wave complexes, less organization of the epileptiform complexes and more fragmentation. Although most are well controlled with antiseizure medication, the majority do not remit with age.[53]

14.12.2 Self-Limited Focal Epilepsy with Centrotemporal Spikes (Formerly Called Benign Epilepsy with Central Temporal Spikes)

Self-limited epilepsy with centrotemporal spikes (formerly called benign epilepsy with central temporal spikes (BECTS), also known as benign rolandic epilepsy), consists of focal motor seizures that may secondarily generalize in young school-age children, most often appearing between 5–8 years of age.[54] The EEG has a characteristic appearance of centrotemporal spikes with a horizontal dipole (Figure 14.31). These spikes are diphasic, high-amplitude, and can be unilateral, bilaterally synchronous, or bilaterally independent (Figure 14.32). They are activated by drowsiness and sleep, often occurring in trains. The spikes can be blocked by contralateral finger tapping or fist clenching in some patients. The background activity is otherwise normal. The classic epileptiform discharges may be present on EEG in 30–50% of persons without seizures and is thus considered a genetic trait on EEG. Patients with clinical seizures should have cessation of their epilepsy by adolescence, and clinical resolution usually precedes EEG normalization. Although considered a "benign" epilepsy, it has been associated with an increased risk of cognitive and behavioral problems. Although most children have a normal IQ, deficits in specific domains such as verbal fluency and other language tasks have been demonstrated.[55]

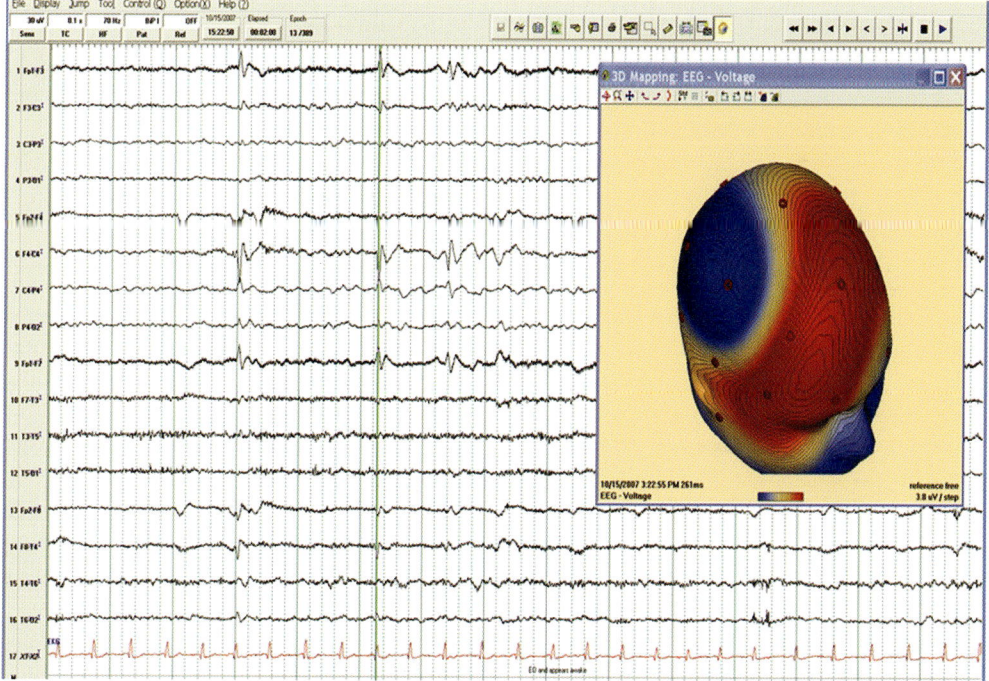

Figure 14.31 Note centrotemporal spikes with a horizontal dipole.

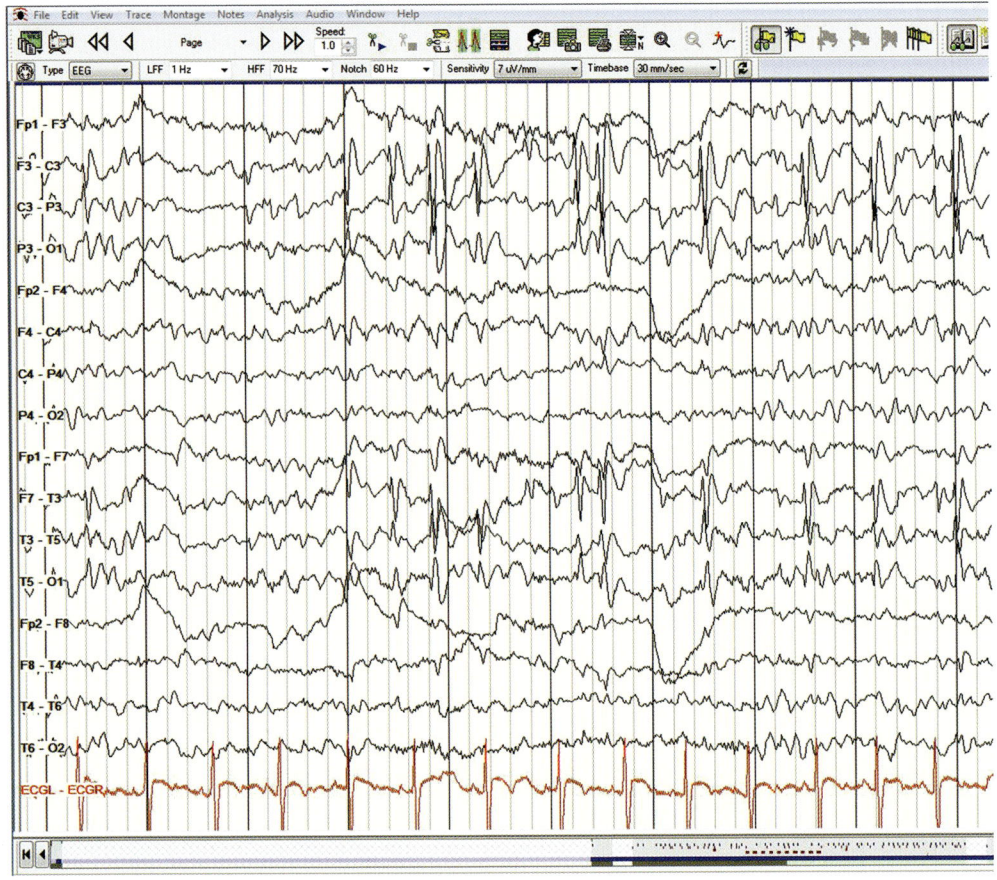

Figure 14.32 Note diphasic, high amplitude centrotemporal spikes on the left.

14.12.3 Self-Limited Occipital Epilepsy of Childhood, Early-Onset Form (Formerly Called Childhood Epilepsy with Occipital Paroxysms)

Self-limited occipital epilepsy of childhood, early-onset form also known as Panayiotopoulos syndrome, or childhood epilepsy with occipital paroxysms, is considered a benign focal epilepsy.[54] The average age of onset is 5 years of age. Seizures typically manifest as autonomic symptoms with impaired awareness during the night with the possibility of duration of over 30 min (i.e., autonomic status epilepticus). The interictal EEG shows multifocal high-voltage epileptiform discharges that may have an occipital predominance and are activated by drowsiness and sleep (Figure 14.33). The background activity is otherwise normal. Seizures typically start posteriorly on EEG with slowing of the background activity with intermixed spikes, and then spread anteriorly. Seizures should resolve by adolescence.

14.12.4 West Syndrome

West syndrome is comprised of a triad of features: epileptic (or "infantile") spasms, developmental delay or regression, and hypsarrhythmia pattern on EEG (Figure 14.34).

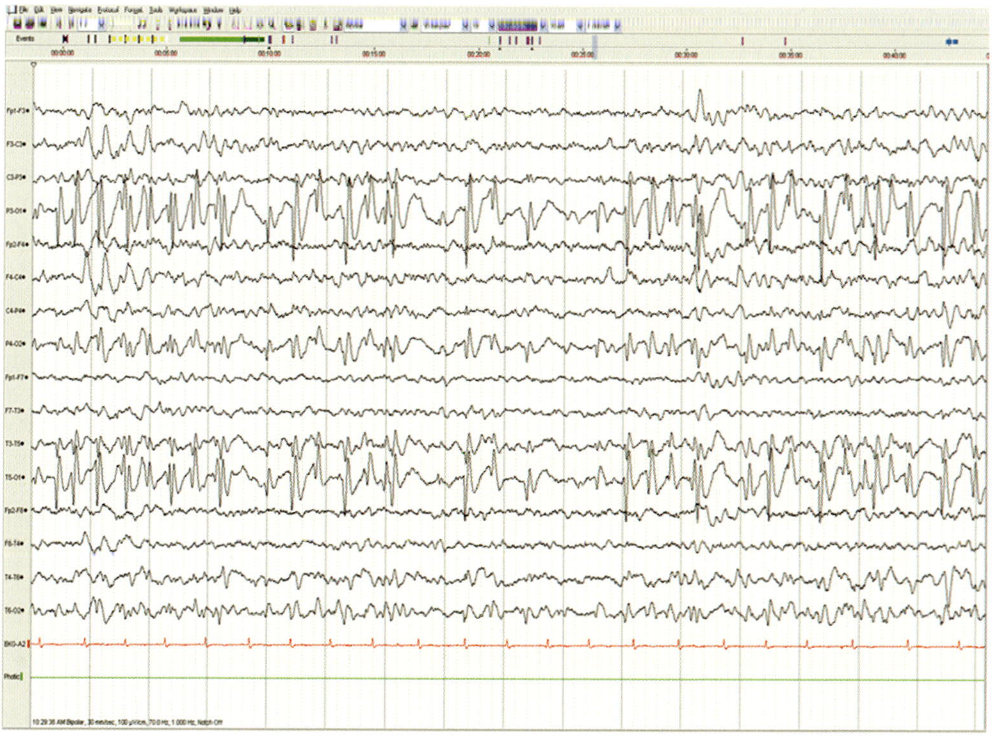

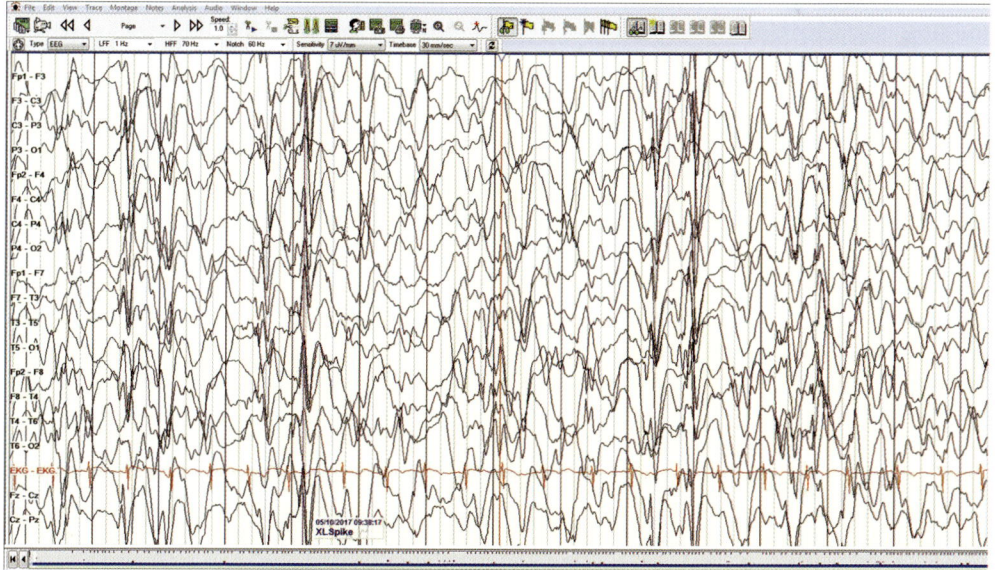

Figure 14.33 Note high-voltage epileptiform discharges with occipital predominance, activated by drowsiness and sleep in occipital epilepsy of childhood.

Figure 14.34 Note hypsarrhythmia pattern with a disorganized appearance of very high-voltage frequent multifocal spikes and slow wave activity in West syndrome.

Onset is usually in the first year of life, with a peak around 4–6 months of age.[56] The potential underlying causes for West syndrome are vast, and include genetic (e.g., tuberous sclerosis complex, Trisomy 21), structural (focal cortical dysplasia, hemimegalencephaly), and previous CNS insult (neonatal stroke, hypoxic ischemic encephalopathy). Patients are divided into unknown (previously "cryptogenic"; ~20%) and structural/metabolic/genetic (previously "symptomatic"; ~80%). Patients classified as unknown have no identified etiology, and are otherwise normal in development and neurologic exam. The spasms themselves consist of a brief myoclonic jerk with tonic extension, flexion, or both extension/flexion of the head, neck, and/or upper extremities. They are brief, lasting 1–2 seconds, but occur in clusters and are most noticeable upon arousal from sleep. The interictal EEG pattern of hypsarrhythmia consists of very high voltage (> 300 μV) frequent multifocal spikes and slow-wave activity with a disorganized appearance. Periods of electrodecrement may also be present, particularly during sleep. Hypsarrhythmia is most pronounced in early non-REM sleep and least obvious during REM sleep. Therefore, in a patient with clinically suspected spasms, the EEG must include sleep to definitively evaluate for hypsarrhythmia. Ictal patterns vary between patients and may consist of a diffuse slow wave, diffuse sharp and slow waves, or relative voltage attenuation with or without superimposed faster frequencies time locked to the spasm event. Focal features such as unilateral hypsarrhythmia may be present in the setting of such entities as hemimegalencephaly, and may manifest with hemispasms. In terms of treatment, high-dose adrenocorticotropic hormone gel and vigabatrin are recommended as first-line treatments.[57] Vigabatrin is preferred in the setting of tuberous sclerosis complex. The developmental outcome in West syndrome is generally poor, with the majority of children going on to be diagnosed with intellectual disability and other seizure types.[58]

14.12.5 Lennox–Gastaut Syndrome

Lennox–Gastaut syndrome (LGS) is an epileptic encephalopathy comprised of a triad of multiple seizures types (atonic, tonic, tonic–clonic, myoclonic, and atypical absence), cognitive impairment, and slow spike-and-wave activity on EEG. Onset is usually 2–6 years of age. West syndrome may evolve into LGS as the child ages. Multiple etiologies exist, including genetic, structural, and metabolic.[59] The spike and slow wave is typically 1.5–2.5 Hz and may be generalized or unilateral (Figure 14.35). The background activity is abnormal and slow for age. Runs of rapid spikes may be seen, especially later in the course. Generalized paroxysmal fast activity (Figure 14.36) (typically in sleep) is often seen and this, along with tonic seizures, helps differentiate LGS from other epilepsy syndromes such as myoclonic atonic epilepsy. Antiseizure medications that may be useful include rufinamide, felbamate, clobazam, lamotrigine, topiramate, and valproate. The ketogenic diet, vagus nerve stimulator, and complete corpus callosotomy have also been used. The outcome is generally poor, with drug-resistant seizures and moderate to severe intellectual disability.

14.12.6 Landau–Kleffner Syndrome and Continuous Spike in Slow-Wave Sleep

Continuous spike in slow-wave sleep (CSWS) refers to the EEG finding of continuous spike in slow-wave sleep (e.g. electrical status epilepticus in sleep or ESES) and resultant epileptic encephalopathy (Figure 14.37). Clinical seizures start in early childhood around 2–4 years of age.[60] ESES develops a bit later on in the course, usually around 4–8 years of age. When it

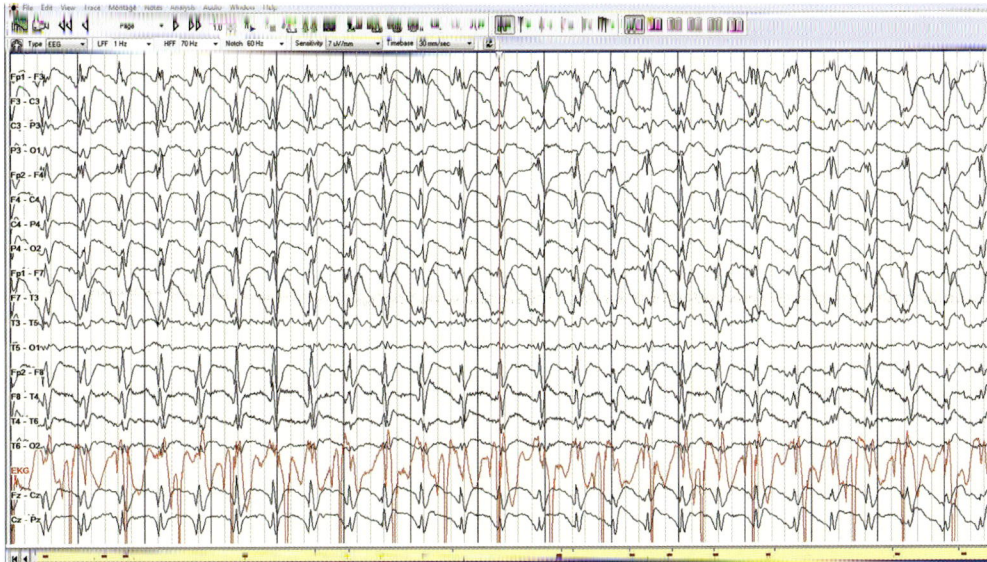

Figure 14.35 Note 1.5–2.5 Hz spike and slow waves in Lennox–Gastaut syndrome.

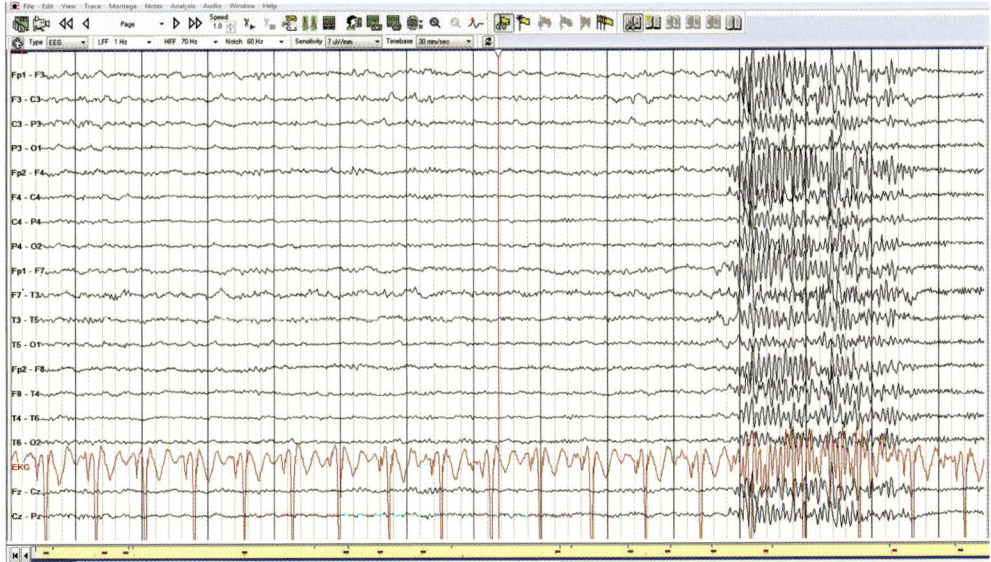

Figure 14.36 Note a burst of generalized paroxysmal fast activity (GPFA) in sleep noted in Lennox–Gastaut syndrome.

does occur, developmental regression sets in. The EEG shows almost continuous generalized spike and slow waves repeating at 1.5–3 Hz during non-REM sleep that occupy 85% or more of the EEG sleep recording. This value is expressed as the spike-and-wave index, which is the percentage of slow-wave sleep occupied by spike and slow waves. This is usually determined by counting the number of 1-s epochs with at least one spike and slow wave

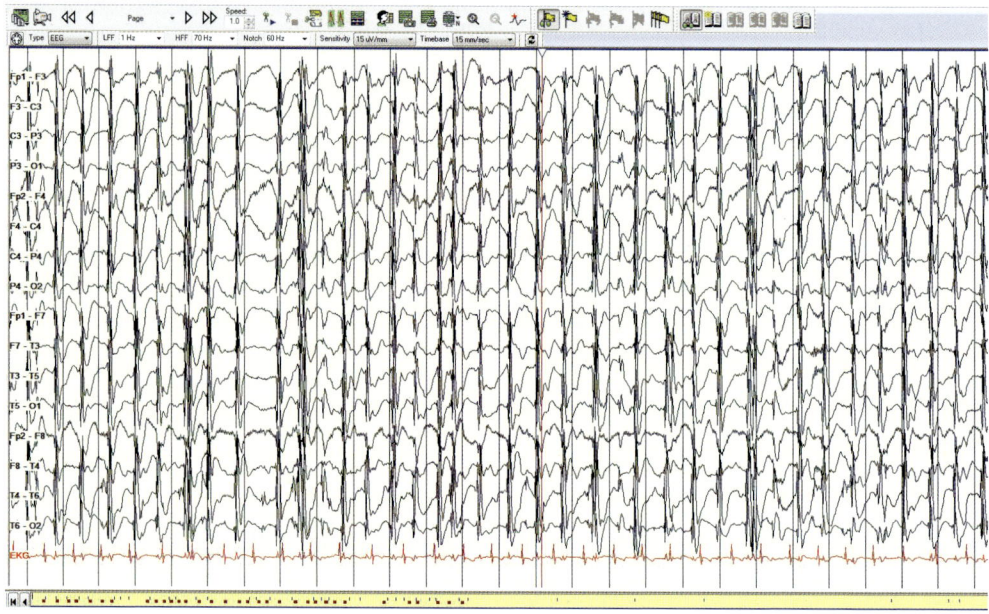

Figure 14.37 Note continuous generalized spike and slow waves repeating at 1.5–3 Hz during non-REM sleep in continuous spike in slow-wave sleep (CSWS).

present. Treatments that have been used include corticosteroids, high-dose benzodiazepines, ethosuximide, and levetiracetam.

In Landau–Kleffner syndrome (LKS), clinical seizures are infrequent or absent and the primary manifestation is in loss of language skills, initially presenting as a verbal auditory agnosia. First receptive language is lost followed by expressive language. In contrast to CSWS, epileptiform discharges are more focal and typically lateralized to one posterior quadrant. These discharges are activated by sleep and become more diffuse. Treatments include corticosteroids, valproate, and benzodiazepines. Multiple subpial transection has also been used.

14.13 Abnormal EEG Patterns in Specific Pediatric Genetic or Infectious Syndromes

Diagnosing a neurologic syndrome in the pediatric population entails an understanding of the genetic and neurophysiologic underpinnings of that particular diagnosis. Prior to the advent of advanced genetic testing, recognizing EEG patterns in association with specific clinical features allowed for proper diagnosis. Knowledge of these EEG patterns continues to provide a deeper understanding of these syndromes and is important to properly treat the associated neurologic symptoms such as epilepsy.

14.13.1 Rett Syndrome

Rett syndrome affects almost exclusively females as it is caused by mutations in the *MECP2* gene on the X chromosome. Typically, development is normal until 6 months to 3 years of age, at which point developmental regression, ataxia, autistic features, microcephaly, and classic "hand-wringing" emerge. Seizures occur in 70–90% of affected patients and typically begin after the period of regression.[61] The seizures may mimic those seen in LGS and include atonic, myoclonic, tonic, atypical absence, and focal; ESES and nonconvulsive status epilepticus have also been described.[62] The EEG progression is divided into four stages,[63] which correlate with clinical stages. In Stage 1, the EEG may be normal or show minimal slowing of the posterior dominant rhythm (PDR). In Stage 2, slowing of the PDR, loss of normal sleep architecture, and focal spikes are seen. Narrow spikes in the bi-central head regions may be seen that react to contralateral hand movement similar to the mu rhythm. In Stage 3, further slowing of the PDR, absence of sleep architecture, and multifocal epileptiform discharges are noted. In addition, the classic feature of 4–6 Hz theta rhythmic activity in the central head regions emerges. Care should be taken not to misinterpret this midline rhythmic activity as a seizure[64] particularly in light of the high incidence of nonepileptic paroxysmal events in Rett syndrome. Finally, Stage 4 consists of absent PDR, multifocal epileptiform discharges, and almost continuous generalized slow spike and waves during sleep. Of note, the mutation type does not appear to correlate with epilepsy severity.[62] Clinically, seizure onset after the age of 5 years is associated with better seizure control. Epilepsy severity does directly correlate with overall disease burden.

14.13.2 Angelman Syndrome

Angelman syndrome is caused by a microdeletion on the maternally inherited chromosome 15. This affects the *UBE3A* gene, which is a ubiquitin–protein ligase E3A. It manifests as developmental delay, spells of unexplained laughter, ataxia, and jerky movements. Seizures occur in 80% of patients. Three characteristic EEG patterns have been described.[65] "Delta pattern" consists of high-amplitude diffuse slow-wave activity, with or without admixed epileptiform discharges. This is typically present during infancy and early childhood. The "theta pattern" consists of monomorphic high-amplitude theta waves with either a generalized distribution or posterior predominance. Finally, posterior discharges, which may occur spontaneously or be facilitated by passive eye closure may occur.

The EEG and seizure types mimic LGS.[66] Slow (2–2.5 Hz) generalized spike and slow waves may be present, although at times without a well-defined spike. An aid in distinguishing between Angelman syndrome and LGS is the lack of generalized paroxysmal fast activity in Angelman syndrome. Seizure types include myoclonic, atypical absence, generalized tonic–clonic, and atonic. Seizures may be triggered by fever and may be quite prolonged.

14.13.3 Progressive Myoclonic Epilepsies

Progressive myoclonic epilepsies (PMEs) are a group of epilepsies with the hallmark of predominant myoclonic seizures, although other seizure types such as generalized tonic–clonic, atonic, and other types may be seen. Ataxia and cognitive deterioration occur. Examples include mitochondrial encephalomyopathy, lactic acidosis, and stroke-like episodes (MELAS), neuronal ceroid lipofuscinosis (NCL), Lafora's disease, and Unverricht–Lundborg progressive familial myoclonic epilepsy. An exaggerated somatosensory-evoked potential amplitude or high-amplitude epileptiform discharges may occur with IPS at low frequencies (0.5–3Hz).[38,67]

14.13.4 Subacute Sclerosing Panencephalitis

Subacute sclerosing panencephalitis (SSPE) is a postinfectious disease following measles infection. The disease is divided into phases. During the first phase, personality changes and cognitive decline are noted. It is during the second phase that the classic EEG finding occurs. Very high-amplitude (>500 µV) diffuse multiphasic complexes comprised of slow waves and spikes occur periodically, every 4–10 s.[68] The complex duration is quite long, lasting 1–3 s. In association with the complex, a myoclonic jerk may occur. Typically, the interdischarge background activity is also abnormal, with slowing of the posterior dominant rhythm and/or relative attenuation. This creates a burst-suppression type appearance. The final clinical phase of SSPE entails unresponsiveness, decerebrate posturing, rigidity, and hypothalamic dysfunction. The onset of SSPE is typically around 5–15 years of age. Risk of SSPE following measles infection is increased by younger age of measles infection and male gender.

References

1. Lamblin MD, de Villepin-Touzery A. EEG in the neonatal unit. *Neurophysiol Clin.* 2015;45(1):87–95.

2. Selton D, Andre M, Hascoet JM. Normal EEG in very premature infants: reference criteria. *Clin Neurophysiol.* 2000;111 (12):2116–2124.

3. Peters JF, Varner JL, Ellingson RJ. Interhemispheric amplitude symmetry in the EEGs of normal full term, low risk premature, and trisomy-21 infants. *Electroencephalogr Clin Neurophysiol.* 1981;51(2):165–169.

4. Lombroso CT. Neonatal polygraphy in full-term and premature infants: a review of normal and abnormal findings. *J Clin Neurophysiol.* 1985;2(2):105–155.

5. Holmes GL, Lombroso CT. Prognostic value of background patterns in the neonatal EEG. *J Clin Neurophysiol.* 1993;10 (3):323–352.

6. Hahn JS, Monyer H, Tharp BR. Interburst interval measurements in the EEGs of premature infants with normal neurological outcome. *Electroencephalogr Clin Neurophysiol.* 1989;73(5):410–418.

7. Grigg-Damberger MM, Coker SB, Halsey CL, Anderson CL. Neonatal burst suppression: its developmental significance. *Pediatr Neurol.* 1989;5(2):84–92.

8. American Electroencephalographic Society Guidelines in electroencephalography, evoked potentials, and polysomnography. *J Clin Neurophysiol.* 1994;11(1):1–147.

9. Lombroso CT. Neurophysiological observations in diseased newborns. *Biol Psychiatry.* 1975;10(5):527–558.

10. Almubarak S, Wong PK. Long-term clinical outcome of neonatal EEG findings. *J Clin Neurophysiol.* 2011;28(2):185–189.

11. Clancy RR, Tharp BR. Positive rolandic sharp waves in the electroencephalograms of premature neonates with intraventricular hemorrhage. *Electroencephalogr Clin Neurophysiol.* 1984;57(5):395–404.

12. Mizrahi EM, Kellaway P. Characterization and classification of neonatal seizures. *Neurology.* 1987;37(12):1837–1844.

13. Clancy RR, Legido A. The exact ictal and interictal duration of electroencephalographic neonatal seizures. *Epilepsia.* 1987;28(5):537–541.

14. Tsuchida TN, Wusthoff CJ, Shellhaas RA, et al. American clinical neurophysiology society standardized EEG terminology and categorization for the description of continuous EEG monitoring in neonates: report of the American Clinical Neurophysiology Society Critical Care Monitoring Committee. *J Clin Neurophysiol.* 2013;30(2):161–173.

15. Clancy R, Malin S, Laraque D, Baumgart S, Younkin D. Focal motor seizures heralding stroke in full-term neonates. *Am J Dis Child.* 1985;139(6):601–606.

16. Scher MS, Painter MJ, Bergman I, Barmada MA, Brunberg J. EEG diagnosos of neonatal seizures: clinical correlations and outcome. *Pediatr Neurol.* 1989;5(1):17–24.

17. Dehan M, Quillerou D, Navelet Y, et al. [Convulsions in the fifth day of life: a new syndrome?]. *Arch Fr Pediatr.* 1977;34 (8):730–742.

18. Kato M, Yamagata T, Kubota M, et al. Clinical spectrum of early onset epileptic encephalopathies caused by KCNQ2 mutation. *Epilepsia.* 2013;54(7):1282–1287.

19. Miles DK, Holmes GL. Benign neonatal seizures. *J Clin Neurophysiol.* 1990;7 (3):369–379.

20. Aicardi J, Gouticres F. [Neonatal myoclonic encephalopathy (author's transl)]. *Rev Electroencephalogr Neurophysiol Clin.* 1978;8(1):99–101.

21. Ohtahara S, Ohtsuka Y, Yamatogi Y, Oka E. The early-infantile epileptic encephalopathy with suppression-burst: developmental aspects. *Brain Dev.* 1987;9 (4):371–376.

22. Westmoreland BF, Klass DW. Unusual EEG patterns. *J Clin Neurophysiol.* 1990;7 (2):209–228.

23. Mizrahi EM. Avoiding the pitfalls of EEG interpretation in childhood epilepsy. *Epilepsia.* 1996;37 Suppl 1(s1):S41–51.

24. Arroyo S, Lesser RP, Gordon B, et al. Functional significance of the mu rhythm of human cortex: an electrophysiologic study with subdural electrodes. *Electroencephalogr Clin Neurophysiol.* 1993;87(3):76–87.

25. Evans CC. Spontaneous excitation of the visual cortex and association areas; lambda waves. *Electroencephalogr Clin Neurophysiol.* 1953;5(1):69–74.

26. Scott DF, Groethuysen UC, Bickford RG. Lambda responses in the human electroencephalogram. *Neurology.* 1967;17 (8 Pt 1):770–778.

27. Vignaendra V, Matthews RL, Chatrian GE. Positive occipital sharp transients of sleep: relationships to nocturnal sleep cycle in man. *Electroencephalogr Clin Neurophysiol.* 1974;37(3):239–246.

28. Brenner RP, Zauel DW, Carlow TJ. Positive occipital sharp transients of sleep in the blind. *Neurology.* 1978;28(6):609–612.

29. White JC, Tharp BR. An arousal pattern in children with organic cerebral dysfunction. *Electroencephalogr Clin Neurophysiol.* 1974;37(3):265–268.

30. Gibbs FA, Rich CL, Gibbs EL. Psychomotor variant type of seizure discharge. *Neurology.* 1963;13(12):991–998.

31. Westmoreland BF, Klass DW. Midline theta rhythm. *Arch Neurol.* 1986;43 (2):139–141.

32. Lombroso CT, Schwartz IH, Clark DM, et al. Ctenoids in healthy youths. Controlled study of 14- and 6-per-second positive spiking. *Neurology.* 1966;16 (12):1152–1158.

33. Silverman D. Fourteen and six per second positive spike pattern in a patient with hepatic coma. *Electroencephalogr Clin Neurophysiol.* 1964;16(4):395–398.

34. Yamada T, Young S, Kimura J. Significance of positive spike burst in Reye syndrome. *Arch Neurol.* 1977;34(6):376–380.

35. Tharp BR. The 6-per-second spike and wave complex. The wave and spike phantom. *Arch Neurol.* 1966;15 (5):533–537.

36. Westmoreland BF. Epileptiform electroencephalographic patterns. *Mayo Clin Proc.* 1996;71(5):501–511.

37. Brigo F, Cicero R, Fiaschi A, Bongiovanni LG. The breach rhythm. *Clin Neurophysiol.* 2011;122(11):2116–2120.

38. Mendez OE, Brenner RP. Increasing the yield of EEG. *J Clin Neurophysiol.* 2006;23 (4):282–293.

39. de Stegge BM, van Putten MJ. A patient with a transient photomyogenic response. *Clin Neurophysiol.* 2010;121(1):118–120.

40. Harding GF, Herrick CE, Jeavons PM. A controlled study of the effect of sodium valproate on photosensitive epilepsy and its prognosis. *Epilepsia.* 1978;19(6):555–565.

41. Verrotti A, Beccaria F, Fiori F, Montagnini A, Capovilla G. Photosensitivity: epidemiology, genetics, clinical

manifestations, assessment, and management. *Epileptic Disord.* 2012;14 (4):349–362.

42. Glick TH. The sleep-deprived electroencephalogram: evidence and practice. *Arch Neurol.* 2002;59 (8):1235–1239.

43. Guilhoto LM, Manreza ML, Yacubian EM. Occipital intermittent rhythmic delta activity in absence epilepsy. *Arq Neuropsiquiatr.* 2006;64(2A):193–197.

44. Desai J, Mitchell WG, Rosser T, et al. Clinical associations of occipital intermittent rhythmic delta activity. *J Child Neurol.* 2012;27(4):503–506.

45. Desai JD, Toczek MT, Mitchell WG. Frontal intermittent rhythmic delta activity (FIRDA): is there a clinical significance in children and adolescents? *Eur J Paediatr Neurol.* 2012;16 (2):138–141.

46. Sunwoo JS, Byun JI, Moon J, et al. Unfavorable surgical outcomes in partial epilepsy with secondary bilateral synchrony: intracranial electroencephalography study. *Epilepsy Res.* 2016;122:102–109.

47. Lombroso CT, Erba G. Primary and secondary bilateral synchrony in epilepsy; a clinical and electroencephalographic study. *Arch Neurol.* 1970;22(4):321–334.

48. Scheffer IE, Berkovic S, Capovilla G, et al. ILAE classification of the epilepsies: position paper of the ILAE Commission for Classification and Terminology. *Epilepsia.* 2017;58(4):512–521.

49. Masur D, Shinnar S, Cnaan A, et al. Pretreatment cognitive deficits and treatment effects on attention in childhood absence epilepsy. *Neurology.* 2013;81 (18):1572–1580.

50. Glauser TA, Cnaan A, Shinnar S, et al. Ethosuximide, valproic acid, and lamotrigine in childhood absence epilepsy. *N Engl J Med.* 2010;362(9):790–799.

51. Guilhoto LM. Absence epilepsy: continuum of clinical presentation and epigenetics? *Seizure.* 2017;44:53–57.

52. Janz D. The idiopathic generalized epilepsies of adolescence with childhood and juvenile age of onset. *Epilepsia.* 1997;38 (1):4–11.

53. Beghi M, Beghi E, Cornaggia CM, Gobbi G. Idiopathic generalized epilepsies of adolescence. *Epilepsia.* 2006;47 Suppl 2 (s2):107–110.

54. Guerrini R, Pellacani S. Benign childhood focal epilepsies. *Epilepsia.* 2012;53 Suppl 4:9–18.

55. Vannest J, Tenney JR, Gelineau-Morel R, Maloney T, Glauser TA. Cognitive and behavioral outcomes in benign childhood epilepsy with centrotemporal spikes. *Epilepsy Behav.* 2015;45:85–91.

56. Pavone P, Striano P, Falsaperla R, Pavone L, Ruggieri M. Infantile spasms syndrome, West syndrome and related phenotypes: what we know in 2013. *Brain Dev.* 2014;36 (9):739–751.

57. Go CY, Mackay MT, Weiss SK, et al. Evidence-based guideline update: medical treatment of infantile spasms. Report of the Guideline Development Subcommittee of the American Academy of Neurology and the Practice Committee of the Child Neurology Society. *Neurology.* 2012;78 (24):1974–1980.

58. Widjaja E, Go C, McCoy B, Snead OC. Neurodevelopmental outcome of infantile spasms: a systematic review and meta-analysis. *Epilepsy Res.* 2015;109:155–162.

59. Mastrangelo M. Lennox-Gastaut syndrome: a state of the art review. *Neuropediatrics.* 2017;48(3):143–151.

60. Hughes JR. A review of the relationships between Landau-Kleffner syndrome, electrical status epilepticus during sleep, and continuous spike-waves during sleep. *Epilepsy Behav.* 2011;20(2):247–253.

61. Moser SJ, Weber P, Lutschg J. Rett syndrome: clinical and electrophysiologic aspects. *Pediatr Neurol.* 2007;36(2):95–100.

62. Nissenkorn A, Gak E, Vecsler M, et al. Epilepsy in Rett syndrome – the experience of a National Rett Center. *Epilepsia.* 2010;51(7):1252–1258.

63. Glaze DG. Neurophysiology of Rett syndrome. *J Child Neurol.* 2005;20 (9).740–746.

64. Weber AR, Ostendorf A. Teaching NeuroImages: a central theta EEG rhythm in Rett syndrome can masquerade as seizure. *Neurology.* 2016;87(3):e29–30.

65. Valente KD, Andrade JQ, Grossmann RM, et al. Angelman syndrome: difficulties in EEG pattern recognition and possible misinterpretations. *Epilepsia.* 2003;44 (8):1051–1063.

66. Thibert RL, Larson AM, Hsieh DT, Raby AR, Thiele EA. Neurologic manifestations of Angelman syndrome. *Pediatr Neurol.* 2013;48(4):271–279.

67. Satishchandra P, Sinha S. Progressive myoclonic epilepsy. *Neurol India.* 2010;58 (4):514–522.

68. Demir N, Cokar O, Bolukbasi F, et al. A close look at EEG in subacute sclerosing panencephalitis. *J Clin Neurophysiol.* 2013;30(4):348–356.

Scalp Video-EEG Monitoring

Maria Stefanidou

15.1 Introduction

The initial evaluation of patients presenting with a seizure includes obtaining a detailed history of the event, a thorough physical examination, identifying risk factors for seizure occurrence, and the use of ancillary tests that help establish the diagnosis, namely laboratory tests, an electroencephalogram (EEG), and neuroimaging. In certain cases a lumbar puncture may also be indicated.

15.2 History and Physical Examination

Obtaining a detailed history of the event is very important. Pertinent information to obtain is the age of onset, presence of a warning sign (aura), a detailed step-by-step description of the semiology of the event, presence or absence of alteration of awareness, duration of the attack, and the patient's behavior in the postictal period. If more than one attack has occurred, it is important to inquire regarding the presence of stereotypy between attacks. Often the physician has to rely on witnesses for a description as patients are amnestic of the event. It is also vital to ask about triggers (detailed medication list, including any recent changes, history of alcohol and illicit drug abuse, sleep deprivation, recent illnesses), as well as risk factors for recurrent unprovoked seizures (history of perinatal insults, prematurity, developmental delay, traumatic brain injury, history of febrile seizures, prior CNS infection, family history). A detailed neurological examination is essential. It is not uncommon for patients with epilepsy to have a normal exam between seizures. Focal deficits on exam could be due to structural brain lesions (tumor, stroke, etc.) responsible for seizure generation, and postictal transient focal deficits may offer an insight into the seizure onset zone. Especially in children, it is important to include a detailed skin examination to rule out signs of neuro-cutaneous syndromes associated with seizures (tuberous sclerosis complex, Sturge–Weber syndrome, etc.).

15.3 Laboratory Tests

Laboratory tests that include blood glucose, blood counts, and electrolyte panels (particularly sodium) are almost always obtained with a first-time seizure. The primary purpose is to rule out metabolic conditions that may provoke seizures (hyponatremia, hyperglycemia, hypoglycemia etc.), as in these cases treating the underlying metabolic disturbance will prevent seizure recurrence. The American Academy of Neurology (AAN) recommends obtaining these tests in the right clinical setting in addition to performing a lumbar puncture and toxicologic serum and/or urine screening when there is high clinical suspicion, but there is insufficient data to support or refute performing these tests routinely.[1]

15.4 Scalp EEG

15.4.1 Routine Scalp EEG

Routine scalp EEG is the most common diagnostic study performed for the diagnosis of epilepsy, and has been available for nearly a century. Its duration varies at different institutions, between 20 min and 1 hour, and can be performed either on an inpatient or an outpatient basis. Given its short duration it focuses mainly on the evaluation of the interictal period. A routine EEG that shows interictal epileptiform discharges (IEDs) (sharps, spikes, or spike-wave discharges) may predict a 30–70% risk for seizure recurrence within the next year,[1] and an initial study has sensitivity to capture such abnormalities in 29% to 55% of cases.[2] Obtaining additional routine EEGs may further increase the yield, with four sequential EEGs identifying up to 92% of seizure cases, but further testing adds little to the diagnosis.[3] The optimal time for obtaining a sleep-deprived EEG is within the first 2–3 days following a seizure,[4,5] as it has been shown to increase its diagnostic potential. One should always keep in mind that a very low proportion of normal adults have epileptiform discharges (0.5%),[2] therefore the findings should always be interpreted in the appropriate clinical context. The American Epilepsy Society (AES) and the International League Against Epilepsy (ILAE) recommend obtaining a routine EEG with hyperventilation, photic stimulation, and sleep deprivation[1,6–8] in patients undergoing evaluation for seizures.

One potential limitation in identifying true epileptiform discharges is over interpretation of either nonspecific abnormalities or epileptiform discharges that can be seen in the context of metabolic encephalopathy or secondary to medications (lithium, clozapine) and do not carry an increased risk for unprovoked seizures.[2] The absence of IEDs on a scalp EEG may either be attributed to their infrequent nature in certain individuals or because they may be generated in areas of the brain not accessible by the scalp EEG recording (deep seated in sulci, interhemispheric location, etc).[2]

15.4.2 Long-Term Scalp EEG Monitoring

15.4.2.1 Ambulatory EEG With or Without Video Recording

It is now possible from a technological standpoint to obtain a prolonged EEG recording lasting a few hours to a few days as an outpatient. Most common indications include:

1. Epilepsy diagnosis/classification by identifying IEDs
2. Characterization of stereotypical events in the patient's home and as they go about their routine daily activities, when they may be more likely to occur
3. Assessment of the efficacy of treatment in known epilepsy cases.

In this setting, it is particularly helpful to rule out subclinical seizures, or evaluate epileptiform activity that is primarily linked to the sleep–wake cycle and requires an overnight record (e.g., continuous spike wave of sleep).[9] The ambulatory nature of the study in addition to being more cost effective,[10] offers less disturbed sleep compared to the inpatient setting.[11] The yield of ambulatory EEG for capturing IEDs has been estimated to be about 25% following a normal routine EEG.[12] Overall, ambulatory EEG has been shown to be diagnostic, either by the identification of epileptiform activity or by ruling it out during habitual events of interest in 65–80% of cases.[13] Significant limitations include potential technical malfunctions and artifacts that may either limit the interpretation of the EEG (muscle artifact) or be confused for abnormal activity (brushing teeth, talking, chewing artifacts) when video is not available. Recently portable cameras recording video that is time-locked and synchronized to the EEG signal acquisition, have also become available for outpatient use, overcoming some of these limitations.[11]

15.4.2.2 Long-Term Video-EEG Monitoring in the Intensive Care Unit (ICU)/Inpatient Floor

The main indications for obtaining a prolonged EEG in ICU or inpatient floor are:

1. Detection of nonconvulsive/electrographic seizures in the setting of unexplained alteration of mental status. This is the most common type of seizure detected in the ICU and risk factors include coma, prior history of seizures, CNS infection, brain tumors, neurosurgical procedures, and presence of periodic epileptiform discharges.[14] It is important to identify subclinical seizures early, as delays in treatment have been linked to worse outcomes and higher mortality rates.[15] The optimal duration of the recording for ruling out epileptic activity varies in different clinical settings. One study showed that lack of IEDs within the first 4 hours of EEG recording is a strong predictor against seizure activity thereafter.[16] Evidence suggests that a 24-hour recording is sufficient when evaluating a noncomatose patient, but may have to be extended to 48 hours in coma cases.[14] When a patient presents in clinical convulsive status epilepticus and there is persistence of impaired consciousness despite initial treatment and resolution of clinical seizure activity, it is essential to obtain continuous EEG, as ongoing seizure activity has been found in 48% and nonconvulsive status epilepticus in 14% of patients.[17] Other clinical scenarios that carry a high risk of seizures are hemorrhagic strokes that are complicated by seizures in one-third of cases, half of which are subclinical,[18] and traumatic brain injury with seizures recorded in 20% of patients, half of which are also subclinical.[19]

2. Management of status epilepticus. The use of continuous EEG has been especially useful in treating status epilepticus, as noted above, as well as in cases of refractory status epilepticus when sedating agents are used for seizure management.[20] The EEG is helpful in the determination of the level of sedation and in achieving burst-suppression patterns.

3. Cardiac arrest. Immediately following cardiac arrest, prolonged EEG is helpful in differentiating postanoxic encephalopathy from status epilepticus. In addition, the evolution of the EEG background in the hours to days post-arrest, as well as the presence of certain EEG patterns may help with prognostication. Persistent isoelectric pattern, low voltage activity, or burst suppression with identical bursts at 24 hours post-arrest predict a poor outcome without false positives. Rapid recovery toward continuous EEG patterns within 12 hours is strongly associated with a good neurological outcome. Predictive values are highest in the first 24 hours, even in the presence of mild therapeutic hypothermia and sedative medication.[21]

4. Another emerging use includes identification of acute ischemic brain injury in the setting of SAH.[22]

15.4.2.3 Long-Term Scalp Video-EEG Monitoring in an Epilepsy Monitoring Unit

An integral part of specialized epilepsy centers is the epilepsy monitoring unit (EMU), which includes an interdisciplinary team of neurologists and neurosurgeons, neuropsychologists, nurse specialists, EEG technologists, and other personnel with special training and experience in the treatment of epilepsy.[23] Patients are admitted to record continuous EEG over a long period of time,[24] with the goal of capturing a patient's typical, recurring event in a monitored setting, and correlating the EEG data with a video recording.[25] In general, the EEG setup in adults should include a minimum of 21 electrodes (FP1, FP2, F3, F4, F7, F8, T3, T4, T5, T6, C3, C4, P3, P4, O1, O2, Fz, Cz, Pz, one ground electrode, and one reference electrode) positioned in the 10-20 system, and one ECG electrode.[9] The EEG signal acquisition is carried out in a referential montage with the potential of reconstruction to other montages. A strict synchronization between the EEG signal and the audiovisual recording is required. One or two high-quality cameras are usually used, with infrared capability for recording during the night.[9]

The most common clinical indications for an EMU admission fall into four categories:

1. Diagnosis of recurrent stereotypical events, mainly differential diagnosis between nonepileptic (psychogenic or physiologic) and epileptic seizures
2. Classification and characterization of seizure types and epilepsy syndromes through the detection of IEDs or capturing seizures
3. Presurgical evaluation in drug-resistant epilepsy for localization of the ictal focus[26]
4. Monitoring seizure quantification following medication adjustments.[9]

Scalp video-EEG recording in the EMU is considered a reliable diagnostic test for differentiating between epileptic and psychogenic nonepileptic spells (PNES).[27] It has been shown to change the diagnosis in 25% of cases, both among those presumed to have epileptic seizures, but also among those with presumed PNES who were proven to have epilepsy.[13] When considering all patients admitted to EMU units, 9–15% have a combination of both epileptic and nonepileptic events.[28] There is great value in recording the clinical semiology of attacks. A recent study that compared accuracy in diagnosis based on description alone of both epileptic and nonepileptic events versus review of video recordings showed that diagnostic accuracy improved from 54% to 85%.[29] A proposed bedside diagnostic tool for differentiating PNES from epileptic seizures in patients with generalized motor events is based on six clinical signs that include side-to-side head movements, forceful eye closure, fluctuating course, asynchronous limb movements, rotation in bed (flailing), and opisthotonus, and have very high specificity in identifying PNES.[30] Conversely, certain reported symptoms and observed behaviors are characteristic of epileptic seizures and help localize and lateralize the seizure onset zone (Table 15.1).[31] In order to increase the diagnostic yield of the audiovisual recording the ILAE recommends standardized testing of patients during their attacks; nurses attending to the patient having an event should first address safety concerns (ABCs, place the patient on their side during a generalized tonic–clonic seizure (GTC), remove covers and ensure the camera is on the patient, describe loudly observations that might be subtle (sweating, pallor, eye deviation, etc.) and perform a battery of tests that assess the patient's responsiveness, speech comprehension, naming, repetition, ictal palsy, and verbal and visual memory.[32] Three potential pitfalls in the evaluation of events with the use of video-EEG are the possible lack of scalp-EEG correlate in frontal onset seizures,[33] the inability to interpret the EEG given extensive muscle artifacts during hyperkinetic seizures, and failure to record the patient's typical event or all of the events in patients who report multiple different semiologies.[13] One important finding during EMU evaluation is that patients with epilepsy may be aware of only a fraction of their seizures and that ranges

Table 15.1 Localizing and lateralizing seizure semiology

	Localization	Lateralization
Somatosensory: tingling, numbness	Primary sensory cortex – unilateral symptoms Supplementary sensory motor area, superior bank of sylvian fissure, posterior insula – bilateral symptoms	Contralateral Nonlateralizing
Visual Flashing lights Complex hallucinations	Broadman's are 17&18 Association cortex (parieto-temporal)	Contralateral when the visual phenomenon is perceived in one visual field
Auditory: buzz, noise	Heschl's gyrus in the superior temoral gyrus	Nonlateralizing
Olfactory: unpleasant smell	Mesial temporal	Nonlateralizing
Gustatory: unpleasant taste	Insula	Nonlateralizing
Autonomic: palpitations, sweating etc.	Probable insula	Nonlateralizing
Abdominal	Temporal lobe and less often insula or frontal lobe	Nonlateralizing
Psychic: autoscopy, déjà vu, jamais vu, etc.	Temporal lobe	Nonlateralizing
Pilomotor	Nonlocalizing	Ipsilateral
Ictal vomiting, retching spitting, cough	Temporal	Nonlateralizing
Ictal hypersalivation	Temporal	Nondominant
Ictal or peri-ictal water drinking	Temporal	Nondominant
Ictal urinary urge	Temporal	Nondominant
Ictal speech	Temporal lobe involvement	Nondominant
Ictal or post-ictal aphasia	Temporal lobe involvement	Dominant hemisphere
Dystonic arm posturing	Temporal>>extra-temporal	Contralateral
Post-ictal nose wipe	Temporal	Ipsilateral
Todd's paralysis	Nonlocalizing	Contralateral
Focal seizures with altered awareness	Mesial temporal lobe – long duration Frontal lobe – shorter duration	Nonlateralizing Motor signs, if present, may help lateralization

Table 15.1 (cont.)

	Localization	Lateralization
Myoclonic seizures	Generalized	Nonlateralizing
Tonic seizures	Supplementary motor area – preservation of awareness Frontal lobe >> temporal lobe	Contralateral when tonic posturing is clearly unilateral
Primary generalized tonic–clonic seizures	Generalized – tonic flexion of the body with shoulder and arm elevation followed by tonic hyperextension of the entire body	Nonlateralizing
Spread to bilateral tonic–clonic seizures from focal onset	Does not localize seizure onset Motor sequence: (a) version, (b) pulling of the face, (c) fencing sign, followed by (d) figure 4 sign	Contralateral when ≥2 signs present
Epileptic spasms	Generalized, but also focal (common parieto-occipital)	Nonlateralizing
Clonic seizures	Primary motor cortex-preservation of awareness Temporal – face, hand, and frontal eye field affected before legs	Contralateral
Versive seizures	Frontal and temporal onset but occur earlier in frontal seizures	Contralateral
Hypermotor seizures	Orbital and mesial frontal, also temporal or insular	Nonlateralizing
Automotor (mouth and hand automatisms)	Temporal lobe >> frontal lobe	Ipsilateral when automatisms are unilateral
Gelastic seizures	Hypothalamic hamartoma 50%, also anterior cingulate, also frontal, parietal, and temporal lobe	Nonlateralizing
Atonic seizures	Symptomatic generalized epilepsies – usually preceded by myoclonus, also frontal and temporal lobe	Nonlateralizing

Data from reference 31

between 40% and 68% of captured events in different studies.[34,35] This may have important clinical implications when following a patient in the outpatient setting, and an EMU admission may be considered in cases when there is clinical suspicion for incomplete seizure control, especially if the patient is in the process of resuming driving. When considering both epileptic and nonepileptic events, a positive diagnosis is possible in 82–90% of patients at the end of an EMU admission.[36,37] There are also data to suggest that repeating the test after an initial failure to capture the event of interest can be successful in about 40% of cases.[38]

Methods to Provoke Seizures in the EMU

During EMU admissions, certain activation procedures are used in order to facilitate seizure occurrence that may be unpredictable or infrequent and in order to decrease the length of stay in the hospital.

1. Tapering and discontinuation of antiseizure drugs (ASDs). There is no universal protocol for performing ASD withdrawal. Rapid withdrawal of ASDs over 4–6 days in refractory temporal lobe epilepsy was effective in triggering seizures, but about 50% of patients experienced seizure clusters defined as three or more focal seizures with impaired awareness in 24 hours.[39] Slower taper on alternate days showed a 40% risk of seizure clustering.[40] A different study that combined fast ASD discontinuation within 24 hours (except barbiturates and high-dose benzodiazepines) and sleep deprivation showed a very high diagnostic yield of 90% with a minor complications rate of only 5%, and the authors argued it was a safe protocol as long as it was performed in a highly specialized and supervised hospital setting (patient:nurse ratio 2:1, 24-hour direct supervision) and IV benzodiazepines to prevent seizure clustering was readily available.[41] Barbiturates carry a higher risk for seizure clustering and secondary generalization, and a slower taper for these agents is recommended.[39] It is also recommended that patients with prior history of status epilepticus also undergo a slower taper.[41] There should be a set protocol for administration of rescue benzodiazepines in the event of seizure clustering and generalized convulsions.

2. Sleep deprivation triggers epileptiform discharges in 30–70% of cases.[42,43] Epileptic abnormalities tend to occur during transition phases between sleep and wakefulness and it has been shown to activate epileptiform discharges even in the absence of obtaining a sleep record.[8] Some authors recommend complete sleep deprivation the night before or partial, ranging from 30–50%, decrease in duration and both techniques have been found to be efficacious without a direct comparison having been performed.[42,44]

3. Hyperventilation is a safe and effective method for seizure provocation, especially in temporal lobe epilepsy, that does not modify any of the seizure characteristics and can also be used for obtaining an ictal single-photon emission computed tomography (SPECT).[45] It is argued that during a prolonged EEG its duration may be extended to 5 minutes and can be repeated throughout the patient's stay in the EMU.[9] However, the effectiveness varies in the literature.[45,46] It can activate epileptiform discharges in both primary generalized and focal epilepsies.[47]

4. Photic stimulation may trigger photoparoxysmal responses, more commonly seen in generalized epilepsies.[48]

Number of Seizures Needed to Capture

The number of seizures needed to capture in the EMU for confirmation of diagnosis is at least one typical event.[49] More seizures are needed in the presurgical evaluation of patients in order to ensure consistency of both the semiology and EEG pattern of the seizures,[50] but the exact number varies in the literature between two and five seizures.[51,52] An analysis of the number of seizures needed to capture for 90% confidence of absence of multifocal seizures with a pretest probability of multifocal epilepsy of 20% (for example unilateral temporal IEDs and concordant hippocampal sclerosis), 50% (bilateral hippocampal changes) and 80% (multifocal interictal discharges, multifocal epileptogenic lesions) was

three seven and nine seizures respectively.[50] It is important during the hospitalization to verify with the patient and relatives that the events recorded are the habitual ones.

Duration of Stay

The mean duration of stay in the EMU reported in the literature is 5–6 days, with 2–3 days average time needed to record a first seizure/event.[39,40,49,53] The length of stay, however, may vary considerably and depends on the indication for admission, epilepsy classification, medication burden, and prior history of invasive management (vagus nerve stimulation (VNS), epilepsy surgery, or both).[54] Those admitted for presurgical evaluation, on three or more ASDs, prior history of invasive management, and with generalized symptomatic epilepsy, all potential markers of higher disease complexity, require longer EMU admissions for completion of the workup. In contrast, admissions in order to distinguish PNES from epileptic seizures usually require capturing a single typical event and the majority can be characterized within the first 2 days of admission.[55]

Safety in the EMU

Most common adverse events (AEs) during EMU admissions are falls and physical injuries, seizure clustering, status epilepticus, and postictal psychosis.[25,53,56,57] Other infrequent AEs include fractures, cardiac arrest, pneumonia, and death.[25] Predictors for the occurrence of AEs are disease duration,[56,58] temporal epilepsy,[58] and focal seizures with alteration of awareness,[58] and overall presence of more severe epilepsy as indicated by history of status epilepticus,[56,58] use of VNS,[58] intellectual disability,[58] and admission for presurgical evaluation.[58] Psychiatric comorbidities are associated with higher risk for psychiatric AEs that persist even after the discharge from the EMU.[56] ASD withdrawal is not a determining factor in the occurrence of AEs.[58] In regards to risk of death, including sudden unexpected death in epilepsy (SUDEP) patients, the MORTality in Epilepsy Monitoring Unit Study (MORTEMUS) conducted a retrospective comprehensive evaluation of cardiorespiratory arrests encountered in EMUs worldwide. Available cardiorespiratory data from 10 cases of SUDEP helped shed light on the pathophysiology of the condition, which appears to follow an early postictal, centrally mediated, severe alteration of respiratory and cardiac function induced by a GTC, either leading to immediate death or to a short period of partly restored cardiorespiratory function followed by terminal apnea and cardiac arrest. Common patient profiles and circumstances of death in these cases included young adults, GTC seizures occurring at night, prone position, suboptimal supervision, and ASD withdrawal. A potential window for life-saving intervention with cardio-pulmonary resuscitation (CPR) starting within 3 min of cardiorespiratory arrest was identified in those successfully resuscitated. In this study SUDEP incidence in EMUs was estimated at 5.1 (95% CI 2.6–9.2) per 1000 patient years, with a risk of 1.2 (0.6–2.1) per 10,000 video-EEGs.[59]

International surveys have shown wide variability in hospital EMU practices,[26,60,61] and highlighted the importance of multidisciplinary care and the need for risk-management strategies to prevent avoidable harm in the EMUs. In 2008, a workgroup of health care professionals from the American Epilepsy Society was convened to address an apparent lack of consensus regarding patient care in the EMU[25] and develop consensus-based recommendations for patient safety in the EMU.[62] The consensus recommendations are summarized in the box.

Consensus recommendations for EMU practices[62]

Patient and family assessment and education	Assess patient prior to or at the time of admission to an EMU in order to determine the plan of observation, types of provocation to be used, and identify risks for injuries, seizure emergencies, and potential comorbid conditions that could be exacerbated Patients and families should receive pre- and upon-admission education in regards to seizure and safety precautions, risk of injury and seizures, action at the start of a seizure, and the impact of provocative techniques
Orientation, training and communication	Pre-established chain of command for communication and decision-making about patient care Staff providing seizure observation should receive appropriate training recognizing changes in behavior or possible seizures An EMU facility should have the resources to manage patients' concurrent medical conditions Family members, companions, health aides, and volunteers who are performing seizure observation should be instructed in observation techniques and patient safety All staff on an EMU should undergo orientation and ongoing training within their scope of practice that includes: (1) seizure recognition/reporting, (2) clinical assessment during a seizure, (3) medication management, (4) first aid, (5) care of seizure emergencies
Seizure observation	Seizure observation should include direct observation or use of closed-circuit camera by dedicated technicians or care providers Automated seizure detection systems may be used, but should not replace direct human observation or video monitoring Cardiac monitoring with a minimum of a single-lead ECG should be used on all patients In some circumstances, family members, friends, and caregivers familiar with patient's seizures or behaviors can assist staff in observation of seizures and behavior Review description of event or video recording of captured events with patient/family/caregivers to confirm typical events recorded Continuous observation is needed for patients with invasive electrode monitoring, patients at high risk for injury, and patients undergoing ASD withdrawal
Daily assessment	Patients should be assessed daily by the patient care team for at least: • Integrity of head wrap, presence of drainage/bleeding on head wrap if implanted electrodes are used • Date and time of last seizure • Date and time of last "prn" or rescue seizure medication

	• Presence, integrity, and functioning of scalp/other electrodes • Mental status and behavior, including symptoms of postictal psychosis
Activity and environment	Heightened safety restrictions may be necessary in patients with implanted electrodes to protect patient from dislodging the electrodes Develop and communicate plans to manage patient activity and safety during EEG monitoring Tailor activity around patient status and seizure activity Use of safe exercise equipment with supervision Personnel in EMUs should assess patient room and bathroom facilities to optimize patient safety. Staff assistance to bathroom
Seizure provocation	Plans to withdraw ASDs should be individualized When tapering or stopping ASDs that affect mood, pain, or other comorbid conditions, patients should be educated about potential changes and the need for observation The use and type of seizure provocation should be considered carefully in patients with a history of seizure clusters or status epilepticus If restarting ASDs, establish therapeutic doses as quickly as possible with attention to ASD pharmacokinetics, drug interactions, side effects, and tolerance The use of ASD withdrawal or other provocation is appropriate in patients with implanted electrodes
Response to acute seizures	EMU staff must have immediate access to emergency medications, including IV preparations of ASDs for treatment of seizure emergencies and CPR Patients should have an individualized plan for managing acute seizures based on reason for admission, seizure history, risk for seizure emergencies, medication allergies, etc Physicians able to manage seizure emergencies available in-house to EMU 24 hours a day Intravenous access or alternative methods for drug administration should be established at the beginning of the monitoring period in all patients
Seizure precautions	EMU staff should implement seizure precautions as clinically indicated and provide seizure first aid for all seizure types. Strategies for seizure first aid should include: • Monitor changes in consciousness, mental status, and behaviors • Monitor vital signs during acute seizures, during and after administration of IV ASDs, and as clinically indicated

	• Turn patient on their side as soon as possible and support head to help keep open airway (for generalized seizures) • Have suction and oxygen available • Use padded side rails • Assess patient frequently after event until return to baseline • Time length of event and document observations
Discharge planning	Ensuring that patients have been seizure-free for 24 hours prior to discharge or that their seizure frequency is stable or at a baseline rate for that patient Discharge teaching should include: • When to call for emergency help • When to contact their epileptologist and/or psychiatrist for changes in seizures, behavior, or mood • ASD changes during monitoring period and medications to be taken after discharge • How to manage seizures after discharge, including use of rescue or "prn" meds for temporary treatment of seizures if clinically indicated • Timing of follow-up appointments • Safety precautions, activity limitations, when to resume normal activity • Recognition and treatment of postictal psychosis or other changes in mood or behavior that may occur after discharge

References

1. Krumholz A, Wiebe S, Gronseth G, et al. Practice parameter: evaluating an apparent unprovoked first seizure in adults (an evidence-based review). Report of the Quality Standards Subcommittee of the American Academy of Neurology and the American Epilepsy Society. *Neurology*. 2007;69(21):1996–2007.

2. Pillai J, Sperling MR. Interictal EEG and the diagnosis of epilepsy. *Epilepsia*. 2006;47 (Suppl 1):14–22.

3. Salinsky M, Kanter R, Dasheiff RM. Effectiveness of multiple EEGs in supporting the diagnosis of epilepsy: an operational curve. *Epilepsia*. 1987;28 (4):331–334.

4. Gandelman-Marton R, Theitler J. When should a sleep-deprived EEG be performed following a presumed first seizure in adults? *Acta Neurol Scand*. 2011;124 (3):202–205.

5. Sundaram M, Hogan T, Hiscock M, Pillay N. Factors affecting interictal spike discharges in adults with epilepsy. *Electroencephalogr Clin Neurophysiol*. 1990;75(4):358–360.

6. Flink R, Pedersen B, Guekht AB, et al. Guidelines for the use of EEG methodology in the diagnosis of epilepsy. International League Against Epilepsy: commission report. Commission on European Affairs: Subcommission on European Guidelines. *Acta Neurol Scand*. 2002;106(1):1–7.

7. Fountain NB, Van Ness PC, Swain-Eng R, et al. Quality improvement in neurology: AAN epilepsy quality measures. Report of the Quality Measurement and Reporting

Subcommittee of the American Academy of Neurology. *Neurology*. 2011;76 (1):94–99.

8. Fountain NB, Kim JS, Lee SI. Sleep deprivation activates epileptiform discharges independent of the activating effects of sleep. *J Clin Neurophysiol*. 1998;15 (1):69–75.

9. Michel V, Mazzola L, Lemesle M, Vercueil L. Long-term EEG in adults: sleep-deprived EEG (SDE), ambulatory EEG (Amb-EEG) and long-term video-EEG recording (LTVER). *Neurophysiol Clin*. 2015;45 (1):47–64.

10. Dash D, Hernandez-Ronquillo L, Moien-Afshari F, Tellez-Zenteno JF. Ambulatory EEG: a cost-effective alternative to inpatient video-EEG in adult patients. *Epileptic Disord*. 2012;14(3):290–297.

11. Kandler R, Ponnusamy A, Wragg C. Video ambulatory EEG: A good alternative to inpatient video telemetry? *Seizure*. 2017;47:66–70.

12. Morris GL, 3rd, Galezowska J, Leroy R, North R. The results of computer-assisted ambulatory 16-channel EEG. *Electroencephalogr Clin Neurophysiol*. 1994;91(3):229–231.

13. Drazkowski JF, Chung SS. Differential diagnosis of epilepsy. *Continuum (Minneap Minn)*. 2010;16(3 Epilepsy):36–56.

14. Hirsch LJ. Continuous EEG monitoring in the intensive care unit: an overview. *J Clin Neurophysiol*. 2004;21(5):332–340.

15. Young GB, Jordan KG, Doig GS. An assessment of nonconvulsive seizures in the intensive care unit using continuous EEG monitoring: an investigation of variables associated with mortality. *Neurology*. 1996;47(1):83–89.

16. Shafi MM, Westover MB, Cole AJ, et al. Absence of early epileptiform abnormalities predicts lack of seizures on continuous EEG. *Neurology*. 2012;79 (17):1796–1801.

17. DeLorenzo RJ, Waterhouse EJ, Towne AR, et al. Persistent nonconvulsive status epilepticus after the control of convulsive status epilepticus. *Epilepsia*. 1998;39 (8):833–840.

18. Claassen J, Jette N, Chum F, et al. Electrographic seizures and periodic discharges after intracerebral hemorrhage. *Neurology*. 2007;69(13):1356–1365.

19. Vespa PM, Nuwer MR, Nenov V, et al. Increased incidence and impact of nonconvulsive and convulsive seizures after traumatic brain injury as detected by continuous electroencephalographic monitoring. *J Neurosurg*. 1999;91 (5):750–760.

20. Krishnamurthy KB, Drislane FW. Depth of EEG suppression and outcome in barbiturate anesthetic treatment for refractory status epilepticus. *Epilepsia*. 1999;40(6):759–762.

21. Hofmeijer J, van Putten MJ. EEG in postanoxic coma: prognostic and diagnostic value. *Clin Neurophysiol*. 2016;127(4):2047–2055.

22. Claassen J, Hirsch LJ, Kreiter KT, et al. Quantitative continuous EEG for detecting delayed cerebral ischemia in patients with poor-grade subarachnoid hemorrhage. *Clin Neurophysiol*. 2004;115(12):2699–2710.

23. Labiner DM, Bagic AI, Herman ST, et al. Essential services, personnel, and facilities in specialized epilepsy centers – revised 2010 guidelines. *Epilepsia*. 2010;51 (11):2322–2333.

24. Tatum WO, 4th. Long-term EEG monitoring: a clinical approach to electrophysiology. *J Clin Neurophysiol*. 2001;18(5):442–455.

25. Shafer PO, Buelow J, Ficker DM, et al. Risk of adverse events on epilepsy monitoring units: a survey of epilepsy professionals. *Epilepsy Behav*. 2011;20(3):502–505.

26. Kobulashvili T, Hofler J, Dobesberger J, et al. Current practices in long-term video-EEG monitoring services: a survey among partners of the E-PILEPSY pilot network of reference for refractory epilepsy and epilepsy surgery. *Seizure*. 2016;38:38–45.

27. Chen DK, LaFrance WC, Jr. Diagnosis and treatment of nonepileptic seizures. *Continuum (Minneap Minn)*. 2016;22(1 Epilepsy):116–131.

28. Benbadis SR, Agrawal V, Tatum WO, 4th. How many patients with psychogenic

nonepileptic seizures also have epilepsy? *Neurology.* 2001;57(5):915–917.

29. Beniczky SA, Fogarasi A, Neufeld M, et al. Seizure semiology inferred from clinical descriptions and from video recordings. How accurate are they? *Epilepsy Behav.* 2012;24(2):213–215.

30. De Paola L, Terra VC, Silvado CE, et al. Improving first responders' psychogenic nonepileptic seizures diagnosis accuracy: development and validation of a 6-item bedside diagnostic tool. *Epilepsy Behav.* 2016;54:40–46.

31. Tufenkjian K, Luders HO. Seizure semiology: its value and limitations in localizing the epileptogenic zone. *J Clin Neurol.* 2012;8(4):243–250.

32. Beniczky S, Neufeld M, Diehl B, et al. Testing patients during seizures: a European consensus procedure developed by a joint taskforce of the ILAE - Commission on European Affairs and the European Epilepsy Monitoring Unit Association. *Epilepsia.* 2016;57 (9):1363–1368.

33. Devinsky O, Sato S, Kufta CV, et al. Electroencephalographic studies of simple partial seizures with subdural electrode recordings. *Neurology.* 1989;39(4):527–533.

34. Tatum WO, 4th, Winters L, Gieron M, et al. Outpatient seizure identification: results of 502 patients using computer-assisted ambulatory EEG. *J Clin Neurophysiol.* 2001;18(1):14–19.

35. Blume WT, Oliver LM. Noninvasive electroencephalography in supplementary sensorimotor area epilepsy. *Adv Neurol.* 1996;70:309–317.

36. Elgavish RA, Cabaniss WW. What is the diagnostic value of repeating a nondiagnostic video-EEG study? *J Clin Neurophysiol.* 2011;28(3):311–313.

37. Logar C, Walzl B, Lechner H. Role of long-term EEG monitoring in diagnosis and treatment of epilepsy. *Eur Neurol.* 1994;34 (Suppl 1):29–32.

38. Robinson AA, Pitiyanuvath N, Abou-Khalil BW, et al. Predictors of a nondiagnostic epilepsy monitoring study and yield of

repeat study. *Epilepsy Behav.* 2011;21 (1):76–79.

39. Yen DJ, Chen C, Shih YH, et al. Antiepileptic drug withdrawal in patients with temporal lobe epilepsy undergoing presurgical video-EEG monitoring. *Epilepsia.* 2001;42(2):251–255.

40. Di Gennaro G, Picardi A, Sparano A, et al. Seizure clusters and adverse events during pre-surgical video-EEG monitoring with a slow anti-epileptic drug (AED) taper. *Clin Neurophysiol.* 2012;123(3):486–488.

41. Rizvi SA, Hernandez-Ronquillo L, Wu A, Tellez Zenteno JF. Is rapid withdrawal of anti-epileptic drug therapy during video EEG monitoring safe and efficacious? *Epilepsy Res.* 2014;108(4):755–764.

42. Ellingson RJ, Wilken K, Bennett DR. Efficacy of sleep deprivation as an activation procedure in epilepsy patients. *J Clin Neurophysiol.* 1984;1(1):83–101.

43. el-Ad B, Neufeld MY, Korczyn AD. Should sleep EEG record always be performed after sleep deprivation? *Electroencephalogr Clin Neurophysiol.* 1994;90(4):313–315.

44. Kubicki S, Scheuler W, Wittenbecher H. Short-term sleep EEG recordings after partial sleep deprivation as a routine procedure in order to uncover epileptic phenomena: an evaluation of 719 EEG recordings. *Epilepsy Res Suppl.* 1991;2:217–230.

45. Guaranha MS, Garzon E, Buchpiguel CA, et al. Hyperventilation revisited: physiological effects and efficacy on focal seizure activation in the era of video-EEG monitoring. *Epilepsia.* 2005;46 (1):69–75.

46. Holmes MD, Dewaraja AS, Vanhatalo S. Does hyperventilation elicit epileptic seizures? *Epilepsia.* 2004;45(6):618–620.

47. Wirrell EC, Camfield PR, Gordon KE, et al. Will a critical level of hyperventilation-induced hypocapnia always induce an absence seizure? *Epilepsia.* 1996;37 (5):459–462.

48. Maganti RK, Rutecki P. EEG and epilepsy monitoring. *Continuum (Minneap Minn).* 2013;19(3 Epilepsy):598–622.

49. Friedman DE, Hirsch LJ. How long does it take to make an accurate diagnosis in an epilepsy monitoring unit? *J Clin Neurophysiol.* 2009;26(4):213–217.

50. Struck AF, Cole AJ, Cash SS, Westover MB. The number of seizures needed in the EMU. *Epilepsia.* 2015;56(11):1753–1759.

51. Rosenow F, Luders H. Presurgical evaluation of epilepsy. *Brain.* 2001;124(Pt 9):1683–1700.

52. Blum D. Prevalence of bilateral partial seizure foci and implications for electroencephalographic telemetry monitoring and epilepsy surgery. *Electroencephalogr Clin Neurophysiol.* 1994;91(5):329–336.

53. Noe KH, Drazkowski JF. Safety of long-term video-electroencephalographic monitoring for evaluation of epilepsy. *Mayo Clin Proc.* 2009;84(6):495–500.

54. Gazzola DM, Thawani S, Agbe-Davies O, Carlson C. Epilepsy monitoring unit length of stay. *Epilepsy Behav.* 2016;58:102–105.

55. Lobello K, Morgenlander JC, Radtke RA, Bushnell CD. Video/EEG monitoring in the evaluation of paroxysmal behavioral events: duration, effectiveness, and limitations. *Epilepsy Behav.* 2006;8 (1):261–266.

56. Dobesberger J, Walser G, Unterberger I, et al. Video-EEG monitoring: safety and adverse events in 507 consecutive patients. *Epilepsia.* 2011;52(3):443–452.

57. Rose AB, McCabe PH, Gilliam FG, et al. Occurrence of seizure clusters and status epilepticus during inpatient video-EEG monitoring. *Neurology.* 2003;60 (6):975–978.

58. Fahoum F, Omer N, Kipervasser S, Bar-Adon T, Neufeld M. Safety in the epilepsy monitoring unit: a retrospective study of 524 consecutive admissions. *Epilepsy Behav.* 2016;61:162–167.

59. Ryvlin P, Nashef L, Lhatoo SD, et al. Incidence and mechanisms of cardiorespiratory arrests in epilepsy monitoring units (MORTEMUS): a retrospective study. *Lancet Neurol.* 2013;12 (10):966–977.

60. Fitzsimons M, Browne G, Kirker J, Staunton H. An international survey of long-term video/EEG services. *J Clin Neurophysiol.* 2000;17(1):59–67.

61. Buelow JM, Privitera M, Levisohn P, Barkley GL. A description of current practice in epilepsy monitoring units. *Epilepsy Behav.* 2009;15(3):308–313.

62. Shafer PO, Buelow JM, Noe K, et al. A consensus-based approach to patient safety in epilepsy monitoring units: recommendations for preferred practices. *Epilepsy Behav.* 2012;25(3):449–456.

Intracranial EEG Monitoring

Marc R. Nuwer, Dawn Eliashiv, and John Stern

16.1 Introduction

More than 3 million individuals in the United States have epilepsy, and over 50 million worldwide. One million in the United States continue to suffer from seizures, despite medication. Their mortality is twice that of the general population, i.e., about 2% mortality per year.[1,2] Surgery for epilepsy has a favorable outcome. Among well-selected patients, 70% are seizure-free after surgery. Many of the remaining patients have seizure frequency greatly reduced, e.g., from twice weekly to twice yearly. Surgical outcome avoids mortality risk, morbidity, and costs of medically refractory seizures, and greatly enhances the patient's quality of life. Yet only 2000 patients per year undergo resective surgery. Surgery for epilepsy is very underutilized.[3]

To qualify for surgery, a patient undergoes an evaluation with electroencephalography (EEG) monitoring and ancillary testing. In the initial testing phase, several-day-long video-EEG recording from the scalp captures a sample of typical seizures. Medications are tapered to increase the yield of seizures, which requires hospitalization for safety. Hospitalization also presents the opportunity for unit nurses to conduct examinations during seizures and auras, enhancing the detailed understanding of the seizure and its behavioral manifestations. Other ancillary tests conducted are brain magnetic resonance imaging (MRI) with thin coronal cuts, positron emission tomography (PET), and neuropsychometric testing to localize the patient's epileptogenic focus, which focus may be associated with mesial temporal sclerosis, cortical dysplasia, or other developmental anomalies. Sometimes specific disorders are present in an MRI, and the region of the seizure onset needs to be determined in comparison to the lesion, e.g., in tuberous sclerosis or with multiple cavernous angiomas.

Concepts used define several zones relevant for invasive epilepsy recordings and surgical planning.[4] The goal of depth and subdural electrode recordings, electrocorticography (ECoG), and functional mapping are to define the *epileptogenic* zone, which is the area necessary and sufficient for resection to stop seizures. This zone should not be confused with other defined zones:

- *Epileptogenic* zone: the area whose resection is necessary and sufficient to abolish further seizures and separate from nearby necessary cortical regions that are not epileptogenic
- *Lesional* zone: the area on imaging or visually that is morphologically altered; the lesional zone may be smaller than or distant from the epileptogenic zone
- *Irritative* zone: the area of interictal spikes, that can appear more widely compared to the epileptogenic zone, even including contralateral regions

- *Symptomatic zone:* an area where activation brings on the presence of symptoms, such as an aura, movement, or sensations
- *Functional deficit* zone: an area whose dysfunction brings on an absence of abilities, such as amnesia or paresis.

Scalp EEG monitoring and ancillary tests sometimes sufficiently define the epileptogenic zone for surgical resection decisions. Surgery is recommended when a concordance of localization is found among localized or lateralized temporal PET hypometabolism, MRI demonstration of hippocampal sclerosis, a series of seizures consistent with mesial temporal onset, and neuropsychological findings suggesting lateralized or localized cognitive deficits. Both MRI lesional and nonlesional temporal lobe onset have the same postoperative prognosis, that is, 70–80% seizure control when PET temporal hypometabolism is clear and unilateral.[5]

When a concordance is lacking or indeterminate among the scalp seizures, imaging and neuropsychometric findings, other ancillary testing may help clarify the localization sufficiently to allow a recommendation for resective surgery. The additional ancillary tests include ictal single-photon emission computed tomography (SPECT), intracarotid amytal testing, spike dipole source localization, or magnetoencephalography, which help when initial testing is indeterminate. Scalp EEG monitoring results with ancillary testing is referred to as *phase 1* evaluation.

When the phase 1 evaluation does not localize the epileptogenic zone sufficiently to recommend respective surgery, a *phase 2* intracranial recording is the usual next option available. The intracranial techniques are available when needed as a more definitive method to define the epileptogenic zone. The phase 2 intracranial methods include the following:

- *Depth electrode* recording using electrodes implanted into deep structures, e.g., mesial temporal
- *Subdural electrode* grid and strip recording using electrodes placed in the subdural space over the cortical surface
- *ECoG*, which records during surgery typically from the cortical surface to refine the limits of resection
- *Functional cortical mapping* using electrical stimulation to define cortical regions involved in language, movement, sensation, or other eloquent functions.

Once a surgical resection is underway, *intraoperative monitoring* helps to assure patient safety. Monitoring watches EEG for seizures or other untoward changes, and evoked potentials can monitor the intact functional status of motor and sensory hemispheric pathways during the resection.

Overall, modern generation clinical neurophysiology brings to bear techniques and options to identify the epileptic focus, refine its margins, reduce risks of resection, and improve patient outcomes. The neurology community still greatly underutilizes this resource for epilepsy surgery.

16.2 Depth Electrodes

16.2.1 Techniques

Depth electrodes are usually thin flexible tubes with multiple electrical contacts near the end. When they are placed, a temporary stiff stilette is inserted to help implant it under

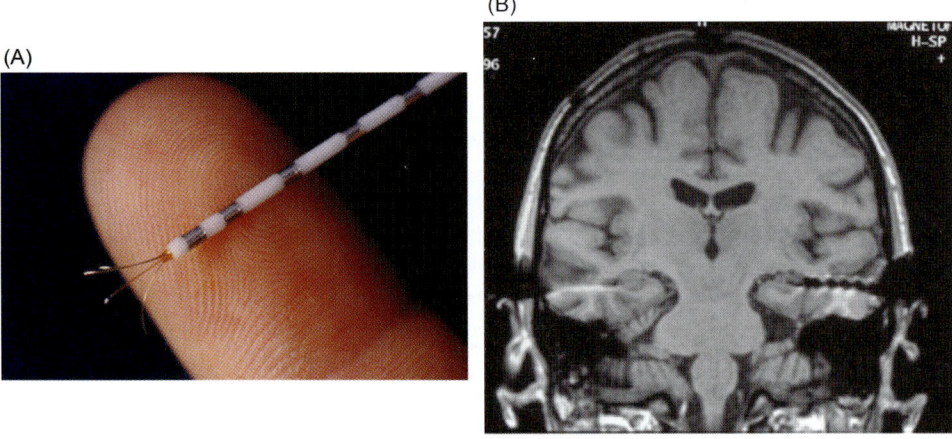

Figure 16.1 (A) Depth electrode showing several recording contacts along the shaft. Also shown are four microwires inserted through its hollow center. (B) Magnetic resonance image demonstrating placement into the hippocampus. The magnetic susceptibility artifact appears much larger than the electrode actually is.

stereotactic guidance. Presurgical targeting aims to place the tips of a dozen such electrodes at specific structures, typically mesial temporal hippocampal region structures. The several electrical contacts spaced 5–10 mm along the electrode shaft are platinum–iridium or nickel–chrome alloys, allowing for MRI if they are made of platinum. Once they are secured to the skull, depth electrodes may be left in place for weeks for chronic seizure recordings on the epilepsy monitoring unit (EMU). Often 120 to 160 channels are recorded in these patients that includes full scalp and many channels of depth recordings.

When scalp recordings and ancillary testing are insufficient to proceed directly to surgery, they may still allow formulation of hypotheses about where seizures may arise. Depth electrodes are placed based on testing these hypotheses.

Depth electrodes (Figure 16.1A) are placed using stereotactic targeting after a three-dimensional reconstruction of MRI and computed tomography angiography with coregistration before and after electrode placement. Electrodes are placed within about 2 mm of the desired target locations. Adding more external fiducial markers improves precision. Electrode artifacts are used to identify their exact localization on imaging (Figure 16.1B).

Intracranial electrodes record from the immediately adjacent tissue but not from tissue a few centimeters away. In this way they differ from scalp recordings that can pick up from a greater distance. Ictal onsets outside a depth electrode's immediate zone appear in that electrode's recording only when the epileptic rhythm propagates to tissue adjacent to the electrode. Since the ictal onsets found with depth recordings are very sensitive to the location of the electrodes, it is critical that depth electrodes are used only when the preimplant localization hypothesis is sufficiently specific.

Depth electrodes lack the muscle artifacts commonly encountered at the scalp.[6] This allows depth recordings to be easier to interpret. Sometimes large head movements affect the external leads causing low-frequency sway in the recordings. Occasional 20- to 40-Hz respiration-linked vibration artifacts from snoring affect limbic depth electrodes.[7]

After the depth electrodes are placed, the stiff stillette is removed, allowing the electrode to move slightly as the brain shifts with edema or cardiac pulses. This flexibility also provides safety in case the electrodes are jarred during seizures. The remaining hollow core presents an opportunity for introduction of microelectrodes or dialysis catheters for research studies.

16.2.2 Risks

Depth electrode implantation runs the risk of intracerebral hemorrhage and infection. Bleeding occurs in 1–4% of implants.[8–10] Improvements in stereotactic targeting and electrode construction keep the rate of life-threatening hemorrhages low. Postoperative imaging identifies bleeds for monitoring and treatment. Reported mortality from implantation has been below 0.1% since 1990.

Antiplatelet drugs are not used during the preoperative period to avoid bleeding risk, which includes avoiding valproic acid, a seizure medication with an antiplatelet effect.

The area around the electrode insertion through the scalp is treated as a sterile region during the monitoring period. This includes keeping the patient from scratching the scalp nearby when the scalp itches under the bandages. Some centers add prophylactic antibiotics. The risk of infection is less than 0.5%. The infection risk is greater when a cerebrospinal fluid leak is detected alongside an electrode implantation site.

The electrodes leave chronic gliotic changes along their insertion channels. These are sufficiently distinct as to be seen in some modern MRI images. The gliosis is considered benign and incidental.

There is a danger of tissue damage when a technologist conducts impedance checks. Electrode contacts have a small surface area touching tissue compared to routine scalp electrodes. The usual amount of impedance test current would exceed safety limits for such a small surface contact area. Too much current through too small a contact area causes local tissue damage. To avoid this risk, a special impedance meter is used to test depth electrode electrical integrity, a meter that uses a safe, greatly reduced test current.

16.2.3 Depth Interpretations

Depth interictal background activity is somewhat similar in content to scalp EEG.[6,11] It is notable that epileptiform spikes seen prominently in depth electrodes may be entirely absent on the scalp channels. These transients may appear sharper and more abundant in depth recordings. Depth channels also can demonstrate very high-frequency oscillations not recordable from the scalp.

Interictal depth epileptiform abnormalities are not uniformly reliable for defining the extent of the epileptogenic region.[6,12] The most frequent, persistent, steady interictal epileptiform activity tends to be within the ictal onset zone. Routine interictal epileptiform activity can lead to incorrect localization.

16.2.3.1 Mesial Temporal Depth Recording

Two types of ictal onset activity occur for mesial temporal lobe seizures associated with hippocampal sclerosis.[13] The low-voltage 10–16 Hz fast pattern increases in amplitude as the seizure progresses. The synchronous 1–3 per second periodic spike or spike and slow-wave pattern persists for 5 s to 2 min before evolving into a low-voltage fast pattern. The periodic spiking pattern is more likely associated with focal rather than regional onsets, seizures that spread contralaterally more slowly, more hippocampus neuronal loss, and better operative outcomes.[14–17] Depth-recorded mesial temporal onsets due to hippocampal sclerosis may vary in onset origin in an individual patient within one temporal lobe,

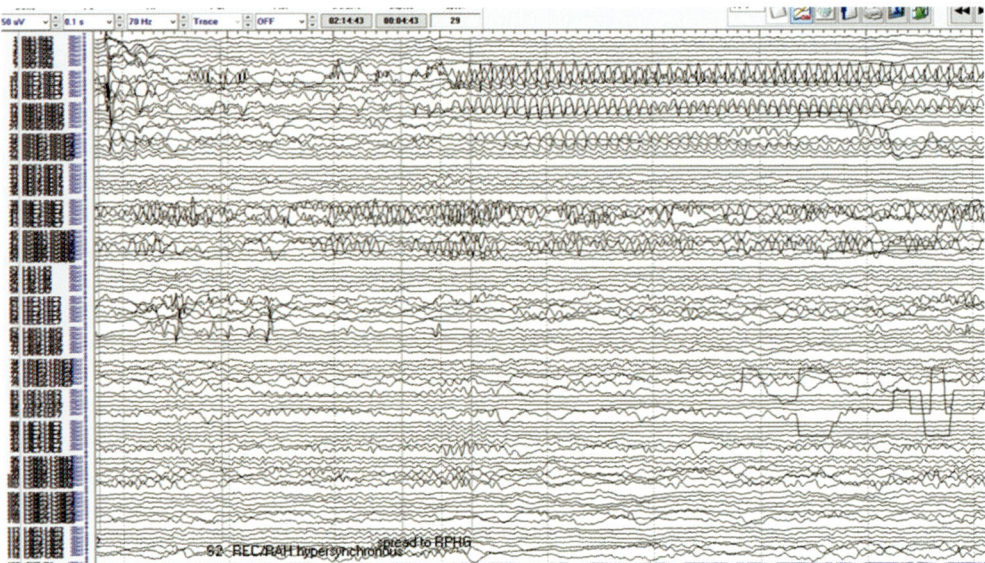

Figure 16.2 Depth-recording of ictal onset with a hypersynchronous onset pattern at the mesial right entorhinal cortex with spread to the right parahippocampal gyrus. Note that the recording contains many channels. Over 160 channels are common in depth-electrode recordings.

spreading within the lobe as the seizure evolves. Figure 16.2 demonstrates two different patterns, one low-amplitude fast and one hypersynchronous. It also emphasizes the complexity of interpreting so many channels of data, which can often exceed 100 simultaneously recorded data channels. Reviewing and comparing all this data takes time, patience, and experience, especially when the overall recording is several weeks long.

Seizures spread outside the originating temporal lobe, whereas auras remain confined to one hippocampus. Auras may remain for as long as 60 s as ictal discharges recorded by electrodes at one temporal depth, and reported behaviorally by the patient, but not seen by scalp electrodes. Typical spread is initially to the ipsilateral neocortex followed by subsequent spread to the contralateral neocortex. Occasionally, initial spread is to the contralateral hippocampus before the ipsilateral neocortex. Long interhippocampal propagation times (i.e., more than 50 s) are associated with good surgical outcome, whereas a short propagation time (i.e., less than 5 s) carries a higher risk of continuing seizures after surgery.[18] Patients with pre-existing ipsilateral neocortical damage may show spread through the contralateral hippocampus to the contralateral neocortex prior to a clear involvement of the ipsilateral neocortex. These patients have false scalp-recorded lateralization of ictal onset, based on this apparent contralateral scalp onset. Depth electrodes reveal the true underlying ictal onset propagation pattern.

16.2.3.2 Frontal Depth Recording

Depth electrodes are sometimes placed in medial and the orbitofrontal cortex and anterior cingulate gyrus to localize extratemporal ictal onsets. Medial or orbital frontal lobe localization-related seizures are often brief (15–60 s) with little postictal confusion, partial responsiveness, or rapid return to contact. With secondary spread to the mesial temporal region, these seizures may last several minutes. Medial and orbitofrontal seizures often are frequent, e.g., 10 per day, and sometimes in clusters with seizure-free periods of days to weeks. Complex motor automatisms may include bilateral coordinated leg movements. Frontal spread patterns vary widely among patients.

Frontal seizure discharges tend to spread quickly and spread through the medial frontal region to the contralateral frontal lobe. The ictal EEG consists of high-frequency activity that may be preceded by a period of initial suppression. These ictal suppressions may contain very high-frequency activity, e.g., 60–100 Hz discharges, too high in frequency to be detected by some standard recording methods. Brief ictal discharges tend to remain within the frontal lobes after such a rapid bilateral spread, which can obscure lateralization. More prolonged seizures are more likely to spread to medial temporal regions.

16.2.3.3 Insular Depth Recording

Seizures arising from the insula can have an aura of a sensation of laryngeal constriction and dysesthesias over large regions, sometimes accompanied by perioral and abdominal sensations. Symptoms may progress to dysarthria or brief mutism. Seizures spreading to the insula may have these symptoms late in the evolution of the seizure. Seizures spreading out of the insula have motor and sensory symptoms of the frontal, parietal, and temporal regions to which they spread.

Insular depth electrode recordings show ictal onsets with a low-voltage fast pattern, or rhythmic spikes or recruiting activity.[19] These are typical of a neocortical type of seizure-onset pattern. Initial insula activity most likely spreads initially to the mesial temporal region, the frontal or temporal operculum, or the superior temporal gyrus.[19]

16.2.3.4 Heterotopia Depth Studies

Heterotopias can give rise to seizures, although many do not do so directly. Many are a sign of cortical dysgenesis, and suggest the presence of further, possibly more subtle, developmental epileptogenic regions nearby. Identifying the epileptogenic region is key, since surgery for a nonepileptogenic heterotopia is futile for control of seizures. Heterotopias often are either subependymal or subcortical regions and may be multiple or bilateral.

Depth electrodes in heterotopic nodules show low-voltage, low-frequency activity with frequent high-amplitude epileptiform spike–wave discharges. This epileptiform activity has been seen as synchronous with epileptiform activity in the overlying neocortex, but independent in different nodules.[20] Ictal onsets involve either the hippocampus or overlying cortex. The depth-recorded ictal onsets may involve nodular heterotopias too. Ictal onset discharges consist of low-voltage 30–35 Hz activity that evolves within several seconds to 5–10 Hz. Surgery to remove the epileptogenic zone has sometimes included part of a nodular heterotopia, but has always included the defined neocortex or hippocampus involved in the epileptogenic zone. Surgical outcomes have been favorable for unilateral nodular heterotopias defined in this way. [20–23]

16.3 Subdural Electrodes

16.3.1 Techniques

Subdural electrodes (Figure 16.3) are strips or arrays of disk electrodes embedded in silastic material. The discs are platinum–iridium, nickel–chrome, or stainless steel alloys, allowing for MRI if they are platinum. These 3 mm discs often are 1 cm apart center-to-center.

(A)

(B)

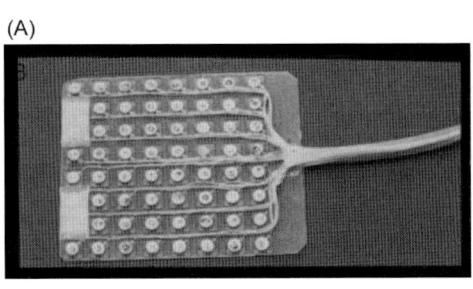
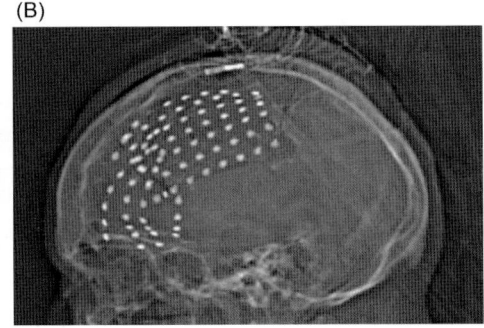

Figure 16.3 (A) A subdural 8 × 8 grid. Individual discs are 10 mm from each other center-to-center. (B) Subdural grid and strips in place imaged on X-ray. These images help document locations. Note a larger 8 × 8 frontal grid plus several smaller 1 × 8 strips.

For a strip electrode the discs are arranged in a line. For a grid electrode, the discs are arranged in a square or rectangle, e.g., 4 × 5 (20 electrodes) or 8 × 8 (64 electrodes). Strip electrodes can be inserted through burr holes. Grids are placed through a craniotomy. Both are placed subdurally on the pia mater. Review of positions by MRI or computed tomography imaging is common to account for shifts after implantation. Figure 16.3B is an example of a subdural grid imaged after implantation. A cable running from one edge of the strip or grid contains wires from each contact. These are plugged into an EEG jackbox for recording.

16.3.2 Indications and Placement

Subdural electrodes precisely locate seizure onset when it occurs within the covered region. Large grid arrays can cover parts of two to three lobes, e.g., posterior frontal, temporal, and parietal. Placement of grids and strips requires a hypothesis of the epileptic focus site. This hypothesis is developed from prior scalp EEG and ancillary test evaluations. When the hypothesis indicates a likely focus over the lateral convexity neocortex, subdural grids and strips are the typical invasive technique for recording seizures. In contrast, when the hypothesis indicates a likely focus in the mesial temporal, anterior cingulate, or mesial or orbital frontal cortex, then depth electrodes are often chosen to record from deep structures. Some epilepsy centers slip strip electrodes into deep locations to survey some deep structures in lieu of depth electrodes. Strips, when used in this way, most commonly are placed under the orbitofrontal cortex or inferior temporal lobe with its furthest contact around the hippocampal gyrus.

16.3.3 Risks

Problems include bleeding, edema, infection, and cerebrospinal fluid leakage. Smaller strips have less risk than larger grids, and combined depth electrodes with a larger number of strips and grids carries the highest morbidity rate. Strip electrodes have a complication rate around 1% that includes infections and bleeding when bridge veins are damaged.[24] For larger grid arrays the significant complication rate is reported to be around 10–20%. Complications are fewer in centers with greater experience. Morbidity is less with close monitoring by specialized personnel in a center with ready access to a scanner and an intensive care unit.

The infection risk is less when the cables exit through a tunnel and a second incision a short distance away from the burr hole or craniotomy. Prophylactic antibiotics lower the incidence of infections in patients with large subdural arrays. Daily monitoring for infections is needed.

Subdural hematoma occurs in about 8% of patients with larger grids[25] up to 5 days after implantation. The risk is higher among patients who have had a prior resection.[26] It is safer to remove the electrodes when significant bleeding occurs.

Larger grid arrays are associated with underlying cortical edema. Patients complain of headache. Proactive pain medication treatment and elevating the head of the bed head are helpful. Severe or fatal raised intracranial pressure is extremely rare, but should be kept in mind. Computed tomography can follow the degree of midline shift and decreased ventricular size. Patients with very narrow lateral ventricles have little room to compensate for edema, placing them at greater risk for more severe consequences of edema. Dexamethasone reduces edema, although it may slightly prolong the time needed to capture sufficient seizures.[27,28] Less pain and nausea also is seen with steroids.

16.3.4 Recording Seizures

Grid and strip ictal EEG patterns from neocortical locations tend to begin with low-amplitude fast beta or gamma activity.[29-33] Figure 16.4 shows an example of a subdural grid ictal onset. Subdural electrodes define these much better than scalp EEG. Well-localized, very fast activity at ictal onset is associated with good postresection outcomes. The frequencies seen in these neocortical ictal onsets are faster than the ictal onsets seen in mesial temporal seizures. Rhythmic alpha–theta spike–wave seizure-onset patterns are associated with developmental anomalies, e.g., cortical dysplasias, at a repetition rate slower than typical very fast neocortical ictal onsets. The seizure onsets associated with dysplasia may arise from only one corner of the anomaly, helping to localize the epileptogenic zone from the rest of the dysplasia. Slower frequencies (e.g., theta) seen at neocortical EEG ictal onset suggests propagation from a focus elsewhere.[34,35] The EEG ictal pattern may spread within seconds to other locations, much faster spread than for mesial temporal seizures. The patient may show behavioral changes promptly upon neocortical ictal onset with automatisms and other behavioral signs of seizure activity.

16.3.5 Neocortical Subdural Recordings and Interpretations

Behavioral manifestations of neocortical seizures vary according to the cortical region involved in the seizure onset. Enumeration of the different behavioral presentations is beyond the scope of this chapter. Electrically, regions of neocortical seizure onset may show in cortical subdural electrodes as an increase in interictal epileptiform spike discharges leading up to a seizure. Neocortical seizure onsets often start with attenuation followed by fast activity greater than 20 Hz. The attenuation may contain much faster activity that is beyond the recording ability of many recording systems, e.g., low amplitude 60–120 Hz activity within the epileptogenic zone.[32,36,37] This is followed quickly by a broad, rapid propagation to other neocortical areas. Behavioral manifestations generally follow the same pattern of propagation as seen in the neocortical subdural electrical recordings, possibly delayed by a few seconds in manifestation. Some of the functional deficit zone may be subtle, since lack of abilities is not always tested unless nurses or others take their time to test for specific abilities or signs during seizures.

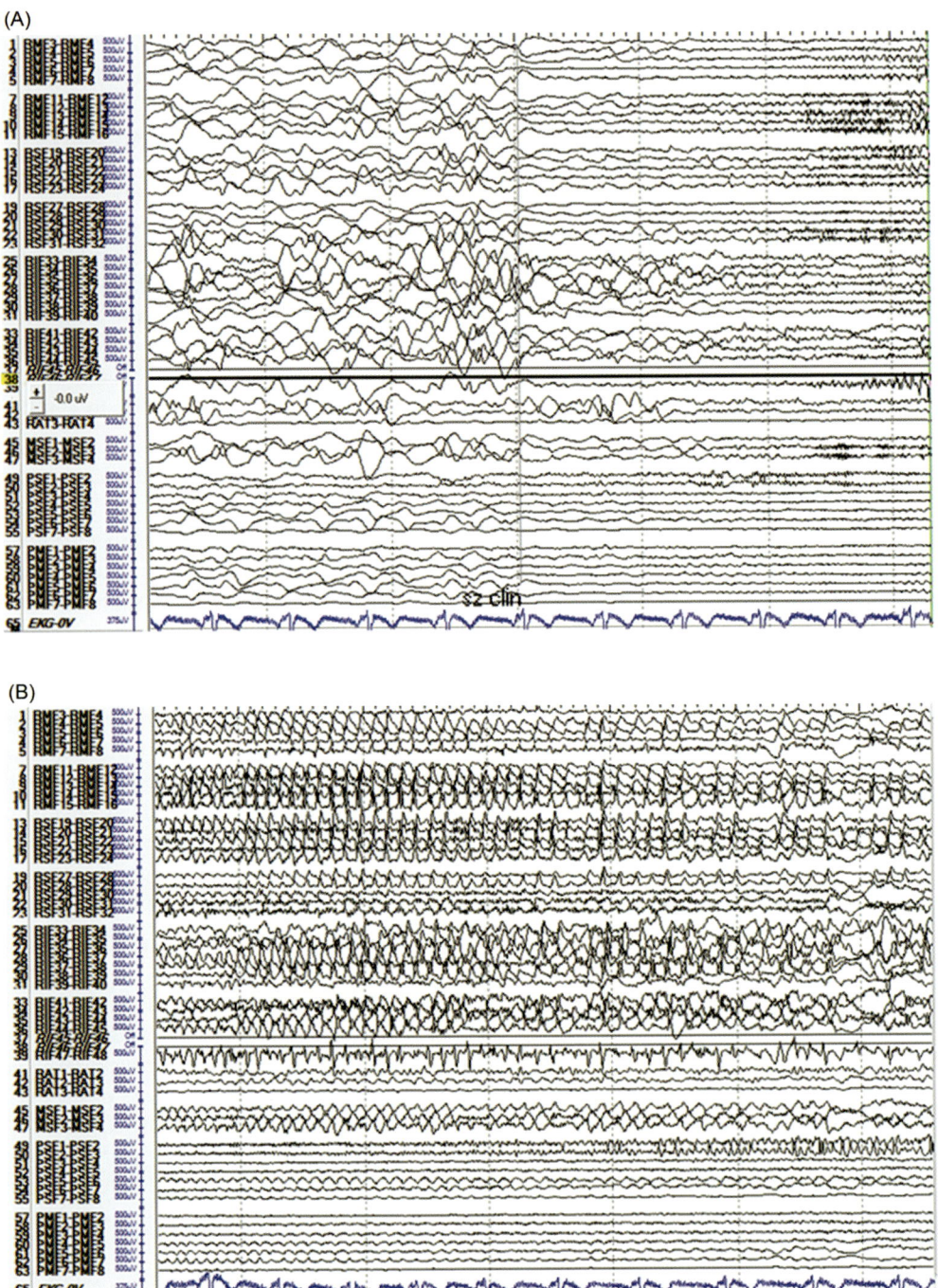

Figure 16.4 Subdural grid ictal onset. (A) Fast activity onset about 1–2 s with the earliest at the superior frontal sites, and with rapid spread to mid-frontal. (B) Ictal pattern evolves broadly across the superior, mid-, and inferior frontal regions. (C) Seizure activity ends followed by a postictal suppression.

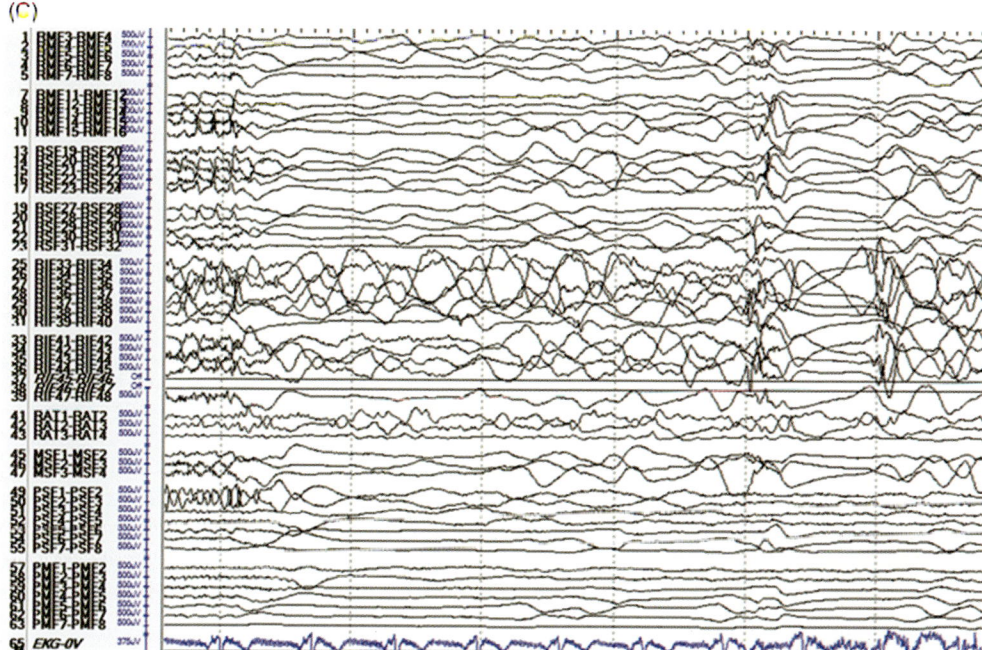

Figure 16.4 (*cont.*)

Seizures associated with structural lesions, e.g., a neoplasm or hamartoma, differ in their subdural manifestation from nonlesional neocortical ictal onsets. More often the lesion-associated subdural grid and strip recordings show an onset with lower-frequency 6-12 Hz activity without a preceding increase in interictal epileptiform spikes.

16.4 Responsive Neurostimulation

The responsive neurostimulation (RNS; NeuroPace, Inc, Mountain View, CA) method involves implanting chronic subdural electrodes that are kept in place for years. A separately implanted programmable battery pack, resembling a pacemaker, powers the device. Signals are recorded, analyzed, and from time to time the device delivers a brief electrical pulse train through the subdural electrodes. The goal is to disrupt incipient seizures before they can spread out of the epileptogenic zone.

Long-term use of RNS is considered for patients for whom resective surgery is not a reasonable option. Resection may be ruled out for a variety of reasons, for example when the epileptogenic zone overlaps with eloquent cortex, e.g., language cortex, or when multiple epileptogenic regions are found. Long-term RNS offers a hope of 50–75% seizure reduction without resection, which is achieved in the majority of patients.

One or two depth or subdural cortical strip leads are surgically placed in the brain at a previously located epileptogenic focus. Each of the four electrodes in a lead can both sense and stimulate, for a total of eight sensing and stimulating electrodes. The device continually records the EEG activity. Because the EEG is recorded directly from the brain surface, it is considered ECoG activity.

The treating physician programs the device to detect specific abnormalities on the ECoG and programs guidance to trigger the stimulation pulses in response to seizure detection. The programming is similar to that of a vagus nerve stimulator or a deep brain stimulator used for Parkinsons. A handheld wand communicates with the battery pack. The physician adjusts each patient's detection and stimulation parameters in order to optimize seizure control. These parameters include stimulus frequency, pulse width, burst duration, current intensity, and which leads were used for detection and stimulation.

Risks of RNS include intracranial bleeding around the time of implant (2%), infection typically soon after implantation (2%), or damage to the electrode leads where they are secured at the burr hole (3%).

16.5 Comparing Depth and Subdural Techniques

Depth electrodes yield better recordings from deep temporal structures rather than using strip electrodes slipped beneath the temporal lobe. Subdural electrodes can identify a mesial temporal focus, but may be too lateral. Subdural contacts lateral to the collateral sulcus may result in a false localization and lateralization due to propagation to orbitofrontal or contralateral temporal cortex before recruitment of the affected mesial temporal structure becomes visible on the subdural electrode.[38]

Depth electrodes are placed bilaterally. They are an elegant method for addressing a hypothesis in which a question remains about which temporal depth generates the seizures. Subdural grids and strips often are placed unilaterally, especially for the larger grid placements. Subdurals are more tuned to answer hypotheses about where seizures arise within a hemisphere. They are a sophisticated method for addressing a hypothesis about a neocortical epileptogenic zone, especially one likely located on the lateral neocortex. In extratemporal lobe epilepsy, subdural electrodes may be preferred over depth electrodes, especially if lateral convexity structures need to be recorded. Subdural grids and strips allow for functional cortical mapping, which can help separately define nearby epileptogenic and eloquent cortex.

Since the actual site of seizure onset is unknown before surgery, sometimes a mixture of techniques is undertaken with some depth electrodes and some strips. Placing both depth electrodes and larger grids is impractical because the craniotomy bone flap can get in the way of the location needed to secure the depth electrode to the bone. The development of edema and movement of the brain after placement of a grid can increase the risks associated with depth electrodes.

High-frequency oscillations (HFOs) of 100–200 Hz, i.e., *ripples*, are seen in depth recording from human hippocampus and entorhinal cortex.[39] Ripples do not clearly localize to seizure onset zones.[40] Higher-frequency oscillations of 250–500 Hz, i.e., *fast ripples*, are associated with the epileptogenic zone in the hippocampal, entorhinal, and neocortical regions.[41,42] This is an area of active research. Figure 16.5 shows an illustration of HFOs.[43]

High-frequency oscillations are recorded in both depth and subdural methods. Recording systems with high EEG sampling rates can capture accurately very fast rhythms in the 30–500 Hz range and above. High-frequency oscillations are seen in the epileptogenic

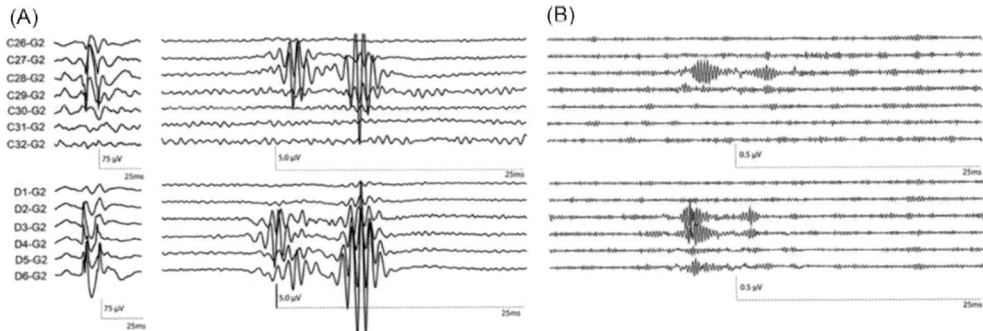

Figure 16.5 Example of high-frequency oscillations taken from an electrocorticography recording. (A) A pair of epileptiform spikes appears as usual with the high filter set to 70 Hz. (B) A pair of ripples is seen with fast sampling and filters set much higher. Time scale is 25 ms in each case (from Zijlmans et al., with permission.[43])

zone. Their physiology and meaning are a matter of current investigation. These are difficult to observe from the scalp. They are seen clearly in depth and subdural recordings when using a high sampling rate, i.e., 2000–5000 samples per second, with a high filter set at 1000 Hz or higher.

High-frequency oscillations are short bursts of high-frequency activity. They usually are divided into *ripples* (60–160 Hz) and *fast ripples* (250–500 Hz).[44] Ripples are found in nonepileptogenic regions. Fast ripples occur predominantly in the epileptogenic zone, either isolated or superposed on an epileptic spike.[45] Fast ripples are more localized and may occur for seconds to minutes preceding ictal onset.[46,47] Ripples and fast ripples are best studied in the temporal lobes, but also appear to occur in extratemporal locations.

16.6 Functional Cortical Mapping

Subdural electrodes allow for electrical stimulation through the electrodes in addition to recording. The aim is to use both techniques to identify the epileptogenic zone, as well as regions of eloquent cortex. The cortical areas associated with language, movement, and sensation, once identified, can be spared from the resection zone if possible. The cortex involved with eloquent functions is identified through functional cortical mapping.

Short 2–5 s intermittent electrical currents are delivered through subdural electrodes. Sensations or involuntary movements may be produced, depending upon the function of the underlying cortex. The primary cortex is easily identified. Other cortical functions, such as language, require greater effort to map.

For many functions, a paradigm to test disruption of function is needed. For language, this tests disruption in one or another language ability. Individual subdural electrode discs are chosen for testing one at a time. Brief 2–5 s stimulus 50 Hz trains are delivered at gradually increasing current intensities until a language task disruption is encountered or not. For safety the stimulation is biphasic, meaning half the time the current flows in one direction and the other half of time it flows in the opposite direction. When finished with functional testing of that task at that site, testing moves on to a different subdural electrode or to testing a different task.

Tasks are presented together with nonstimulation control trials. For example, a task may be presented four times and only the third trial uses electrical cortical stimulation. In that way the tester can assess if the stimulation caused any change from baseline ability. A task is repeated like this several times after achieving high stimulus intensities and finding no disruptions. If a disruption of language or the presence of a movement, sensation, or aura is encountered, a note is made of that finding at that intensity at that site. Then the process moves on to another site, or to another task, and repeats.

Tasks include a variety of language abilities. The patient looks at flash cards for object naming. The patient listens to clues for auditory naming, e.g., "What is the color of grass?" The patient reads clues from a flash card for reading naming, e.g., a printed card: "tall pink bird." Sentence judgment asks about the meaning of similar or passive tense sentences. Overall, these several tasks cover comprehension, expression, and naming in several ways. Conjunction analysis is the assessment of these abilities, and where multiple tasks demonstrate a concurrence of similar findings at the same sites. In this way, a map is drawn of the sites where language abilities lie, which can be compared to the map of the epileptogenic zone. Figure 16.6 shows a map of functional areas defined from cortical mapping with stimulation studies.

Functional cortical mapping can be carried out on the epilepsy monitoring unit. It also can be carried out in the operating room during a craniotomy. When carried out during surgery, the technique is performed with the patient awake to test language abilities. This requires a co-operative patient. The patient's head is stabilized and pinned with a Mayfield device. Neuromuscular blockade is avoided. Local anesthesia is used around the craniotomy incision. The patient is initially anesthetized without intubation during opening of the craniotomy, awakened for the functional cortical mapping, then returned to deeper anesthesia during closing. The surgeon holds a bipolar wand touching various cortical sites instead of using the grip or strip contacts when testing in the operating room. The typical stimulating wand is 30 cm long, with two round metal ball tips separated by a few

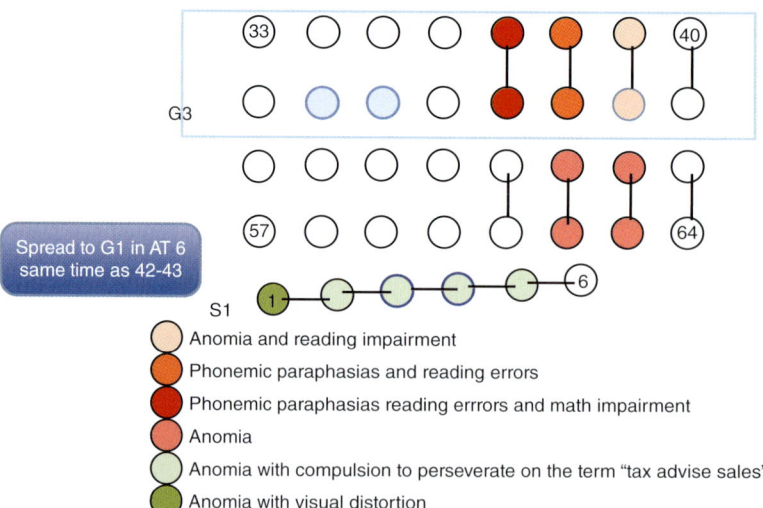

Figure 16.6 Functional cortical localization. Language abilities were disrupted with stimulation of the more anterior contacts, to the reader's right, color-coded in reds and greens. Seizure onset was localized 2–4 cm more posteriorly, color coded light blue.

millimeters. Sometimes the patient is kept awake during resection to continue testing abilities during the resection.

While stimulations are delivered, EEG is observed for epileptiform discharges known as *afterdischarges*. Afterdischarges appear as rhythmic, repetitive high-voltage spikes or polyspike–wave complexes lasting seconds or occasionally minutes. These are provoked by the stimulation and occur especially in the region stimulated. They can spread outside the stimulated region, affecting other nearby or distant sites. They may evolve into seizures, although most are self-limited to 5-20 s of repetitive discharges. Afterdischarges disallow consideration of that stimulation trial, because one cannot be sure how far the disruption event spread, and therefore, any functional disruption found in that trial may have been from the effect of the spread at another site. Afterdischarges also warn that higher-intensity stimulations may be unwise at or near that site, for fear of provoking seizures. Once seizures occur, further functional cortical localization is usually discontinued, because the whole region will be postictal for a while.

Simple *direct cortical stimulation* of the motor cortex may be carried out with the patient still under anesthesia. This uses a technique similar to the language method. For motor testing, muscles are monitored with surface or needle electromyography leads over the face and limbs. Sometimes simple observation is used to watch for movement. Stimulation is delivered to presumed motor cortex, either at 50 Hz or 5 Hz in brief 5-s trains. In the motor cortex, muscle responses are elicited at corresponding peripheral sites.

16.7 Electrocorticography (ECoG)

ECoG is operating room EEG recorded directly from the cerebral cortex (Figure 16.7). It is used to locate epileptic regions prior to resection. The goal is to find regions suitable for surgical resection.[48]

16.7.1 Techniques

ECoG often uses strips and grids with a total of 20 to 40 cortical disc electrodes. Edges are weighted down with saline wetted surgical cottonoid to make good electrical contact with the cortex. The strips and grids are moved about to various cortical regions as needed. ECoG amplitude is several times higher than scalp EEG.

16.7.2 Interpretation

ECoG seeks epileptogenic cortex. Many features seen are similar to scalp EEG. Fronto-central fast activity, low-amplitude generalized slowing and fronto-polar triangular slow waves are common under anesthesia. More fast activity is seen above the Sylvian fissure than below. Impaired cortex may have decreased fast and increased slow activity.

ECoG helps refine resection limits in those patients where limits were uncertain by preoperative methods. Interictal spike discharges may also extend to the cortex beyond the epileptogenic zone, so not all areas of spikes are resected. More severe, persistent spiking is more suggestive of an epileptogenic zone.

After resection, follow-up ECoG may show epileptiform discharges at the resection margins. These may be "injury potentials," not the location of actual epileptic tissue. More concerning would be epileptic spikes distant from the resection margin since the more spikes at a greater distance from the resection, the greater the risk of seizure recurrence.

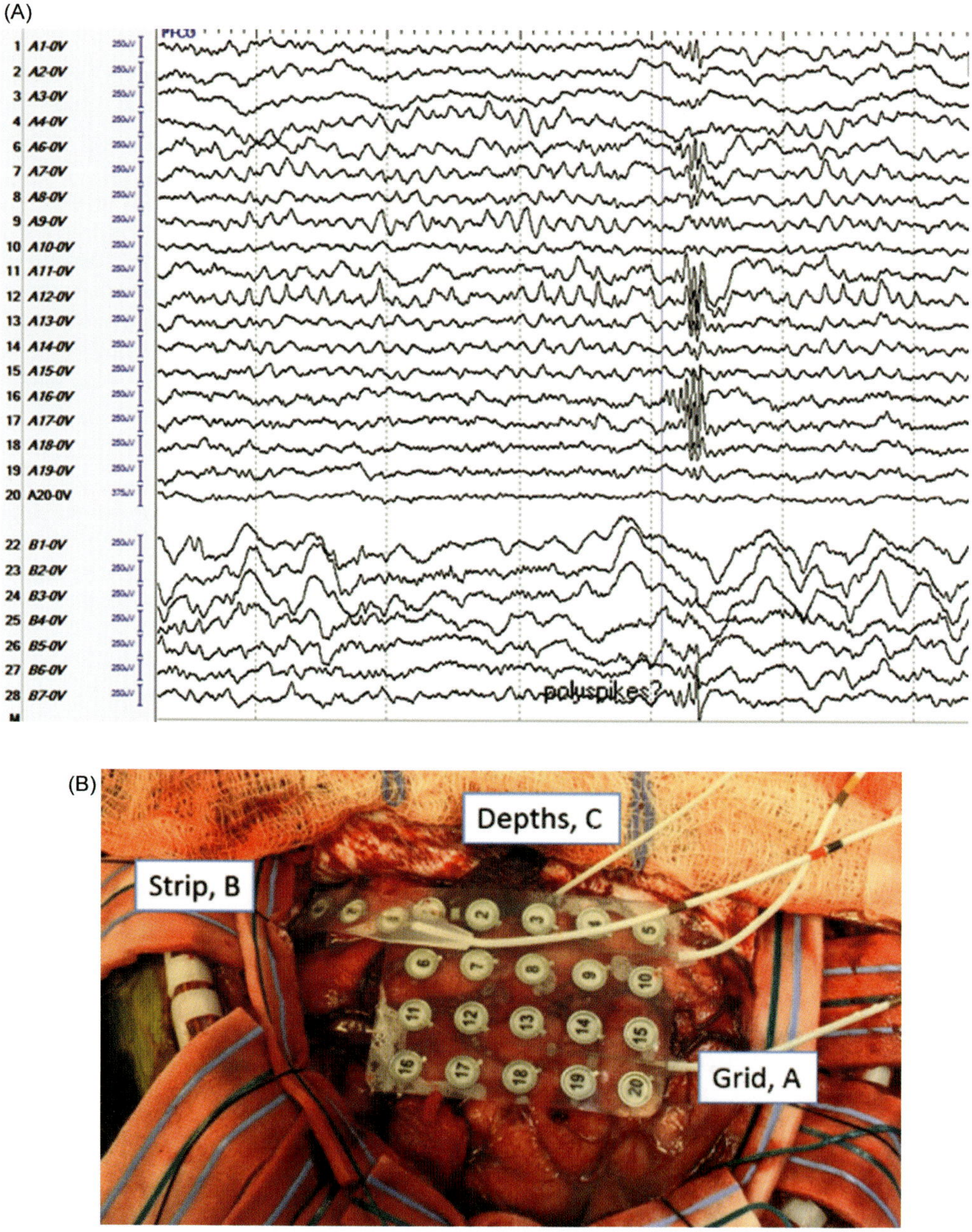

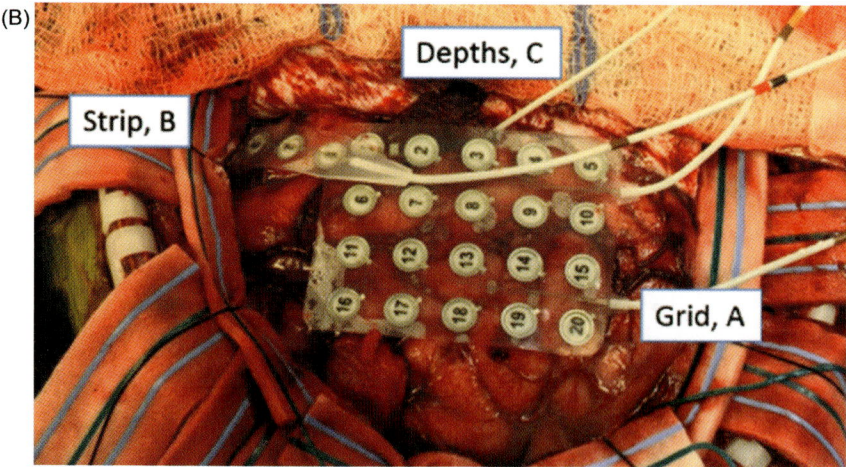

Figure 16.7 This young man had persistent seizures despite a prior resection of a posterior temporal low-grade tumor and suspected cortical dysplasia. The patient was maintained on nitrous and narcotic anesthesia for testing. Electrocorticography demonstrated slowing and lack of fast beta activity at the anterior to mid-temporal cortex with occasional spikes and polyspikes especially at the right superior temporal gyrus. (A) Electrocorticography tracings showing recording from the grid and strip electrodes. A polyspike discharge is seen. (B) A 4 × 5 grid and a 1 × 8 strip are shown in place. A 1 × 4 strip was lowered into the prior resection cavity, labeled *depths*.

16.7.3 Anesthetic Effects

Light or minimal anesthesia is preferred during ECoG because anesthetics can alter epileptiform discharges. Propofol, an activating anesthetic, can be effective relatively quickly, which allows for adequate ECoG. Activating anesthetics inhibit brainstem arousal mechanisms, producing an EEG state more resembling sleep. Inhalation anesthetic agents cause rhythmic fronto-central fast activity. These agents can reduce or increase epileptiform discharges at standard anesthetic levels. Barbiturates produce fronto-central fast activity at low doses and burst suppression at higher doses. The short-acting barbiturate methohexital (0.5 mg/kg) activates ECoG epileptic spiking, which has been used to identify seizure foci. Narcotic drugs can increase epileptiform spiking, including spiking or seizures from sites outside the epileptogenic area. Light anesthesia is preferred during ECoG.

16.7.4 Application in Epilepsy Surgery

Spikes occur in the irritative zone, well beyond the epileptogenic zone. ECoG does not aim to resect the entire irritative zone. Even the most active spiking area may not coincide with the epileptogenic zone. Interictal epileptic disturbances recorded at ECoG in patients with temporal lobe epilepsy often involve adjacent regions. Mesial temporal resection in nonlesional patients is often performed without ECoG, since identifying spikes at the margin of the resection may not have a bearing on the outcome. ECoG recording after a mesial temporal resection remains controversial.

Extratemporal interictal ECoG epileptiform spiking may be widespread, even for patients with a well-defined lesion. The distribution and abundance of ECoG interictal spiking recorded in neocortical recording is a prognostic indicator of postsurgical seizure control. Pre-excision epileptiform activity within two gyri of proposed excision along with relative lack of postexcision spiking distant from the resection are signs favorable for postresection outcome. Residual spiking around the resection borders are not necessarily of great concern.

16.8 Intraoperative Neurophysiologic Monitoring

Intraoperative neurophysiologic monitoring aims to detect impending injury to the nervous system during surgery. Monitoring during epilepsy surgery can forewarn of imminent complications in time for the surgeon to intervene and prevent complications from becoming worse or permanent.

Intraoperative neurophysiologic monitoring in epilepsy surgery includes EEG, and somatosensory and motor-evoked potentials (SEPs and MEPs). A baseline is established early in a procedure and is subsequently compared to changes in SEP or MEP amplitude and latencies, or to EEG frequency content or discharges. Adverse changes raise alerts. Typical thresholds for alerts are set at predetermined levels. EEG and evoked potential modalities are monitored simultaneously.

The type of monitoring needed depends on the surgical plan. MEP is used for surgery near motor tracks. SEP is used more in general to assess the hemisphere and brainstem function, as well as to assess the postcentral cortex in particular. EEG assesses the hemisphere and screens for seizures during surgery. Pre-existing conditions may influence choice and expectations about neurophysiologic intraoperative testing.

16.8.1 Electroencephalography

Monitoring EEG during surgery for patients with epilepsy checks for seizures under anesthesia with neuromuscular blockade. The recording also assesses for occasional unexpected adverse effects such as bleeding, compression, ischemia, edema, hypoxia, or vasospasm. When sufficiently great, these effects change the EEG.

16.8.1.1 Recording

EEG is easily recorded with the standard electrode sites of the 10-20 electrode placement system, modified to delete or move electrodes where a craniotomy itself is conducted. Filters and montages are set at as typical for outpatient recordings. Digital equipment allows side-by-side display of two EEG segments, the current data and a baseline segment used for visual comparison.

16.8.1.2 Interpreting Changes

EEG under anesthesia typically consists of fronto-central fast activity with mixed background slow waves. Inhalation anesthetic can produce fronto-polar triangular waves. EEG is sensitive to depth of anesthesia, and deeper levels can produce burst suppression. Medication boluses affect the EEG transiently.

Ischemia causes decreased fast activity, and greater degrees of ischemia cause increased slowing. Major ischemia produces a global decrease in EEG amplitude that can progress to isoelectric.

EEG in patients with epilepsy is monitored continuously to observe for seizures, especially when the patient is under neuromuscular blockade. During a craniotomy, partial seizures can be treated locally with cool saline applied directly to the cortex.

16.8.2 Somatosensory Evoked Potentials

SEPs are typically recorded from the median and posterior tibial nerves and at the scalp or from electrodes in the surgical site.

16.8.2.1 Stimulation

Median nerve stimulation is applied through needle electrodes at the wrist above motor threshold, e.g., 20–40 mA. The posterior tibial nerve is stimulated just posterior to the medial malleolus. Stimulation is delivered at several per second, up to 5 Hz. Faster stimulation is desirable to produce completed evoked potential trials more quickly, i.e., to complete averaging the desired 300–500 repetitions needed for a new SEP tracing.

16.8.2.2 Recordings

Several scalp and neck channels record SEP signals from the cervical spinal cord, brainstem, and primary somatosensory cortex. Scalp sites are over the central region when possible, although they have to be relocated depending upon a craniotomy flap. Scouting for the best sites early in the case will determine the best locations for monitoring in individual patients, typically 2 cm behind scalp sites C3, C4, and Cz. The low filter is set to 30 Hz and the high filter to 500–1500 Hz. A 50-Hz or 60-Hz notch filter is avoided because it may reduce the SEP peak and produce a ringing stimulus artifact.

16.8.2.3 Interpreting Changes

The primary upper extremity SEP peak is the N20 from the cortical somatosensory cortex. The primary lower extremity SEP peak is the P37 from the cortical somatosensory cortex. Some earlier peaks are also recorded from the cervical spinal cord and brainstem. Classically a 50% amplitude drop is an alarm criterion. A 10% latency increase is a secondary alarm criterion.

The monitoring team must quickly decide whether any significant change encountered is due to technical problems, anesthesia or systemic issues, or surgical problems. A variety of technical problems can occur. Systemic factors considered include hypothermia, hypotension, and hypoxia. Inhalation anesthesia can reduce amplitude, an effect that gradually increases over time. An anesthesia bolus can cause an abrupt amplitude loss. The surgeon and anesthesiologist are alerted to SEP changes.

The surgeon reviews actions, especially what surgical activity has occurred in the past 20–30 minutes that may have led to the observed change. Some surgical maneuvers or actions may take time to cause gradually accumulating effects of bleeding, compression, ischemia, edema, or vasospasm. A search is undertaken to determine the cause of the change. A wide variety of surgical or anesthesia interventions may be taken to reverse any cause of persistent SEP change, details of which are beyond the scope of this chapter.

Not all amplitude decreases predict an adverse neurologic outcome. Several minutes of a 50–80% amplitude decrease poses only a small risk of postoperative deficits, especially if the SEP subsequently returns to baseline. The highest risk of postoperative deficits occurs when the SEPs are abruptly completely lost and remain absent for the remainder of the case. Even in such serious circumstances, the risk of a new postoperative neurologic impairment may be 50–75%.

16.8.3 Motor Evoked Potentials

MEPs monitor the corticospinal tracts, important for preserving motor function during epilepsy surgery. This is important, especially in resection or implantation near the motor cortex or corticospinal tracts. The corticospinal tract pyramids lay anatomically just beneath the hippocampus.

16.8.3.1 Stimulation

Transcranial electrical (tce) stimulation is applied at the scalp through corkscrew needle electrodes located near the motor cortex over each hemisphere. A stimulating anode electrode is located anterior to C3 or C4 electrode sites and a cathode electrode at Cz. Typical stimulation is a train of five to seven individual brief 250–400 mA pulses. Such a stimulus train discharges spinal cord anterior horn cells, resulting in recordable limb muscle activity. Too strong an intensity is avoided because these can discharge axons at too deep a level, possibly as deep as the brainstem. If MEPs are performed during a hemispheric epilepsy resection, too strong a stimulus may initiate corticospinal tract conduction below the surgical level.

16.8.3.2 Recording

Typical recordings are made of limb muscles. Electrodes are placed at several sites in each limb since tceMEPs may provoke good results in just one muscle group in a limb.

Polyphasic complex compound muscle action potentials (CMAPs) are sought at each muscle. These recordings should be stable during surgery.

16.8.3.3 Risk

The most common injury is a tongue or lip laceration[49] caused by brisk jaw muscle contraction. A mouth guard is a precaution. Seizures from cortical electrical stimulation are very rare, and more often a patient with epilepsy has a seizure during surgery spontaneously related to his or her underlying condition – not the stimulation. Minor scalp burns are rare. The tceMEP techniques are not used when a patient has intracranial implanted depth electrodes or vascular aneurysm clips.

16.8.3.4 Interpretation

Major losses of CMAP amplitude are considered as alerts, e.g., 80% or greater decreases. The loss of a small baseline potential may be of no clinical significance. Signals fade with inhalation anesthesia. Decisions to raise a tceMEP alert integrate which muscles changed, how many muscles changed, how big the amplitude change was, and how robust were those recordings at baseline.

16.9 Summary

Invasive and intraoperative techniques supplement routine EEG techniques for capturing epileptiform abnormalities and safeguarding normal cortex when considering epilepsy surgery. In the population at large, epilepsy surgery is greatly underutilized, to the detriment of many patients whose epilepsy could be cured or greatly improved by using these techniques and surgery.

Recording over days to weeks involves depth electrodes or implanted grid and strip electrodes. Recordings wait for a series of typical seizures. Large numbers of recording channels are used to identify the epileptogenic zone.

ECoG traditionally uses acute recordings in the operating room to find spikes that reveal the epileptogenic zone, not just an irritative zone. More recently, chronically recorded ECoG has been developed with stimulation to abort seizures with long-term implanted electrodes.

Functional cortical mapping assesses the regions of movement, sensation, language, or occasionally other functional areas. The goal of these exercises is to spare those areas whenever possible when defining the limits of resection.

Intraoperative monitoring is used to guide the surgeon during resection. This helps to assess that the hemisphere remains free of significant ischemia, compression, hypoxia, hypotension, edema, or other adverse effects during resection. This includes nonconvulsive seizures or convulsive seizures occurring in epilepsy patients who are in surgery under neuromuscular blockade. If adverse events are encountered, the surgeon and anesthesiologist are promptly alerted in time to intervene and reverse incipient complications.

References

1. Devinsky O, Friedman D, Cheng JY, et al. Underestimation of sudden deaths among patients with seizures and epilepsy. *Neurology.* 2017;89(9):886–892.

2. Fazel S, Wolf A, Langstrom N, Newton CR, Lichtenstein P. Premature mortality in epilepsy and the role of psychiatric comorbidity: a total population study. *Lancet.* 2013;382(9905):1646–1654.

3. Engel J, Jr. What can we do for people with drug-resistant epilepsy? The 2016 Wartenberg Lecture. *Neurology*. 2016;87(23):2483–2489.

4. Rosenow F, Luders H. Presurgical evaluation of epilepsy. *Brain*. 2001;124(Pt 9):1683–1700.

5. Carne RP, O'Brien TJ, Kilpatrick CJ, et al. MRI-negative PET-positive temporal lobe epilepsy: a distinct surgically remediable syndrome. *Brain*. 2004;127(Pt 10):2276–2285.

6. Sperling MR. Clinical challenges in invasive monitoring in epilepsy surgery. *Epilepsia*. 1997;38(Suppl 4):S6–12.

7. Engel J, Jr. Respiration-linked 'limbic spindles': vibration artifact recorded from nasopharyngeal and intracerebral electrodes. *Electroencephalogr Clin Neurophysiol*. 1980;49(3–4):366–372.

8. Van Buren JM. Complications of surgical procedures in the diagnosis and treatment of epilepsy. In: Engel J, Jr. ed., *Surgical Treatment of the Epilepsies*. New York: Raven Press; 1987:465–475.

9. Sansur CA, Frysinger RC, Pouratian N, et al. Incidence of symptomatic hemorrhage after stereotactic electrode placement. *J Neurosurg*. 2007;107 (5):998–1003.

10. Tanriverdi T, Ajlan A, Poulin N, Olivier A. Morbidity in epilepsy surgery: an experience based on 2449 epilepsy surgery procedures from a single institution. *J Neurosurg*. 2009;110(6):1111–1123.

11. Sperling MR. *Intracranial Electroencephalography*. New York: Elsevier; 1993.

12. Spencer SS, Sperling MR, Shewmon DA, Kahane P. Inracranial electrodes. In: Engel J, Jr. Pedley TA, eds., *Epilepsy: A Comprehensive Textbook* 2nd edn. Philadelphia: Lippincott Williams & Wilkins; 2008:1791–1815.

13. Spencer SS, Spencer DD. Entorhinal-hippocampal interactions in medial temporal lobe epilepsy. *Epilepsia*. 1994;35 (4):721–727.

14. Spencer SS. Substrates of localization-related epilepsies: biologic implications of localizing findings in humans. *Epilepsia*. 1998;39(2):114–123.

15. Velasco AL, Wilson CL, Babb TL, Engel J, Jr. Functional and anatomic correlates of two frequently observed temporal lobe seizure-onset patterns. *Neural Plast*. 2000;7 (1–2):49–63.

16. Schuh LA, Henry TR, Ross DA, et al. Ictal spiking patterns recorded from temporal depth electrodes predict good outcome after anterior temporal lobectomy. *Epilepsia*. 2000;41(3):316–319.

17. Spencer SS, Marks D, Katz A, Kim J, Spencer DD. Anatomic correlates of interhippocampal seizure propagation time. *Epilepsia*. 1992;33(5):862–873.

18. Lieb JP, Babb TL. Interhemispheric propagation time of human hippocampal seizures: II. Relationship to pathology and cell density. *Epilepsia*. 1986;27(3):294–300.

19. Isnard J, Guenot M, Sindou M, Mauguiere F. Clinical manifestations of insular lobe seizures: a stereo-electroencephalographic study. *Epilepsia*. 2004;45(9):1079–1090.

20. Tassi L, Colombo N, Cossu M, et al. Electroclinical, MRI and neuropathological study of 10 patients with nodular heterotopia, with surgical outcomes. *Brain*. 2005;128(Pt 2):321–337.

21. Aghakhani Y, Kinay D, Gotman J, et al. The role of periventricular nodular heterotopia in epileptogenesis. *Brain*. 2005;128(Pt 3):641–651.

22. Francione S, Kahane P, Tassi L, et al. Stereo-EEG of interictal and ictal electrical activity of a histologically proved heterotopic gray matter associated with partial epilepsy. *Electroencephalogr Clin Neurophysiol*. 1994;90(4):284–290.

23. Engel J, Jr. Outcome with respect to epileptic seizures. In: Engel J, Jr., ed., *Surgical Treatment of the Epilepsies*. New York: Raven Press; 1987:553–571.

24. Wyler AR, Walker G, Somes G. The morbidity of long-term seizure monitoring using subdural strip electrodes. *J Neurosurg*. 1991;74(5):734–737.

25. Lee WS, Lee JK, Lee SA, Kang JK, Ko TS. Complications and results of subdural grid

electrode implantation in epilepsy surgery. *Surg Neurol.* 2000;54(5):346–351.

26. Onal C, Otsubo H, Araki T, et al. Complications of invasive subdural grid monitoring in children with epilepsy. *J Neurosurg.* 2003;98(5):1017–1026.

27. Araki T, Otsubo H, Makino Y, et al. Efficacy of dexamathasone on cerebral swelling and seizures during subdural grid EEG recording in children. *Epilepsia.* 2006;47(1):176–180.

28. Sahjpaul RL, Mahon J, Wiebe S. Dexamethasone for morbidity after subdural electrode insertion – a randomized controlled trial. *Can J Neurol Sci.* 2003;30(4):340–348.

29. Wetjen NM, Marsh WR, Meyer FB, et al. Intracranial electroencephalography seizure onset patterns and surgical outcomes in nonlesional extratemporal epilepsy. *J Neurosurg.* 2009;110 (6):1147–1152.

30. McGonigal A, Bartolomei F, Regis J, et al. Stereoelectroencephalography in presurgical assessment of MRI-negative epilepsy. *Brain.* 2007;130(Pt 12):3169–3183.

31. Spencer SS, Guimaraes P, Katz A, Kim J, Spencer D. Morphological patterns of seizures recorded intracranially. *Epilepsia.* 1992;33(3):537–545.

32. Fisher RS, Webber WR, Lesser RP, Arroyo S, Uematsu S. High-frequency EEG activity at the start of seizures. *J Clin Neurophysiol.* 1992;9(3):441–448.

33. Schiller Y, Cascino GD, Busacker NE, Sharbrough FW. Characterization and comparison of local onset and remote propagated electrographic seizures recorded with intracranial electrodes. *Epilepsia.* 1998;39(4):380–388.

34. Lee SA, Spencer DD, Spencer SS. Intracranial EEG seizure-onset patterns in neocortical epilepsy. *Epilepsia.* 2000;41 (3):297–307.

35. Blumenfeld H, Rivera M, McNally KA, et al. Ictal neocortical slowing in temporal lobe epilepsy. *Neurology.* 2004;63 (6):1015–1021.

36. Allen PJ, Fish DR, Smith SJ. Very high-frequency rhythmic activity during SEEG suppression in frontal lobe epilepsy. *Electroencephalogr Clin Neurophysiol.* 1992;82(2):155–159.

37. Worrell GA, Parish L, Cranstoun SD, et al. High-frequency oscillations and seizure generation in neocortical epilepsy. *Brain.* 2004;127(Pt 7):1496–1506.

38. Eisenschenk S, Gilmore RL, Cibula JE, Roper SN. Lateralization of temporal lobe foci: depth versus subdural electrodes. *Clin Neurophysiol.* 2001;112(5):836–844.

39. Bragin A, Engel J, Jr., Wilson CL, Fried I, Mathern GW. Hippocampal and entorhinal cortex high-frequency oscillations (100–500 Hz) in human epileptic brain and in kainic acid–treated rats with chronic seizures. *Epilepsia.* 1999;40(2):127–137.

40. Urrestarazu E, Chander R, Dubeau F, Gotman J. Interictal high-frequency oscillations (100–500 Hz) in the intracerebral EEG of epileptic patients. *Brain.* 2007;130(Pt 9):2354–2366.

41. Staba RJ, Wilson CL, Bragin A, Fried I, Engel J, Jr. Quantitative analysis of high-frequency oscillations (80-500 Hz) recorded in human epileptic hippocampus and entorhinal cortex. *J Neurophysiol.* 2002;88(4):1743–1752.

42. Jirsch JD, Urrestarazu E, LeVan P, et al. High-frequency oscillations during human focal seizures. *Brain.* 2006;129(Pt 6):1593–1608.

43. Zijlmans M, Worrell GA, Dumpelmann M, et al. How to record high-frequency oscillations in epilepsy: a practical guideline. *Epilepsia.* 2017;58(8):1305–1315.

44. Bragin A, Wilson CL, Staba RJ, et al. Interictal high-frequency oscillations (80–500 Hz) in the human epileptic brain: entorhinal cortex. *Ann Neurol.* 2002;52 (4):407–415.

45. Engel J, Jr., Bragin A, Staba R, Mody I. High-frequency oscillations: what is normal and what is not? *Epilepsia.* 2009;50 (4):598–604.

46. Staba RJ, Wilson CL, Bragin A, et al. High-frequency oscillations recorded in human

medial temporal lobe during sleep. *Ann Neurol.* 2004,56(1):108–115.

47. Khosravani H, Mehrotra N, Rigby M, et al. Spatial localization and time-dependant changes of electrographic high frequency oscillations in human temporal lobe epilepsy. *Epilepsia.* 2009;50(4):605–616.

48. Fernandez IS, Loddenkemper T. Electrocorticography for seizure foci mapping in epilepsy surgery. *J Clin Neurophysiol.* 2013;30(6):554–570.

49. Reuber M, Kral T, Kurthen M, Elger CE. New-onset psychogenic seizures after intracranial neurosurgery. *Acta Neurochir (Wien).* 2002;144(9):901–907; discussion 907.

Neuroimaging in Epilepsy

Andrew Zillgitt

17.1 Structural Brain Imaging in Seizures and Epilepsy

The use of neuroimaging in the evaluation of epilepsy dates back to X-ray radiography, which was obtained in the early temporal lobe surgical evaluations.[1,2] In the 1940s the first temporal lobectomy was performed and skull X-ray, along with air encephalography, was obtained to detect findings such as dilatation of the horns of the lateral ventricles, as well as changes in the middle cranial fossa curvature.[2,3] Although with further evaluations these findings were not substantiated, dilatation of the temporal horns on brain magnetic resonance imaging (MRI) can be a finding in mesial temporal sclerosis (MTS).[4]

Today, skull X-rays are rarely obtained in the evaluation of epilepsy. However, a skull X-ray is beneficial in evaluating skull fractures in acute trauma, in assessing calcified intrauterine infections such as toxoplasmosis and cytomegalovirus, or calcified hamartomata in tuberous sclerosis and the classic tram-track sign in Sturge–Weber syndrome.[1]

By the 1970s, computed tomography (CT) of the head emerged as the neuroimaging modality of choice in the evaluation of epilepsy.[2] It is readily available and inexpensive, and has a significant role in acute and emergent settings.[4] In individuals who present with a first, or new, seizure, CT may be beneficial in identifying acute lesions, e.g., intracerebral hemorrhage, subarachnoid hemorrhage, or subdural or epidural hematoma.[4] It also has utility in detecting calcifications and large vascular malformations, as seen in Sturge–Weber syndrome or arteriovenous malformations.[4,5]

However, lesions near the skull base, in the orbitofrontal region and mesial temporal lobe, may be obscured by bone and are not easily detected.[4] Additionally, CT has low sensitivity in differentiating tissues such as gray and white matter, and may only identify focal epileptic lesions in approximately 30% of cases.[5,6]

MRI was first used in a human in 1977 and the first brain MRI was obtained in 1980. By 1997 the Commission of Neuroimaging of the International League Against Epilepsy (ILAE) had concluded that MRI is superior to CT in sensitivity and specificity with regard to epileptic lesions.[7] As the magnetic field strength of MRI has increased from 0.15 tesla (T) to 1.5 T and 3 T, with 7 T and 9.4 T on the horizon, the identification of epileptic lesions continues to improve with time.[6,8,9]

As the use of brain MRI has become ubiquitous in the evaluation of seizures, imaging protocols have become standardized. With the increasing availability of 3 T MRI, the ability to identify subtle epileptic lesions has improved.

An epilepsy MRI brain protocol should contain 3D, T1-weighted volumetric acquisition with isotropic voxel size of 1 or 1.5 mm.[4] A T1-weighted spin-echo acquisition as a scout image is necessary to position brain slices of other pulse sequences.[10] In addition to T1-weighted sequences that generally provide detailed anatomical differentiation,

T2-weighted sequences that often illustrate underlying structural abnormalities, including fluid-attenuated inversion recovery (FLAIR), should be obtained.

One advantage of T2-weighted sequences in the evaluation of potential epileptic lesions is the clear delineation of brain tissue and cerebral spinal fluid (CSF). Areas of T2 hyperintensity can be present in a variety of disease states and pathological processes including MTS, malformations of cortical development (MCD), e.g., focal cortical dysplasia (FCD), vascular malformations, neoplasms, both primary and metastatic, and even from frequent or recent seizures.[5] However, T2 hyperintensities from surrounding CSF may obscure abnormal pathologic signals, as can be the case in MTS.[10] In this setting, high signal intensity from neighboring CSF in the temporal horns of the lateral ventricle may obstruct visualization of hyperintensities within the hippocampus.[10] As such, FLAIR sequences, which are regarded as predominant T2-weighted images with darkened CSF, are valuable in accentuating brain pathology near CSF. In a study from 1996 comparing FLAIR with T2-weighted imaging in people with mesial temporal lobe epilepsy (MTLE) and MTS, FLAIR sequences accurately identified increased signal within the hippocampus in 97% of cases compared to 91% for T2 sequences ($p < 0.02$).[11] FLAIR sequences may offer other advantages over T2-weighted sequences, specifically by identifying subtle hyperintensities at the gray–white interface, better visualization of subcortical foci of gliosis within regions of encephalomalacia and the extent of infiltration of low-grade brain tumors.[10]

T1-weighted sequences have unique advantages over T2-weighted and FLAIR images. Typically, T2-weighted and FLAIR sequences have slice thicknesses of 4–5 mm, which may lead to failure in identifying less obvious lesions. To reduce this limitation, T1 sequences are often obtained at 1 mm contiguous slices, enhancing the visualization of normal anatomy and potential epileptic lesions. T1-weighted sequences, such as fast spoiled gradient-recalled echo, magnetization-prepared rapid acquisition gradient echo, and gradient-recalled acquisition in a steady state, are common sequences in epilepsy protocols. These images provide clear delineation of the gray and white matter and can be used to qualitatively assess the volume and morphology of the hippocampus. Due to the thin slices, identification of other subtle MCD and neoplasms may be more obvious with these T1-weighted sequences. However, the hypointensity of gray matter is similar to that of CSF and abnormalities in the gray matter may be less obvious.[10]

Diffusion-weighted imaging (DWI) may be beneficial in the evaluation of epilepsy and DWI sequences are usually included in most epilepsy protocols. Areas of restricted diffusion and decreased apparent diffusion coefficient have been described in peri-ictal changes in people with focal epilepsies.[12] In addition, areas of restricted diffusion have been reported in prolonged focal status epilepticus.[13] Similarly, in people with temporal lobe epilepsy (TLE), increased apparent diffusion coefficient (ADC) signal is described in the ictogenic hippocampus and postictal DWI changes are attributed to the origin and propagation of the preceding seizure.[14]

Despite these techniques, up to 30% of TLE cases are MRI-negative and up to 40% of drug-resistant epilepsy cases may have "normal" brain MRI.[15,16] Moreover, approximately 30% of histopathologically verified FCDs are not identifiable on standard brain MRI.[17] To improve detection of epileptic lesions the use of a 3 T MRI scanner over a 1.5 T may be beneficial.[18]

From a clinical perspective, the identification of potential epileptic lesions from a brain MRI can be dichotomized into MTLE and neocortical epilepsy.[4] MTLE is the most common adult focal epilepsy (Table 17.1, Figure 17.1).[19] Epilepsy MRI brain protocols should include

Table 17.1 Mesial temporal sclerosis (MTS) findings on structural brain MRI[4]

MRI finding	MRI features
Hippocampal atrophy	Most specific and reliable finding The normal hippocampal shape is oval, but in hippocampal sclerosis it becomes flattened and inclined Hippocampal atrophy is defined by comparing the hippocampus circumference on each side on all coronal slices[*]
Increased T2/FLAIR signal	As an isolated finding, T2/FLAIR hyperintensity may not be adequate to diagnosis MTS Relaxometry is an objective measurement of abnormal T2 signal and may be employed when visualization is subtle
Loss of internal architecture	This finding is due to neuronal loss and gliosis with a collapse of pyramidal cell layers Often associated with atrophy and T2/FLAIR signal intensity
Miscellaneous	Asymmetry of the temporal horn of the lateral ventricles (variable and could lead to false lateralization) Atrophy of the anterior temporal lobe (nonspecific) Atrophy of the fornix and mammillary body ipsilateral to MTS

FLAIR, fluid-attenuated inversion recovery; MRI, magnetic resonance imaging.
* Small hippocampal asymmetries may be present from normal variation and/or head tilt in the scanner. These should not be interpreted as abnormal.

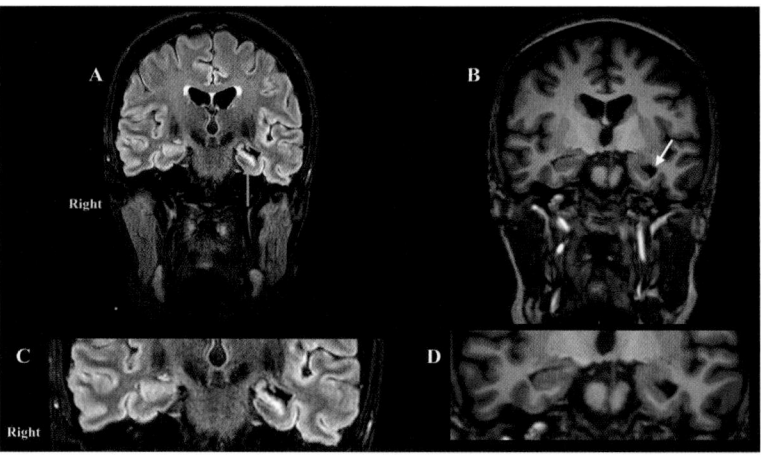

Figure 17.1 MRI brain in left MTLE with MTS. The patient is a 57-year-old right-handed woman with drug-resistant focal epilepsy. Her noninvasive diagnostic studies implicated an epileptogenic zone within the left temporal lobe. (A) and (C) are coronal FLAIR and IRSPGR sequences, respectively, that reveal loss of internal architecture within the left hippocampus with hippocampal atrophy and increased FLAIR signal. (B) and (D) zoom in to further detail these abnormalities.

T1, T2, and FLAIR sequences with thin slices of at least 3 mm or less (preferably 1 mm slices). Coronal MRI slices perpendicular to the longitudinal axis of the hippocampus are imperative when assessing for MTS.[20] Hippocampal volume, shape, and internal architecture may be best evaluated through T1 inversion recovery sequences (e.g., IRSPGR), while

T2 and FLAIR sequences provide qualitative assessment of signal intensity.[20] In regard to FLAIR images, abnormalities on these sequences, e.g., signal hyperintensity, have revealed 97% accuracy for abnormalities associated with hippocampal sclerosis (HS) verified on histopathology.[21]

Other MRI abnormalities may be associated with MTS as well. For example, asymmetry of the temporal horn of the lateral ventricle has been associated with MTS.[4] There may also be atrophy of the anterior temporal lobe, which can be viewed on both coronal and axial MRI sequences.[5] Finally, atrophy within the ipsilateral fornix and mammillary body may be present in recurrent hippocampal onset seizures in MTS.[4] Most often the brain MRI findings in MTS are unilateral, but some cases may demonstrate bilateral findings.[4]

Unlike the well-characterized clinical, electrographic, and neuroimaging features of MTLE, neocortical TLE and extratemporal lobe epilepsy (ETLE) often have diverse clinical presentations with a broad spectrum of neuroimaging findings ranging from MRI-negative to subtle blurring of the gray–white matter junction to obvious MCD, such as schizencephaly.[4,17,20] The diversity in clinical presentation and neuroimaging is due to the diversity in etiology of these epilepsies. One of the most common, and at times under-recognized, causes of neocortical TLE and ETLE are MCD, in particular FCD. The identification of FCD on structural brain MRI can be challenging,

Since 1971 there have been several attempts at classifying FCD, and in 2011 a consensus classification of FCD was provided by the ILAE.[22–24] FCD was defined as disorganized cortical lamination with bizarre neurons, including balloon cells, and divided into three types: FCD Type I, FCD Type II, and FCD Type III.[24]

With FCD Type Ia–c brain MRI findings may include mild hemispheric hypoplasia, thinning of the cortex, blurring of the gray–white matter junction, and abnormally shaped sulci at times with deepened sulci.[4,24,25] FCD Type IIa may be MRI-negative and FCD Type IIb may have a variety of abnormalities.[24]

Some FCD may have subtle MRI findings, while other FCD, e.g. FCD type IIb, have more obvious MRI signal changes, such as transmantle sign (Figure 17.2).[5] The transmantle sign has been associated with FCD Type IIb.[4,24,26] Overall, it can be characterized by tapering of T2 and FLAIR hyperintensity from the cortex to the ventricular surface.[4]

MRI findings in FCD Type IIIa–d may include any of the features described above, with the associated principal lesion usually within the same lobe or region.[4,24]

Many MCDs have more obvious MRI findings. In lissencephaly ("smooth brain"), an MCD due to defective neuronal migration during 12–24 weeks of gestation resulting in no development of gyri or sulci, brain MRI shows a smooth cortex with highly simplified or absent gyri.[5] Brain MRI in polymicrogyria may reveal a thickened cortex with numerous gyri often accompanied by T2 and FLAIR signal abnormalities and blurring of the gray–white junction on T1-weighted sequences.[5]

Hemimegalencephaly is another MCD that is characterized by an abnormally enlarged and dysplastic cerebral hemisphere (Figure 17.3).[27] Brain MRI demonstrates hemispheric enlargement, always within the cerebral hemisphere and at times within the cerebellum and brainstem.[5]

Yakovlew and Wadsworth introduced the term schizencephaly in 1946. Schizencephaly can be classified as open-lipped, in which the walls of the cleft do not oppose each other, and closed-lipped, where the clefts are opposed and often fused.[27] These lesions can be unilateral or bilateral and are present in the frontal and parietal lobes in 65% of cases.[27] On brain MRI there is "puckering" or a "dimple" outward of the lateral ventricle at the point

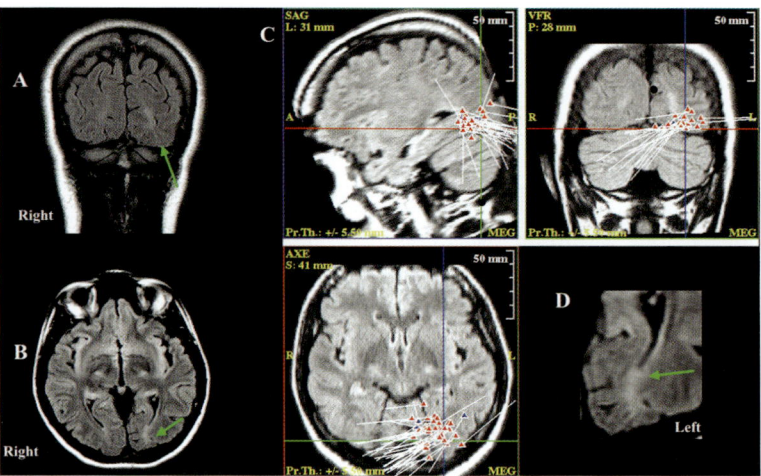

Figures 17.2 MRI brain in left occipital lobe epilepsy due to FCD. The patient is 36-year-old woman with drug-resistant focal epilepsy. Her seizures would begin with an abdominal sensation or elementary visual hallucinations within the right upper visual quadrant. (A) and (B) are coronal and axial FLAIR images, respectively, revealing hyperintensity extending from the posterior horn of the left lateral ventricle into the adjacent cortex consistent with a transmantle sign. (C) reveals a cluster of MEG ECD corresponding to the MRI abnormality. (D) is zoomed into the transmantle sign to further delineate the area of interest.

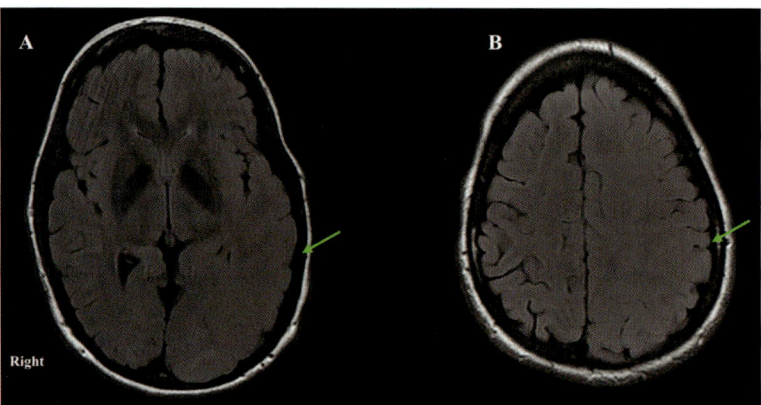

Figure 17.3 MRI brain in a patient with drug-resistant focal epilepsy. The patient is a 31-year-old woman with drug-resistant focal epilepsy and hemimegalencephaly. Note the abnormally enlarged and dysplastic left cerebral hemisphere (green arrows). (A) and (B) – axial FLAIR.

the cleft reaches the ventricular margin.[27] The cleft is lined by gray matter that may look similar to polymicrogyria.[27] Increased T2 signal within the white matter should give pause and may be more consistent with porencephaly than schizencephaly.[27] Often, in up to 30% of cases, schizencephaly is associated with agenesis of the septum pellucidum and hypoplasia of the optic nerves.[27] Therefore, schizencephaly may be on the spectrum of septo-optic dysplasia (Figure 17.4).[27]

Heterotopias are a group of cells in an inappropriate location, but within the correct tissue of origin,[27] most commonly present in the periventricular region and within the

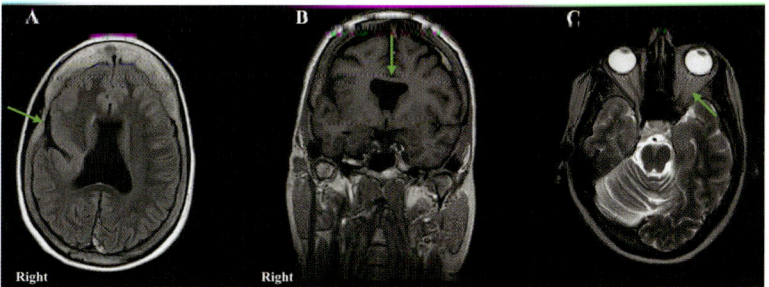

Figure 17.4 MRI brain in a patient with drug-resistant focal epilepsy. The patient is a 54-year-old right-handed woman with drug-resistant epilepsy. Her brain MRI findings included schizencephaly (A), agenesis of the septum pellucidum (B), and hypoplasia of the optic nerves (C). These findings are consistent with septo-optic dysplasia. (A) – axial FLAIR; (B) – coronal IRSPGR; (C) – axial T2.

subcortical white matter.[27] Subcortical laminar heterotopias, or double cortex, consist of continuous, or near continuous, ectopic bands of gray matter below the cortical mantle.[4] On structural brain MRI heterotopias appear isointense to the cortex regardless of the pulse sequence.[5]

Tuberous sclerosis complex is a common neurocutaneous disorder[28] and abnormalities include cortical hamartomas (tubers), subependymal nodules, and subependymal giant cell astrocytoma (SEGA).[27] Although brain MRI may reveal multiple cortical hamartomata, not all hamartomata are epileptogenic.[4] Recently studies have documented diffusion tensor imaging (DTI) abnormalities in ADC and radial diffusivity in epileptogenic hamartomata.[29,30] Correlation of structural brain MRI to functional neuroimaging may be necessary to accurately identify epileptogenic hamartomata. 11C-alpha-methyl-L-tryptophan (AMT) positron emission tomography (PET) has routinely demonstrated accuracy in identifying epileptogenic tubers and magnetoencephalography (MEG) may also be useful in delineating epileptogenic and nonepileptogenic tubers.[31–35]

Brain tumor-related seizures and epilepsy are common. The most common brain tumors are metastatic cancers arising from primary lung, breast, renal, and gastrointestinal cancers, as well as melanoma. On brain MRI these lesions usually appear isointense or hypointense on T1 sequences, and hyperintense on T2 and FLAIR sequences. When a brain tumor, either primary or metastatic, is suspected, gadolinium injection is necessary. In the case of metastatic brain tumors, there is robust postcontrast enhancement.[5]

Meningiomas are benign extra-axial tumors that are often epileptogenic. These tumors are isointense on both T1 and T2 sequences.[5]

Hypothalamic hamartomas are frequently associated with gelastic seizures, cognitive impairments, and behavioral disturbances. On structural brain MRI, these tumors are isointense on T1 imaging and reveal variable T2/FLAIR hyperintensity.[20]

Cerebral vascular malformations may cause seizures and epilepsy. There are five major types of cerebral parenchymal vascular malformations: (1) cavernomas, (2) developmental venous anomalies, (3) capillary telangiectasias, (4) arteriovenous malformations, and finally (5) leptomeningeal angiomatosis (Sturge–Weber syndrome).[36] Cavernomas, cavernous hemangiomas, or cavernous angiomas, do not contain true blood vessels and are located within the bed of the parenchyma.[5,36] These multicystic lesions contain blood products of various ages and a rim of hemosiderin.[36] On T2 and FLAIR sequences cavernomas display dark susceptibility artifact rings with a "popcorn" shape on gradient echo (GRE) and susceptibility weight images (SWI).[5,36] Arteriovenous malformations are characterized by abnormal arterioles connecting to atypical venuoles.[36]

Over time, MRI has become the imaging modality of choice for both ischemic and hemorrhagic stroke. On brain MRI acute ischemic strokes exhibit diffusion restriction that appears bright on DWI and dark on ADC. As the ischemic stroke evolves T2 and FLAIR hyperintensities become more prominent and are often associated with surrounding gliosis and encephalomalacia. Hemorrhagic strokes are hyperintense on T2 and FLAIR sequences. Additionally, gradient echo (GRE) may be beneficial for the identification of microhemorrhages.[5]

Autoimmune epilepsy, once thought to be relatively uncommon, has been recognized with increasing regularity. Rasmussen encephalitis may be the most classic form of auto-immune epilepsy. This is a T-cell-mediated condition that presents in childhood with hemiplegia, neurodevelopmental regression, and epilepsia partialis continua.[5] Atrophy within the affected cerebral hemisphere is best visualized on T2 and FLAIR sequences and may be most prominent in the insula and operculum.[5,20] In addition, T2 and FLAIR hyperintensities may be present within the affected hemisphere. In other autoimmune epilepsy cases, brain MRI findings are variable and may consist of increased T2 and FLAIR signals as well as postcontrast enhancement.[5,37,38] In the correct clinical setting, otherwise unexplained T2 and FLAIR hyperintensities within the temporal lobes should raise concern for an autoimmune process.

The majority of this chapter has been dedicated to neuroimaging in focal epilepsy, in which the identification of epileptic lesions is crucial for accurate diagnosis, treatment, and prognosis. However, neuroimaging may play a role in generalized epilepsies. Structural abnormalities are common in structural/metabolic (previously symptomatic) generalized epilepsies and may be the prevailing etiology in up to 75% of Lennox–Gastaut syndrome cases.[39] Additionally, up to 24% of people with genetic (idiopathic) generalized epilepsy may have structural abnormalities on brain MRI.[40] Although the majority of these are nonspecific, neuropathologic findings may suggest atypical neuronal organization within the frontal cortex.[41,42] Finally, with advanced neuroimaging techniques, such as DTI connectivity, EEG-functional MRI (fMRI), and MEG, network analyses in generalized epilepsy may be possible.[43–50]

17.2 Functional Brain Imaging in Seizures and Epilepsy

Functional neuroimaging in epilepsy encompasses a variety of modalities, including nuclear medicine studies (PET and single-photon emission computed tomography or SPECT), fMRI, and MEG. These imaging modalities are complementary techniques to structural imaging and primarily used in the epilepsy presurgical evaluation to delineate epileptogenic regions, functional defect zones, and eloquent cortices. Functional neuroimaging may also accentuate underlying normal, or abnormal, structural or network connections. For example, pre- and post-epilepsy surgery PET scans have demonstrated dynamic changes within regions connected, but distant from the epileptic focus.[51] Functional MRI, through a variety of techniques, has well established its ability to localize language centers in the brain and more recent studies have revealed EEG-fMRI may identify seizure onset zones (SOZs).[52–55] Finally, MEG, a neurophysiology and neuroimaging modality that is a direct measurement of neuronal function, has documented capability of detecting irritative zones (IZs) as well as possibly the epileptogenic zone (EZ) in addition to eloquent cortices, including the somatosensory cortex, visual cortex, and language regions.[56–67]

Perhaps the most frequently used functional neuroimaging modality in the epilepsy presurgical evaluation is the PET scan. PET utilizes tracers labeled with positron emitters to visualize and quantify cerebral metabolism.[52] There are multiple PET ligands used in clinical epilepsy that are obtained from cyclotrons, including 11C-flumazenil (11C-FMZ), AMT, and the most common clinically utilized tracer, 2-deoxy-2-[^{18}F] fluoroglucose PET scan (FDG-PET).[52] In general, PET is an interictal study and displays superior spatial resolution when compared to other nuclear medicine imaging modalities, such as SPECT scans.[52]

When obtaining a PET scan, specifically an FDG-PET scan, the patient should be seizure-free for at least 12, preferably 24 hours prior to the study. Continuous EEG may be obtained during the PET scan to avoid an "ictal study." In general, in adults during the interictal state areas of hypometabolism (reduced FDG uptake) are likely to contain the EZ. However, it is important to note that in children hypermetabolism may be present in the EZ. In adults with TLE, it is challenging to distinguish MTLE from neocortical TLE on FDG-PET due to spatial resolution, volume averaging, and diffuse temporal lobe hypometabolism. Additionally, the hypometabolism often extends beyond the epileptic lesion and the volume and severity may increase over the duration of epilepsy.[52]

In general, FDG-PET in MTLE reveals reduced FDG uptake in the ipsilateral mesial and anterolateral temporal lobe, basal ganglia, thalamus, and at times the frontal cortex (insula, inferior frontal lobe, orbitofrontal region, and prefrontal cortex) and parietal lobe (Figure 17.5).[52] Bilateral temporal lobe hypometabolism may be present in bilateral MTLE or ETLE.[52] The use of other PET ligands, such as ^{11}C-FMZ, may aid in distinguishing MTLE from NTLE with restricted hypometabolism present on ^{11}C-FMZ compared to that of FDG-PET.[68,69] In addition, ^{11}C-FMZ may identify occult MCD in people with non-lesional TLE.[68]

The sensitivity of FDG-PET in people with TLE, particularly lesional TLE, e.g., TLE due to MTS, ranges from 80–90%.[52] Some authors have suggested the absence of hypometabolism within the temporal lobe in MTLE should raise questions as to the diagnosis of

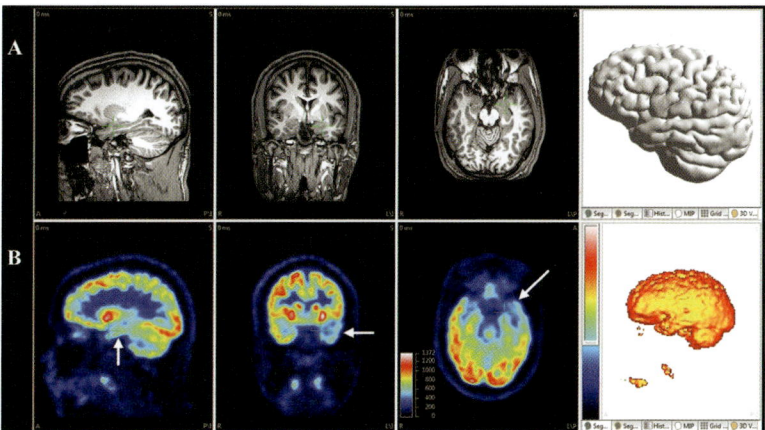

Figure 17.5 FDG-PET in a brain MRI-negative patient with focal epilepsy. The patient is a 25-year-old right-handed man with drug-resistant focal epilepsy. His seizures manifest as focal hyperkinetic seizures with impaired awareness. (A) Brain MRI did not demonstrate an obvious epileptic lesion. (B) FDG-PET revealed marked hypometabolism within the left temporal lobe (white arrow)

MTLE.[70] Furthermore, reduced FDG metabolism by 15–40% has been correlated with seizure freedom following surgery in TLE.[71] Although sensitivity of FDG-PET in lesional TLE is high, the sensitivity falls to 44% in nonlesional TLE and possibly lower in ETLE cases.[52]

As previously noted, functional imaging techniques may augment previously unidentified epileptic lesions.[20,68,72–78] With FDG-PET this can be accentuated by coregistering FDG-PET with structural brain MRI.[52] One study reported that, with FDG-PET/MRI coregistration, localization of an epileptogenic focus was obtained in 33% of subjects with MRI-negative scans or discordant MRI and EEG data.[74]

Although FDG may be the most common clinically used ligand, the utility of ^{11}C-FMZ and AMT in clinical epilepsy has been well documented.[31–33,68,75,79] Specifically, in people with tuberous sclerosis complex and epilepsy, including Lennox–Gastaut syndrome, epileptogenic cortical hamartomata may be hypermetabolic on AMT-PET with reduced metabolism on conventional FDG-PET.[31,32,52] In these patients improved seizure control may be obtained following resection of the epileptogenic tuber.[80] Additionally, in children with nonlesional brain MRI and infantile spasms or West syndrome, PET scans, including ^{11}C-FMZ and AMT, may identify abnormalities and resection of these regions may alleviate seizures and prevent further neurocognitive decline.[52,81]

Whereas PET is a functional imaging modality that measures cerebral metabolism primarily in the interictal state, SPECT is a nuclear medicine study that measures regional cerebral perfusion (rCP) and can be completed in both the interictal and ictal states. Although the advantage of SPECT over PET is the ability to obtain a scan during a seizure, the spatial resolution for SPECT is poorer compared to PET. There are three US Food and Drug Administration-approved radiopharmaceuticals, isopropyl-iodo-amphetamine and two Tc-99m radionucleotides, hexamethylpropylamine oxime (HMPAO) and ethyl cysteinate dimer (ECD). These compounds will bind to specific regions in the brain and remain for hours. Typically, SPECT scans are obtained during an admission to the epilepsy monitoring unit. A pre-existing IV is necessary to inject the radionucleotide as close to seizure onset as possible. Injection of the compound should be completed within 20 s of the seizure onset and the seizure duration should be over 5–10 s. The precise times of the clinical and EEG seizure onsets should be recorded in addition with the time of tracer injection. When obtaining an interictal study, the patient should be seizure-free for at least 30 minutes prior to the study. In general, a SOZ will demonstrate increased rCP (hyperperfusion), while IZs in the interictal state will reveal reduced rCP (hypoperfusion).

The time of injection for an ictal SPECT scan is imperative, because these studies may reveal seizure propagation patterns. In TLE there is propagation to the ipsilateral insula, basal ganglia, and frontal lobe, and propagation to the contralateral temporal lobe may also be present. With MTLE, ictal SPECT findings may be more localized when compared to NTLE and exhibit hyperperfusion medially with reduced rCP in the lateral temporal lobe up to 15 min after the seizure onset. Ictal SPECT may be more challenging in ETLE, because the seizures are often shorter in duration. In these cases early injection of the radionucleotide is crucial in identifying the seizure onset and propagation pattern (Figure 17.6).

Overall, for focal impaired-awareness seizures, ictal SPECT scans have a sensitivity ranging from 71–93% and approximately 90% for temporal lobe seizures.[52] The sensitivity for identifying an EZ in focal impaired-awareness seizures of extratemporal onset is somewhat lower with a sensitivity of approximately 75%.[52] Interictal SPECT scans are less sensitive than ictal studies and in TLE lateralize the EZ in 35–80% of cases.[82] The sensitivity

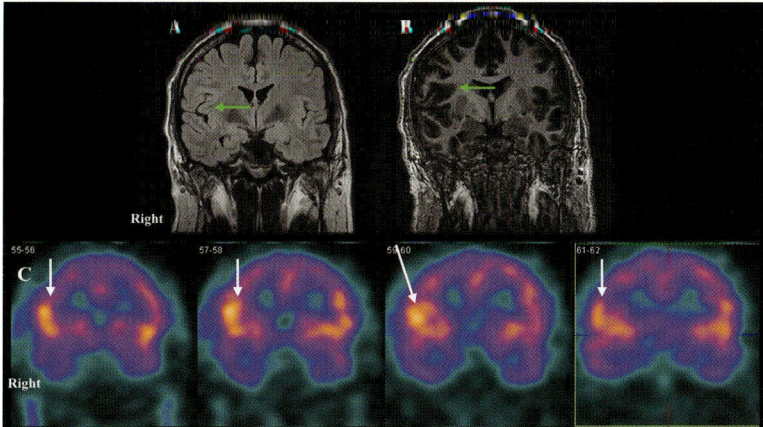

Figures 17.6 Ictal SPECT in a patient with frontal lobe epilepsy. The patient is a 33-year-old right-handed man with a history of drug-resistant focal epilepsy. His seizures begin with an arousal from sleep with throat parathesias that are followed by hyperkinetic movements without an overt loss of awareness. His scalp EEG was nonlocalizing and his brain MRI was initially reported as normal. (A) and (B) Brain MRI showing abnormal gyri and sulci within the right insula and operculum (arrows). (C) An ictal SPECT injected at seizure onset demonstrating hyperperfusion within the right insula and frontal operculum (arrows).

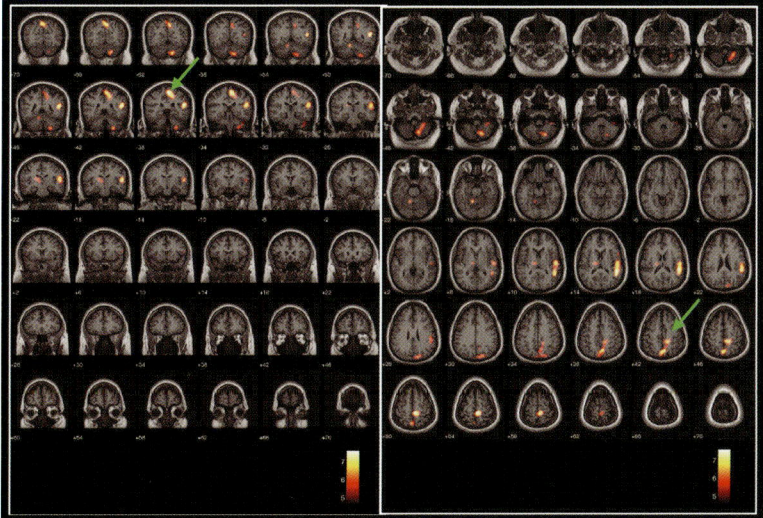

Figure 17.7 SISCOM in a patient with frontal lobe epilepsy. The patient is a 37 year old right handed woman with drug-resistant focal epilepsy. Her seizures begin with a nondescript sensation followed by urinary urgency and a subsequent loss of awareness. She also experiences focal evolving to bilateral tonic–clonic seizures. Her noninvasive diagnostic studies were initially nonlocalizing, but SISCOM demonstrated a focal area of hyperperfusion within the left rostral cingulate gyrus (arrows). Responsive neural stimulator implantation in this region resulted in marked improvement in her seizure frequency and severity.

of interictal SPECT in identifying the EZ in ETLE is even lower, ranging from 15–30%.[82] In general, ictal and interictal SPECT scans may be most beneficial for guidance of intracranial EEG (icEEG) implantation.[52]

Subtracted ictal SPECT coregistered to MRI (SISCOM) may provide improved localization of an EZ and further guide icEEG implantation strategies (Figure 17.7).[52,82] A SISCOM image is produced by coregistering the difference between ictal and interictal SPECT studies with the patient's structural brain MRI and may be most beneficial in MRI-negative cases, multiple epileptic lesions, discordant structural imaging and EEG findings, and seizure recurrence following epilepsy surgery.[82] Early studies of SISCOM demonstrated localization of an EZ in 86% of patients with dysplasia who were MRI-negative.[83] A more recent meta-analysis of SISCOM in the epilepsy presurgical evaluation reported positive and concordant rates of 85.9% and 65.3%, respectively, including an 83.8% SISCOM-positive rate in MRI-negative patients.[84] Additionally, of 178 surgical patients with concordant SISCOM, the pooled positive predictive value was 56%.[84] Finally, concordant SISCOM was associated with a higher seizure-free odds ratio compared to discordant SISCOM.[84]

Another functional neuroimaging modality is proton magnetic resonance spectroscopy (MRS). This imaging technique differs from SPECT and PET in that PET and SPECT cover the entire brain, while MRS primarily covers limited large voxels. Proton-MRS measures proton metabolite concentrations in the brain, providing an assessment of neuronal integrity through quantification of the N-acetylaspartate (NAA) peak compared to concentrations of choline or creatine peaks. Reductions in signal intensity of NAA can lateralize and localize an epileptogenic focus in focal epilepsies, particularly MTLE. Additionally, NAA may be a marker of epileptogenicity.[4] There are several limitations with proton-MRS. Clinically, in regard to findings in MTLE, NAA changes are frequently present bilaterally. Although NAA may be a marker of epileptogenic activity, it is also a measurement of neuronal density. These findings may cloud clinical decision-making. Technically, there is poor signal-to-noise ratio with proton-MRS and perhaps most importantly only a small area of brain is analyzed.[4]

PET, SPECT, and proton-MRS are predominantly used to approximate the IZ, SOZ, and possibly the EZ, while fMRI is a functional imaging modality primarily utilized to identify eloquent cortices.[52–54,82] However, EEG-fMRI may be employed to detect IZs as well as SOZs in people with focal epilepsy[55,85–87] and may provide insight into the generation of generalized epileptiform discharges.[41,42,45,88] Currently the standard fMRI technique is blood-oxygen-level dependent (BOLD) imaging. This measurement detects signal changes in venous flow as a result of excessive deoxyhemoglobin after an increase in perfusion during brain activation.[82] The BOLD changes appear bright on fMRI, but are small and require high-field MRI scanners, preferably 3 T MRI.[52]

In people with drug-resistant focal epilepsy, epilepsy surgery may be a viable treatment option. For individuals who may undergo resective surgery, localization of eloquent cortices, e.g., language centers, somatosensory cortex, primary visual cortex, etc., is imperative to minimize postoperative complications. Resective surgeries, such as anterior temporal lobectomy, may place patients at risk for postoperative memory and language impairments.[89,90] The use of fMRI can reduce the risk of these potential complications.

Language lateralization and localization is the most common clinical indication for fMRI.[82] However, the identification of language centers in the brain can be complex. The majority of people are primarily left-hemisphere dominant for expressive and receptive language, but people with epilepsy, particularly those with an epilepsy onset prior to the age of 7 years or with developmental lesions, e.g., MCD, may exhibit atypical language representation.[52]

A 2011 meta-analysis outlining the utility of fMRI in lateralizing and localizing language centers revealed a high correlation between fMRI language mapping and the Wada procedure, with a sensitivity of 83.5% and specificity of 88.1% for the identification of atypical

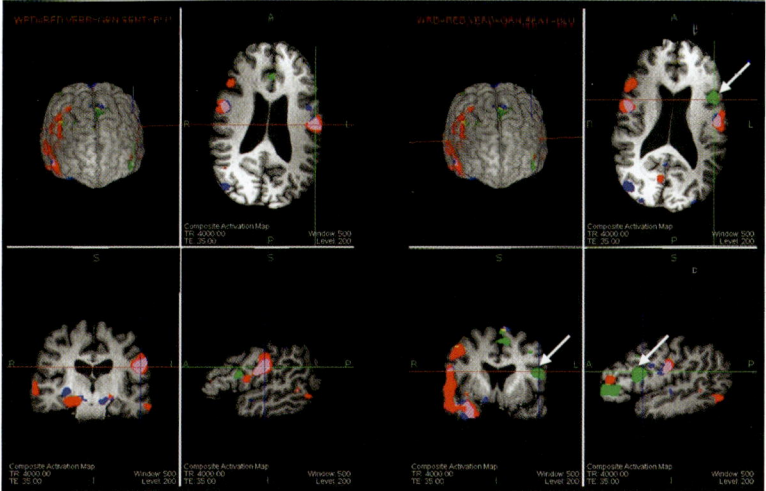

Figure 17.8 fMRI language testing in a patient with right MTLE. The patient is a 47-year-old right-handed woman with drug-resistant MTLE. Her seizures consist of impaired awareness, often with speech arrest. Language testing revealed bilateral language representation with a possible suggestion of left lateralization for expressive speech (arrow).

language lateralization with fMRI.[91] A more recent meta-analysis compared fMRI with the Wada procedure and demonstrated similar findings across 31 studies with a sensitivity for fMRI of 88.7% and specificity of 74.1% (Figure 17.8).[92] Functional MRI has also been used in combination with DTI to lateralize language function.[54] In one study, a logistic regression model incorporating DTI of the arcuate fasciculus, fMRI activity in Broca's area, and handedness correctly identified language lateralization according to their Wada score in 95.6% of cases.[54] The use of DWI tractography with maximum a posteriori probability (DWI-MAP) in language lateralization was studied in conjunction with fMRI language areas and electrical stimulation mapping.[53] DWI-MAP predicted language-activation areas on fMRI in normal developing children and children with focal epilepsy with an accuracy of 77% and up to 82%, respectively.[53] In addition, decreased volumes in DWI-MAP-defined pathways after epilepsy surgery were associated with postoperative language deficits.[53]

Motor and sensory cortex localization may be obtained with fMRI as well. These studies can be completed quickly with finger tapping (motor localization) or finger tapping and/or a hand squeeze (sensory localization) and typically demonstrate activation around the central sulcus. In addition, visual and auditory brain regions can be localized with fMRI via flashing checkerboard or tones, respectively.[52]

MEG is a neurophysiology study included as a functional imaging technique based primarily on magnetic source imaging (MSI). It is a noninvasive test that directly measures neuronal signaling by recording the magnetic flux created from dendritic, intracellular, electrical currents from the surface of the head. In this regard, MEG offers unique advantages over other functional imaging modalities that measure brain activity via cerebral metabolism or rCP. It also has excellent temporal and spatial resolution with a temporal resolution of less than 1 ms and spatial resolution primarily within millimeters.[93–99]

The most accepted and widely used MEG measurement is the single equivalent current dipole (ECD).[96–99] With the implementation of various parameters, e.g., confidence volume

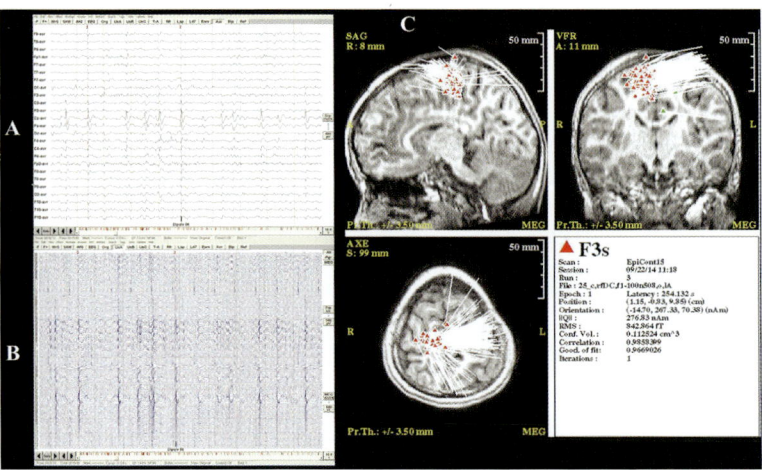

Figure 17.9 MEG ECD cluster in mesial frontal lobe epilepsy. The patient is a 9-year-old ambidextrous girl with drug-resistant focal epilepsy. Her seizures manifested as rhythmic clonic movements of the left lower extremity with left leg and hip flexion. On other occasions she would experience dizziness without a loss of awareness. Her EEG (A) and concomitant MEG (B) demonstrated nearly continuous midline sharp-and-wave discharges. Single ECD analysis revealed a cluster of dipoles within the right mesial frontal lobe (C, triangles).

and goodness of fit,[100] the ECD is coregistered to the patient's brain MRI to reveal the estimated source localization.[101] Therefore, MEG/MSI with the ECD is most clinically useful and appropriate when there is a reason to believe that the measured field at a particular time point is generated by a single source (Figure 17.9).[56]

Several studies have illustrated the utility of MEG/MSI with ECD in localizing the IZ and EZ. In one case series published in 2003, MSI localization agreed with the resected lobe in 89% of cases.[57] In a prospective study comparing MEG/MSI with icEEG, MEG/MSI localized the EZ at nearly the same proportion as icEEG, 65.3% compared to 69.4%, respectively.[59] More recently a retrospective cohort study of people with focal epilepsy who underwent MEG and surgical resection reported concordant and specific MEG findings predicting seizure freedom with an odds ratio of 5.11.[61] A retrospective study of 50 patients who underwent MEG followed by stereotactic EEG (sEEG) demonstrated one single tight cluster of ECDs were more likely to become seizure-free after surgery compared to patients without a tight cluster.[62]

As noted above, MEG has clinical value in the noninvasive presurgical mapping of eloquent cortices for people preparing for surgical interventions.[63,96–99] The somatosensory evoked fields from the somatosensory cortex can be reliably and reproducibly mapped with MEG/MSI.[99] Localization of the auditory cortex via MEG was illustrated in the early 1980s and the use of auditory evoked fields has aided in the localization of the primary auditory cortex on the superior temporal gyrus.[99] Visual evoked fields may be measured when attempting to localize the primary visual cortex and can be used to guide intracranial surgeries.[64,99,102–104]

Another promising area of MEG is in regard to lateralizing, and possibly localizing, language centers in the brain.[99] In a study of 100 epilepsy surgical patients, MEG/MSI using an ECD was compared to the Wada procedure and displayed a high degree of concordance (87%).[105] Bowyer et al. demonstrated similar results using a current distribution technique (in place of FCD).[106] More recently, a study of 10 right handed adolescents compared MEG with fMRI and revealed MEG and fMRI were 100% concordant with picture verb generation and 75% concordant with word verb generation.[107] Overall, the literature suggests MEG provides results comparable to the Wada procedure, and possibly fMRI, in language lateralization.[99,105–109]

17.3 New Frontiers in Neuroimaging

If the 1990s were designated the decade of the brain, the 2000s could be considered the era of neuroimaging. From the initiation of the Human Connectome Project in July 2009 to the launch of the Brain Research through Advancing Innovative Neurotechnologies (BRAIN Initiative) in April 2013, there has been considerable investment in research and development in the expansion of neuroimaging capabilities.[110,111] Perhaps one of the most clinically promising developments and emerging frontiers in brain imaging in people with epilepsy is in postprocessing techniques, which increase the sensitivity of identifying subtle epileptic lesions in otherwise MRI-negative focal epilepsy.

Voxel-based morphometry (VBM) is a postprocessing technique that may augment regions of abnormality in individuals with identifiable epileptic lesions, as well as distinguish previously unidentified epileptic lesions. In MTLE, VBM has routinely demonstrated gray matter reductions in MTLE outside the hippocampus, involving the adjacent limbic structures and the frontal and temporal lobes.[77] In ETLE, VBM may increase the ability to identify previously unidentified epileptic lesions. In MRI-negative patients, VBM has revealed a 43% detection rate for previously unidentified lesions.[112–114]

Other postprocessing techniques, such as volumetry, cortical thickness, and shape analysis may aid in the augmentation or identification of potentially epileptic lesions. In addition, computational models of FCD may be employed. These models, first introduced by Bernasconi, quantify cortical thickening and signal hyperintensity with the evaluation of the gray–white matter transition. This may provide a more comprehensive analysis of the variable morphologic features related to different forms of FCD and may also increase the sensitivity of detecting FCD.[77]

Another post-processing technique, sulcal morphometry, may increase the identification of bottom-of-the-sulcus dysplasia.[77] Recall that deepened sulci may be a sign of FCD and some studies have noted up to 85% of small FCD eluding visual detection are present at the bottom of an abnormally deep sulcus.[115] Identification of these abnormalities is imperative, because the chance for seizure freedom increases significantly if identified and resected, especially in bottom-of-the-sulcus dysplasia.[116]

Beyond the identification of epileptic lesions, advanced neuroimaging techniques may be employed to localize eloquent cortices. More detailed fMRI studies applying DTI or DWI may aid in detection of eloquent brain centers and pathways.[53,54] A growing area of research has focused on the use of fMRI in the assessment of memory and cognitive functions, although it remains challenging at this time.

17.4 Conclusions

Neuroimaging provides invaluable information in the diagnosis and management of epilepsies. Structural brain MRI is the standard of care in people with epilepsy. Functional neuroimaging techniques, such as PET, SPECT, fMRI, and MEG, have augmented structural brain MRI in identifying epileptic lesions and expanded the understanding of epileptic networks and eloquent cortices. The implementation of MRI postprocessing techniques has further improved the ability to detect subtle brain abnormalities and increased the understanding of the EZ. Continued investment toward research and development of neuroimaging techniques will further bolster its utility in the evaluation and better management of patients with epilepsy.

References

1. Chugani HT, Kumar A. Historical perspectives of neuroimaging in epilepsy. In: Chugani HT, ed., *Neuroimaging in Epilepsy*. Oxford: Oxford University Press; 2010:3–7.

2. Shorvon S. The surgical therapy of epilepsy. In: Shorvon S, ed., *Handbook of Epilepsy Treatment*. 3rd edn. Oxford: Wiley-Blackwell; 2010:314–364.

3. Falconer MA. Place of surgery for temporal lobe epilepsy during childhood. *Br Med J.* 1972;2(5814):631–635.

4. Cendes F. Neuroimaging in investigation of patients with epilepsy. *Continuum (Minneap Minn).* 2013;19(3 Epilepsy):623–642.

5. Luedke MW, Gallentine WB. Structural neuroimaging. In: Husain AM, ed., *Practical Epilepsy*. New York: Demos Medical Publishing; 2016:200–218.

6. Sostman HD, Spencer DD, Gore JC, et al. Preliminary observations on magnetic resonance imaging in refractory epilepsy. *Magn Reson Imaging.* 1984;2(4):301–306.

7. Commission on Neuroimaging of the International League Against Epilepsy. Recommendations for neuroimaging of patients with epilepsy. *Epilepsia.* 1997;38 (11):1255–1256.

8. Budde J, Shajan G, Hoffmann J, Ugurbil K, Pohmann R. Human imaging at 9.4 T using T(2) *-, phase-, and susceptibility-weighted contrast. *Magn Reson Med.* 2011;65 (2):544–550.

9. van der Kolk AG, Hendrikse J, Zwanenburg JJ, Visser F, Luijten PR. Clinical applications of 7 T MRI in the brain. *Eur J Radiol.* 2013;82(5):708–718.

10. Moosa ANV, Ruggieri PM. Magnetic resonance imaging in evaluation for epilepsy surgery. In: Wyllie E, ed., *Wyllie's*

Treatment of Epilepsy: Principles and Practice. 6th edn. Philadelphia: Wolters Kluwer; 2015:794–809.

11. Jack CR, Jr., Rydberg CH, Krecke KN, et al. Mesial temporal sclerosis: diagnosis with fluid-attenuated inversion-recovery versus spin-echo MR imaging. *Radiology.* 1996;199(2):367–373.

12. Diehl B, Najm I, Ruggieri P, et al. Periictal diffusion-weighted imaging in a case of lesional epilepsy. *Epilepsia.* 1999;40 (11):1667–1671.

13. Katramados AM, Burdette D, Patel SC, et al. Periictal diffusion abnormalities of the thalamus in partial status epilepticus. *Epilepsia.* 2009;50(2):265–275.

14. Hufnagel A, Weber J, Marks S, et al. Brain diffusion after single seizures. *Epilepsia.* 2003;44(1):54–63.

15. Muhlhofer W, Tan YL, Mueller SG, Knowlton R. MRI-negative temporal lobe epilepsy-what do we know? *Epilepsia.* 2017;58(5):727–742.

16. So EL, Ryvlin P. Scope and implications of MRI-negative refractory focal epilepsy. In: So EL, Ryvlin P, eds., *MRI-Negative Epilepsy: Evaluation and Surgical Management*. Cambridge: Cambridge University Press; 2015:1–5.

17. Hauptman JS, Mathern GW. Surgical treatment of epilepsy associated with cortical dysplasia: 2012 update. *Epilepsia.* 2012;53(Suppl 4):98–104.

18. Knake S, Triantafyllou C, Wald LL, et al. 3T phased array MRI improves the presurgical evaluation in focal epilepsies: a prospective study. *Neurology.* 2005;65(7):1026–1031.

19. Tatum WO, IV. Mesial temporal lobe epilepsy. *J Clin Neurophysiol.* 2012;29 (5):356–365.

20. Cendes F, Theodore WH, Brinkmann BH, Sulc V, Cascino GD. Neuroimaging of

epilepsy. *Handb Clin Neurol* 2016;136:985–1014.

21. Kuzniecky RI, Bilir E, Gilliam F, et al. Multimodality MRI in mesial temporal sclerosis: relative sensitivity and specificity. *Neurology*. 1997;49(3):774–778.

22. Mischel PS, Nguyen LP, Vinters HV. Cerebral cortical dysplasia associated with pediatric epilepsy. Review of neuropathologic features and proposal for a grading system. *J Neuropathol Exp Neurol*. 1995;54(2):137–153.

23. Palmini A, Najm I, Avanzini G, et al. Terminology and classification of the cortical dysplasias. *Neurology*. 2004;62(6 Suppl 3):S2–8.

24. Blumcke I, Thom M, Aronica E, et al. The clinicopathologic spectrum of focal cortical dysplasias: a consensus classification proposed by an ad hoc task force of the ILAE Diagnostic Methods Commission. *Epilepsia*. 2011;52(1):158–174.

25. Lapalme-Remis S, Cascino GD. Imaging for adults with seizures and epilepsy. *Continuum (Minneap Minn)*. 2016;22(5, Neuroimaging):1451–1479.

26. Barkovich AJ, Kuzniecky RI, Bollen AW, Grant PE. Focal transmantle dysplasia: a specific malformation of cortical development. *Neurology*. 1997;49 (4):1148–1152.

27. Leventer RJ, Guerrini R, Dobyns WB. Malformations of cortical development and epilepsy. *Dialogues Clin Neurosci*. 2008;10 (1):47–62.

28. DiMario FJ, Jr., Sahin M, Ebrahimi-Fakhari D. Tuberous sclerosis complex. *Pediatr Clin North Am*. 2015;62(3):633–648.

29. Gallagher A, Grant EP, Madan N, et al. MRI findings reveal three different types of tubers in patients with tuberous sclerosis complex. *J Neurol*. 2010;257(8):1373–1381.

30. Yogi A, Hirata Y, Karavaeva E, et al. DTI of tuber and perituberal tissue can predict epileptogenicity in tuberous sclerosis complex. *Neurology*. 2015;85 (23):2011–2015.

31. Chugani DC, Chugani HT, Muzik O, et al. Imaging epileptogenic tubers in children with tuberous sclerosis complex using alpha-[11C]methyl-L-tryptophan positron emission tomography. *Ann Neurol*. 1998;44 (6):858–866.

32. Batista CEA, Chugani DC, Chugani HT. Alpha-[11C]methyl-L-tryptophan positron emission tomography. In: Chugani HT, ed., *Neuroimaging in Epilepsy*. Oxford: Oxford University Press; 2010:186–198.

33. Chugani DC. Alpha-methyl-L-tryptophan: mechanisms for tracer localization of epileptogenic brain regions. *Biomark Med*. 2011;5(5):567–575.

34. Wu JY, Sutherling WW, Koh S, et al. Magnetic source imaging localizes epileptogenic zone in children with tuberous sclerosis complex. *Neurology*. 2006;66(8):1270–1272.

35. Shukla G, Kazutaka J, Gupta A, et al. Magnetoencephalographic identification of epileptic focus in children with generalized electroencephalographic (EEG) features but focal imaging abnormalities. *J Child Neurol*. 2017;32(12):981–995.

36. Rosenow F, Alonso-Vanegas MA, Baumgartner C, et al. Cavernoma-related epilepsy: review and recommendations for management – report of the Surgical Task Force of the ILAE Commission on Therapeutic Strategies. *Epilepsia*. 2013;54 (12):2025–2035.

37. Quek AM, Britton JW, McKeon A, et al. Autoimmune epilepsy: clinical characteristics and response to immunotherapy. *Arch Neurol*. 2012;69 (5):582–593.

38. Hoftberger R, van Sonderen A, Leypoldt F, et al. Encephalitis and AMPA receptor antibodies: novel findings in a case series of 22 patients. *Neurology*. 2015;84 (24):2403–2412.

39. Camfield PR. Definition and natural history of Lennox-Gastaut syndrome. *Epilepsia*. 2011;52(Suppl 5):3–9.

40. Betting LE, Mory SB, Lopes-Cendes I, et al. MRI reveals structural abnormalities in patients with idiopathic generalized epilepsy. *Neurology*. 2006;67(5):848–852.

41. Meencke HJ. Neuron density in the molecular layer of the frontal cortex in

primary generalized epilepsy. *Epilepsia*. 1985;26(5):450–454.

42. Meencke HJ, Janz D. Neuropathological findings in primary generalized epilepsy: a study of eight cases. *Epilepsia*. 1984;25 (1):8–21.

43. Benuzzi F, Mirandola L, Pugnaghi M, et al. Increased cortical BOLD signal anticipates generalized spike and wave discharges in adolescents and adults with idiopathic generalized epilepsies. *Epilepsia*. 2012;53 (4):622–630.

44. Benuzzi F, Ballotta D, Mirandola L, et al. An EEG-fMRI study on the termination of generalized spike-and-wave discharges in absence epilepsy. *PLoS One*. 2015;10(7): e0130943.

45. Vollmar C, O'Muircheartaigh J, Symms MR, et al. Altered microstructural connectivity in juvenile myoclonic epilepsy: the missing link. *Neurology*. 2012;78 (20):1555–1559.

46. Wandschneider B, Thompson PJ, Vollmar C, Koepp MJ. Frontal lobe function and structure in juvenile myoclonic epilepsy: a comprehensive review of neuropsychological and imaging data. *Epilepsia*. 2012;53(12):2091–2098.

47. Zhang CH, Sha Z, Mundahl J, et al. Thalamocortical relationship in epileptic patients with generalized spike and wave discharges – a multimodal neuroimaging study. *Neuroimage Clin*. 2015;9:117–127.

48. Stefan H, Paulini-Ruf A, Hopfengartner R, Rampp S. Network characteristics of idiopathic generalized epilepsies in combined MEG/EEG. *Epilepsy Res*. 2009;85 (2–3):187–198.

49. Elshahabi A, Klamer S, Sahib AK, Lerche H, Braun C, Focke NK. Magnetoencephalography reveals a widespread increase in network connectivity in idiopathic/genetic generalized epilepsy. *PLoS One*. 2015;10(9): e0138119.

50. de Leon SC, Niso G, Canuet L, et al. Praxis-induced seizures in a patient with juvenile myoclonic epilepsy: MEG-EEG coregistration study. *Epilepsy Behav Case Rep*. 2016;5:1–5.

51. Spanaki MV, Kopylev L, DeCarli C, et al. Postoperative changes in cerebral metabolism in temporal lobe epilepsy. *Arch Neurol*. 2000;57(10):1447–1452.

52. Oldan J, Wong T, Petrella J. Functional neuroimaging. In: Husain AM, ed., *Practical epilepsy*. New York: Demos Medical Publishing; 2016:219–228.

53. Jeong JW, Asano E, Juhasz C, Chugani HT. Localization of specific language pathways using diffusion-weighted imaging tractography for presurgical planning of children with intractable epilepsy. *Epilepsia*. 2015;56(1):49–57.

54. Ellmore TM, Beauchamp MS, Breier JI, et al. Temporal lobe white matter asymmetry and language laterality in epilepsy patients. *Neuroimage*. 2010;49 (3):2033–2044.

55. Khoo HM, Hao Y, von Ellenrieder N, et al. The hemodynamic response to interictal epileptic discharges localizes the seizure-onset zone. *Epilepsia*. 2017;58(5):811–823.

56. Papanicolaou AC. Basic concepts. In: Papanicolaou AC, ed. *Clinical Magnetoencephalography and Magnetic Source Imaging*. New York: Cambridge University Press; 2009:3–6.

57. Stefan H, Hummel C, Scheler G, et al. Magnetic brain source imaging of focal epileptic activity: a synopsis of 455 cases. *Brain*. 2003;126(Pt 11):2396–2405.

58. Fischer MJ, Scheler G, Stefan H. Utilization of magnetoencephalography results to obtain favourable outcomes in epilepsy surgery. *Brain*. 2005;128(Pt 1):153–157.

59. Knowlton RC, Elgavish R, Howell J, et al. Magnetic source imaging versus intracranial electroencephalogram in epilepsy surgery: a prospective study. *Ann Neurol*. 2006;59(5):835–842.

60. Almubarak S, Alexopoulos A, Von-Podewils F, et al. The correlation of magnetoencephalography to intracranial EEG in localizing the epileptogenic zone: a study of the surgical resection outcome. *Epilepsy Res*. 2014;108(9):1581–1590.

61. Englot DJ, Nagarajan SS, Imber BS, et al. Epileptogenic zone localization using magnetoencephalography predicts seizure

freedom in epilepsy surgery. *Epilepsia*
2015;56(6):949–958.

62. Murakami H, Wang ZI, Marashly A, et al.
Correlating magnetoencephalography to
stereo-electroencephalography in patients
undergoing epilepsy surgery. *Brain*.
2016;139(11):2935–2947.

63. Burgess RC, Funke ME, Bowyer SM, et al.
American Clinical
Magnetoencephalography Society clinical
practice guideline 2: presurgical functional
brain mapping using magnetic evoked
fields. *J Clin Neurophysiol*. 2011;28
(4):355–361.

64. Nakasato N, Seki K, Fujita S, et al. Clinical
application of visual evoked fields using an
MRI-linked whole head MEG system.
Front Med Biol Eng. 1996;7(4):
275–283.

65. Simos PG, Breier JI, Zouridakis G,
Papanicolaou AC. Identification of
language-specific brain activity using
magnetoencephalography. *J Clin Exp
Neuropsychol*. 1998;20(5):706–722.

66. Bowyer SM, Moran JE, Mason KM, et al.
MEG localization of language-specific
cortex utilizing MR-FOCUSS. *Neurology*.
2004;62(12):2247–2255.

67. Baumgartner C, Doppelbauer A, Deecke L,
et al. Neuromagnetic investigation of
somatotopy of human hand somatosensory
cortex. *Exp Brain Res*. 1991;87(3):641–648.

68. Koepp MJ. [11C]flumazenil positron
emission tomography. In: Chugani HT, ed.,
Neuroimaging in Epilepsy. Oxford: Oxford
University Press; 2010:174–185.

69. Burdette DE, Sakurai SY, Henry TR, et al.
Temporal lobe central benzodiazepine
binding in unilateral mesial temporal lobe
epilepsy. *Neurology*. 1995;45(5):934–941.

70. Spencer SS. Neural networks in human
epilepsy: evidence of and implications for
treatment. *Epilepsia*. 2002;43(3):219–227.

71. Horky LL, Treves ST. PET and SPECT in
brain tumors and epilepsy. *Neurosurg Clin
N Am*. 2011;22(2):169–184, viii.

72. Moore KR, Funke ME, Constantino T,
Katzman GL, Lewine JD.
Magnetoencephalographically directed

review of highspatialresolution surface-
coil MR images improves lesion detection
in patients with extratemporal epilepsy.
Radiology. 2002;225(3):880–887.

73. Funke ME, Moore K, Orrison WW, Jr.,
Lewine JD. The role of
magnetoencephalography in "nonlesional"
epilepsy. *Epilepsia*. 2011;52(Suppl 4):10–14.

74. Salamon N, Kung J, Shaw SJ, et al. FDG-
PET/MRI coregistration improves
detection of cortical dysplasia in patients
with epilepsy. *Neurology*. 2008;71
(20):1594–1601.

75. Chugani HT, Kumar A, Kupsky W, et al.
Clinical and histopathologic correlates of
11C-alpha-methyl-L-tryptophan (AMT)
PET abnormalities in children with
intractable epilepsy. *Epilepsia*. 2011;52
(9):1692–1698.

76. Perissinotti A, Setoain X, Aparicio J, et al.
Clinical role of subtraction ictal SPECT
coregistered to MR imaging and (18)
F-FDG PET in pediatric epilepsy. *J Nucl
Med*. 2014;55(7):1099–1105.

77. Wang ZI, Jones SE, Bernasconi A. MRI
postprocessing techniques and clinical
applications. In: Wyllie E, ed., *Wyllie's
Treatment of Epilepsy: Principles and
Practice*. New York: Wolters Kluwer;
2015:848–854.

78. Brinkmann BH, Sulc V. Multimodality
image coregistration for MRI-negative
epilepsy surgery. In: So EL, Ryvlin P, eds.,
*MRI-Negative Epilepsy: Evaluation and
Surgical Management*. Cambridge:
Cambridge University Press;
2015:80–89.

79. Chugani DC, Muzik O. Alpha[C-
11]methyl-L-tryptophan PET maps brain
serotonin synthesis and kynurenine
pathway metabolism. *J Cereb Blood Flow
Metab*. 2000;20(1):2–9.

80. Chugani HT, Luat AF, Kumar A, et al.
Alpha-[11C]-Methyl-L-tryptophan – PET
in 191 patients with tuberous sclerosis
complex. *Neurology*. 2013;81(7):674–680.

81. Chugani HT, Ilyas M, Kumar A, et al.
Surgical treatment for refractory epileptic
spasms: the Detroit series. *Epilepsia*.
2015;56(12):1941–1949.

82. Bargallo Alabart N, Setoain Parego X. [Imaging in epilepsy: functional studies]. *Radiologia (Roma)*. 2012;54(2):124–136.

83. O'Brien TJ, So EL, Cascino GD, et al. Subtraction SPECT coregistered to MRI in focal malformations of cortical development: localization of the epileptogenic zone in epilepsy surgery candidates. *Epilepsia*. 2004;45(4):367–376.

84. Chen T, Guo L. The role of SISCOM in preoperative evaluation for patients with epilepsy surgery: a meta-analysis. *Seizure*. 2016;41:43–50.

85. Watanabe S, Dubeau F, Zazubovits N, Gotman J. Temporal lobe spikes: EEG-fMRI contributions to the "mesial vs. lateral" debate. *Clin Neurophysiol*. 2017;128 (6):986–991.

86. Coan AC, Campos BM, Beltramini GC, et al. Distinct functional and structural MRI abnormalities in mesial temporal lobe epilepsy with and without hippocampal sclerosis. *Epilepsia*. 2014;55(8):1187–1196.

87. An D, Fahoum F, Hall J, et al. Electroencephalography/functional magnetic resonance imaging responses help predict surgical outcome in focal epilepsy. *Epilepsia*. 2013;54(12):2184–2194.

88. Kay B, Szaflarski JP. EEG/fMRI contributions to our understanding of genetic generalized epilepsies. *Epilepsy Behav*. 2014;34:129–135.

89. Wiebe S, Jette N. Pharmacoresistance and the role of surgery in difficult to treat epilepsy. *Nat Rev Neurol*. 2012;8 (12):669–677.

90. Sherman EM, Wiebe S, Fay-McClymont TB, et al. Neuropsychological outcomes after epilepsy surgery: systematic review and pooled estimates. *Epilepsia*. 2011;52 (5):857–869.

91. Dym RJ, Burns J, Freeman K, Lipton ML. Is functional MR imaging assessment of hemispheric language dominance as good as the Wada test?: a meta-analysis. *Radiology*. 2011;261(2):446–455.

92. Massot-Tarrus A, Mousavi SR, Mirsattari SM. Comparing the intracarotid amobarbital test and functional MRI for the presurgical evaluation of language in epilepsy. *Curr Neurol Neurosci Rep*. 2017;17 (7):54.

93. Cohen D. Magnetoencephalography: evidence of magnetic fields produced by alpha-rhythm currents. *Science*. 1968;161 (3843):784–786.

94. Cohen D. Magnetoencephalography: detection of the brain's electrical activity with a superconducting magnetometer. *Science*. 1972;175(4022):664–666.

95. Rosenow F, Luders H. Presurgical evaluation of epilepsy. *Brain*. 2001;124(Pt 9):1683–1700.

96. ACMEGS Position Statement Committee: Bagic A, Funke ME, Ebersole J. American Clinical MEG Society (ACMEGS) position statement: the value of magnetoencephalography (MEG)/magnetic source imaging (MSI) in noninvasive presurgical evaluation of patients with medically intractable localization-related epilepsy. *J Clin Neurophysiol*. 2009;26 (4):290–293.

97. ACMEGS Clinical Practice Guideline Committee: Bagic AI, Knowlton RC, Rose DF, Ebersole JS. American Clinical Magnetoencephalography Society clinical practice guideline 1: recording and analysis of spontaneous cerebral activity. *J Clin Neurophysiol*. 2011;28(4):348–354.

98. ACMEGS Clinical Practice Guideline Committee: Bagic AI, Barkley GL, Rose DF, Ebersole JS. American Clinical Magnetoencephalography Society clinical practice guideline 4: qualifications of MEG-EEG personnel. *J Clin Neurophysiol*. 2011;28(4):364–365.

99. ACMEGS Position Statement Committee: Bagic AI, Bowyer SM, Kirsch HE, Funke ME, Burgess RC. American Clinical MEG Society (ACMEGS) position statement #2: the value of magnetoencephalography (MEG)/magnetic source imaging (MSI) in noninvasive presurgical mapping of eloquent cortices of patients preparing for surgical interventions. *J Clin Neurophysiol*. 2017;34(3):189–195.

100. Krupa K, Bekiesinska-Figatowska M. Artifacts in magnetic resonance imaging. *Pol J Radiol*. 2015;80:93–106.

101. Bowyer SM, Mason K, Tepley N, Smith D, Barkley GL. Magnetoencephalographic validation parameters for clinical evaluation of interictal epileptic activity. *J Clin Neurophysiol.* 2003;20(2):87–93.

102. Bagic AI. Disparities in clinical magnetoencephalography practice in the United States: a survey-based appraisal. *J Clin Neurophysiol.* 2011;28(4):341–347.

103. Grover KM, Bowyer SM, Rock J, et al. Retrospective review of MEG visual evoked hemifield responses prior to resection of temporo-parieto-occipital lesions. *J Neurooncol.* 2006;77(2):161–166.

104. Pang EW, Chu BH, Otsubo H. Occipital lobe lesions result in a displacement of magnetoencephalography visual evoked field dipoles. *J Clin Neurophysiol.* 2014;31 (5):456–461.

105. Papanicolaou AC, Simos PG, Castillo EM, et al. Magnetocephalography: a noninvasive alternative to the Wada procedure. *J Neurosurg.* 2004;100(5):867–876.

106. Bowyer SM, Moran JE, Weiland BJ, et al. Language laterality determined by MEG mapping with MR-FOCUSS. *Epilepsy Behav.* 2005;6(2):235–241.

107. Pang EW, Wang F, Malone M, Kadis DS, Donner EJ. Localization of Broca's area using verb generation tasks in the MEG: validation against fMRI. *Neurosci Lett.* 2011;490(3):215–219.

108. Stefan H, Rampp S, Knowlton RC. Magnetoencephalography adds to the surgical evaluation process. *Epilepsy Behav.* 2011;20(2):172–177.

109. Barkley GL, Baumgartner C. MEG and EEG in epilepsy. *J Clin Neurophysiol.* 2003;20(3):163–178.

110. Mark and Mary Stevens Neuroimaging and Informatics Institute, University of Southern California. Human Connectome Project. http:// www.humanconnectomeproject.org/. Accessed April 3, 2019.

111. National Institute of Health, US Department of Health and Human Services. The BRAIN initiative. https:// www.braininitiative.nih.gov/. Accessed April 3, 2019.

112. Privitera M. Epilepsy treatment: a futurist view. *Epilepsy Curr.* 2017;17(4):204–213.

113. Wang ZI, Jones SE, Jaisani Z, et al. Voxel-based morphometric magnetic resonance imaging (MRI) postprocessing in MRI-negative epilepsies. *Ann Neurol.* 2015;77 (6):1060–1075.

114. Wang ZI, Jones SE, Ristic AJ, et al. Voxel-based morphometric MRI post-processing in MRI-negative focal cortical dysplasia followed by simultaneously recorded MEG and stereo-EEG. *Epilepsy Res.* 2012;100(1–2):188–193.

115. Besson P, Andermann F, Dubeau F, Bernasconi A. Small focal cortical dysplasia lesions are located at the bottom of a deep sulcus. *Brain.* 2008;131(Pt 12):3246–3255.

116. Harvey AS, Mandelstam SA, Maixner WJ, et al. The surgically remediable syndrome of epilepsy associated with bottom-of-sulcus dysplasia. *Neurology.* 2015;84 (20):2021–2028.

Chapter 18

The Role of Neuropsychology in Epilepsy Surgery

Brent A. Funk and Dana R. Connor

18.1 General Neuropsychology

Broadly speaking, clinical neuropsychology is an applied science concerned with the behavioral expression of brain dysfunction. A thorough clinical interview aimed at understanding previous and current functioning, as well as current factors that may influence the patient's performance on testing, is the foundation of a neuropsychological evaluation.[1] Comprehensive neuropsychological assessments aim to identify the patient's cognitive strengths and weaknesses, as well as to evaluate the status of overall brain function, different brain regions, and networks. Although there is no standard neuropsychological test battery, the following domains are typically assessed: performance validity, premorbid and intellectual functioning, attention and working memory, processing speed, language abilities, visuospatial skills, verbal and nonverbal learning and memory, executive functioning, and motor abilities. Objective measures of personality and affective functioning are also commonly administered.

18.2 Neuropsychology in Epilepsy

The histories of neuropsychology and epilepsy are fundamentally intertwined. As epilepsy surgery became a viable treatment option for medically intractable epilepsy in the early twentieth century, neurodiagnostics were limited to EEG alone, which at the time had a maximum of eight channels. Thus, close collaborations between neurosurgery, neurology, and neuropsychology were essential to characterize the nature of epilepsy, establish surgical candidacy, and guide surgical treatment. It was within this context of early epilepsy surgery that neuropsychology was first recognized to play a valuable diagnostic role clinically.[2]

In the tragic and now infamous case of patient H.M., neuropsychological assessment was essential in detailing the role of hippocampi in memory function following bilateral temporal lobectomy. Though H.M. was certainly not the first to undergo this drastic surgery, previous surgical cases had only been reported in terms of seizure control, rather than cognitive outcomes.[3] It was only in light of these neuropsychological findings that significant memory deficits were retrospectively identified in earlier bilateral temporal lobectomy patients. Consequently, in documenting the cognitive risks of epilepsy surgery, neuropsychology prompted the major topics of cognitive outcomes and quality of life issues in epilepsy, which continues today.[4]

18.2.1 Neuropsychology Roles in Epilepsy

In this new era of neurodiagnostic technologies, in which brain imaging and EEG efficiently and accurately assess anatomical or neurophysiological abnormalities, clinical neuropsychologists no longer serve the primary purpose of diagnosing a patient's type of epilepsy or seizure etiology. Rather, as it has been consistently shown that even the most homogenous neurologic syndromes with well-demonstrated lesions on neuroimaging can differ widely across individuals, neuropsychology plays the unique role of quantifying the functional impact of epilepsy and its treatment on a patient's cognition and behavior. Although the role of neuropsychology in epilepsy has undoubtedly evolved, it remains a vital component of the comprehensive epilepsy program.

Neuropsychology is especially valuable in treatment planning, as the assessment can assist in ascertaining an individual's functional abilities and disabilities, detecting focal dysfunction, identifying potential risks and benefits of treatment options, and providing nonmedical treatment recommendations, within the context of an individual's neurocognitive and psychosocial status. Furthermore, neuropsychological assessment may find cognitive abilities that are inconsistent with what would be expected based on anatomic findings. Such discrepancies are significant as they may indicate, for example, an unsuspected atypical representation of language. Therefore, integrating neuropsychological findings with data from multiple sources allows for the most comprehensive picture for individual patients.[5] Finally, clinical neuropsychologists' expertise in brain–behavior relationships can assist in distinguishing between epileptic versus psychogenic nonepileptic seizures (PNES), which make up 15–30% of referrals to tertiary epilepsy centers.[6]

18.2.2 Factors Associated with Cognitive Decline in Epilepsy

It is well known that cognitive impairment can be associated with chronic epilepsy. However, studies examining cognition in children with epilepsy have found that cognitive deficits often predate the first seizure, implicating a pre-existent neuropathology associated with underlying epileptogenesis.[7,8] With the exception of an episode of status epilepticus, which can immediately damage the brain and result in stepwise cognitive declines, a single seizure does not permanently impair intellectual or behavioral abilities. Only frequent, poorly controlled seizures have been shown to result in morphological and functional changes within the brain.[9,10]

Neuropsychological impairments in individuals with epilepsy are the result of a synergistic combination of numerous reversible and irreversible factors. Potentially reversible factors affecting cognition in individuals with epilepsy include postictal dysfunction, effects of epilepsy treatment, and psychiatric comorbidity.[11] Irrevocable factors that may influence cognition are the etiology of epilepsy and the location of the epileptogenic focus. However, even largely homogenous epileptic syndromes, including mesial temporal lobe epilepsy, can exhibit varied neurocognitive symptoms across individuals. Other fixed factors associated with greater cognitive declines are seizure severity, higher frequency and lifetime number of seizures, longer duration of seizure disorder, younger age of seizure onset, and older current age.[12–14] Women with epilepsy are also at greater risk than their male counterparts for widespread cognitive deficits, though the reasons for this are unclear.[15]

18.2.3 Common Cognitive Deficits in Epilepsy

Naming and word-finding difficulties are the most frequently reported subjective cognitive complaint of patients with epilepsy.[16] Memory impairments, attentional difficulties, and mental slowness are also commonly reported in adults with epilepsy.[17] An individual's pattern of cognitive and functional deficits is, in part, dependent on the neurological pathophysiology of his or her epilepsy. For example, naming complaints are particularly prevalent in patients with temporal seizures originating in the language-dominant hemisphere.[18,19] Temporal lobe epilepsy (TLE) often leads to memory impairments, given the involvement of the hippocampus and the mesial temporal lobe, with the severity and form of memory impairment largely related to the extent and site of hippocampal atrophy.[11,20] Commonly known as the material-specific memory model, it was once largely accepted that left temporal lobe seizures were invariably related to deficits in verbal memory processes and right temporal lobe seizures resulted in visuospatial memory impairments.[21-23] However, it is now understood that the type of memory impairments exhibited is related to the language-dominant hemisphere, as individuals with lesions in the language-dominant temporal lobe experience impairments in the learning and retention of verbal material and those with lesions of the nondominant temporal lobe evidence impairments in nonverbal memory.[24-27]

In other epilepsies, changes in the thalamocortical network are associated with attention, language, and executive functioning deficits. Individuals with frontal lobe epilepsy often exhibit impaired executive functions and may also show deficits in memory, processing speed, and language. Epilepsies that impact the Sylvian and Rolandic regions of the brain primarily influence language abilities, and may also result in impaired attention and executive functioning.[11]

18.2.4 Other Factors Affecting Cognitive Performances Common in Epilepsy

18.2.4.1 Postictal State

Following a seizure, many individuals experience a period of poor memory, decreased concentration, and fatigue. As this postictal period can last from several minutes to hours, it is important for the neuropsychologist to assess for recent seizure activity and consider possible postictal effects on cognitive testing.

18.2.4.2 Antiseizure Drugs

Antiseizure drugs (ASDs) prevent seizure activity by decreasing membrane excitability, increasing postsynaptic inhibition, and altering synchronization of neural networks. Thus, by their very nature, virtually all ASDs have the potential for cognitive side effects, including psychomotor slowing, poor attention, and distractibility. Other side effects may include sedation, somnolence, insomnia, dizziness, and poor coordination, which can further impact cognitive efficiency and performance on neuropsychological assessment.[1,2,28] Among the various factors affecting cognitive functioning in patients with epilepsy, ASDs are unique, since medication choice is under the control of the physician and the patient. Fortunately, these adverse cognitive effects usually abate after dose reduction or cessation.[3,11]

Of older-generation ASDs, phenobarbital and phenytoin have evidenced the most significant cognitive side effects. The newer ASDs are less problematic in terms of their cognitive side-effect profile, impacting only about 5% of patients. In fact, certain newer medications are associated with subjective improvements in cognition for some patients (e.g., carbamazepine, clobazam, lamotrigine, levetiracetam). The exception to this is topiramate. Despite being highly effective in managing focal seizures, topiramate has been implicated in frontal lobe dysfunction, including reduced cognitive speed, verbal fluency, and short-term memory.[4]

18.2.4.3 Psychiatric Factors

Individuals with epilepsy experience greater rates of anxiety and depression than the greater population.[29] Comorbid psychiatric disorders and cognitive impairments are generally thought to be independent symptoms of epilepsy. However, it is widely accepted that depression can exacerbate cognitive inefficiencies, and psychological symptoms can be aggravated by awareness of cognitive impairments and their related psychosocial obstacles.

Depression is the most frequent psychiatric comorbidity of epilepsy[4] and has been found to result in poor attention, reduced memory performances, and slowed motor speed in some individuals. There is some research to suggest that depression has the greatest impact on cognition of individuals with left lateralized temporal lobe epilepsy.[30] Involvement of the left frontal lobe is also implicated in the convergence of depression, attention, and memory deficits in some individuals with epilepsy.[4]

18.3 Neuropsychology in Surgical Epilepsy

18.3.1 Purposes of Presurgical Evaluations

Despite advancements in the diagnosis and pharmacological treatment of epilepsy, approximately 30–40% of epilepsy patients remain resistant to AEDs to some degree.[31] For those individuals for whom seizures remain refractory to medical therapy, surgery is an increasingly viable treatment option. In conjunction with other exploratory techniques, neuropsychological evaluation is indicated for patients who are being considered for epilepsy surgery. This assessment serves multiple purposes including: (1) assisting in determining the site of cerebral dysfunction and functional correlates, (2) identifying possible lateralization of impairment, (3) assessing for risks of postsurgical cognitive impairment, (4) establishing a cognitive baseline, (5) assisting in predicting seizure control, and (6) identifying other risk factors for surgery. These functions will be discussed further in the sections below.

Localization and Lateralization

Neuropsychologists use multiple measures to evaluate for lateralization and localization of seizure focus, including language (e.g., naming), visuospatial, and verbal and visual memory measures to assess temporal lobe involvement. Patterns of sensory and fine motor impairment are also considered. Frontal lobe involvement is assessed with special consideration given to patterns of higher-order executive functioning performances.

Among temporal lobe epilepsy patients, the accuracy of neuropsychological assessment in lateralizing the seizure focus is found to be between 80% and 90%, which is similar to the accuracy rates of EEG and neuroimaging.[32–34] The sensitivity of neuropsychological assessment in localizing the epileptogenic zone is lower, ranging from 66% to 73%.[18,33] Overall, neuropsychological assessment is not sufficient alone in lateralizing and localizing the seizure focus, but can provide valuable information when taken together with results of EEG and MRI.

Identify Risks of Cognitive Impairment

Epilepsy surgery holds both the possibility of significant reduction of seizures and improved quality of life, as well as the risk of cognitive decline following surgery. Despite substantial variability in cognitive outcomes after epilepsy surgery, it is important to identify patients who are at a particularly high risk of postoperative declines.[35,36]

Postoperative cognitive declines can be thought of as the product of the functional adequacy of the resected tissue during surgery and the functional reserve of the remaining structures.[37] Thus, individuals who are at greatest risk of cognitive decline after temporal lobe surgery are those with resection of the language-dominant hemisphere and those in which the dysfunctional temporal lobe still actively contributes to memory functioning.[4] Not surprisingly, there is a greater risk for cognitive decline with more extensive resections.[38–40]

For patients undergoing language-dominant temporal lobe resection, immediate post-operative changes in language function, word-finding, and naming abilities are common.[41–43] Significant language deficits may persist in as many as 25% of these patients.[44] There is also a greater risk of verbal memory dysfunction postoperatively for these individuals.[45] In contrast, resection in the language nondominant hemisphere appears to have fewer neuropsychological consequences.[46]

The factors associated with postoperative memory decline are often indirect indicators of ipsilateral or contralateral hippocampal integrity in temporal lobe epilepsy. For instance, one of the most consistent risk factors for postsurgical cognitive decline is the presence of intact memory functioning preoperatively.[47] Likewise, individuals without hippocampal sclerosis have been found to be at greater risk of memory decline and naming deficits postsurgically.[48,49] Nonetheless, those individuals with stronger preoperative memory generally demonstrate better postoperative cognitive abilities than their low-baseline counterparts, given the reserve capacity of their preserved tissue. Put more simply, patients who have already "lost" memory function stand to lose far less postsurgically than their counterparts with largely intact memory and cognition. Importantly, individuals with low levels of cognitive reserve are more likely to experience functional declines.

Postoperative memory functioning also depends on a network of factors beyond those associated with hippocampal integrity.[3] Specifically, older age at time of surgery, lower baseline functioning, lower intellectual capacity, poorer seizure control, and female gender have been found to be associated with greater risk for cognitive decline.[4,15,40,50,51] Several of these factors have been found to have a primary effect on the neocortex and higher-order aspects of cognition, suggesting that the bilaterally disposed and less-specialized mesial structures are better able to compensate each other over a longer period than are cortical structures.[40,52]

Finally, results of neuropsychological assessment may be utilized to assist in determining whether an individual is a good candidate for surgical treatment. For example, if a right temporal lobectomy candidate exhibited significant verbal compared to nonverbal learning and memory deficits on testing, the patient would be at risk of limited memory capacity following resection of the presumably more functional right temporal lobe, and thus may be found inappropriate for surgery.

Establish Cognitive Baseline

The importance of establishing a cognitive baseline is twofold. First, given that an individual's reserve capacity preoperatively is significantly associated with postoperative cognitive risk, baseline neuropsychological performances should be considered in presurgical evaluations.[39,40] Second, obtaining a valid baseline of neurocognitive functioning assists in evaluating and interpreting postsurgical cognitive outcomes.[1,53]

Predict Seizure Control

Seizure freedom has been demonstrated to be an important factor in neuropsychological outcomes, including long-term memory functioning.[38,54] As many as 25% of patients demonstrate postoperative improvements in memory functioning,[55–57] which is thought to be, at least in part, secondary to seizure control. Cognitive improvements after a patient becomes seizure-free are conceptualized as a hierarchical release of extratemporal functions within the first year of surgery. Improvement of temporal lobe functioning can also be seen in longer-term follow-up.[58] Moreover, seizure freedom is associated with improved psychosocial outcomes, better quality of life, and better emotional functioning. Unfortunately, freedom from seizures is not obtained for all individuals who undergo epilepsy surgery.

There are few neurocognitive indicators that reliably predict seizure control. Nonetheless, patients found to have greater general dysfunction, multilobar focus, or extratemporal dysfunction tend to have worse seizure control outcomes. Individuals whose neuropsychological weaknesses are consistent with medical predictions for lateralization and localization of dysfunction are more likely to experience seizure control postoperatively.

Identify Substance and Psychiatric Risks

Although there are no clear psychiatric contraindications to epilepsy surgery, a preoperative psychiatric history is associated with greater risk of postoperative psychiatric disorders, including depression and anxiety.[59] In individuals with premorbid depression, approximately 50% will experience worsening depressive symptoms within a month after surgery.[58,60] Additionally, patients with preoperative personality disorders or traits are at greater risk of poor psychosocial outcomes.[61,62] Clinical neuropsychologists also assess for substance abuse history, as individuals who abuse alcohol or drugs postoperatively are at a greater risk of seizure recurrence, given that many substances of abuse lower the threshold for seizures and may also be related to poor medication compliance.[63]

18.3.2 Intracarotid Amobarbital (Wada) Procedure

In specialty epilepsy centers, neuropsychologists may also be involved in performing and interpreting the cognitive portions of specialty evaluations such as functional magnetic resonance imaging, intraoperative mapping of higher-order cognitive functions, and the Wada procedure. The Wada procedure was initially developed in the late 1940s and early 1950s to establish language laterality,[64] though has expanded over time to include prediction of postsurgical risk of memory loss. The procedure is multidisciplinary and only the neuropsychological sections are covered here. The Wada procedure involves direct injection of a fast-acting barbiturate (i.e., sodium amobarbital or methohexital) into each carotid artery separately, resulting in brief inactivation of the tissues served by the anterior and middle cerebral arteries. During this time, screening of cognitive domains (oftentimes language and memory) is attempted to determine the functional reserve of the hemisphere contralateral to the side that was injected.

Unlike other neuropsychological evaluation procedures, the procedures used during the Wada are not standardized, though various authors have presented their test batteries (as an example see the text by Lee[65]). Given the unstandardized nature, there is debate in the available literature about the clinical interpretations of findings. Grossly, language laterality may appear obvious if aphasia is present after the injection of one hemisphere and not another. However, some studies have shown that atypical language representation (e.g., mixed or right hemisphere representation) on Wada testing can be relatively common.[66] Clinically, information about language representation from the Wada test is most likely to be used to assist in determining the extent of a proposed surgical resection, particularly the extent to which lateral neocortex can be safely resected. Additionally, when Wada testing reveals atypical language lateralization, caution is advised when interpreting cognitive performances on neuropsychological measures. For instance, in these cases there is limited interpretability of lateralization of memory functioning based on the modality of presentation (i.e., auditory or visual) or based on assumptions of typical language and visuospatial representation.[67]

Memory assessment during the Wada test can serve the functions of predicting post-surgical memory loss, confirming side of seizure onset, and predicting postsurgical seizure control. Generally, the more functionally adequate the to-be-resected hippocampus is, the more likely there will be material specific postoperative memory decline.[37] Wada memory assessment also allows for the measurement of functional reserve of the contralateral hippocampus.[68] Wada memory testing may assist in predicting seizure control, as greater asymmetries in performance between hemispheres have been linked to higher rates of seizure freedom (for example, see Loring et al.[69]).

18.3.3 Purpose of Postoperative Evaluations

Postoperative neuropsychological evaluations are a critical component in assessing the effects of epilepsy surgery on an individual patient's cognition and behavior, as well as to assess for emotional disturbances and low mood, which can have a significant impact on memory function.[63,70] As some initial deficits following surgery may be transient, post-operative assessments should be conducted no earlier than 3 to 6 months following surgery.

Cognitive functioning after epilepsy surgery can change over time. For some individuals, memory abilities continue to improve more than 1 year postoperatively, as there is thought to be a release of functions and reserve capacities that were previously suppressed or irritated by seizures. For others, particularly those with left temporal lobe epilepsy who do not experience seizure remission, progressive memory declines can be seen.[38,71] For these reasons, additional follow-up evaluations can be performed at 1- to 2-year intervals to track recovery.[5]

18.4 Future of Neuropsychology Research

As new measures of brain structure and function continue to evolve, the role of neuro-psychology will remain vital in characterizing functional impairments and disease severity in epilepsy. There is nevertheless a continued need to strengthen normative test data among epilepsy cohorts, particularly for those currently under-represented, including patients with intellectual disabilities, left-handedness, and right-hemisphere language dominance. Innovative test development which improves sensitivity to detect slight changes in neurocognitive functioning is also indicated.[72] The National Institute of Neurological Disorders and Stroke (NINDS) established a Common Data Elements (CDE) Project in 2008. The CDE Project aims to standardize data collection across studies, including common measures and constructs, to facilitate aggregation of information and direct comparisons across studies. This is one promising avenue for the future of neuropsychology epilepsy research.

References

1. Baker GA, Goldstein LH. The dos and don'ts of neuropsychological assessment in epilepsy. *Epilepsy Behav*. 2004;5(Suppl 1): S77–80.

2. Loring DW. History of neuropsychology through epilepsy eyes. *Arch Clin Neuropsychol*. 2010;25(4):259–273.

3. Baxendale S. The impact of epilepsy surgery on cognition and behavior. *Epilepsy Behav*. 2008;12(4):592–599.

4. Helmstaedter C. Neuropsychological aspects of epilepsy surgery. *Epilepsy Behav*. 2004;5 Suppl 1:S45–55.

5. Jones-Gotman M, Smith ML, Risse GL, et al. The contribution of neuropsychology to diagnostic assessment in epilepsy. *Epilepsy Behav*. 2010;18(1–2):3–12.

6. Bodde NM, Brooks JL, Baker GA, et al. Psychogenic non-epileptic seizures – diagnostic issues: a critical review. *Clin Neurol Neurosurg*. 2009;111(1):1–9.

7. Hermann B, Jones J, Sheth R, et al. Children with new-onset epilepsy: neuropsychological status and brain structure. *Brain*. 2006;129(Pt 10):2609–2619.

8. Dutch Study Group of Epilepsy in Childhood: Oostrom KJ, Smeets-Schouten A, Kruitwagen CL, Peters AC, Jennekens-Schinkel A. Not only a matter of epilepsy: early problems of cognition and behavior in children with "epilepsy only" – a prospective, longitudinal, controlled study starting at diagnosis. *Pediatrics*. 2003;112(6 Pt 1):1338–1344.

9. Sutula TP, Hagen J, Pitkanen A. Do epileptic seizures damage the brain? *Curr Opin Neurol*. 2003;16(2):189-195.

10. Vingerhoets G. Cognitive effects of seizures. *Seizure*. 2006;15(4):221-226.

11. Greener M. Beyond seizures: understanding cognitive deficits in epilepsy. *Prog Neurol Psychiatry*. 2013;17 (3):31-32.

12. Dodrill CB. Neuropsychological effects of seizures. *Epilepsy Behav*. 2004;5(Suppl 1): S21–24.

13. Lodhi S, Agrawal N. Neurocognitive problems in epilepsy. *Advances in Psychiatric Treatment*. 2012;18(3):232-240.

14. Jokeit H, Schacher M. Neuropsychological aspects of type of epilepsy and etiological factors in adults. *Epilepsy Behav*. 2004;5 (Suppl 1):S14–20.

15. Baxendale S, Heaney D, Thompson PJ, Duncan JS. Cognitive consequences of childhood-onset temporal lobe epilepsy across the adult lifespan. *Neurology*. 2010;75(8):705-711.

16. Thompson PJ, Corcoran R. Everyday memory failures in people with epilepsy. *Epilepsia*. 1992;33(Suppl 6):S18–20.

17. van Rijckevorsel K. Cognitive problems related to epilepsy syndromes, especially malignant epilepsies. *Seizure*. 2006;15 (4):227–234.

18. Ogden-Epker M, Cullum CM. Quantitative and qualitative interpretation of neuropsychological data in the assessment of temporal lobectomy candidates. *Clin Neuropsychol*. 2001;15(2):183–195.

19. Schefft BK, Testa SM, Dulay MF, Privitera MD, Yeh HS. Preoperative assessment of confrontation naming ability and interictal paraphasia production in unilateral temporal lobe epilepsy. *Epilepsy Behav*. 2003;4(2):161–168.

20. Squire LR, Zola SM. Structure and function of declarative and nondeclarative memory systems. *Proc Natl Acad Sci USA*. 1996;93 (24):13515–13522.

21. Binnie CD, Kasteleijn-Nolst Trenite DG, Smit AM, Wilkins AJ. Interactions of epileptiform EEG discharges and cognition. *Epilepsy Res*. 1987;1(4):239–245.

22. Helmstaedter C, Pohl C, Hufnagel A, Elger CE. Visual learning deficits in nonresected patients with right temporal lobe epilepsy. *Cortex*. 1991;27(4):547–555.

23. Milner B. Psychological aspects of focal epilepsy and its neurosurgical management. *Adv Neurol*. 1975;8:299–321.

24. Baxendale SA. The role of the hippocampus in recognition memory. *Neuropsychologia*. 1997;35(5):591–598.

25. Ivnik RJ, Sharbrough FW, Laws ER, Jr. Effects of anterior temporal lobectomy on cognitive function. *J Clin Psychol*. 1987;43 (1):128–137.

26. Miller LA, Munoz DG, Finmore M. Hippocampal sclerosis and human memory. *Arch Neurol*. 1993;50(4):391–394.

27. Thompson PJ, Trimble MR. Neuropsychological aspects of epilepsy. In: Grant I, Adams KM, eds., *Neuropsychological Assessment of Neuropsychiatric Disorders*. New York, NY: Oxford University Press; 1996:263–287.

28. Ortinski P, Meador KJ. Cognitive side effects of antiepileptic drugs. *Epilepsy Behav*. 2004;5(Suppl 1):S60–65.

29. Hermann BP, Whitman S. Behavioral and personality correlates of epilepsy: a review, methodological critique, and conceptual model. *Psychol Bull*. 1984;95(3):451–497.

30. Paradiso S, Hermann BP, Blumer D, Davies K, Robinson RG. Impact of depressed mood on neuropsychological status in temporal lobe epilepsy. *J Neurol Neurosurg Psychiatry*. 2001;70(2):180–185.

31. Kwan P, Brodie MJ. Early identification of refractory epilepsy. *N Engl J Med*. 2000;342 (5):314–319.

32. Akanuma N, Alarcon G, Lum F, et al. Lateralising value of neuropsychological protocols for presurgical assessment of temporal lobe epilepsy. *Epilepsia*. 2003;44 (3):408–418.

33. Fargo JD, Schefft BK, Szaflarski JP, Howe SR, Yeh HS, Privitera MD. Accuracy of clinical neuropsychological versus statistical prediction in the classification of seizure types. *Clin Neuropsychol*. 2008;22 (2):181–194.

34. Moser DJ, Bauer RM, Gilmore RL, et al. Electroencephalographic, volumetric, and neuropsychological indicators of seizure focus lateralization in temporal lobe epilepsy. *Arch Neurol*. 2000;57 (5):707–712.

35. Baxendale S, Thompson P, Harkness W, Duncan J. Predicting memory decline following epilepsy surgery: a multivariate approach. *Epilepsia*. 2006;47 (11):1887–1894.

36. Stroup E, Langfitt J, Berg M, et al. Predicting verbal memory decline following anterior temporal lobectomy (ATL). *Neurology*. 2003;60(8):1266–1273.

37. Chelune GJ. Hippocampal adequacy versus functional reserve: predicting memory functions following temporal lobectomy. *Arch Clin Neuropsychol*. 1995;10 (5):413–432.

38. Helmstaedter C, Kurthen M, Lux S, Reuber M, Elger CE. Chronic epilepsy and cognition: a longitudinal study in temporal lobe epilepsy. *Ann Neurol*. 2003;54 (4):425–432.

39. Jokeit H, Ebner A. Long-term effects of refractory temporal lobe epilepsy on cognitive abilities: a cross sectional study. *J Neurol Neurosurg Psychiatry*. 1999;67 (1):44–50.

40. Helmstaedter CA. Prediction of memory reserve capacity. *Adv Neurol*. 1999;81:271–279.

41. Bell BD, Davies KG, Hermann BP, Walters G. Confrontation naming after anterior temporal lobectomy is related to age of acquisition of the object names. *Neuropsychologia*. 2000;38(1):83–92.

42. Saykin AJ, Stafiniak P, Robinson LJ, et al. Language before and after temporal lobectomy: specificity of acute changes and

relation to early risk factors. *Epilepsia.*
1995;36(11):1071–1077.

43. Schwarz M, Pauli E, Stefan H. Model-based
    prognosis of postoperative object naming
    in left temporal lobe epilepsy. *Seizure.*
    2005;14(8):562–568.

44. Langfitt JT, Rausch R. Word-finding
    deficits persist after left anterotemporal
    lobectomy. *Arch Neurol.* 1996;53(1):72–76.

45. Milner B. Disorders of learning and
    memory after temporal lobe lesions in
    man. *Clin Neurosurg.* 1972;19:421–446.

46. Mintzer S, Sperling MR. When should a
    resection sparing mesial structures be
    considered for temporal lobe epilepsy?
    Epilepsy Behav. 2008;13(1):7–11.

47. Baxendale SA. Neuropsychologic outcomes
    after epilepsy surgery in adults. In:
    Schachter SC, Holmes GL, Kasteleijn-Nost
    Trenité DGA, eds., *Behavioral Aspects of
    Epilepsy: Principles and Practice.* New York,
    NY: Demos; 2008:311–317.

48. Hermann BP, Wyler AR, Somes G, Berry
    AD, 3rd, Dohan FC, Jr. Pathological status
    of the mesial temporal lobe predicts
    memory outcome from left anterior
    temporal lobectomy. *Neurosurgery.* 1992;31
    (4):652–656.

49. Hermann BP, Wyler AR, Somes G,
    Clement L. Dysnomia after left anterior
    temporal lobectomy without functional
    mapping: frequency and correlates.
    Neurosurgery. 1994;35(1):52–56.

50. Baxendale S, Thompson PJ, Duncan JS.
    Neuropsychological function in patients
    who have had epilepsy surgery: a long-term
    follow-up. *Epilepsy Behav.* 2012;23
    (1):24–29.

51. Jokeit H, Ebner A. Effects of chronic
    epilepsy on intellectual functions. *Prog
    Brain Res.* 2002;135:455–463.

52. Helmstaedter C, Reuber M, Elger CC.
    Interaction of cognitive aging and memory
    deficits related to epilepsy surgery. *Ann
    Neurol.* 2002;52(1):89–94.

53. Jones-Gotman M, Smith ML, Zatorre RJ.
    Neuropsychological testing for localizing
    and lateralizing the epileptogenic region.
    In: Engel J, Jr., ed., *Surgical Treatment of*

the *Epilepsies.* 2nd edn. New York, NY:
Raven Press; 1993:245–261.

54. Tellez-Zenteno JF, Dhar R, Hernandez-
    Ronquillo L, Wiebe S. Long-term outcomes
    in epilepsy surgery: antiepileptic drugs,
    mortality, cognitive and psychosocial
    aspects. *Brain.* 2007;130(Pt 2):334–345.

55. Cukiert A, Buratini JA, Machado E, et al.
    Seizure-related outcome after
    corticoamygdalohippocampectomy in
    patients with refractory temporal lobe
    epilepsy and mesial temporal sclerosis
    evaluated by magnetic resonance imaging
    alone. *Neurosurg Focus.* 2002;13(4):ecp2.

56. Leijten FS, Alpherts WC, Van Huffelen AC,
    Vermeulen J, Van Rijen PC. The effects on
    cognitive performance of tailored resection
    in surgery for nonlesional mesiotemporal
    lobe epilepsy. *Epilepsia.* 2005;46
    (3):431–439.

57. Sanyal SK, Chandra PS, Gupta S, et al.
    Memory and intelligence outcome
    following surgery for intractable temporal
    lobe epilepsy: relationship to seizure
    outcome and evaluation using a
    customized neuropsychological battery.
    Epilepsy Behav. 2005;6(2):147–155.

58. Altshuler L, Rausch R, Delrahim S, Kay J,
    Crandall P. Temporal lobe epilepsy,
    temporal lobectomy, and major depression.
    J Neuropsychiatry Clin Neurosci. 1999;11
    (4):436–443.

59. Malmgren K, Starmark JE, Ekstedt G,
    Rosen H, Sjoberg-Larsson C. Nonorganic
    and organic psychiatric disorders in
    patients after epilepsy surgery. *Epilepsy
    Behav.* 2002;3(1):67–75.

60. Blumer D, Wakhlu S, Davies K, Hermann
    B. Psychiatric outcome of temporal
    lobectomy for epilepsy: incidence and
    treatment of psychiatric complications.
    Epilepsia. 1998;39(5):478–486.

61. Inoue Y, Mihara T. Psychiatric disorders
    before and after surgery for epilepsy.
    Epilepsia. 2001;42(Suppl 6):13–18.

62. Koch-Stoecker S. Personality disorders as
    predictors of severe postsurgical psychiatric
    complications in epilepsy patients
    undergoing temporal lobe resections.
    Epilepsy Behav. 2002;3(6):526–531.

63. Foong J, Flugel D. Psychiatric outcome of surgery for temporal lobe epilepsy and presurgical considerations. *Epilepsy Res.* 2007;75(2–3):84–96.

64. Wada J, Rasmussen T. Intracarotid injection of sodium amytal for the lateralization of cerebral speech dominance. *J Neurosurg.* 1960;17(2):266–282.

65. Lee GP. *Neuropsychology of Epilepsy and Epilepsy Surgery*. New York, NY: Oxford University Press; 2010.

66. Snyder PJ, Novelly RA, Harris LJ. Mixed speech dominance in the intracarotid sodium amytal procedure: validity and criteria issues. *J Clin Exp Neuropsychol.* 1990;12(5):629–643.

67. Loring DW, Meador KJ, Lee GP, et al. Crossed aphasia in a patient with complex partial seizures: evidence from intracarotid amobarbital testing, functional cortical mapping, and neuropsychological assessment. *J Clin Exp Neuropsychol.* 1990;12(2):340–354.

68. Kneebone AC, Chelune GJ, Dinner DS, Naugle RI, Awad IA. Intracarotid amobarbital procedure as a predictor of material-specific memory change after anterior temporal lobectomy. *Epilepsia.* 1995;36(9):857–865.

69. Loring DW, Meador KJ, Lee GP, et al. Wada memory performance predicts seizure outcome following anterior temporal lobectomy. *Neurology.* 1994;44(12):2322–2324.

70. Dulay MF, York MK, Soety EM, et al. Memory, emotional and vocational impairments before and after anterior temporal lobectomy for complex partial seizures. *Epilepsia.* 2006;47(11):1922–1930.

71. Dodrill CB. Progressive cognitive decline in adolescents and adults with epilepsy. *Prog Brain Res.* 2002;135:399–407.

72. Raspall T, Donate M, Boget T, et al. Neuropsychological tests with lateralizing value in patients with temporal lobe epilepsy: reconsidering material-specific theory. *Seizure.* 2005;14(8):569–576.

Principles of Antiseizure Drug Management

Georgia Montouris

19.1 Introduction

Seizures are categorized as unprovoked or provoked, and the former may lead to the diagnosis of epilepsy. The term unprovoked seizure refers to a seizure of unknown etiology or that occurs in relation to a presenting brain lesion or progressive nervous system disorder. Provoked seizures are due to an acute condition such as toxic or metabolic disturbance, head trauma, or acute stroke. About 30% of patients with unprovoked seizures, which are nearly always generalized tonic–clonic convulsions, are seen by physicians after only a single attack. Studies have now established high-risk groups for recurrence after a single unprovoked seizure. The risk for epilepsy is greatly increased in the presence of an abnormal electroencephalogram (EEG), history of brain injury, and family history of epilepsy.[1] Age of onset may impact the choice of antiseizure drug (ASD). Etiologies often vary with age of onset. Prognosis, consequences of etiology, and response to treatment may vary depending on age and comorbid conditions.

19.2 Special Populations for ASD therapy

19.2.1 Neonates

The overall goal of treatment in neonates is to minimize brain injury that may be associated with or caused by recurrent seizures.[2] Rational selection of ASD for neonatal seizures is limited by a number of uncertainties, including a clinical classification, the wide variety of possible etiologies, and lack of suitable studies comparing the efficacy of ASDs in well-defined subcategories of neonatal seizures. Thus, the drug selection is largely based on empiric and pharmacological considerations. Favorable pharmacological properties make phenobarbital the drug of first choice in the treatment of neonatal seizures.[3–6] The volume of distribution is 1 l/kg irrespective of gestational age. Initial loading dose is 20 mg/kg intravenously over 10 min yielding a serum level of 20–24 µg/ml.[5,7]

One-third of neonates will respond to this dose[5,8]; 60% of infants respond to the loading dose. Caution is required for rapid administration of the loading dose as it can cause apnea. If seizures persist after the loading dose, additional 5 mg/kg intravenous doses need to be given until seizures stop, or 40 mg/kg dose has been given.[9]

If seizures persist, the second drug of choice in neonatal seizures is phenytoin.[8,10] The use of phosphenytoin would be preferred, given that the solution of phenytoin is alkaline, thus avoiding the risk of extravasation and impact on vessels.

Diazepam has been employed successfully as a continuous infusion for periods of 1–18 days.[11] Lorazepam has been used as adjunctive in successful management of severe refractory neonatal seizures due to asphyxia.

Over the course of the second and third postnatal weeks, increase in glomerular filtration rate, induction of hepatic metabolites, reduction in body water and fall in serum protein levels results in faster elimination of all anticonvulsants. Near adult values are achieved by the second and third postnatal weeks and clearance exceeds those of adults by the fourth to fifth postnatal weeks, requiring adjustment of dosage.[12–15]

As for phenytoin, during the first week of life, the hepatic mechanism of the neonate is partially saturated. This results in nonlinear kinetics for drug elimination and an increase in half-life (T½) as serum concentration increases.[16,17]

The higher the risk for developing epilepsy, the longer treatment should be considered. The presence of underlying etiology, abnormal interictal EEG findings, and neurological deficits in the neonatal period increase the risk for developing epilepsy in the future. Watanabe's large series[18] found a 30% risk of epilepsy among infants surviving neonatal seizures after perinatal hypoxia, intracranial trauma, or meningitis. The overall risk for developing chronic epilepsy ranges from 2–22% for infants surviving the neonatal period after neonatal seizures.[1,3,12,19,20] Neonates whose seizure occurred in 1 day had 1.1% risk for epilepsy, compared to a 10% risk if the seizure persisted for more than 3 days.[21]

The goal of treating neonatal seizures is to prevent long-term central nervous system (CNS) dysfunction. While it is not definitely determined that either recurring seizures or acute or chronic ASDs have adverse effects on the developing brain, evidence suggests both may have unwanted sequelae.

19.2.2 Elderly Age Group

Treating elderly patients can be complicated as there are often age-related changes in liver, kidney, and gastrointestinal functions. Concomitant medical conditions also add to the equation, as most elderly patients are being treated with multiple other medications. The polypharmacy can have effects on the pharmacokinetics of the ASDs.

Age-related changes in physiology can affect absorption, distribution, metabolism, and elimination. Alterations in serum proteins with age can have a significant effect on total serum concentrations of highly protein-bound ASDs such as carbamazepine, phenytoin, and valproic acid. Total serum concentrations correlate well with therapeutic and toxic response when protein binding is stable or the fraction of the drug bound is relatively low.[22] Age-related reductions in liver volume, hepatic blood flow, and glomerular filtration rate are responsible for a decline in drug elimination in the elderly.[22] Elderly patients require smaller doses given less frequently to maintain desired unbound ASD concentrations. Serum concentrations at the upper limits of proposed ASD therapeutic ranges may frequently cause side effects.[22] Administration of any medication to an elderly patient is complicated by both complex and specific pharmacokinetics, polypharmacy, concomitant illness, and unusual sensitivity to drug effects with a narrowing of the therapeutic range of drugs. Elderly patients with declining cognitive function, motor impairment, or altered sensory function may be especially susceptible to dose-related side effects of ASDs. Decline in mental function may be seen as a result of drug-induced delirium or intensifying of underlying dementia.[23] Given the risks of any of the above, careful consideration must be given to the choice of ASD to be prescribed. Simplicity in dosing regimen also needs to be considered.

19.3 Starting an ASD

It is important to consider the risk of seizure recurrence. As per the guidelines, adults with unprovoked seizures should be informed that risk of seizure recurrence is greatest within the first 2 years (21–45%).[24] Clinical variables associated with increased risk of recurrence may include prior brain insult, abnormal EEG, significant brain imaging abnormality, and nocturnal seizures. Age is also a factor, noting that the risk of recurrent seizure in patients whose seizures begin over the age of 65 is 75% within the first 6 months, and 90% within the first year if untreated. Immediate ASD therapy compared to waiting for the second seizure, is likely to reduce recurrence risk within the first 2 years.[24]

Patients should be informed of potential adverse effects of the ASD and that most are mild and reversible. In those patients with a first seizure who are found to have a CNS abnormality, such as a tumor, CNS infections, or scar tissue from trauma, the risk of recurrence is high. In these cases, most physicians would initiate treatment. These patients meet the new ILAE guidelines, defined by a single unprovoked seizure with an estimated risk of recurrence of >60% over 10 years, as having epilepsy. Once the second unprovoked seizure occurs, ASDs should be started if not initiated earlier.

Patients with seizures that occur in the setting of acute neurologic illness or injury (e.g., stroke, TBI, meningitis, anoxic encephalopathy) are often treated with ASDs in the acute setting because of the risk of prolonged recurrent seizures or aggravation of a systemic injury.

Cases of acute symptomatic seizures that occur in the setting of acute medical illness or metabolic disturbance are not felt to be at risk for future epilepsy, but are at risk of seizure recurrence in the acute setting.[25] Short-term therapy may be indicated.

19.4 Important Factors When Choosing an ASD

19.4.1 Dosing Frequency

Most ASDs are prescribed in twice daily doses. The frequency with which a drug must be taken is an important factor in compliance and seizure control. ASDs that require more frequent dosing include immediate release, such as carbamazepine and tiagabine, and regular and delayed release, such as valproate, gabapentin, and pregabalin. Once daily dosing may be possible with phenobarbital, phenytoin, extended-release valproate, zonisamide, eslicarbazepine, perampanel, and extended-release formulations of levetiracetam, lamotrigine, topiramate, and oxcarbazepine.

19.4.2 Drug Interactions

ASDs with hepatic enzyme induction or inhibition properties have the greatest potential for interaction. Enzyme induction occurs with the majority of the older ASDs that include phenytoin, phenobarbital, and carbamazepine. ASDs that are inducers increase the metabolism of other medications that are broken down in the same pathway. Phenytoin induces the metabolism of warfarin, potentially leading to a subtherapeutic international normalized ratio or an increased dose requirement for warfarin. Commonly prescribed drugs with the potential to interact with enzyme-inducing drugs include statins, calcium channel blockers, serotonin reuptake inhibitors, antipsychotics, tricyclic antidepressants, hormone contraceptive therapy, warfarin, and many anticancer drugs.[26] In contrast, valproate is a hepatic enzyme inhibitor and may cause a significant increase in serum concentration of medications that are metabolized by the liver.

With some ASDs, interactions are related to protein binding. Addition of a highly protein-bound drug will displace another protein-bound drug, increasing the free fraction. In the setting of reduced serum albumin, the effect is amplified. An example of this is lamotrigine serum concentration being reduced by estrogen-containing hormonal contraceptives.[24]

19.4.3 Side Effects of ASDs

Many potential side effects can occur and need to be recognized upon occurrence or noted as potential occurrence given the patients' comorbid conditions or concomitant medications, as well as allergies or history of medication intolerance. It is of great importance that monitoring of potential side effects is undertaken for patient compliance and successful treatment.

The various subsets of adverse effects are discussed in the following sections.

19.4.3.1 Neurocognitive Problems

Most ASDs are associated with a negative impact on cognition.[27] Older drugs, such as phenobarbital, are associated with the greatest impairment as compared to carbamazepine, valproate, and phenytoin, which have similar but more modest negative effects.[28,29] Negative cognitive effects are seen in exposure to topiramate, some to carbamazepine and oxcarbazepine, and less with gabapentin and lamotrigine.

19.4.3.2 Hypersensitivity

Hypersensitivity is seen as TEN (toxic epidermal necrolysis), Stevens–Johnson syndrome, and DRESS (drug rash with eosinophilia and systemic symptoms). Although these conditions are rare, they are severe. These reactions are more often seen with exposure to carbamazepine, oxcarbazepine, lamotrigine, and phenobarbital, and less commonly with topiramate and valproate. However, almost all of the ASDs have been associated with this reaction.[30,31]

19.4.3.3 Weight Gain/Loss

Weight gain has been associated with valproate, gabapentin, carbamazepine, vigabatrin, and perampanel, and loss with felbamate, topiramate, and zonisamide. It is important to keep this in mind as complications of weight gain and loss can be very detrimental. In addition the risk of polycystic ovarian syndrome and diabetes with weight-gaining agents should be monitored.

19.4.3.4 Suicidality

ASDs as a class have been associated with an approximate twofold increased relative risk of suicidal behavior ideation based on pooled analyses of placebo-controlled trials.[24]

19.4.3.5 Depression and Anxiety

As depression and anxiety are known comorbidities of epilepsy, patients with these conditions may be at risk for exacerbation of depression with some ASDs, which may influence the choice of medication and will require close supervision.

19.4.4 Cost of Medication

This can play a significant role in the choice of ASDs. Generic substitution can be of benefit, but not always. Generics may be effective; however, they also may be associated with a change in seizure control or tolerability.[24]

19.4.5 Seizure-Related Considerations

Treatment is diverse from narrow-spectrum to broad-spectrum agents. Broad-spectrum agents work for both focal and generalized epilepsy, whereas narrow-spectrum medications work only for focal and may actually exacerbate generalized seizures if prescribed in some patients. Examples of this are oxcarbazepine,[32] carbamazepine, phenytoin, vigabatrin, and gabapentin,[33] which have all been reported to worsen certain seizures types in generalized epilepsy syndromes.

19.4.6 Specific Etiologies

Poststroke epilepsy is generally easily controlled with ASD monotherapy.[24] The choice of agent needs to take into consideration drug–drug interactions (for example with warfarin and salicylates) and the impact on poststroke functional recovery as well. Brain tumors account for the etiology of epilepsy in 30–70% patients. As such, the choice of ASD needs to take into account possible drug interactions with chemotherapy agents. There is also a risk of allergic cutaneous reactions when ASDs are used during radiotherapy.[34,35]

19.4.7 Syndromes

The advent of rufinamide and clobazam has been effective in treatment of Lennox–Gastaut syndrome, which includes not only multiple seizure types, but also developmental delays and cognitive impairment. Behavioral issues often accompany this syndrome, especially as the patient ages. These patients are often treated with polypharmacy.

19.4.8 Comorbidities

Comorbid conditions need to be considered when choosing the appropriate ASD.

19.4.8.1 Renal and Hepatic Conditions

Renal excretion may impact certain medications and hepatic disease will impact agents metabolized by the liver.

ASDs that are renally excreted include gabapentin, topiramate, zonisaminde, lacosamide, levetiracetam, brivaracetam and pregabalin. Doses should be lowered in the presence of renal impairment.[36–38] In patients with hemodialysis, adding a low dose of the ASD after dialysis may be warranted to yield therapeutic levels. Albuminuria may lead to an increased fraction of free drug as it reduces protein binding fraction and binding affinity. Renal stones are associated with topiramate and zonisamide as well as occurrence of renal acidosis. Monitoring serum bicarbonate levels is warranted.[39]

Caution is needed in potential interactions between ASDs and immunosuppressive therapy. Enzyme inducers may lower serum concentration of immunosuppressant levels, while inhibitors may increase levels.[24] Avoid valproate and felbamate, which are associated with hepatic toxicity.[38,40]

19.4.8.2 Psychiatric Comorbidities

Some of the ASDs are known to have some mood-stabilizing effects, so in patients with this comorbid condition, ASDs may have dual benefits. Others that potentiate gamma-aminobutyric acid neurotransmission can cause or exacerbate a depressed mood (phenobarbital, tiagabine, vigabatrin, and topiramate). Some have been reported to cause psychosis, such as levetiracetam, perampanel, zonisamide, ethosuximide, topiramate, and vigabatrin.[41]

An added benefit of selective antiseizure therapy using topiramate or valproate may be related to treatment of migraines in patients with epilepsy. As such, this may limit polypharmacy.

19.4.8.3 Osteoporosis Risk

ASDs in chronic use have been associated with bone loss. Initially bone loss was thought to be related to enzyme-inducing drugs, but it has been found to extend to valproate and some of the newer agents.[42-44] Monitoring of bone density, supplementation with calcium and vitamin D, along with weight-bearing exercise is warranted.

19.4.8.4 Cardiovascular Disease

Potential drug interactions between enzyme-inducing ASDs and statins, calcium channel blockers, and warfarin should be considered.

As the cytochrome P450 enzymes are involved in cholesterol synthesis, it is possible that enzyme-inducing ASDs may affect vascular risk.

19.4.9 Gender-Related Issues

Treatment in women requires consideration of various factors, including hormonal impact on menstruation as well as on contraception and age, as related to childbearing and menopausal issues. Issues related to medication in the childbearing years include risk of teratogenicity from ASDs, risk of miscarriage, and the impact of seizures on the developing fetus, to mention a few.

Part of the treatment plan should include folic acid supplementation at a dose of 4 mg per day if on carbamazepine or valproate, whereas for those not on these agents less folic acid would be required. In the case of catamenial epilepsy (seizures related to the menstrual cycle) intermittent adjunctive therapy is often required to control the increased seizure frequency.

Selecting an appropriate ASD in this subset of patients is extremely important to avoid major malformations to the offspring of women with epilepsy.

Valproate presents with a higher risk among the ASDs. In addition to congenital malformation risk, including spina bifida, the risk of cognitive impairment has been shown in offspring exposed to 1000 mg or more of valproate daily. Seizure control is extremely important during pregnancy to avoid complications to both mother and fetus. Serum concentrations need to be monitored throughout the pregnancy as levels drop. Those ASDs that are highly protein bound, such as phenytoin and carbamazepine, decrease most in the third trimester. Lamotrigine is affected by glucuronidation, and levels drop frequently during pregnancy. The levels of agents that are renally excreted drop as renal clearance increases in pregnancy. Often adjustments need to be made to maintain seizure control. Monthly monitoring of serum concentrations of ASDs during pregnancy is recommended.

Adjustment in dosage may need to be made upon delivery, especially if raised during pregnancy. Otherwise levels may increase significantly, and toxicity, glucuronidation, protein binding, and renal clearance revert to the pregestational state. ASD levels should be drawn on the day of delivery and minimally 1 day postpartum. Breastfeeding is also not contraindicated.

19.5 Monotherapy versus Polypharmacy

When patients do not become seizure free on their first or second ASD, the options for treatment include add-on therapy or sequential monotherapy substitution. Substitution can involve the risk of worsening the condition, and sometimes physicians and patients opt to add a second drug. The concept of polypharmacy was once frowned upon, but currently with the advent of newer agents, especially with fewer side effects compared to older agents and more novel mechanisms, it is acceptable and often most effective.

19.6 When to Start Treatment with an ASD after the First Seizure

Definitely:

- With structural lesion:

  · brain tumor, such as meningioma, glioma, or neoplasia
  · arteriovenous malformations
  · infections such as abscess and herpes encephalitis

- Without structural lesion:

  · history of epilepsy in sibling (not parents)
  · EEG with definite epileptic pattern
  · history of previous brain injury, stroke, CNS infection, significant head trauma
  · status epilepticus at onset

Possibly:

- Unprovoked seizure with some of the above risk factors[45]

19.7 Discontinuation of ASDs

ASDs do not offer a cure to epilepsy, but they may yield success in controlling seizures or they may cause side effects. This raises the question of when is it in the patient's best interest to discontinue ASD therapy. Perspectives from the patient and family as well as the physician must be acknowledged.

Consequences of the discontinuation of treatment include the risk of recurrence and the consequences thereof. In adults, discontinuation poses a greater impact on the individual, specifically on driving, work, and emotionally. In children, academic and developmental milestones can be impacted.

A number of factors need to be considered when discontinuing ASDs.

19.7.1 Duration of Epilepsy and Duration of Seizure Control

Longer duration of seizure freedom is associated with a decrease in the relapse rate. Various studies report varying timelines, with 70% of children who were seizure free for 1–4 years and had stopped ASDs and remained seizure free,[46] about 30% had recurrence and 1% became refractory. Other studies have used a 2-year seizure-free duration to initiate discontinuation.[47–49]

19.7.2 Age of Patient

In adults, discontinuation poses a greater impact on the individual, specifically on driving, work, and emotionally. In children, academic and developmental milestones can be impacted by discontinuation of medication. Seizure recurrences may be due to lack of protection after discontinuation and may not appear for years, although most occur within a year and treatment needs to be restarted.[50]

19.7.3 Predictors of Discontinuation Failure

Many factors have been described as predictors of discontinuation failure including severity of disease along with seizure-free period.[48] One study demonstrated evidence that waiting to discontinue ASDs for 2 or more seizure-free years in the presence of abnormal EEG and partial seizures reduced the relapse rate.[51]

ASD withdrawal after 1 year of seizure freedom has led to 29–40% seizure recurrence,[52,53] while withdrawal after 6–12 months of treatment led to seizure recurrence in approximately half of all patients, regardless of the duration of therapy.[54]

19.7.4 Rate of Withdrawal/Reduction of ASDs

This remains controversial. One study demonstrated that 149 patients were randomized to either a 6-week taper or a 9-month taper and had seizure recurrences of 40% with no difference between the groups.[53]

Rapid withdrawal of benzodiazepines and barbiturates is known to cause withdrawal seizures.

Carbamazepine was shown to demonstrate an increase in seizure frequency, as reported by Duncan et al.,[55] but not enough to support withdrawal symptoms. Standard of care dictates that a slower withdrawal of carbamazepine is warranted unless serious adverse effects suggest otherwise.

19.7.5 Syndromic Epilepsy

Syndromic epilepsy can influence the continuation or discontinuation of ASDs. Childhood absence along with benign rolandic epilepsy are two syndromes that generally remit at puberty, suggesting discontinuation of medication is acceptable, whereas juvenile myoclonic epilepsy appears likely to require lifelong therapy.

19.8 Success with Restarting ASD

A meta-analysis showed that reinitiating ASD therapy led to control in 80% of patients with seizure recurrence who had earlier discontinued ASDs, and in half of these patients, it took up to 1–5 years to achieve seizure control, while 20% remained refractory.[56]

The decision to start or discontinue ASDs in patients with epilepsy is very complex, requiring a thorough discussion of the risks and benefits, concerns, and ability to cope with outcomes, between the patient/family and the physician.

References

1. Freeman JM, Pedley TA. Indications for treatment. In: Engel J, Jr., Pedley TA, eds., *Epilepsy: A Comprehensive Textbook*. 2nd edn. Philadelphia: Lippincott Williams & Wilkins; 2008:1119–1123.

2. Rust RS, Volpe JJ. Neonatal seizures. In: Dodson WE, Pellock JM, eds., *Pediatric Epilepsy: Diagnosis and Therapy*. New York: Demos Publications; 1993:107–128.

3. Volpe JJ. Neonatal seizures. In: Volpe JJ, ed., *Neurology of the Newborn*. Philadelphia: Saunders; 1987:129–158.

4. Aicardi J. Neonatal and infantile seizures. In: Morselli PL, Pippenger CE, Penry JK, eds., *Antiepileptic Drug Therapy in Pediatrics*. New York: Raven Press; 1983:103–117.

5. Lockman LA, Kriel R, Zaske D, Thompson T, Virnig N. Phenobarbital dosage for control of neonatal seizures. *Neurology*. 1979;29(11):1445–1449.

6. Rust RS, Dodson WE. Phenobarbital: absorption, distribution and excretion. In: Levy RH, Dreifuss FE, Mattson RH, Meldrum BS, Penry JK, eds., *Antiepileptic Drugs*. 3rd edn. New York: Raven Press; 1989.

7. Fischer JH, Lockman LA, Zaske D, Kriel R. Phenobarbital maintenance dose requirements in treating neonatal seizures. *Neurology*. 1981;31(8):1042–1044.

8. Painter MJ, Pippenger C, Wasterlain C, et al. Phenobarbital and phenytoin in neonatal seizures: metabolism and tissue distribution. *Neurology*. 1981;31 (9):1107–1112.

9. Gilman JT, Gal P, Duchowny MS, Weaver RL, Ransom JL. Rapid sequential phenobarbital treatment of neonatal seizures. *Pediatrics*. 1989;83(5):674–678.

10. Gal P, Toback J, Boer HR, Erkan NV, Wells TJ. Efficacy of phenobarbital monotherapy in treatment of neonatal seizures – relationship to blood levels. *Neurology*. 1982;32(12):1401–1404.

11. Thong YH, Abramson DC. Continuous infusion of diazepam in infants with severe recurrent convulsions. *Med Ann Dist Columbia*. 1974;43(2):63–65.

12. Dodson WE. Antiepileptic drug use in newborns and infants. In: Pedley TA, Meldrum BS, eds., *Recent Advances in Epilepsy*. Edinburgh: Churchill Livingstone; 1983:231–249.

13. Morselli PL. Development of physiological variables important for drug kinetics. In: Morselli PL, Pippenger CE, Penry JK, eds., *Antiepileptic Drug Therapy in Pediatrics*. New York: Raven Press; 1983:1–12.

14. Bourgeois BF, Dodson WE. Phenytoin elimination in newborns. *Neurology*. 1983;33(2):173–178.

15. Morselli PL, Baruzzi A. *Serum Levels and Pharmokinetics of Anticonvulsants in the Management of Seizure Disorders*. Chicago: Year Book Medical Publishers; 1978.

16. Dodson WE. Phenytoin elimination in childhood: effect of concentration-dependent kinetics. *Neurology*. 1980;30 (2):196–199.

17. Dodson WE. Nonlinear kinetics of phenytoin in children. *Neurology*. 1982;32 (1):42–48.

18. Watanabe K, Kuroyanagi M, Hara K, Miyazaki S. Neonatal seizures and subsequent epilepsy. *Brain Dev*. 1982;4 (5):341–346.

19. Holden KR, Mellits ED, Freeman JM. Neonatal seizures. I. Correlation of prenatal and perinatal events with outcomes. *Pediatrics*. 1982;70(2):165–176.

20. Bergman I, Painter MJ, Crumrine PK. Neonatal seizures. *Semin Perinatol*. 1982;6 (1):54–67.

21. Mizrahi EM, Kellaway P. Characterization and classification of neonatal seizures. *Neurology*. 1987;37(12):1837–1844.

22. Cloyd J. *Commonly Used Antiepileptic Drugs: Age-Related Pharmacokinetics*. Woburn, MA: Butterworth-Heinemann; 1997.

23. Willmore J. Commonly used antiepileptic drugs: age related efficacy. In: Rowan AJ, Ramsay E, eds., *Seizures and Epilepsy in the*

Elderly. Woburn, MA: Butterworth-Heinemann; 1997:229–238.

24. Krumholz A, Wiebe S, Gronseth GS, et al. Evidence-based guideline: Management of an unprovoked first seizure in adults. Report of the Guideline Development Subcommittee of the American Academy of Neurology and the American Epilepsy Society. *Neurology*. 2015;84(16):1705–1713.

25. Fields MC, Labovitz DL, French JA. Hospital-onset seizures: an inpatient study. *JAMA Neurol*. 2013;70(3):360–364.

26. Gidal BE, French JA, Grossman P, Le Teuff G. Assessment of potential drug interactions in patients with epilepsy: impact of age and sex. *Neurology*. 2009;72(5):419–425.

27. Hessen E, Lossius MI, Gjerstad L. Antiepileptic monotherapy significantly impairs normative scores on common tests of executive functions. *Acta Neurol Scand*. 2009;119(3):194–198.

28. Motamedi G, Meador K. Epilepsy and cognition. *Epilepsy Behav*. 2003;4 Suppl 2: S25–38.

29. Meador KJ. Cognitive and memory effects of the new antiepileptic drugs. *Epilepsy Res*. 2006;68(1):63–67.

30. Yang CY, Dao RL, Lee TJ, et al. Severe cutaneous adverse reactions to antiepileptic drugs in Asians. *Neurology*. 2011;77(23):2025–2033.

31. Mockenhaupt M, Messenheimer J, Tennis P, Schlingmann J. Risk of Stevens-Johnson syndrome and toxic epidermal necrolysis in new users of antiepileptics. *Neurology*. 2005;64(7):1134–1138.

32. Gelisse P, Genton P, Kuate C, et al. Worsening of seizures by oxcarbazepine in juvenile idiopathic generalized epilepsies. *Epilepsia*. 2004;45(10):1282–1286.

33. Perucca E, Gram L, Avanzini G, Dulac O. Antiepileptic drugs as a cause of worsening seizures. *Epilepsia*. 1998;39(1):5–17.

34. Vecht CJ, van Breemen M. Optimizing therapy of seizures in patients with brain tumors. *Neurology*. 2006;67(12 Suppl 4): S10–13.

35. Michelucci R. Optimizing therapy of seizures in neurosurgery. *Neurology*. 2006;67(12 Suppl 4):S14–18.

36. Bazil CW. Antiepileptic drugs in the 21st century. *CNS Spectr*. 2001;6(9):756–762, 765.

37. Lacerda G, Krummel T, Sabourdy C, Ryvlin P, Hirsch E. Optimizing therapy of seizures in patients with renal or hepatic dysfunction. *Neurology*. 2006;67(12 Suppl 4):S28–33.

38. Israni RK, Kasbekar N, Haynes K, Berns JS. Use of antiepileptic drugs in patients with kidney disease. *Semin Dial*. 2006;19 (5):408–416.

39. Sheth RD. Metabolic concerns associated with antiepileptic medications. *Neurology*. 2004;63(10 Suppl 4):S24–29.

40. Ahmed SN, Siddiqi ZA. Antiepileptic drugs and liver disease. *Seizure*. 2006;15(3):156–164.

41. Mula M, Hesdorffer DC, Trimble M, Sander JW. The role of titration schedule of topiramate for the development of depression in patients with epilepsy. *Epilepsia*. 2009;50(5):1072–1076.

42. Pack AM, Morrell MJ, Marcus R, et al. Bone mass and turnover in women with epilepsy on antiepileptic drug monotherapy. *Ann Neurol*. 2005;57 (2):252–257.

43. Pack A. Effects of treatment on endocrine function in patients with epilepsy. *Curr Treat Options Neurol*. 2005;7(4):273–280.

44. Pack AM, Morrell MJ, Randall A, McMahon DJ, Shane E. Bone health in young women with epilepsy after one year of antiepileptic drug monotherapy. *Neurology*. 2008;70(18):1586–1593.

45. Dulac O, Leppick IE, Chadwick DW, Specchio L. Starting and stopping treatment. In: Engel J, Pedley TA, Aicardi J, eds., *Epilepsy: A Comprehensive Textbook*. 2nd edn. Philadelphia: Wolters Kluwer Health/Lippincott Williams & Wilkins; 2008:1301–1310.

46. Camfield P, Camfield C. The frequency of intractable seizures after stopping AEDs in seizure-free children with epilepsy. *Neurology*. 2005;64(6):973–975.

47. Nakazawa Y, Ishida S, Maeda H, Sakurai S, Motooka H. Prognosis of epilepsy withdrawn from antiepileptic drugs. *Psychiatry Clin Neurosci.* 1995;49 (3):163–168.

48. Specchio LM, Tramacere L, La Neve A, Beghi E. Discontinuing antiepileptic drugs in patients who are seizure-free on monotherapy. *J Neurol Neurosurg Psychiatry.* 2002;72(1):22–25.

49. So NK. Recurrence, remission, and relapse of seizures. *Cleve Clin J Med.* 1993;60 (6):439–444.

50. Armijo JA, Adin J. [Pharmacological basis for withdrawal of antiepileptic drugs]. *Rev Neurol.* 2000;30(4):336–350.

51. Sirven JI, Sperling M, Wingerchuk DM. Early versus late antiepileptic drug withdrawal for people with epilepsy in remission. *Cochrane Database Syst Rev.* 2001(3):Cd001902.

52. Berg AT, Shinnar S. Relapse following discontinuation of antiepileptic drugs: a meta-analysis. *Neurology.* 1994;44 (4):601–608.

53. Tennison M, Greenwood R, Lewis D, Thorn M. Discontinuing antiepileptic drugs in children with epilepsy: a comparison of a six-week and a nine-month taper period. *N Engl J Med.* 1994;330(20):1407–1410.

54. Peters AC, Brouwer OF, Geerts AT, et al. Randomized prospective study of early discontinuation of antiepileptic drugs in children with epilepsy. *Neurology.* 1998;50 (3):724–730.

55. Duncan JS, Shorvon SD, Trimble MR. Withdrawal symptoms from phenytoin, carbamazepine and sodium valproate. *J Neurol Neurosurg Psychiatry.* 1988;51 (7):924–928.

56. Schmidt D, Loscher W. Uncontrolled epilepsy following discontinuation of antiepileptic drugs in seizure-free patients: a review of current clinical experience. *Acta Neurol Scand.* 2005;111(5):291–300.

Gender Issues in Epilepsy

Patricia E. Penovich

20.1 Introduction

All individuals deal with decisions regarding sexuality, reproduction, and family. Men with epilepsy (MWE) and women with epilepsy (WWE) also consider additional factors: effects of seizures, effects of antiseizure drugs (ASDs), psychological and psychiatric barriers such as self-image, anxiety, and depression.

With the onset of puberty and menarche, sex steroid hormones (SSH) exert effects on cortical excitability and sexual and reproductive functioning.[1,2] The major production of SSH is gonadal, with some contribution from the adrenals and brain. Feedback loops exist between the gonads and hypothalamus (Figure 20.1). SSH are neuroactive with identified receptors: estrogen receptor stimulation being proconvulsant, while progesterone is inhibitory due to its $GABA_A$ receptor binding. Testosterone's (T) effect is twofold: excitatory due to its hepatic metabolism to estrogen via aromatase, and inhibitory due to its three metabolites (5α-androstane-3α-diol, androsterone, and etiocholanolone).

These functions can be disrupted by the effects of seizures on the feedback loops between the cerebral cortex and the hypothalamic–pituitary–gonadal axis. Some ASDs alter the concentrations of active SSH by inducing hepatic SSH metabolism or by increasing hepatic production of sex hormone binding globulin (SHBG), thus reducing free active SSH.[3] Seizures also affect the levels of these neurosteroids.

20.2 Catamenial Epilepsy

For postpubertal women, the primary estrogen is the metabolite estradiol. Evaluation of hormonal levels reveals a normal cyclical pattern of ovarian SSH production (Figure 20.2). Increased estrogen levels occur with ovulation, while progesterone increases by corpus luteum secretion at days 13–24. A fall in estradiol and progesterone results in menstruation if there is no fertilization and implantation around day 25. At both of these times, the estrogen/progesterone ratio is elevated. If there is no ovulation, the progesterone surge does not develop and the estradiol effects are greater. Herzog defined three patterns of seizure clusters in WWE during reproductive years, termed catamenial epilepsy.[4] The C_1 pattern occurs in the perimenstrual period, days –3 to +3, the C_2 pattern occurs at the periovulatory time, days 10 to –13; and the C_3 pattern occurs in anovulatory cycles when estrogen and seizure frequencies are elevated through all phases with lowest seizure frequency being days 3–10.[4,5]

The reported frequency of catamenial patterns varies, between 30% and 50%. The definition of a catamenial pattern ranges from any increase in seizures to a more rigorous requirement of an increase in seizure frequency of ≥3 times the follicular rate, yielding an incidence of 33% of WWE having at least one of the patterns.

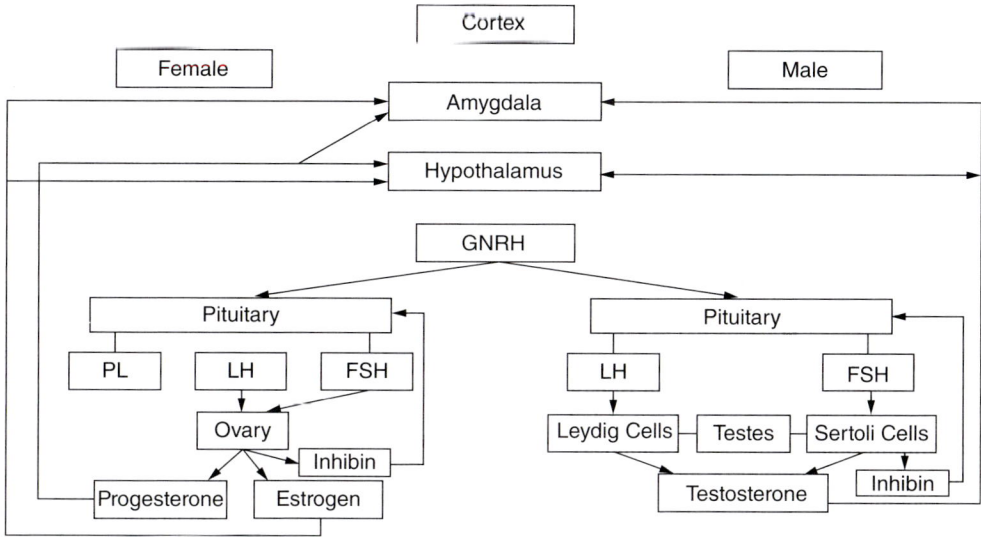

Figure 20.1 Feedback loops between the gonads and hypothalamus

Various attempts to improve seizure control by manipulating this hormonal pattern have been attempted (Table 20.1).[6–9] A placebo-controlled multicenter study of natural progesterone compared each woman's baseline 3-month pattern to a 3-month treatment period. There was no difference between progesterone and placebo percentage responder rates overall, for seizure freedom or for any seizure type except for women with C_1 patterns who had a seizure increase >3.10. Ganaxolone, a synthetic derivative of allopregnanolone, which modulates the $GABA_A$ receptor complex and has no hormonal activity, may have efficacy in catamenial epilepsy and is being studied.[11,12] To date, there is no well-defined treatment guideline.

20.3 Menstrual Disorders

Up to 50% of WWE have menstrual disorders with 20% being amenorrheic.[13] In WWE, up to 35% have anovulatory cycles compared to 8% in controls. This may be more frequent in temporal lobe epilepsy (TLE).[14,15] Anovulatory cycles result in infertility, defined as failure to conceive after 1 year of regular unprotected sexual intercourse. Reasons for anovulatory cycles include hypothalamic and pituitary etiologies and polycystic ovarian syndrome (PCO syndrome), defined as chronic oligomenorrhea (menstrual cycle >35 days) or amenorrhea (no menses for >6 months) with hyperandrogenemia. Other features of PCO syndrome include obesity, hirsutism, acne, hyperlipidemia, insulin resistance, and male balding pattern. The presence of polycystic ovaries on ultrasound is not required. PCO syndrome prevalence in the general population is 4–6%, while in women with TLE it occurs at 10–25%.[3,16–18] Most anovulatory cycles occur in women who do not express the full syndrome.

Valproate (VPA) appears to be causal in the development of PCO with or without full syndromic expression or hyperandrogenism. Up to 80% of WWE who received VPA prior to age 20 had PCO and/or hyperandrogenism.[19] In girls on VPA for 0.8–10.3 years, hyperandrogenism was seen in one-third of prepubertal and in one-half of postpubertal

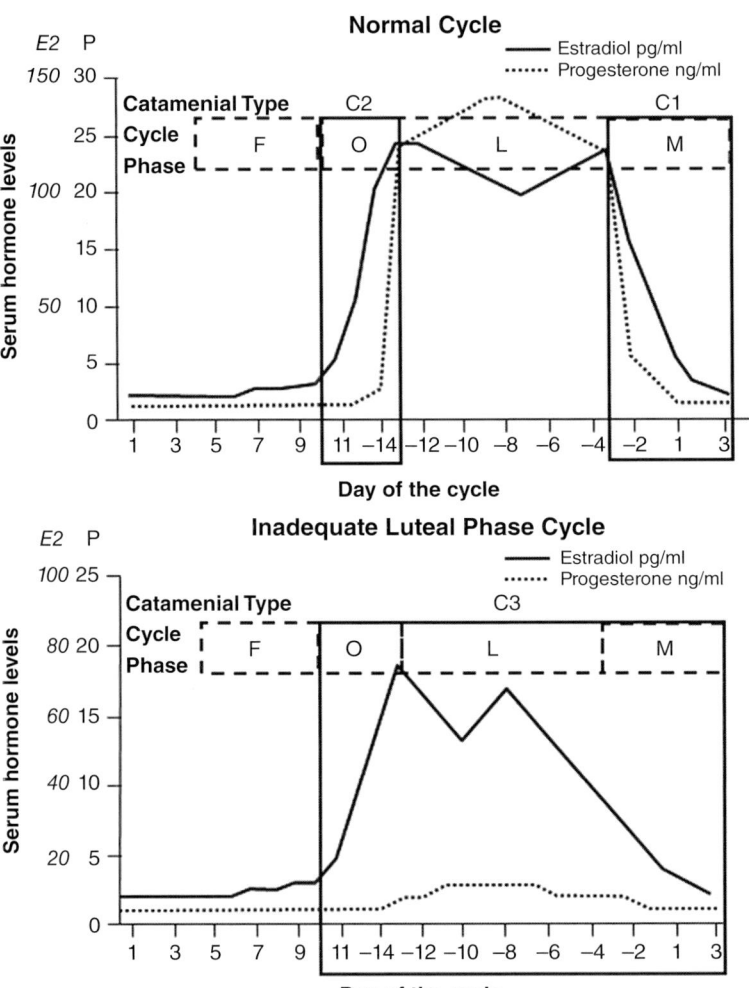

PATTERNS OF CATAMENIAL EPILEPSY

Figure 20.2 Phases in the menstrual cycle, and patterns in catamenial epilepsy: C_1 in the perimenstrual phase, C_2 in the ovulatory phase, and C_3 in anovulatory cycle.

girls. In postpubertal girls with epilepsy with menstrual irregularity, 75% had hyperandrogenism. Obesity did not correlate with hyperandrogenism.[20] Other studies suggest that PCOS seen with VPA is correlated with the presence of obesity.[19,21,22] When VPA-treated women were compared to those only ever on carbamazepine (CBZ) or lamotrigine (LTG), only the VPA patients had evidence of PCO syndrome.[23] In one prospective study, WWE were randomized to VPA or LTG therapy.[24] More women on VPA developed ovulatory dysfunction (54% versus 38%), PCO syndrome (9% versus 2%), and hyperandrogenism if <26 years old (44% versus 23%). Another study evaluated women with hyperandrogenism and obesity and found that these abnormalities reversed when VPA was changed to LTG.[25] This association of PCO syndrome with VPA is also seen in treatment of bipolar disease.[26]

Table 20.1 Open-labeled, noncontrolled hormonal trials in catamenial epilepsy [6-9]

	Depo-medroxyprogesterone[6]	Progesterone[7,8]		Clomiphene[9]
Regimen	120–150 mg IM q 6–12 weeks	100–200 tid,Days 15–28 cycle		25–100 mg q day
Months	12	3	36	3
Subjects	14	25	15	12
Number improved		18 (72%)	75 (100%)	10 (83%)
Reduction in seizure frequency	39%	54–58% CPS SGMS		87%

IM, intramuscular; CPS, complex partial seizures or focal impaired awareness seizures; SGMS. Secondarily generalized motor seizure or focal to bilateral tonic–clonic seizures

20.4 Contraception

Effective contraception is possible for WWE. The failure rate does increase from 1% in the general population to as high as 6% for WWE. For most women, estrogen-based contraceptives do not affect seizure frequency. The progestin component is the active contraceptive agent while estrogen affects the bleeding.[27] ASDs that induce hepatic enzymes result in a decrease in both of the active hormones thus decreasing the efficacy.[27,28] It is generally suggested that higher hormone-concentration pills be prescribed with these ASDs or to use an additional barrier method. Progestin only (mini pills) and subdermal implants are also induced by ASDs and are not recommended. The hormonal effects of intrauterine devices occur locally at the uterus and are not affected by ASDs.[27]

20.5 Fertility

There is conflicting information regarding fertility rates in people with epilepsy. Retrospective evaluation of MWE and WWE reports decreased fertility compared to same-sex siblings without epilepsy not attributable to marriage rates.[29] A population-based Finnish cohort study compared live births for epilepsy patients and controls. They found decreased birth rates over a 9-year period for both MWE (hazard ratio 0.58) and WWE (hazard ratio 0.88).[30] Another Finnish study based on questionnaires, hospital discharges, and medication records found that compared to a reference group, WWE had fewer deliveries and pregnancies, particularly if the epilepsy was not in remission before age 20. MWE also had fewer children, particularly if not in remission before age 20. Both MWE and WWE also had lower rates of marriage/cohabitation than the reference population.[31] An Icelandic study found no difference compared to controls for number of children born to patients with idiopathic/cryptogenic epilepsy or remote symptomatic patients when patients with mental retardation or cerebral palsy were removed.[32] An Indian study showed significantly decreased marriage rates, particularly if epilepsy began <20 years and lower fertility rates in people with epilepsy.[33] The Indian Kerala registry reported increased infertility in women exposed to ASDs, with highest risk in polytherapy and if exposed to phenobarbital.[34]

20.6 Pregnancy and Obstetric Outcomes

About half a million WWE in the United States of America are of childbearing age and experience 3–5 births per 1000. Medical management involves prepregnancy counseling, increased management of ASDs, prevention of seizures during pregnancy, and obstetric management.

American Academy of Neurology Practice Parameters and the Maternal Outcomes and Neurodevelopmental Effects of Antiepileptic Drugs (MONEAD) study confirm there is no increased risk for cesarean section, pre-eclampsia, peripartum hemorrhage, small-for-gestational-age infants, or other major OB complications.[35,36] Polytherapy is associated with a higher rate of premature rupture of membranes, prematurity, and NICU admission rates.[36] Miscarriages occurred in 3% of WWE compared to 0% in women without epilepsy in the MONEAD trial; both rates being low.[37] Although very low at 80/100,000, the risk of death in WWE at delivery was 10-fold greater than nonepileptic pregnancies, at 6/100,000.[38]

Seizure frequency in pregnancy remains stable in 64% of women; 93% of these women were seizure-free throughout pregnancy and more likely had primary generalized epilepsy.[39] The rate of remaining seizure-free during pregnancy is 84–92% if seizure-free for 9–12 months prior to pregnancy.[35] Optimization of treatment prior to pregnancy is important, aiming for monotherapy and seizure freedom. Loss of seizure control is attributed to change in ASD levels due to altered pharmacokinetics, particularly for lamotrigine and oxcarbazepine. This increase in clearance begins in the first trimester and persists until delivery. It is recommended that monthly ASD levels be monitored and doses adjusted to maintain seizure control. Post delivery prompt readjustment of doses is needed to prevent toxicity.

The goal is to maintain seizure control to maximize maternal and fetal safety. Fetal monitoring of infants exposed to focal seizures and generalized seizures has shown both prolonged uterine contractions and marked decrease in fetal heart rates with prolonged recovery period.[40–42] Infants exposed to repeated seizures have a higher risk for being small for gestational age (SGA), low birth weight, and preterm delivery.[43] Seizures during delivery are rare.

20.7 Teratogenesis

Every WWE and her family have concerns over the risk she subjects her baby to by taking ASDs during pregnancy versus the risk of having seizures while pregnant. The mechanisms of teratogenesis are probably multiple and incompletely understood. Animal models have not fully reproduced or predicted the human responses. Folate deficiency, ischemia, reactive metabolites such as free radicals, genotypic susceptibility, and neuronal apoptosis induced by ASDs have been suggested. Fetal exposure is dependent on multiple factors.[44] Birth registries provide some evidence. Single-drug registries frequently lack control populations and have small numbers of exposures with limited demographic data. Different international registries employ different registration techniques, but when taken together offer helpful guidance, despite limitations.[45] At the time of initial drug approval, information is not available for direct applicability to human use. Monotherapy exposure of >700 is needed to get meaningful data for low-incidence occurrences, even without controlling for any other factors, such as maternal age, nutrition, family history of major congenital malformations (MCM), and dose. Over all ASDs and combinations, MCM rates for WWE range between 4% and 9% compared to control populations and untreated epilepsy patients with rates of 1.6–2.8%.[46,47]

Table 20.2 Prevalence of major malformations in ASD monotherapy use

	North American[49]		United Kingdom[50]	NEAD[51]
Enrolled pregnancies	9294		5206	333[c]
	% (CI) N		**% (CI)**	
External control[a]	1.6 (1.5–1.7)	69277	None	None
Internal control[b]	1.5 (0.47–2.5)	532	None	None
Lamotrigine	2.1 (1.7–2.8)	1994	2.3 (1.8–3.1)	1.0 (0.03–5.6)
Carbamazepine	3.0 (2.1–4.2)	1094	2.7 (1.9–3.5)	8.2 (3.8–15.0)
Levetiracetam	2.0 (1.1–3.2)	769	N/A	N/A
Topiramate	4.4 (2.7–6.8)	451	N/A	N/A
Phenytoin	2.8 (1.5–4.9)	422	N/A	10.7 (4.0–21.9)
Valproate	8.9 (6.1–12.5)	336	6.7 (5.5–8.3)	20.3 (11.6–31.7)
Oxcarbazepine	1.7 (0.5–4.4)	230	N/A	N/A
Phenobarbital	5.9 (3.1–10.2)	202	N/A	N/A
Gabapentin	1.2 (0.1–4.2)	169	N/A	N/A
Zonisamide	1.5 (0.2–5.2)	136	N/A	N/A
Clonazepam	2.3 (0.3–8.1)	87	N/A	N/A

Results refer to major malformations only
a External controls are from the Active Malformation Surveillance Program at Brigham and Women's Hospital
b Internal controls are friends and family of participants
c Includes major malformations and fetal death

Rates are significantly higher with ASD polytherapy, particularly with valproate use, 6.2–17.1%.[47] Higher MCM risks may be associated with higher doses of valproate and lamotrigine.[48] This report does not correlate dose and serum levels and others do not see this dose/risk correlation for lamotrigine.

Incidence rates derived from monotherapy exposures provide the closest exposure/ causation relationship. Published results from two large registries are seen in Table 20.2.[49 51] Unfortunately, the largest registry EURAP has not yet published its monotherapy results from its >2300 enrollees of women taking ASDs for any reason.

In general, registry results raise concern for use of phenobarbital and valproate, with relative safety observed for lamotrigine and levetiracetam. One report of increased clefts with lamotrigine has not been substantiated by other registries.[52,53] There is one report of increased MCM with topiramate.[54] Reports with larger exposure groups which include data for other medical uses of topiramate report an increased odds ratio (OR) of 3.6 for cleft lip and palate.[55,56] Other ASDs and newer ASDs have not had sufficient use in monotherapy in pregnancy to make full recommendations, however.

Valproate monotherapy exposure has shown a 12–16 times higher risk over the general population for spina bifida and 2–7 times risk for atrial septal defect, cleft palate, hypospadias, polydactyly, craniosynostosis, and limb reduction.[57] Although the adjusted odds ratio for these are high, the absolute risks are 0.6% for spina bifida and lower still for the other conditions.[57]

Table 20.3 ASDs in breast milk[63–66]

ASD	Infant serum µM/l	T½ Infant (h)	% M level	Infant dosing	Milk/P level
Carbamazepine	20				0.1–0.7
Ethotoin	285		24.75		0.8–1.0
Gabapentin	1.9				0.5–2
Levetiracetam	0–77				0.8–1.3
Lamotrigine	1–2 µg/ml–11 µM/l		20.4	0.5 mg/kg/ day	0.1–1.4
Oxcarbazepine	0.5				0.5
Phenobarbital	39				0.3–0.5
Pregabalin			8		
Phenytoin	<1				0.1–0.6
Topiramate	2.1				0.7–1.1
Valproate	28				0.01–0.3
Zonisamide	N/A	100			0.9

ASD, antiseizure drug; M, maternal; P, maternal plasma level
Inconsistent methods and measurements prevent cross report assessments
Empty cells imply no data reported.

Besides MCM, minor anomalies appear increased with phenotypic expression including glue ear, joint laxity, and myopia. Facial dysmorphic features include epicanthal folds, infraorbital grooves, flat nasal bridge, widely spaced eyebrows, short nose with anteverted nares, shallow philtrum, long thin upper lip, thick lower lip, and small downturned mouth.[58]

Infants exposed to ASDs may be small with lower weights, lengths, and head circumferences, and may meet SGA criteria.[59] This has been reported in particular with topiramate and zonisamide.[60]

20.8 Breastfeeding

Infants born to WWE are exposed to ASDs throughout pregnancy. The mother also faces the decision about exposing the infant to ASDs during breastfeeding. Breastfeeding is recommended by the American Academy of Pediatrics for the first 6 months for nutrition, protection from infectious and immunological diseases, and promotion of development and bonding.[61] Practice parameter recommendations by American Academy of Neurology and American Epilepsy Society recommend it.[62] Lack of safety data leads to conflicting advice. ASDs do enter the breast milk. The amount is small and typically clinically insignificant. Multiple factors complicate the assessment of the infant exposure: maternal plasma levels, volume amount of milk ingested, infant serum levels at time of feeding related to maternal peak or trough time, ASD milk concentration at beginning versus end of feeding session, changes in infant hepatic metabolism, and maturity of infant metabolic pathways.[63] There are no large series of infants on various individual ASDs. Table 20.3 summarizes what has been reported. [63–66]

One prospective evaluation of 30 infants exposed to lamotrigine found high intra- and interindividual variability in the infant/maternal total level (18.3%) and free level (30.9%), reflecting low infant binding. No adverse outcomes were reported. The calculated dose exposure was 0.51 mg/kg/day.[65]

One review of breastfeeding classifies phenytoin, valproate, and carbamazepine as safe, and lamotrigine, oxcarbazepine, levetiracetam, topiramate, gabapentin, and pregabalin as moderately safe.[67] Possibly hazardous ASDs are phenobarbital, primidone, benzodiazepines, ethosuximide, and zonisamide, most likely attributable to long plasma half-life accumulation.

Infant development in breastfed infants at 6 months was more favorable than in infants who did not breastfeed or discontinued it.[68] By age 36 months the difference between breastfed and nonbreastfed groups disappeared. The Neurodevelopmental Effects of Antiepileptic Drugs (NEAD) study evaluated infants who were exposed to carbamazepine, lamotrigine, phenytoin, and valproate monotherapy and breastfed for a mean of 7.2 months.[69] The IQ at age 6 did not differ across groups, except for valproate with a worse IQ by 7–13%. Breastfed infants scored 4 IQ percentage points higher in the verbal cognitive domain.

20.9 Infant Cognitive Outcomes

Developmental delay, behavioral abnormalities, and cognitive dysfunction are described in children of mothers who took ASDs. The mechanism for these deficits is not clearly known. Given that learning and cognitive skills develop in the third trimester, neuronal apoptosis may be responsible. In rat pups, monotherapy with levetiracetam, lamotrigine, topiramate, and carbamazepine did not produce cell death. Cell death caused by phenytoin was not enhanced by topiramate or levetiracetam but was by carbamazepine.[70,71] This may suggest that monotherapy and polytherapy choices should consider cognitive as well as structural teratogenetic effects and risks.

It is recognized that there may be increased risk of neurodevelopmental disorders in children exposed to ASDs.[68] Children born to MWE perform on testing as well as control group children.[72] In the NEAD monotherapy study at age 3, verbal abilities were lower than nonverbal abilities for children exposed to carbamazepine, phenytoin, lamotrigine, and valproate. Statistical significance was only seen for valproate for both verbal and nonverbal abilities and found to be dose dependent. Children exposed to folate preconceptually had higher verbal outcomes.[73] By age 6, IQ improved but the valproate differences persisted with additional effects on executive and memory scores.[74]

Fine motor skills and social skills were impaired in ASD-exposed children compared to a reference group, but less so if breastfed. By 36 months these children remained impaired, even if breastfed.[68] Lower IQs found at age 2 persisted and predicted lower IQ at adolescence in another report.[75]

Valproate in monotherapy or polytherapy is identified as a causative for developmental delay in multiple studies.[76-78] An analysis of 11 studies found only valproate statistically significant for cognitive delay compared to unexposed controls. Psychomotor delay, occurrence of autism/dyspraxia, and language delay were also noted.[79] In one community study, 62% of valproate-exposed children required educational support, compared to 15% of carbamazepine-exposed children and nonexposed children.[80] Attention and verbal working memory were significantly decreased for valproate-exposed children in monotherapy or polytherapy compared to children of WWE not on ASDs, of mothers on other ASDs, or control children.[78]

Some studies show no increased risks with levetiracetam or lamotrigine. Polytherapy itself appears to be a factor producing lower scores for IQ, language and motor skills, and memory.[68,77,79,81]

20.9.1 Autism

Autism spectrum disorders present with impaired social interactions and communication skills and exhibit stereotypical behaviors. The clinical expression may be mild to severe. Autism spectrum disorders limit academic and occupational performance, social interactions, and personal organization.[82,83]

The prevalence of autism spectrum disorders in United States children aged 3–17 years is 1.1%.[84,85] A Danish registry of all children born between 1996 and 2006 found that for children exposed to valproate for any diagnosis there was an absolute risk of 4.42% for autism spectrum disorders, and 2.50% for childhood autism.[86] If use was for epilepsy alone, the absolute risk was 4.15% for autism spectrum disorders, and 1.0% for childhood autism. There was no increased risk seen with oxcarbazepine, lamotrigine, carbamazepine or clonazepam monotherapy. Autism and fetal valproate syndrome may occur simultaneously.[87,88] It has also been noted that the autism spectrum disorders male>female ratio is equalized, unlike the unexposed reference ratio of 4.6. Autistic behaviors in animals exposed to valproate in pregnancy are described but the mechanism producing the clinical picture is not known.[86]

20.10 Menopause

Menopause, defined as the time period after 1 year of amenorrhea, shows low stable estrogen and progesterone levels. The cyclical monthly fluctuations seen in younger women have ceased and catamenial patterns have ended. During the preceding perimenopause, the estrogen and progesterone levels fluctuate erratically. For WWE and particularly those exhibiting prior catamenial patterns, seizures may increase.[88] Supplementing WWE who experience severe perimenopausal symptoms with hormone replacement therapy results in increased seizures in 60% of women.[89]

In the United States of America, the mean age of natural menopause is 51.3 years. In WWE the mean age of menopause is 46–47 years and may be related to past lifetime seizure frequency, early seizure onset, and use of enzyme-inducing ASDs.[90] Premature ovarian failure, defined as menopause before age 40, occurs in 1% of the general population and 4.8% of WWE, again correlated with early onset of seizures and intractable seizures, and with focal epilepsy in another study.[91,92]

20.11 Men with Epilepsy

The effects of male hormones on epilepsy and the effects of epilepsy and ASDs on male function has not been as extensively or prospectively studied as the issues for women. The results have been contradictory at times due to study methods as well as what hormone has been measured.

Testosterone (T) secretion by the Leydig cells of the testes is regulated directly by pituitary luteinizing hormone (LH) secretion, which in turn is regulated by hypothalamic

GNRH secretion (Figure 20.1). The hypothalamus receives feedback regulation mainly from gonadal T and the circulating metabolite of T, estradiol.[93] T is bound weakly to albumin and strongly to SHBG. The functional effects of T are then related to free testosterone (FT) and the free androgen index (FAI) (FAI = 100 × T ÷ SHBG). The metabolism of T occurs by two pathways: (1) inducible oxidation by aromatase to estradiol and (2) reduction by 5-alpha-reductase to 5-alpha-dihydrotestosterone (DHT), which then is converted to 3-alpha-androstanediol (3A). These two pathways provide antagonistic effects on cellular excitability in animal models: estradiol being proconvulsant, while DHT and 3A exhibit anticonvulsant properties through $GABA_A$ receptor modulation.[94]

Human sexual response is a combination of desire and arousal, as well as function. Toone et al. found lower FT levels in men with low sexual activity.[95] Rodin et al. found low sexual arousal scores on the Bear–Fedio Personality Inventory in men with low T levels.[96] Enzyme-inducing ASDs result in increased SHBG, decreased FT, and decreased FAI.[97,98] The changes seen in MWE are seen within 1 year of therapy.[97] Polytherapy produces the same results.[98]

Herzog found reduced biologically active testosterone (BAT) (BAT = FT + albumin bound T) and decreased BAT/LH ratio, a measure of gonadal efficiency.[99] Sexual dysfunction occurred in 20% of MWE. Of MWE who had low sexual function scores, 70.6% had low BAT compared to controls. MWE on a noninducing ASD, lamotrigine, had hormone results similar to controls. MWE switched from carbamazepine, an inducing ASD, to noninducing oxcarbazepine normalized function.[100]

A major question not completely answered is the effect of the epilepsy itself on sexual function and hormone levels. Most of the studies report patients with localization-related epilepsy. Some studies eliminated patients with valproic acid therapy, presumably some of whom had primary generalized epilepsy. Bauer et al. evaluated 117 men with TLE, 39 other focal epilepsies, and 22 with idiopathic generalized epilepsy.[101] They found FT low in all groups and lower in TLE than extratemporal focal epilepsy. Patients with TLE on VPA rather than CBZ had higher total T.

Evaluation of 22 men who had temporal lobectomy without change in CBZ therapy revealed that in the 14 patients who became seizure-free, T, FT, and androstendione (A) normalized to control levels.[102]

Erectile dysfunction is reported in up to 56% MWE compared to 20–22% in the general population.[103] Guldner and Morrell evaluated eight patients with TLE and one patient with nonepileptic events as a control.[104] They measured desire, tumescence, determined vascular function, and rigidity, a neurogenic function. All had normal desire, but 75% of the patients with TLE had decreased rigidity.

Brain pathology, effects of ASDs, and social factors may all contribute to sexual dysfunction in men. Talbot et al. compared 60 MWE from outpatient clinics to 60 control men using serum hormone levels (T, estrogen, SHBG, BAT, FT, androgen) and multiple questionnaires (Hospital Anxiety and Depression scale United Kingdom, Sexual Desire Inventory, Sexual Response Inventory, Sexual Self-Efficacy Scale-Erectile functioning).[105] MWE reported 3:1 reduced sexual desire and 2:1 for reduced erectile function. The Hospital Anxiety and Depression scale scores significantly correlated with desire and erectile functioning scores. The hormone differences were not significant for T, FT, and BAT although the BAT was significantly higher in nonenzyme inducers compared to inducers. The MWE in general had higher SHBG than controls.

Table 20.4 Effects of ASDs on male fertility (Data from[106])

	Sperm counts	Morphology	Motility	Testicular volume
Carbamazepine	DECR	ABN	DECR	NL
Oxcarbazepine		ABN		NL
Phenytoin	DECR	ABN	DECR	DECR
Valproate		ABN	DECR	DECR

Data from [106]; ASD, antiseizure drug; ABN, abnormal; DECR, decreased; NL, normal

Table 20.5 Goals of epilepsy care through a woman's lifetime

	Menarche	Woman of childbearing potential		Menopausal
		Prepregnancy	Pregnant	
Seizure freedom	✓	✓	✓	✓
Folate supplementation	✓	✓	✓	
Assess need for continued ASD	✓	✓		✓
Confirm ASD choice[a] and make changes	✓	✓	b	✓
Consider contraception interaction, adjusted doses, and alternative method	✓	✓	N/A	
Counsel on compliance and adverse effects	✓	✓	✓	✓
Counsel regarding effects of epilepsy on pregnancy and effects of pregnancy on seizures and ASDs		✓	✓	
Counsel on ASD choice and teratogenesis		✓	✓	
Counsel on breastfeeding		✓	✓	
Vitamin D level	✓	✓		✓
DEXA scan if inducing ASD	✓	✓		✓
Vitamin D ± calcium supplement	✓	✓	✓	✓
Avoid valproate	✓	✓	✓	
Avoid polytherapy	✓	✓	✓	✓

ASD, antiseizure drug
[a] Monotherapy if possible
[b] Adjust doses as needed for levels. Readjust at delivery

Recommendations and counseling for care of pregnant women with epilepsy

- Communication with obstetric provider
- Counseling – maintain compliance with antiseizure drugs
- Maintain monotherapy if possible
- Seizure freedom predicted by course of seizures in past 9 months
- Continue folate
- Monthly levels with dose adjustment to maintain prepregnancy levels and avoid high peaks
- Daily dosing will likely be increased, especially if on lamotrigine or oxcarbazepine. Free levels should be evaluated
- Level 2 high-definition ultrasound week 18–20
- Create delivery/postdelivery down-titration plan to get to baseline doses postdelivery
- Sleep requirements – avoid sleep deprivation and nap when baby naps
- Breastfeeding is generally safe and recommended
- Infant safety:
    - Bathe infant with another person present
    - Avoid a changing surface at heights
    - Carry infant in a carrier pouch or use a stroller

Fertility for males is related to sperm count and motility. Isojärvi et al. evaluated 60 MWE and 41 controls.[106] Focal epilepsy occurred in 33: 15 on carbamazepine and 18 on oxcarbazepine; 27 were on valproate for generalized epilepsy. Compared to controls, ASD-treated men showed multiple differences (Table 20.4).[106]

MWE may experience changes in sexuality, both in desire and performance, and fertility. Evaluation of MWE should assess anxiety and depression, psychosocial stressors, seizure control and epilepsy type, comedications, ASD effects, comorbidities, and primary sex organ dysfunction. Referral to a urology specialist may be indicated. Supplementation with testosterone may be useful in men with T levels below 12 nM/l.[105] Pharmacological therapies with phosphodiesterase type-5 inhibitors is useful for some. Some patients may benefit from devices.[107]

20.12 Guidelines and Recommendations

The American Academy of Neurology and the American Epilepsy Society jointly released evidence-based guidelines for the care of WWE.[62,108] They are currently being revised. Following guidelines should improve patient care and outcomes. Guidelines are a starting point and may not always be followed; particular circumstances may require deviations. Guidelines are also a measurement tool that providers and health outcome evaluators can use to assess and improve care. A practical longitudinal approach is suggested in Table 20.5.

Caring for WWE during pregnancy calls for additional commitment and increased patient education. This is outlined in the box.

Caring for MWE and WWE requires a comprehensive grasp of their overall health. In addition to seizure control, this means assessment of psychological health. Comorbid anxiety and depression are common. Clinicians should be comfortable addressing this and make referrals to an appropriate specialist as indicated.

Every clinician managing epilepsy should communicate well with other providers and specialists to insure that all are aware of ASD–drug interactions and be mindful of interventions that may lower seizure threshold.

In summary, while many clinical challenges are common to both genders, there is a growing body of knowledge about clinical issues that are specifically distinctive to women and to men. Every epilepsy specialist needs to be familiar with them, a challenge that will mean ongoing attention from all of us.

References

1. Pennell PB. Hormonal aspects of epilepsy. *Neurol Clin.* 2009;27(4):941–965.

2. Penovich PE. The effects of epilepsy and its treatment on sexual and reproductive function. *Epilepsia.* 2000;41(Suppl 2): S53–61.

3. Harden CL, Pennell PB. Neuroendocrine considerations in the treatment of men and women with epilepsy. *Lancet Neurol.* 2013;12(1):72–83.

4. Herzog AG. Catamenial epilepsy: definition, prevalence pathophysiology and treatment. *Seizure.* 2008;17 (2):151–159.

5. Herzog AG, Klein P, Ransil BJ. Three patterns of catamenial epilepsy. *Epilepsia.* 1997;38(10):1082–1088.

6. Frederiksen MC. Depot medroxyprogesterone acetate contraception in women with medical problems. *J Reprod Med.* 1996;41(5 Suppl):414–418.

7. Herzog AG. Progesterone therapy in women with epilepsy: a 3-year follow-up. *Neurology.* 1999;52(9):1917–1918.

8. Herzog AG. Progesterone therapy in women with complex partial and secondary generalized seizures. *Neurology.* 1995;45 (9):1660–1662.

9. Herzog AG. Clomiphene therapy in epileptic women with menstrual disorders. *Neurology.* 1988;38(3):432–434.

10. Herzog AG, Fowler KM, Smithson SD, et al. Progesterone vs placebo therapy for women with epilepsy: a randomized clinical trial. *Neurology.* 2012;78(24):1959–1966.

11. Nohria V, Giller E. Ganaxolone. *Neurotherapeutics.* 2007;4(1):102–105.

12. Reddy DS, Rogawski MA. Neurosteroid replacement therapy for catamenial epilepsy. *Neurotherapeutics.* 2009;6 (2):392–401.

13. Herzog AG. Psychoneuroendocrine aspects of temporolimbic epilepsy. Part II: epilepsy and reproductive steroids. *Psychosomatics.* 1999;40(2):102–108.

14. Cummings LN, Giudice L, Morrell MJ. Ovulatory function in epilepsy. *Epilepsia.* 1995;36(4):355–359.

15. Herzog AG, Seibel MM, Schomer DL, Vaitukaitis JL, Geschwind N. Reproductive endocrine disorders in women with partial seizures of temporal lobe origin. *Arch Neurol.* 1986;43(4):341–346.

16. Herzog AG, Schachter SC. Valproate and the polycystic ovarian syndrome: final thoughts. *Epilepsia.* 2001;42(3):311–315.

17. Bilo L, Meo R, Nappi C, et al. Reproductive endocrine disorders in women with primary generalized epilepsy. *Epilepsia.* 1988;29(5):612–619.

18. Knochenhauer ES, Key TJ, Kahsar-Miller M, et al. Prevalence of the polycystic ovary syndrome in unselected black and white women of the southeastern United States: a prospective study. *J Clin Endocrinol Metab.* 1998;83(9):3078–3082.

19. Isojarvi JI, Laatikainen TJ, Pakarinen AJ, Juntunen KT, Myllyla VV. Polycystic ovaries and hyperandrogenism in women

taking valproate for epilepsy. *N Engl J Med.* 1993;329(19):1383-1388.

20. Vainionpaa LK, Rattya J, Knip M, et al. Valproate-induced hyperandrogenism during pubertal maturation in girls with epilepsy. *Ann Neurol.* 1999;45(4):444-450.

21. Isojarvi JI, Tauboll E, Tapanainen JS, et al. On the association between valproate and polycystic ovary syndrome: a response and an alternative view. *Epilepsia.* 2001;42(3):305–310.

22. Isojarvi JI, Laatikainen TJ, Knip M, et al. Obesity and endocrine disorders in women taking valproate for epilepsy. *Ann Neurol.* 1996;39(5):579–584.

23. Lofgren E, Mikkonen K, Tolonen U, et al. Reproductive endocrine function in women with epilepsy: the role of epilepsy type and medication. *Epilepsy Behav.* 2007;10(1):77–83.

24. Morrell MJ, Hayes FJ, Sluss PM, et al. Hyperandrogenism, ovulatory dysfunction, and polycystic ovary syndrome with valproate versus lamotrigine. *Ann Neurol.* 2008;64(2):200–211.

25. Isojarvi JI, Rattya J, Myllyla VV, et al. Valproate, lamotrigine, and insulin-mediated risks in women with epilepsy. *Ann Neurol.* 1998;43(4):446–451.

26. Joffe H, Cohen LS, Suppes T, et al. Valproate is associated with new-onset oligoamenorrhea with hyperandrogenism in women with bipolar disorder. *Biol Psychiatry.* 2006;59(11):1078–1086.

27. Cramer JA, Gordon J, Schachter S, Devinsky O. Women with epilepsy: hormonal issues from menarche through menopause. *Epilepsy Behav.* 2007;11(2):160–178.

28. Reimers A, Brodtkorb E, Sabers A. Interactions between hormonal contraception and antiepileptic drugs: clinical and mechanistic considerations. *Seizure.* 2015;28:66–70.

29. Schupf N, Ottman R. Reproduction among individuals with idiopathic/cryptogenic epilepsy: risk factors for reduced fertility in marriage. *Epilepsia.* 1996;37(9):833–840.

30. Artama M, Isojarvi JI, Raitanen J, Auvinen A. Birth rate among patients with epilepsy: a nationwide population-based cohort study in Finland. *Am J Epidemiol.* 2004;159(11):1057–1063.

31. Lofgren E, Pouta A, von Wendt L, et al. Epilepsy in the northern Finland birth cohort 1966 with special reference to fertility. *Epilepsy Behav.* 2009;14(1):102–107.

32. Olafsson E, Hauser WA, Gudmundsson G. Fertility in patients with epilepsy: a population-based study. *Neurology.* 1998;51(1):71–73.

33. Agarwal P, Mehndiratta MM, Antony AR, et al. Epilepsy in India: nuptiality behaviour and fertility. *Seizure.* 2006;15(6):409–415.

34. Sukumaran SC, Sarma PS, Thomas SV. Polytherapy increases the risk of infertility in women with epilepsy. *Neurology.* 2010;75(15):1351–1355.

35. Harden CL, Hopp J, Ting TY, et al. Practice parameter update. Management issues for women with epilepsy – focus on pregnancy (an evidence-based review): obstetrical complications and change in seizure frequency. Report of the Quality Standards Subcommittee and Therapeutics and Technology Assessment Subcommittee of the American Academy of Neurology and American Epilepsy Society. *Neurology.* 2009;73(2):126–132.

36. Pennell PB, Meador KJ, May R, et al. Obstetric and neonatal outcomes in the MONEAD study [Abst. 1.217]. *American Epilepsy Society 71st Annual Meeting; December 1-5, 2017; Washington, DC.* 2017.

37. Meador KJ, Pennell PB, May RC, et al. Miscarriages in pregnant women with epilepsy: findings from the MONEAD Study. *32nd International Epilepsy Congress; Barcelona, Spain.* 2017.

38. MacDonald SC, Bateman BT, McElrath TF, Hernandez-Diaz S. Mortality and morbidity during delivery hospitalization among pregnant women with epilepsy in the United States. *JAMA Neurol.* 2015;72(9):981–988.

39. EURAP Study Group. Seizure control and treatment in pregnancy: observations from the EURAP epilepsy pregnancy registry. *Neurology.* 2006;66(3):354–360.

40. Nei M, Daly S, Liporace J. A maternal complex partial seizure in labor can affect fetal heart rate. *Neurology.* 1998;51 (3):904–906.

41. Ramus RM, Cantrell DC, Cunningham FG, Leveno K, Riela AR. Effects of partial seizures on the infants of women with epilepsy [abstract]. *Epilepsia.* 1997;38 (S8):230.

42. Teramo K, Hiilesmaa V, Bardy A, Saarikoski S. Fetal heart rate during a maternal grand mal epileptic seizure. *J Perinat Med.* 1979;7(1):3–6.

43. Chen YH, Chiou HY, Lin HC, Lin HL. Effect of seizures during gestation on pregnancy outcomes in women with epilepsy. *Arch Neurol.* 2009;66(8):979–984.

44. Hovinga CA, Pennell PB. Antiepileptic drug therapy in pregnancy II: fetal and neonatal exposure. *Int Rev Neurobiol.* 2008;83:241–258.

45. Meador KJ, Pennell PB, Harden CL, et al. Pregnancy registries in epilepsy: a consensus statement on health outcomes. *Neurology.* 2008;71(14):1109–1117.

46. Artama M, Auvinen A, Raudaskoski T, Isojarvi I, Isojarvi J. Antiepileptic drug use of women with epilepsy and congenital malformations in offspring. *Neurology.* 2005;64(11):1874–1878.

47. Morrow J, Russell A, Guthrie E, et al. Malformation risks of antiepileptic drugs in pregnancy: a prospective study from the UK Epilepsy and Pregnancy Register. *J Neurol Neurosurg Psychiatry.* 2006;77 (2):193–198.

48. Tomson T, Battino D, Bonizzoni E, et al. Dose-dependent risk of malformations with antiepileptic drugs: an analysis of data from the EURAP epilepsy and pregnancy registry. *Lancet Neurol.* 2011;10 (7):609–617.

49. North American Antiepileptic Drug Pregnancy Registry. Update on montherapy findings: comparative safety of 11 antiepileptic drugs used during pregnancy. *North American Antiepileptic Drug Pregnancy Registry Newsletter.* 2016; Winter 2016:1–2.

50. Campbell E, Kennedy F, Russell A, et al. Malformation risks of antiepileptic drug monotherapies in pregnancy: updated results from the UK and Ireland Epilepsy and Pregnancy Registers. *J Neurol Neurosurg Psychiatry.* 2014;85 (9):1029–1034.

51. Meador KJ, Baker GA, Finnell RH, et al. In utero antiepileptic drug exposure: fetal death and malformations. *Neurology.* 2006;67(3):407–412.

52. Holmes LB, Wyszynski DF, Baldwin EJ, et al. Increased risk for non-syndromic cleft palate among infants exposed to lamotrigine during pregnancy [abstract]. *Birth Defects Res Part A Clin Mol Teratol.* 2006;76(5):318.

53. EUROCAT Antiepileptic Drug Working Group: Dolk H, Jentink J, Loane M, Morris J, de Jong-van den Berg LT. Does lamotrigine use in pregnancy increase orofacial cleft risk relative to other malformations? *Neurology.* 2008;71 (10):714–722.

54. Hunt S, Russell A, Smithson WH, et al. Topiramate in pregnancy: preliminary experience from the UK Epilepsy and Pregnancy Register. *Neurology.* 2008;71 (4):272–276.

55. Green MW, Seeger JD, Peterson C, Bhattacharyya A. Utilization of topiramate during pregnancy and risk of birth defects. *Headache.* 2012;52(7):1070–1084.

56. Margulis AV, Mitchell AA, Gilboa SM, et al. Use of topiramate in pregnancy and risk of oral clefts. *Am J Obstet Gynecol.* 2012;207(5):405.e1–7.

57. Jentink J, Loane MA, Dolk H, et al. Valproic acid monotherapy in pregnancy and major congenital malformations. *N Engl J Med.* 2010;362(23):2185–2193.

58. Moore SJ, Turnpenny P, Quinn A, et al. A clinical study of 57 children with fetal anticonvulsant syndromes. *J Med Genet.* 2000;37(7):489–497.

59. Veiby G, Daltveit AK, Engelsen BA, Gilhus NE. Fetal growth restriction and birth defects with newer and older antiepileptic drugs during pregnancy. *J Neurol.* 2014;261 (3):579–588.

60. Hernandez-Diaz S, Mittendorf R, Smith CR, et al. Association between topiramate and zonisamide use during pregnancy and

low birth weight. *Obstet Gynecol*. 2014;123 (1):21–28.

61. Johnston M, Landers S, Noble L, Szucs K, Viehmann L; Section on Breastfeeding. Breastfeeding and the use of human milk. *Pediatrics*. 2012;129(3):e827–841.

62. Harden CL, Pennell PB, Koppel BS, et al. Practice parameter update. Management issues for women with epilepsy – focus on pregnancy (an evidence-based review). Vitamin K, folic acid, blood levels, and breastfeeding: report of the Quality Standards Subcommittee and Therapeutics and Technology Assessment Subcommittee of the American Academy of Neurology and American Epilepsy Society. *Neurology*. 2009;73(2):142–149.

63. Tomson T. Gender aspects of pharmacokinetics of new and old AEDs: pregnancy and breast-feeding. *Ther Drug Monit*. 2005;27(6):718–721.

64. Zonisamide use while breastfeeding. https://www.drugs.com/breastfeeding/zonisamide.html. Accessed April, 2019.

65. Liporace J, Kao A, D'Abreu A. Concerns regarding lamotrigine and breast-feeding. *Epilepsy Behav*. 2004;5(1):102–105.

66. Newport DJ, Pennell PB, Calamaras MR, et al. Lamotrigine in breast milk and nursing infants: determination of exposure. *Pediatrics*. 2008;122(1):e223–231.

67. Veiby G, Bjork M, Engelsen BA, Gilhus NE. Epilepsy and recommendations for breastfeeding. *Seizure*. 2015;28:57–65.

68. Veiby G, Engelsen BA, Gilhus NE. Early child development and exposure to antiepileptic drugs prenatally and through breastfeeding: a prospective cohort study on children of women with epilepsy. *JAMA Neurol*. 2013;70 (11):1367–1374.

69. Meador KJ, Baker GA, Browning N, et al. Breastfeeding in children of women taking antiepileptic drugs: cognitive outcomes at age 6 years. *JAMA Pediatr*. 2014;168 (8):729–736.

70. Kim J, Kondratyev A, Gale K. Antiepileptic drug-induced neuronal cell death in the immature brain: effects of carbamazepine, topiramate, and levetiracetam as monotherapy versus polytherapy.

J Pharmacol Exp Ther. 2007;323 (1):165–173.

71. Meador KJ, Baker G, Cohen MJ, Gaily E, Westerveld M. Cognitive/behavioral teratogenetic effects of antiepileptic drugs. *Epilepsy Behav*. 2007;11(3):292–302.

72. Veiby G, Daltveit AK, Schjolberg S, et al. Exposure to antiepileptic drugs in utero and child development: a prospective population-based study. *Epilepsia*. 2013;54 (8):1462–1472.

73. Meador KJ, Baker GA, Browning N, et al. Foetal antiepileptic drug exposure and verbal versus non-verbal abilities at three years of age. *Brain*. 2011;134(Pt 2):396–404.

74. Meador KJ, Baker GA, Browning N, et al. Fetal antiepileptic drug exposure and cognitive outcomes at age 6 years (NEAD study): a prospective observational study. *Lancet Neurol*. 2013;12(3):244–252.

75. Titze K, Koch S, Helge H, et al. Prenatal and family risks of children born to mothers with epilepsy: effects on cognitive development. *Dev Med Child Neurol*. 2008;50(2):117–122.

76. Bromley RL, Mawer GE, Briggs M, et al. The prevalence of neurodevelopmental disorders in children prenatally exposed to antiepileptic drugs. *J Neurol Neurosurg Psychiatry*. 2013;84(6):637–643.

77. Thomas SV, Ajaykumar B, Sindhu K, et al. Motor and mental development of infants exposed to antiepileptic drugs in utero. *Epilepsy Behav*. 2008;13(1):229–236.

78. Veroniki AA, Rios P, Cogo E, et al. Comparative safety of antiepileptic drugs for neurological development in children exposed during pregnancy and breast feeding: a systematic review and network meta-analysis. *BMJ Open*. 2017;7(7): e017248.

79. Kantola-Sorsa E, Gaily E, Isoaho M, Korkman M. Neuropsychological outcomes in children of mothers with epilepsy. *J Int Neuropsychol Soc*. 2007;13 (4):642–652.

80. Viinikainen K, Eriksson K, Monkkonen A, et al. The effects of valproate exposure in utero on behavior and the need for educational support in school-aged

children. *Epilepsy Behav.* 2006;9
(4):636–640.

81. Thomas SV, Sukumaran S, Lukose N,
George A, Sarma PS. Intellectual and
language functions in children of mothers
with epilepsy. *Epilepsia.* 2007;48
(12):2234–2240.

82. Autism Speaks. DSM-5 Diagnostic Criteria.
https://www.autismspeaks.org/what-
autism/diagnosis/dsm-5-diagnostic-
criteria. Accessed April 3, 2019.

83. Carpenter L. DSM-5 autism spectrum
disorder: guidelines and criteria exemplars.
https://depts.washington.edu/dbpeds/
Screening%20Tools/DSM-5%
28ASD.Guidelines%29Feb2013.pdf.
Accessed April 3, 2019.

84. Kogan MD, Blumberg SJ, Schieve LA, et al.
Prevalence of parent-reported diagnosis of
autism spectrum disorder among children
in the US, 2007. *Pediatrics.* 2009;124
(5):1395–1403.

85. Autism and Developmental Disabilities
Monitoring Network Surveillance Year
2006 Principal Investigators, Centers for
Disease Control and Prevention.
Prevalence of autism spectrum disorders –
Autism and Developmental Disabilities
Monitoring Network, United States,
2006. *MMWR Surveill Summ.* 2009;58
(10):1–20.

86. Christensen J, Gronborg TK, Sorensen MJ,
et al. Prenatal valproate exposure and risk
of autism spectrum disorders and
childhood autism. *JAMA.* 2013;309
(16):1696–1703.

87. Rasalam AD, Hailey H, Williams JH, et al.
Characteristics of fetal anticonvulsant
syndrome associated autistic disorder. *Dev
Med Child Neurol.* 2005;47(8):551–555.

88. Harden CL, Pulver MC, Ravdin L, Jacobs
AR. The effect of menopause and
perimenopause on the course of epilepsy.
Epilepsia. 1999;40(10):1402–1407.

89. Pennell PB. More is not better: hormones
for menopausal women with epilepsy?
Epilepsy Curr. 2007;7(3):68–70.

90. Harden CL, Koppel BS, Herzog AG,
Nikolov BG, Hauser WA. Seizure
frequency is associated with age at

menopause in women with epilepsy.
Neurology. 2003;61(4):451–455.

91. Serje A, Klein P. Premature ovarian failure
in women with epilepsy [abstract].
Epilepsia. 2000;41(Suppl 7):198.

92. Tran TA. B.01 Premature ovarian failure in
women with epilepsy [abstract]. *Epilepsia.*
2006;47(S4):7.

93. Winters SJ, Janick JJ, Loriaux DL, Sherins
RJ. Studies on the role of sex steroids in the
feedback control of gonadotropin
concentrations in men. II. Use of the
estrogen antagonist, clomiphene citrate.
J Clin Endocrinol Metab. 1979;48
(2):222–227.

94. Reddy DS. Testosterone modulation of
seizure susceptibility is mediated by
neurosteroids 3alpha-androstanediol and
17beta-estradiol. *Neuroscience.* 2004;129
(1):195–207.

95. Toone BK, Wheeler M, Nanjee M, Fenwick
P, Grant R. Sex hormones, sexual activity
and plasma anticonvulsant levels in male
epileptics. *J Neurol Neurosurg Psychiatry.*
1983;46(9):824–826.

96. Rodin E, Subramanian MG, Gilroy J.
Investigation of sex hormones in male
epileptic patients. *Epilepsia.* 1984;25
(6):690–694.

97. Isojarvi JI, Repo M, Pakarinen AJ,
Lukkarinen O, Myllyla VV.
Carbamazepine, phenytoin, sex hormones,
and sexual function in men with epilepsy.
Epilepsia. 1995;36(4):366–370.

98. Duncan S, Blacklaw J, Beastall GH, Brodie
MJ. Antiepileptic drug therapy and sexual
function in men with epilepsy. *Epilepsia.*
1999;40(2):197–204.

99. Herzog AG, Drislane FW, Schomer DL,
et al. Differential effects of antiepileptic
drugs on sexual function and hormones in
men with epilepsy. *Neurology.* 2005;65
(7):1016–1020.

100. Isojarvi JI, Pakarinen AJ, Rautio A,
Pelkonen O, Myllyla VV. Serum sex
hormone levels after replacing
carbamazepine with oxcarbazepine. *Eur
J Clin Pharmacol.* 1995;47(5):461–464.

101. Bauer J, Stoffel-Wagner B, Flugel D, et al.
Serum androgens return to normal after

temporal lobe epilepsy surgery in men. *Neurology*. 2000;55(6):820–824.

102. Bauer J, Blumenthal S, Reuber M, Stoffel-Wagner B. Epilepsy syndrome, focus location, and treatment choice affect testicular function in men with epilepsy. *Neurology*. 2004;62(2):243–246.

103. Hellmis E. Sexual problems in males with epilepsy – an interdisciplinary challenge! *Seizure*. 2008;17(2):136–140.

104. Guldner GT, Morrell MJ. Nocturnal penile tumescence and rigidity evaluation in men with epilepsy. *Epilepsia*. 1996;37 (12):1211–1214.

105. Talbot JA, Sheldrick R, Caswell H, Duncan S. Sexual function in men with epilepsy: how important is testosterone? *Neurology*. 2008;70(16):1346–1352.

106. Isojarvi JI, Lofgren E, Juntunen KS, et al. Effect of epilepsy and antiepileptic drugs on male reproductive health. *Neurology*. 2004;62(2):247–253.

107. Isidori AM, Giannetta E, Gianfrilli D, et al. Effects of testosterone on sexual function in men: results of a meta-analysis. *Clin Endocrinol (Oxf)*. 2005;63(4):381–394.

108. Harden CL, Meador KJ, Pennell PB, et al. Practice parameter update. Management issues for women with epilepsy – focus on pregnancy (an evidence-based review): teratogenesis and perinatal outcomes. Report of the Quality Standards Subcommittee and Therapeutics and Technology Assessment Subcommittee of the American Academy of Neurology and American Epilepsy Society. *Neurology*. 2009;73(2):133–141.

Antiseizure Drugs

Sidrah Mahmud and Richard H. Mattson

21.1 History of Antiseizure Drug Development

In 1857 in England, Charles Locock reported that bromides helped control seizures. Others confirmed this efficacy, and it continued as the only true antiseizure drug (ASD) used chronically until the report of efficacy of phenobarbital (PHB) by Hauptman in 1912. Putnam and Merritt developed phenytoin (PHT) in the 1930s and brought it to market with improved side effects and somewhat greater efficacy than phenobarbital. Carbamazepine (CBZ), chemically unrelated to PHB or PHT but having comparable efficacy, was introduced in the 1960s in Europe, and the United States in the 1970s. Both CBZ and PHT were primarily effective against focal- or partial-onset seizures, with or without associated tonic–clonic attacks. No improvement was noted when used for absence, atonic, tonic, and myoclonic seizures. Ethosuximide was effective for absence seizures, but not focal-onset or tonic–clonic seizures. The introduction of valproate in the 1960s in Europe and in 1978 in the United States dramatically improved the ability to control these seizures. Despite these available antiepileptic drugs, approximately two-thirds of patients did not realize full control. Under the leadership of J. Kiffin Penry, MD, Director of the NIH Epilepsy Branch, and Harvey Kupferberg, PhD, the Antiepileptic Drug Development Program was initiated in a collaborative effort from government, industry, and academia. Since that time many new ASDs have become available. Many brought new mechanisms of action, pharmacokinetic properties, and improved safety or tolerability. Unfortunately, these drugs did not provide greater efficacy in comparative clinical trials than the older standard ASDs, carbamazepine, phenytoin, and valproate. However, in individual cases one of the new ASDs can dramatically improve seizure control, even after many failures with other ASDs.

21.2 Individual Antiseizure Drugs

An ASD can be described as possessing many characteristics, such as clinical indication, chemical properties, and population targets, among other groupings. This overview will describe the primary characteristics of each ASD.

21.2.1 Brivaracetam

Brivaracetam (Briviact) is a member of the racetam family of drugs and an analog of levetiracetam (Keppra). It was developed using a screening process of 12,000 compounds by UCB with the goal of finding drugs with binding affinity to the synaptic vesicle protein (SV2A) similar to levetiracetam, but with greater efficacy and fewer side effects.[1]

Brivaracetam is a pyrrolidone derivative, which in addition to similarly inhibiting negative modulators gamma-aminobutyric acid (GABA)$_A$ and glycine receptors, was found to possess an affinity for SV2A that was tenfold greater. In testing, brivaracetam was found to have proportionally greater antiseizure efficacy in animal models with audiogenic seizures. It also surpassed levetiracetam in its ability to exert protection against seizures induced in normal animals by electroshock therapy and several chemoconvulsants, including Metrazol threshold testing. With such a remarkable difference in efficacy, it was surmised that there might also be mechanisms beyond those related to SV2A. Therefore, subsequent studies found brivaracetam to also exhibit some inhibitory activity on neuronal voltage-gated sodium channels. However, unlike levetiracetam, it did not inhibit high-voltage Ca^{2+} channels and AMPA (alpha-amino-3-hydroxyl-5-methyl-4-isoxazole-propionate) receptors.

Pharmacokinetics were similar to levetiracetam with little protein binding, extensive renal metabolism, and renal elimination. It differed in being partially hepatically metabolized via the CYP 2C19 isoenzyme. In addition, unlike levetiracetam, modest interactions can result, with decreased levels, when coadministered with ASDs using this pathway, including carbamazepine, phenobarbital, phenytoin, clobazam, and cannabidiol, though typically in a nonclinically significant manner.[2]

The clinical efficacy has been established for focal-onset seizures.[3] In patients with photosensitive epilepsy, brivaracetam has also shown a dose-dependent effect in suppressing or attenuating the photoparoxysmal response.[4] It can be assumed that efficacy will be found for generalized seizures also in view of the similarity to levetiracetam.

Adverse effects are not significant, with sedation being the most common. In clinical trials, affective or behavioral effects did not seem common, which might prove a major advantage over levetiracetam. However, such problems were also not prominent in early trials of levetiracetam, so a longer period of observation may be needed. Safety and tolerability have been good thus far. No major organ toxicity has been reported, and skin hypersensitivity has been rare. Brivaracetam is currently available in 50 mg tablets and in liquid form, as well as in parenteral form.

In summary, brivaracetam, an analog of levetiracetam, shows promise in being a valuable addition to choices for ASD therapy, but further experience will be needed to define its ultimate role.

21.2.2 Carbamazepine

Carbamazepine (Tegretol), a dibenzazepine, carboxamide tricyclic compound, has been used for many years for the successful treatment of epilepsy, trigeminal neuralgia (tic douloureux), and bipolar disorders. In the 1950s, Geigy, a pharmaceutical company in Switzerland, developed carbamazepine in search of a neuroleptic similar to chlorpromazine. The drug was tested in Europe in the 1960s for the treatment of symptomatic epilepsy with focal and generalized tonic–clonic seizures. It was introduced for use in the United States in 1974.

Carbamazepine is almost completely metabolized in the liver, with only about 5% excreted unchanged. This is done primarily via CYP3A4 and CYP2B6, producing the pharmacodynamically active metabolite, carbamazepine-10,11-epoxide. Carbamazepine stimulates the transcriptional upregulation of genes, involved in its own metabolism, through a process of autoinduction. As days and weeks go on, the liver becomes more capable of metabolizing the drug, and a steady dose of 600–800 mg/day or more can be taken and simultaneously eliminated.

Simultaneously taking carbamazepine with phenobarbital or phenytoin increases the conversion to this epoxide, and if taken with valproate, inhibits the clearance and conversion of the metabolite to inactive structures, therefore causing a buildup of this compound. Certain medications taken for high blood pressure, as well as antibiotics such as erythromycin, can interfere with the clearance of carbamazepine and cause it to build up in the blood, causing adverse effects.

Carbamazepine is a highly effective, well-tolerated broad ASD. Effectiveness has been extensively studied in trials in large numbers of patients. Overall, carbamazepine produces complete control of tonic–clonic seizures in approximately 80% of patients. Success with treating focal seizures is somewhat less, with only two-thirds being completely controlled.[5] Among the older drugs, only phenytoin is equally effective.

Although carbamazepine is well tolerated by most people, adverse effects can arise, particularly upon initiation. It may cause sleepiness, dizziness, stomach upset, and blurred or double vision, especially within the first few days. This is almost always a result of too much drug taken too quickly. Although most people can take 600–800 mg daily long term without side effects, this is not true when treatment has only just begun. There are two reasons for this. First, the brain needs to develop tolerance to the drug and this may take a week or two, although in most cases it takes only a few days. Second, the amount in the blood and brain at initiation is higher than that found after regular long-term treatment due to autoinduction of the CYP3A4 isoenzyme.

Another type of adverse effect that often occurs when first starting carbamazepine (or within the first few months) is the appearance of an allergic rash. It is usually located over the face, trunk, arms, and legs, but may be more limited or even more extensive. The rash occurs in between 5% and 10% of patients, and if it occurs, it will spontaneously clear on its own in approximately half the time and will not return. This is particularly true if the medication is not taken for a day or two and then restarted. However, more serious reactions may develop, including Stevens–Johnson syndrome or toxic epidermal necrolysis, so the safest course is to just stop the drug. Studies have shown a strong association with these carbamazepine-induced severe cutaneous adverse reactions in Asian patients with the HLA B-1502 allele.

Neutropenia often occurs with the use of carbamazepine, but is rarely of clinical consequence. There is an initial decrease in the number of white blood cells. However, the lowering of the white blood cell count seen with carbamazepine is rarely significant enough to have any clinical importance. Physicians unfamiliar with this laboratory finding have unnecessarily taken many patients off the drug.

Very rare cases of aplastic anemia were reported in the 1960s when carbamazepine was first introduced to clinical use. Leukopenia is fairly common, but almost never of clinical significance. The sodium concentration in the blood is found to be lower than normal in people taking this drug. It is rarely low enough to be of importance (< 125 mIg/L) in terms of causing any symptoms, although older patients taking sodium-depleting diuretics may sometimes have problems resulting in increased susceptibility to seizure recurrence.

In summary, carbamazepine is one of the reference standards for efficacy in the treatment of focal and tonic–clonic seizures and is the most often prescribed ASD in developed countries. Adverse effects and complex pharmacokinetics are the limitations, but many can be dealt with.

21.2.3 Clobazam

A steady stream of benzodiazepines began after their discovery by Leo Sternbach, with chlordiazepoxide (Librium) in 1959 and diazepam (Valium) in 1963. Boasting anxiolytic and muscle-relaxing properties in addition to broad-spectrum seizure efficacy, benzodiazepines have remained the drug of choice for management of acute seizures.[6] Unfortunately, due to tolerance, which develops along with the side effect of sedation, their use as chronic therapy is limited. Clobazam was then developed more than a decade after the first generation of benzodiazepines. It became approved in Australia in 1970 to treat anxiety, and in France in 1974 to treat epilepsy and anxiety.[7] In the United States, it was later in 2008 that clobazam was granted orphan drug status by the US Food and Drug Administration (FDA) for treatment of Lennox–Gastaut syndrome, and then in 2011, as an adjunctive treatment in people older than 2 years.

Clobazam boasts a unique chemical structure. Unlike other benzodiazepines that have a nitrogen in the 1,4 sites of the B ring of the molecule and a 4,5-imine structure, clobazam has a nitrogen in the 1,5 position of the B ring of the molecule and it does not possess an imine structure. It binds to somewhat different subunits of the $GABA_A$ receptor. These differences confer more antiseizure efficacy and less sedation.

Clobazam is a lipophilic drug that becomes evenly distributed throughout the body. A significant proportion, 85%, becomes protein bound. It is then hepatically metabolized via CYP3A4, and to a lesser extent CYP2C19, which demethylates clobazam to the pharmacodynamically active N-desmethylclobazam. At 50 hours, the half-life of N-desmethylclobazam is remarkably longer than clobazam's, which is 18 hours. Though less involved in clobazam's metabolism, CYP2C19 may play a more clinically significant role in Asian populations, in which it is estimated that 35% of people carry the mutated allele of this enzyme, therefore leading to increased risk of side effects.

Clobazam is typically safe to use with other ASDs. Some CYP3A4 and CYP2C19 inducers, such as carbamazepine, phenobarbital, and phenytoin, may increase clobazam metabolism. However, these medications have been shown to also increase levels of the therapeutically active N-desmethylclobazam, negating the possible reduction of clinical efficacy. It is important to note that concomitant use with cannabidiols also leads to significantly increased levels of clobazam, reported to be as much as a 60–80% increase in children.[8]

Clobazam was specifically approved for use in Lennox–Gastaut syndrome. In the Lennox–Gastaut trial, early responders were still benefiting on 3-year follow-up.[9] However, like other benzodiazepines, its broad-spectrum properties make it suitable for most epilepsy and seizure types. In addition, its anxiolytic properties are also quite significant when given at 30–80 mg/day, superior to diazepam given at 15–40 mg/day, with fewer side effects.[10] In fact, it has been successfully used in most parts of the world except the United States for more than four decades. The late introduction to the United States is likely more due to economic rather than medical reasons.

Clobazam is generally safe to use, with mild side effects when compared to other ASDs. Sedation is the most common side effect seen with clobazam, though less often seen than that caused by diazepam.[9] Tolerance also seems much less common than with use of the 1,4-benzodiazepines. Other rare side effects that have been reported are rash and hypothermia.

In adults, 10–30 mg/day is usually administered, although smaller and larger amounts have also been used. Unlike other benzodiazepines, it is not available for parenteral administration.

In conclusion, clobazam is a very useful option for those with Lennox–Gastaut or multiple seizure types, especially those with concurrent anxiety. Careful monitoring of levels should be performed in those concomitantly taking cannabidiols.

21.2.4 Eslicarbazepine

Eslicarbazepine (Aptiom) is a member of the dibenzapine carboxamine family that includes carbamazepine and oxcarbazepine. It was specifically designed to resemble its two fore-fathers, but with a 5-carboxamide substitute at the 10,11-position, with the aim of having a more effective, better tolerated drug, more able to cross the blood–brain barrier.[11]

The mechanism of action of the oxcarbazepine itself, as well as carbamazepine, is primarily exerted by affecting fast inactivation of the sodium channel, whereas eslicarbazepine has a primary action on slow inactivation.[12] Both decrease excitability, but in somewhat different ways.

Unlike carbamazepine, eslicarbazepine is not metabolized into the carbamazepine 10,11-epoxide, an active and potentially toxic compound. It also has very low enzyme-inducing activity of the cytochrome P450 enzymatic system and does not induce its own metabolism. It is metabolized almost exclusively to the (S)-enantiomer (designated as S-licarbazepine). The drug is the pharmacodynamically active dehydroxy L-enantiomer metabolite of oxcarbazepine. Although eslicarbazepine is the principal metabolite of oxcarbazepine (70%), the R-enantiomer accounts for most of the remaining 30% and is pharmacodynamically minimally active. It is primarily excreted unchanged in the kidney. About a third is conjugated before excretion. The latter step in inducible by carbamazepine, phenobarbital (as well as primidone) and phenytoin, thereby lowering levels by about a third. This might be clinically relevant and warrant dosage changes.[13,14]

Eslicarbazepine is a weak inducer, but lowers levels of oral hormone contraceptives in a potentially meaningful way. Statin metabolism can also be induced, but the clinical relevance depends on lipid levels. The effect on warfarin metabolism is variable, but this would be monitored by the international normalized ratio (INR). Eslicarbazepine also inhibits CYP2C19, which can elevate phenytoin levels. Due to the complex pharmacokinetics of phenytoin metabolism with saturation kinetics, this effect could easily be clinically meaningful.

Eslicarbazepine has demonstrated clear efficacy in treatment of refractory focal-onset seizures, as well as in monotherapy in newly diagnosed patients[15,16] with maximal efficacy seen at 1600 mg/day. The half-life of eslicarbazepine is 18–24 hours in the blood and 24 hours in the cerebrospinal fluid. This property makes once daily dosing feasible and clinical studies have confirmed this efficacy using this dosing.[14]

Adverse effects are similar to the other dibenzapine carboximide relatives, namely dizziness, sedation, diplopia (and related visual symptoms). These are usually dose related and clear with time or reduced dose. Serious adverse effects are few. A hypersensitivity rash seems much less frequent than with carbamazepine and possibly oxcarbazepine. However, a rare drug rash with eosinophilia and systemic symptoms (DRESS) has been reported. Hyponatremia occurs with about the same frequency as oxcarbazepine, but is infrequently of clinical significance.[17]

In summary, eslicarbazepine is the newest analog to the dibenzapine carboxamide family, which has a long history as the "gold standard" in treatment of focal-onset seizures. Eslicarbazepine has the promise of improved pharmacokinetics and fewer adverse effects.

21.2.5 Ethosuximide

Ethosuximide is a drug developed by Parke-Davis (now Pfizer), which was first described for the control of "petit mal epilepsy" by Zimmerman and Burgemeister in 1958. It was one of three succinimides used at the time for epilepsy, including phensuximide (Milontin), methsuximide (Celonitin), and ethosuximide (Zarontin). Its mechanism of action is through the reduction of thalamic low-threshold calcium currents.

Ethosuximide is rapidly and almost completely absorbed. It is then metabolized hepatically through CYP3A4 before being eliminated through the urine. Ethosuximide has a highly specific and selective effect in controlling absence (petit mal) seizures. Approximately 80–85% of absence seizures can be improved or totally controlled with the use of ethosuximide. The success in treatment of atypical absence seizures in infancy and childhood is somewhat less than for patients with typical childhood absence epilepsy. A recent double-blinded randomized clinical trial was completed evaluating the efficacy and tolerability of ethosuximide versus valproic acid versus lamotrigine in the treatment of childhood absence seizures.[18] The conclusion of the study was that ethosuximide and valproic acid are more effective than lamotrigine; however, ethosuximide was associated with fewer adverse attentional effects than valproate.

Ethosuximide is generally well tolerated. The most prominent side effect is gastrointestinal distress. Taking the medication with or after meals can sometimes alleviate this. If the dose is given too quickly or excessively, the usual ASD side effects can be seen, including drowsiness, dizziness, and unsteadiness. Paradoxically, occasional complaints of irritability, hyperactivity, and even hiccups have been reported. Much less commonly, serious toxicity occurs with skin rash and organ involvement, such as liver, kidney, and bone marrow dysfunction. The latter can lead to possibly fatal effects. These complications are rare, but occasional monitoring of blood and liver tests are appropriate. Rarely ethosuximide has also been reported in association with drug-induced lupus erythematosus.[19] Injury to the developing fetus has been observed in animal models with about the same frequency as with other older ASDs. However, the experience is somewhat limited and the risk is not entirely clear. Because absence seizures do not constitute a serious health risk to the patient, some consideration may be given to discontinuation of ethosuximide if pregnancy is planned. It can subsequently be reinstituted.

Ethosuximide is available as a 250 mg capsule and as a syrup containing 250 mg of ethosuximide in each 5 ml of syrup.

In conclusion, ethosuximide is a highly effective and overall very safe ASD to use in those with absence epilepsy, with better tolerability profile than many of its counterparts.

21.2.6 Felbamate

Felbamate (Felbatol) is a chemical compound in the carbamate family and closely related to meprobamate (Miltown), the original "tranquilizer." Though similar in structure, it has few sedative or tranquilizing properties at therapeutic levels. Studies in animal models suggested that it was a compound that would be effective for many types of seizures. Indeed, it was introduced for testing in the early 1990s, and after trials in multiple seizure types, including severe epilepsy syndromes in infants and children, the drug was approved for use. However, it was found to have numerous side effects, some of a very serious nature, which has led to its limited use at the present time.

Felbamate exerts it action through several different mechanisms. It inhibits glycine-enhanced, N-methyl-D-aspartate (NMDA)-induced intracellular calcium currents. At high levels, it leads to the inhibition of excitatory NMDA responses. It also leads to the potentiation of GABA transmission.

Felbamate is well absorbed after oral administration. It is to a small degree hepatically metabolized, resulting in liver enzyme induction and causing plasma levels of felbamate to decline with longer duration of drug administration. However, approximately 70% of orally administered felbamate is excreted unchanged in the urine.

The most common side effects experienced during the early use of felbamate include nausea, vomiting, weight loss, headache, and insomnia. Very gradual administration and avoiding combinations with other ASDs minimize these problems. The primary problem that was recognized after approximately 100,000 patients had been treated with this drug was suppression of the bone marrow, (i.e., aplastic anemia), which occurred in 1 in 2000–5000 people being given the drug. In approximately one-third of the patients, this process could not be reversed and led to a fatal outcome. It was also found that serious, sometimes fatal, liver damage occurred in approximately 1 in 20,000 people taking the drug. It is not clear whether prompt recognition of decreasing white counts or abnormal liver function tests would give sufficient warning to stop the drug and allow recovery without catastrophic outcome. As a consequence, the use of felbamate has been limited. Studies indicate that the damage may be due to a breakdown product of felbamate that is limited to a few certain susceptible individuals, and this may eventually be detectable by a urine test, which could be performed to screen out people at risk for this complication.

Although usually considered adverse effects, the loss of appetite and difficulty in sleeping that occurs in some patients taking this drug has proved to be beneficial to some. Providing that the loss of appetite is not excessive, there is often weight loss, which for some individuals is desirable. Patients also tend to remain quite alert rather than being sleepy, in contrast to the use of most other ASDs.

Felbamate is not available for administration by intravenous or intramuscular injection. It is available in 400 mg and 600 mg tablets. If the drug is administered together with other ASDs, it may result in complex interactions. Whenever possible, it should be taken by itself.

In summary, felbamate is a drug that is effective in treatment of many types of seizures and often exhibits considerable effectiveness for seizures poorly responsive to other drugs, such as atonic seizures characterized by head drops or tonic seizures in infants and children. A Cochrane Review[20] failed to find evidence of efficacy as an add-on agent, yet expert opinion and my personal experience indicates felbamate can be dramatically effective in selective patients. With long-term use, felbamate is often well tolerated, and many patients are especially pleased with the alerting, nonsedating properties, decreased appetite, and the associated weight loss.

21.2.7 Gabapentin

Gabapentin (Neurontin) was invented by Gerhard Satsinger, a medicinal chemist, in the 1960s at Godecke, a division of Parke-Davis in Freiberg, Germany.

The chemical closely resembled GABA chemically, the major neurotransmitter in the central nervous system. Although assumed to exert its action through GABAergic mechanisms, the later studies indicated most action resulted from action at the alpha-2 binding site of the calcium-modulating flow of excitatory transmission.

Gabapentin is handled by the body in a way that makes it very easy to use. It is absorbed by an active process in the intestine and the brain that to some extent limits how much drug gets in, but once absorbed, it is not changed by the liver. It is eliminated through the kidneys and passed into the urine. As a consequence of this form of elimination, it does not cause any effect on other ASDs, nor medications used for other medical problems such as anticoagulants, antibiotics, or oral contraceptives. However, due to its relatively short half-life of about 8 hours, it requires multiple daily dosing, which can often be difficult for some.

Extensive studies have been carried out over the past 50 years on gabapentin, and it has clearly been found to be effective in improving the control of partial and tonic–clonic seizures when used as an adjunct as well as alone. It has no value in the treatment of absence or myoclonic seizures. It has also been found to be a very effective medication for the treatment of chronic neuropathic pain. In fact, the majority of the sales of gabapentin are now made for purposes other than the treatment of epilepsy.

In terms of tolerability, gabapentin also has an excellent record. It rarely produces a rash or other hypersensitivity adverse effects and has almost never been reported to be associated with any toxicity to other organs in the body. A high dose given rapidly, or an excessive dose, may lead to some sleepiness, dizziness, and unsteadiness, but reducing the dose and simply allowing the patient to become accustomed to the gabapentin over time results in clearing of these symptoms in most people. Weight gain is more often reported than patients receiving placebo in clinical trials. The gabapentanoids (including gabapentin and pregabalin) have a very low, but documented, risk of dependence in those with a history of substance abuse.[21] However, overall gabapentin is certainly one of if not the safest drugs used in treatment of any medical problem.

Gabapentin is available in 100, 300, 400, 600, and 800 mg capsules or oral solution. There is no available intravenous or intramuscular injection for this drug.

In conclusion, gabapentin is an effective and safe drug to use, particularly for those on multiple medications, or with concomitant neuropathic pain.

21.2.8 Lacosamide

Lacosamide (Vimpat) is a newer ASD invented by Dr. Harold Kohn, then at the University of Houston, and patented in 1998. It was then developed by Schwartz Pharma, which was acquired by UCB and formerly known as Harkoseride.

Lacosamide acts on the sodium channel, but unlike many other ASDs, it affects slow rather than fast inactivation of the sodium channel. This may help normalize activation thresholds and decrease pathophysiological neuronal activity. Despite its action, it is also effective as an additive to other sodium channel drugs including carbamazepine, lamotrigine, and phenytoin. To a lesser degree, lacosamide also contributes to the modulation of collapsin response mediator protein-2 (CRMP-2), which is involved in the signal transduction cascade of neurotrophic factors and subsequently may convey neuroprotective effects.[22]

Lacosamide is indicated for adjunctive treatment of focal seizures as well as monotherapy. A large Class 1 trial compared lacosamide with carbamazepine extended release.[23] No significant differences were noted in overall efficacy or adverse effects after 6 months into the trial.

Adverse effects are sedation and dizziness. This can be minimized by slow escalation of dose. Safety appears to be very good, but it is sometimes recommended to obtain a baseline electrocardiogram prior to use if any cardiac conduction defect is a risk. A rare side effect that has been observed is PR interval prolongation on the electrocardiogram. More experience is needed as to whether this has any clinical significance.

It comes in 50, 100, 150, and 200 mg oral tablets and solutions. An intravenous formulation is also available.

Overall, lacosamide is a safe, fairly well-tolerated medication that is effective as an adjunctive and monotherapy treatment of partial-onset seizures. The availability of an intravenous formulation is an added benefit.

21.2.9 Lamotrigine

Lamotrigine (Lamictal) was developed in the early 1970s by Dr. Alistair Miller and colleagues at GlaxoWellcome (now GlaxoSmithKline), a pharmaceutical company in the United Kingdom. This drug was one of a group of antimicrobials that had properties that counteracted the effects of folic acid. Though folic acid was found to be in low concentrations in epilepsy patients as a result of taking phenobarbital and phenytoin, early studies suggested folate administration seemed to aggravate seizures (not later proven). On this basis, antifolate compounds were explored for antiseizure properties. One of these was lamotrigine, which actually was found to have very weak antifolate properties. However, screening tests revealed it to be a quite potent drug against seizures of multiple types.

The pharmacokinetics were generally favorable with a half-life as monotherapy of almost 20 hours. It does not induce nor inhibit hepatic CYP450 enzymes, unlike many earlier ASDs. However, it is metabolized by glucuronide conjugation, which is inducible by enzyme-inducing drugs such as the barbiturates, phenytoin, and the dibenzapine carboxamide family.

Lamotrigine is conjugated before being excreted by the kidney. This clearance can be altered by other ASDs as well as estrogen. Valproate significantly inhibits the conjugation, causing increased blood levels, and therefore, making it much more likely that a rash would occur. On the other hand, carbamazepine, phenytoin, and phenobarbital all increase the rate at which lamotrigine is changed and eliminated in the body, so that higher doses may need to be given to achieve the desired effect. Lamotrigine does not, however, change other drugs, such as other ASDs or medicines used for other purposes. Finally, lamotrigine is eliminated more rapidly in women taking estrogen-containing oral contraceptives. Similarly, the marked rise of estrogens during pregnancy significantly lowers lamotrigine levels and may increase the risk of seizure breakthrough, requiring more frequent monitoring of blood levels and dose adjustment.

It was first introduced as adjunctive treatment for focal and secondarily generalized tonic–clonic seizures, but did not appear to be a potent drug in clinical trials. This later proved to be incorrect, and the seizure control in comparative monotherapy studies ultimately indicated that by many measures it was similarly effective to the older standard drugs. Lamotrigine has been found to have broad-spectrum properties, making it useful for the treatment of primary generalized (idiopathic) epilepsies with tonic–clonic, absence, and myoclonic seizures.[24] It has also been helpful for difficult epilepsy syndromes in children with tonic, tonic–clonic, atonic, myoclonic, and absence seizures (as occurs in Lennox–Gastaut syndrome). Lamotrigine has increasingly been used as a substitute for, or in combination with, valproate for these seizure/epilepsy types for safety and tolerability reasons. Although used for absence seizures, it has less efficacy than ethosuximide or valproate.

The medication first appeared to have many side effects similar to carbamazepine, but when used alone, it proved to have very few problems in terms of tolerance.[25] Most importantly, it was not sedating, in contrast to many of the older drugs. It resulted in no cognitive slowing and proved to be generally well liked by patients.

A major problem that did arise, however, was the occurrence of rash in approximately 5–10% of people. In some groups of patients who were also taking valproate (together with rapid dose escalation), the possibility of rash at times rose to 30%. However, in groups treated very slowly at low doses, who were not taking any other medication, the probability of rash was closer to 3–5%. Indeed, it was somewhat less frequent than the occurrence of rash associated with carbamazepine. Nonetheless, occasionally, these allergic reactions progressed on to Stevens–Johnson syndrome or DRESS affecting multiple organs, including the joints and skin, and these infrequently led to the necessity of hospitalization and a potentially fatal outcome. Although this proved to be very uncommon, it is not an adverse effect that can be ignored. Experience has demonstrated that very slow administration, especially when the patient is also receiving valproate, will result in minimal risk. The immediate discontinuation of lamotrigine with apparent onset of a hypersensitivity response is advised.

Specific kits have been developed by the manufacturer (GlaxoSmithKline) to help define the way the drug should be administered. A consequence of the rate of buildup of the drug is that it may take 2 months to achieve an amount in the blood that would be expected to provide seizure control. This is a limitation in patients needing a prompt effect from an added drug.

Like other new ASDs, it is several times more expensive than the older products. It is available in chewable 2, 5, and 25 mg tablets, regular tablets of 25, 100, 150, and 200 mg doses, and oral disintegrating tablets. If it is medically appropriate, the 200 mg dose is more economical. There is a new extended release (XR) formulation that can be given once daily. There is no oral solution or intravenous formulation of this drug available.

In summary, lamotrigine is a newer drug that has very many positive characteristics. It is a broad-spectrum agent effective for most seizure types, similar to valproate among the older drugs. In addition, it has few side effects when used alone and does not cause sleepiness. In general, it is very well liked by the patients taking the drug. Unfortunately, a rash may result, and rarely there may be an allergic reaction of serious consequence in patients who increase the dose too rapidly or are taking valproate at the same time the lamotrigine is started. Careful dosing patterns can minimize this problem.

21.2.10 Levetiracetam

Levetiracetam (Keppra) is a compound developed by UCB in Belgium with a unique mechanism of action binding to synaptic vesicle proteins (SV2A). Unlike most of the older, standard ASDs, this compound showed little effectiveness in preventing seizures, electro-shock or chemical agents causing convulsions, but when given to animals with spontaneous genetic epilepsy, it proved to be highly effective.[26]

The pharmacokinetics are quite favorable. Unlike the older ASDs, it is not hepatically cleared and is primarily renally eliminated. Protein binding is minimal as well, so drug–drug interactions are not a problem.

The serum half-life is rather short, being approximately 8 hours, but clinical trials demonstrated efficacy when administered twice daily. It is water soluble and is easily used for parenteral administration. When given for acute seizure control it carries no risk of respiratory or cardiovascular depression, even when given as a bolus in high dose.

In clinical trials, it was tested against focal and secondarily generalized seizures and proved to be comparably effective to most other new ASDs. A large European trial found it to be equally effective as monotherapy compared with carbamazepine, the "gold standard."[27]

Clinical trials have tested the efficacy as adjunctive therapy in patients with primary generalized epilepsy. In these results, levetiracetam has been shown to be effective as adjunctive therapy in the treatment of myoclonic and generalized tonic–clonic seizures; however, with the treatment of absence seizures, only modest efficacy has been shown. In animal models, levetiracetam showed promise of being able to prevent the development of epilepsy in addition to controlling seizures; however, this has not been proven in humans.

Levetiracetam is unusually free of serious adverse effects, other than some sleepiness or dizziness, which were minimal. Only rarely have a rash or other organ safety problems occurred.

Psychiatric and behavioral adverse events (agitation, depression, emotional lability, and irritability) can be a problem and are noted in possibly a quarter of patients treated with levetiracetam in clinical experience. Curiously, such adverse effects were much less frequent in the original controlled trials.

Based on animal studies and pregnancy registries, levetiracetam has proven to be one of the safest, with very little evidence of teratogenicity.

The dosage range is from 1000 mg to 3000 mg, daily administered in a tablet or oral solution form. An extended release formulation is available for easy daily use.

In summary, levetiracetam is a drug that has unique properties in experimental models, including some evidence that it can prevent the development of epilepsy. It also has a broad-spectrum effectiveness, excellent safety, good tolerability, and overall excellent pharmacokinetic properties. Levetiracetan has been proven to be a safe and effective ASD, which, combined with other features, have led to it being a drug of choice in focal seizures and an alternative for seizures of generalized onset.

21.2.11 Oxcarbazepine

Oxcarbazepine (Trileptal) has been extensively used in Europe for many years. Oxcarbazepine is a drug closely related to carbamazepine. It differs slightly from carbamazepine chemically, but these differences produce changes that are clinically important.

The drug is almost fully absorbed and widely distributed throughout the body. It undergoes rapid metabolism by the liver to the active metabolite mono-hydroxycarbazepine (MHD), which is subsequently eliminated in the urine.

Most importantly, and in contrast to its close relative carbamazepine, it does not affect the concentration of other ASDs or medically used drugs, with the exception of some modest reduction in the effectiveness of oral contraceptives. However, when given together with carbamazepine, phenytoin, and probably phenobarbital, the liver metabolism is increased and oxcarbazepine and its metabolite are more rapidly eliminated from the body. This leads to lower concentrations in the body. In this case, higher doses of drug are needed to obtain the same effect, and to maintain constant blood levels, more frequent dosing may be necessary.

Oxcarbazepine has demonstrated effectiveness against focal and generalized tonic–clonic seizures, equal to that of carbamazepine, phenytoin, or valproate. Although it is chemically very similar to carbamazepine, a significant number of patients whose epilepsy was not well controlled by carbamazepine were better controlled on oxcarbazepine. This may occur because there is some selective difference in efficacy or because oxcarbazepine is better tolerated and can be given in higher and more effective doses. Oxcarbazepine has no benefit for the treatment of absence or myoclonic seizures and may actually aggravate them. Like carbamazepine, it is effective in the treatment of trigeminal neuralgia.

In general, the side effects of oxcarbazepine are relatively few. It is less likely to produce dizziness and visual disturbance or sedation upon initiation, even when the dose is advanced much more rapidly than with carbamazepine. Hypersensitivity can be seen, but appears to be less than what is seen with the use of carbamazepine. Greater tolerability has also been seen in comparative trials with carbamazepine and phenytoin, with fewer patients on oxcarbazepine stopping treatment due to side effects.

The drug is supplied in tablets of 150, 300, and 600 mg or oral solution. An extended release formulation (Oxtellar) minimizes peak and trough effects of immediate release. The metabolite of oxcarbazepine, MHD (eslicarbazepine), which is quite water soluble, is also approved by the Food and Drug Administration (FDA) as adjunctive and monotherapy treatment for focal onset seizures.

In conclusion, oxcarbazepine is a safe, effective, and well-tolerated ASD for the treatment of partial and secondarily generalized tonic–clonic seizures.

21.2.12 Phenobarbital

Bromide salts had been used for the treatment of epilepsy since their efficacy was first reported in 1857 by Sir Charles Locock (Queen Victoria's obstetrician). Therefore, phenobarbital is often considered the first true ASD. It was one of a group of barbiturates developed in the late 1800s by the pharmaceutical company Bayer in Germany. Hauptman first reported on the effectiveness of phenobarbital in 1912, with results closely approximating those obtained for new ASDs in clinical trials today. Much higher doses were administered at that time, often resulting in sedation. Nevertheless, the effectiveness was quite striking, tolerability compared to bromides was a significant improvement.

Phenobarbital has been used since that time and is the most frequently prescribed treatment for epilepsy in the world. This does not necessarily reflect its superior properties, but rather the fact that it is by far the least expensive ASD. Treatment with one of the new ASDs may cost 20–40 times more than that by phenobarbital over the span of 1 year.

Phenobarbital is well absorbed in the body and distributed to all tissues. It is a little more slowly transported into the brain than other ASDs. It is changed in the liver to an inactive by-product, but only very slowly the half life being about 4 days. Ultimately, some of the phenobarbital is excreted directly into the urine, and some of it is converted by the liver to an inactive form.

Phenobarbital induces the metabolism of some of the other ASDs such as carbamazepine, valproate, lamotrigine, tiagabine, and topiramate. The addition of valproate to a patient's treatment when already taking phenobarbital may slow the elimination of the phenobarbital and cause mental dullness and sedation due to rising levels of phenobarbital.

The effectiveness of phenobarbital was demonstrated in the initial reports by Hauptman and have been repeated countless times. The first large-scale double-blinded comparative trial proved phenobarbital to be comparably effective in preventing tonic–clonic seizures when compared with carbamazepine, phenytoin, and primidone over a 2-year period of study. However, it was somewhat less effective than carbamazepine and probably phenytoin for preventing focal seizures. Phenobarbital has also been used for many years as a method for stopping repeated frequent seizures, or status epilepticus, when given intravenously. Indeed, in recent studies of status epilepticus, phenobarbital was found to be as effective as any other drug used for this purpose. In experimental models, phenobarbital appears to be effective for most seizure types, but in clinical use, it is not helpful for absence or myoclonic seizures, and at times may increase the frequency of these attacks.

Phenobarbital is often limited by adverse effects proportional to increases in dose. Although many patients will tolerate a low to medium dose, many will become sleepy as the amount of phenobarbital is increased, and it can also lead to cognitive slowing. In the pediatric age group and in the elderly, the opposite effect may take place, with excitement and hyperactivity occurring rather than sleepiness. In the aforementioned comparative Veterans Administration trial, phenobarbital was administered in moderate dose, averaging 120 mg/day, and the overall tolerability was quite good. When given at such modest doses, phenobarbital can be given quite rapidly, built up quickly, and is better tolerated under these circumstances than carbamazepine, phenytoin, or primidone. However, when the dose is increased to 150–180 mg or more, most individuals experience side effects that commonly compromise the ability to optimally carry out school work or other intellectual tasks. In addition, depression may be aggravated by the use of phenobarbital. A small but significant number of men will experience a loss of libido and potency with the use of phenobarbital, which may be reversed when switched to another agent, such as carbamazepine, phenytoin, or valproate. Because there is some adaptation of the brain to the continual administration of phenobarbital, it is advisable when stopping the drug to taper it over many weeks to avoid a withdrawal rebound effect on seizures. Some concern has been raised about the potential for habituation or addiction to phenobarbital, but this problem is exceedingly rare.

In general, phenobarbital is a safe drug. Allergic rash is associated with the drug in approximately 5–10% of people, similar to carbamazepine and phenytoin, and rarely this goes on to serious involvement of other body organs. Occasionally, patients who have taken phenobarbital for many years, especially at high doses, develop aches and pain in their joints, some thickening of the pads of their palms and soles of their feet, some stiffening of the joints (frozen shoulder), and gradual contraction of the fingers of the hand (Dupuytren's contracture). Because these complaints are relatively common in people not on ASDs, the problem may be underdiagnosed. Again as sedation is an effect of increasing dose of phenobarbital, if the amount becomes too high due to accidental or purposeful overdose, life-threatening depression of breathing may occur.

Phenobarbital is available as a liquid elixir for use in the pediatric group, and in 15, 30, 60, and 100 mg tablets. It is also available in an injectable form. In fact due to its ready availability and multiple forms of administration, phenobarbital has long been used as a primary drug for administration to infants and children.

In summary, phenobarbital is the oldest ASD. Because of its overall adequate effectiveness and its affordability, it is the most widely used ASD in the world. In developed countries, other compounds are preferred because of the sedating and mental slowing effects of phenobarbital when given in moderate to high doses.

21.2.13 Phenytoin

Phenytoin (Dilantin) was developed in the 1930s by Merritt and Putnam, who were working at Harvard University and Boston City Hospital. Putnam had been searching for a drug similar to phenobarbital but having less sedative side effects. He theorized the chemical structure that might provide these characteristics, and then made a systematic inquiry of an extensive number of pharmaceutical companies. He finally obtained several compounds from Parke-Davis and carried out tests in animals for their possible protective effect. The very first compound he happened to test was phenytoin, which proved to have marked effectiveness in preventing electrically induced convulsive seizures in animals. Working together, Putnam and Merritt brought this drug to the clinical setting and confirmed that phenytoin was highly effective in the treatment of focal and generalized tonic–clonic seizures. They also confirmed that it was less sedating than phenobarbital. Phenytoin has been widely used since that time.

The pharmacokinetics of phenytoin is somewhat complex. Although it is well absorbed and extensively distributed in the body after being taken by mouth, its elimination is more complicated. It is changed in the liver via CYP2C19 and CYP2C9 to an inactive by-product, which is excreted in the kidney. Unlike phenobarbital, however, the rate of change is not constant and may lead to unexpected changes in blood concentration. The higher the dose of phenytoin, the less rapidly it is converted to an inactive product. For example, if the patient is taking 400 mg of phenytoin daily and somewhat greater control is wanted with higher blood levels, and the dose is increased to 500 mg/day, it might be assumed that the amount in the blood would increase by 20%. In fact, however, the liver begins to lose its ability to convert phenytoin, so that this increase, in some people, may actually result in a doubling of the amount in the blood and brain and lead to overdose effects. The dose at which the liver is less able to change phenytoin varies from patient to patient and is difficult to predict. This change in the rate of phenytoin breakdown is of great importance because small increments of 25 or 30 mg may be necessary to realize the optimal dose for control while avoiding side effects. This problem with "fine tuning" is not sufficiently appreciated, and treatment with phenytoin is sometimes abandoned before it has been optimally prescribed.

The metabolism of phenytoin to an inactive product can be slowed not only by increasing the concentration of phenytoin itself but also by the added administration of carbamazepine, felbamate, and, at times, antibiotics such as erythromycin. However, phenytoin is perhaps one of if not the most potent hepatic enzyme inducers. As a consequence, adding phenytoin to the treatment of someone on carbamazepine, lamotrigine, oxcarbazepine, topiramate, or valproate may double the speed with which these drugs are eliminated from the body. Of potentially significant consequence is that phenytoin causes more rapid elimination of blood thinners, such as warfarin (Coumadin), or drugs given to protect transplants, such as cyclosporin. Thus, phenytoin administration may decrease the effectiveness of these compounds. This can be rectified by increasing the dose of concomitant medications, but awareness of the effect is of great clinical importance. Likewise if phenytoin is discontinued, the levels of other medications can be expected to rise to supratherapeutic levels. This can again be hazardous if someone is taking a blood thinner such as warfarin. Abrupt discontinuation of phenytoin without monitoring of both levels can potentiate the effect and lead to bleeding.

Phenytoin is as effective as, or more effective than, other ASDs for the treatment of focal and secondarily generalized tonic–clonic seizures. In multiple comparative trials, phenytoin was similar to carbamazepine in providing complete control of partial seizures in patients at 1 year of follow-up treatment. Efficacy can be further enhanced by very careful changes and increases in dose. Phenytoin has no value in the treatment of absence or myoclonic seizures, and in this way, it again appears very similar to carbamazepine.

Phenytoin is usually well tolerated at standard doses and is less sedating than phenobarbital at doses required to provide comparable effectiveness. As dose increases, however, phenytoin may cause sedation and slowing of thinking, as is true with excessive dose of most of the ASDs. In addition, as the dose becomes high, incoordination and unsteady gait may occur, as well as dizziness. For the most part, however, phenytoin is very well tolerated, even with rapid administration of the drug by mouth or by intravenous injection, in contrast to carbamazepine. In early development, it was noticed that phenytoin can produce the side effect of gingival hyperplasia, especially if oral hygiene is not carefully followed. In addition, some increase in body hair growth has been associated with its use. Some coarsening of facial tissue has also been observed occasionally with chronic use. These cosmetic side effects are especially problematic in children and women.

On the whole, phenytoin is a safe ASD. Allergic rash and other more serious organ damage occurs with approximately the same frequency as carbamazepine, lamotrigine, or phenobarbital. If a rash develops, it may spontaneously disappear in approximately 50% of patients, but in a small number it may progress to serious skin, joint, or organ involvement, with potentially serious and even fatal outcomes. Phenytoin is associated with some increase in abnormalities of the developing fetus, especially in the first 3 months of pregnancy. Originally, phenytoin was thought to carry the highest risk of this problem. Fortunately, these complications are rare.

Infrequently, but of possible importance, there are some chronic side effects with long-term administration of phenytoin. These include neuropathy, particularly in the legs, and at times even cause some interference with balance. This may improve or disappear if the drug is stopped. Another long-term side effect is damage to the cerebellum. An effect of this is slowly worsening balance and unsteady gait. Recent studies suggest that it actually may be safer than valproic acid or phenobarbital.

Phenytoin has been a standard drug given intravenously for rapid treatment of seizures, but it is increasingly being replaced for this purpose by other parenterally available ASDs, including fosphenytoin and levetiracetam. Fosphenytoin is a nonirritating compound that is rapidly changed to phenytoin once administered into the blood or muscle.

Phenytoin is available in a wide variety of formulations. It is available as a liquid suspension (it is important to vigorously shake the bottle before each use to assure adequate mixing), a 50 mg triangular tablet that can be divided into two 25 mg segments and is also chewable, 30 and 100 mg capsules, and as a generic formulation. Phenytoin is also available as liquid for intravenous injection. This is an irritating toxic substance, but an alternative form, fosphenytoin (Cerebyx), is nontoxic and can be given by vein or into the muscle for prompt effect.

In summary, phenytoin is one of the least expensive, oldest, and most established of the ASDs. Phenytoin and carbamazepine act as potent drugs for the treatment of partial and tonic clonic seizures, equal to or more so than any other drug. It has multiple formulations, allowing it to be used under many circumstances, and is generally well tolerated. For some populations, the cosmetic and teratogenetic side effects of phenytoin make carbamazepine a preferable product. In addition, the pharmacokinetics of phenytoin are complex, and best use, especially in difficult control problems, may require expert understanding. Nonetheless, in these cases, phenytoin may prove to be the most effective compound.

21.2.14 Pregabalin

Pregabalin (Lyrica) is one of the newer ASDs that was designed to be comparable to gabapentin (Neurontin), but with greater efficacy and potency. It was invented by medicinal chemists Richard Silverman and Ryszard Andruszkiewicz at Northwestern University in the United States in 1989. It was then marketed by Parke-Davis (Pfizer), and approved in the European Union in 2003, and soon after in the United States in 2004 for adjunctive therapy of focal seizures in adults.

Like gabapentin, pregabalin also binds to alpha-2-delta protein, an auxiliary subunit of voltage-gated calcium channels, which subtly reduces the synaptic release of several neurotransmitters.

Pregabalin is rapidly and well absorbed with high bioavailability. It does not bind to plasma proteins and is eliminated through the kidneys virtually unchanged. It does not involve hepatic liver enzymes, and there is no known interaction with other medications at this time.

It has been shown to be effective in the treatment of focal and secondarily generalized seizures as adjunctive therapy. Recent studies have shown that pregabalin is also effective at treating chronic pain in disorders such as fibromyalgia and spinal cord injury. In June 2007, pregabalin became the first medication approved by the FDA for the treatment of fibromyalgia. Besides its use for treating neuropathic pain and seizures, pregabalin is an effective anxiolytic and is approved in the European Union for the treatment of generalized anxiety disorder as well.

It is considered to have a low potential for abuse and is a safe and well-tolerated medication. Adverse effects such as drowsiness and dizziness can occur. Among the more worrisome side effects are weight gain and peripheral edema. At this time, pregabalin is too new a drug for there to be sufficient data for complications during pregnancy.

Pregabalin is available in 25, 50, 75, 100, 150, 200, 225, and 300 mg capsules, and an oral solution has been developed. Overall, pregabalin is an effective adjunctive treatment for partial and secondary generalized seizures that is well tolerated and safe.

21.2.15 Primidone

Primidone (Mysoline) was introduced in the 1950s by Ayerst and developed as a drug closely related to phenobarbital, and to possess properties that might convey greater effectiveness and better tolerability.

Its mechanism of action is primarily via enhanced inhibition through action at the GABA receptor similar to phenobarbital. However, it exerts separate anti-seizure action. In experimental studies of mice, primidone suppresses fluorothyl induced myoclonic seizures before any phenobarbital has accumulated in the animals.

Primidone is well absorbed over a few hours and widely distributed in the body. It is metabolized in the liver to phenobarbital. If primidone is administered alone, the amount of primidone in the blood is eventually somewhat less than the amount of phenobarbital. This is variable among individuals, and in some people the primary drug found in the blood is primidone, with comparatively little phenobarbital. It has a half-life of approximately 9–12 hours. After being changed in the liver, primidone is renally eliminated. The amount changed to phenobarbital follows the same pathway of elimination as noted for phenobarbital earlier.

If primidone and carbamazepine are given simultaneously with phenytoin it causes the liver to convert a greater percentage of the primidone to phenobarbital, so that the amount of phenobarbital in the blood is approximately three times greater than the amount of primidone. It is likely that the effect of giving primidone is essentially comparable to taking phenobarbital alone. Taking valproic acid may increase both the primidone and the phenobarbital concentrations, as noted for phenobarbital above

Primidone has been demonstrated to be effective for tonic–clonic seizures, but in the Veterans Administration study, it was somewhat less effective than carbamazepine and phenytoin for the treatment of focal seizures.[28] In addition to tonic–clonic and focal seizures, primidone has also been used with some success in the treatment of myoclonic, but not absence, seizures. In low doses, it is also effective for tremor of benign type.

With chronic use, the side effects of primidone are very similar to those of phenobarbital. However, when beginning treatment, primidone often causes dizziness, nausea and vomiting, excessive sleepiness, and dizziness. This is clearly a side effect of the primidone itself, because almost no conversion to phenobarbital has occurred during the first few days. If the medication is started very slowly, at doses of 25 or 50 mg, and is only gradually increased as tolerated, most of these side effects can be avoided. With chronic use, the drug is well tolerated. Some men complained of a decrease in sexual interest and ability. This was found to occur in approximately 15% of people, similar to phenobarbital. Connective tissue problems reported with chronic use pf phenobarbital have been observed with primidone use. Primidone is a relatively safe drug, comparable again to phenobarbital.

Primidone is available in 50 and 250 mg tablets. No liquid formulation is available for injection, but if substitution is needed and oral intake is not possible, the physician may choose to substitute phenobarbital.

In summary, primidone is a second-order drug among the older drugs after carbamazepine, phenytoin, phenobarbital, and valproate, as well as many of the newer ones. This is due to primidone's poorly tolerated side effects during initiation of treatment, along with the absence of evidence that it offers any additional benefit, other than it being less expensive and more easily administered than its relative, phenobarbital. However, it has been observed that the occasional patient will do very well, tolerate primidone better than the other drugs, and will not experience any adverse effects.

21.2.16 Rufinamide

Rufinamide (Banzel) is a novel ASD designed by Novartis Pharmaceuticals, which is structurally distinguished as a triazole derivative. Although originally intended as a broad-spectrum ASD, it was granted orphan drug status in 2004. Rufinamide received approval for use in Europe in 2007 and later by the FDA in 2008 for adjunctive treatment of seizures associated with Lennox–Gastaut syndrome in children 4 years of age or older.

In rodent models, rufinamide was found to prolong the inactivation of voltage-gated sodium channels, resulting in a decrease of frequency of sustained repetitive firing.[29]

Rufinamide is well absorbed and has even distribution throughout the body. However, with chronic administration, rufinamide absorption decreases progressively by more than 50% with increasing doses from 800 to 7200 mg daily. Early studies have shown that there is better absorption of this medication when taken with food. It is extensively metabolized by the liver without induction of CYP45, but via hydrolysis of the carboxyl-amidic group, into inactive metabolites, which are then renally excreted. There have been some minor drug-to-drug interactions reported. In particular, valproate can decrease rufinamide clearance (up to 70%) leading to a significant increase in plasma rufinamide levels. To a lesser extent, inducers such as phenobarbital, primidone, phenytoin, and carbamazepine, can decrease plasma rufinamide levels by up to 40–50%.[30] However, overall it is considered to be an ASD with limited interactions with other agents.

Rufinamide is commonly used for Lennox–Gastaut syndrome, a severe form of generalized epilepsy that develops in early childhood and is characterized by multiple seizure types that are typically resistant to medications. Rufinamide is particularly effective in the reduction of atonic seizures or drop attacks. More recently, evidence from clinical trials, clinical practice studies, and individual case reports suggest benefit in those with childhood-onset refractory epileptic encephalopathies and in the treatment of partial-onset seizures.[31]

Rufinamide is generally well tolerated. Common adverse effects include gastrointestinal problems such as vomiting, nausea, and loss of appetite. These effects are usually self-limiting, and seen during initiation, rather than maintenance. In some cases, QTC interval shortening can occur. Therefore, familial short QT syndrome is a contraindication to rufinamide use. Otherwise, rufinamide is usually a very well-tolerated medication, and often appreciated for its favorable cognitive profile.

Rufinamide is available in 200 and 400 mg oral tablets and also as an oral solution. It can be titrated up relatively quickly if clinically necessary. No intravenous formulation is yet available.

Overall, rufinamide is a new ASD with a novel mechanism of action that is effective as an adjunctive treatment for patients with devastating epileptic syndromes such as Lennox–Gastaut syndrome. There have been studies showing that rufinamide is an effective treatment for partial seizures in pediatric and adult populations. However, its use has been limited and it is too soon to know its role in the treatment of partial epilepsy.

21.2.17 Tiagabine

Tiagabine (Gabitril) is an ASD that was developed by Novo-Nordisk in Denmark as what might be called a rationally designed drug. The drug was developed as an analog of nicotinic acid, a GABA reuptake inhibitor used in experimental studies.

Tiagabine selectively blocks GABA reuptake at glia and neurons, resulting in an increased concentration of GABA in the synaptic cleft and prolonging the duration of inhibitory synaptic currents in the cortex and hippocampus.

The metabolism of tiagabine is very similar to that of the older drugs. It is extensively, and fairly rapidly, metabolized by the liver by cytochrome P4503A enzymes to an inactive form. Its metabolism is particularly enhanced if given concomitantly with phenytoin or carbamazepine, with half the tiagabine being eliminated from the body in approximately 6 hours. Although this would predict a short period of effectiveness and indicate a need for frequent daily dosing, studies have indicated that good effectiveness is possible, even if the drug is given only twice daily. After metabolism in the liver, it is renally eliminated. Due to it being significantly (~96%) protein bound, unlike gabapentin and vigabatrin, its elimination is accelerated by drugs like carbamazepine and phenytoin. Tiagabine itself, however, does not increase or affect the elimination of other ASDs or medications used for other purposes.

Tiagabine has been demonstrated to be effective in decreasing the frequency of seizures of focal and secondarily generalized tonic–clonic types when given to patients whose seizures were not controlled on carbamazepine, phenytoin, and/or valproate.[32] Use for other seizure types, such as absence and myoclonic seizures, has not been sufficiently studied to know the possible role of this drug. In addition, like gabapentin, tiagabine may have an additional benefit for concomitant neuropathic pain.

The adverse effects of tiagabine are relatively moderate. Dizziness, sleepiness, and, infrequently, gastrointestinal disturbance accompany administration, particularly if the dose is increased too rapidly and is too high. Some cognitive slowing may occur under these circumstances as well. However, when given as an add-on to carbamazepine or phenytoin, it is better tolerated than when carbamazepine or phenytoin are added in comparative trials. In addition, the safety of tiagabine appears to be very favorable. There is no evidence of a hypersensitivity reaction, as seen with carbamazepine, phenobarbital, phenytoin, and lamotrigine, and no cases of more serious organ damage have been reported. Thus, it appears to be very well tolerated and safe for adjunctive therapy.

Tiagabine is available in 4, 12, 16, and 20 mg tablets, but not as an injectable formulation.

In summary, tiagabine is an ASD designed specifically to have action in the brain to increase the nervous system's own method of decreasing excitability. It is effective in helping control difficult focal and secondarily generalized tonic–clonic seizures. It is usually well tolerated and appears to be very safe; however, its use in the treatment of epilepsy has been limited.

21.2.18 Topiramate

Topiramate (Topamax) was developed by Ortho-McNeil as a member of a family of drugs taken orally for the control of diabetes. Topiramate is a fructose derivative and was synthesized as part of a search for compounds with hypoglycemic activity. However, it proved to have minimal effectiveness for this purpose. Instead, during screening studies it was found to have broad-spectrum effects on preventing seizures in many animal models.

Topiramate's broad spectrum of activity may be attributed to its multiple mechanisms of action. It inhibits both voltage-gated sodium channel and kainate-type glutamate receptors, reduces L-type voltage-sensitive calcium currents, increases the frequency of GABA-mediated chloride channel opening, inhibits carbonic anhydrase, and increases potassium conductance. It is not known which of these proposed mechanisms is most important for the antiseizure effects.

Topiramate has near complete absorption and linear pharmacokinetics. About 60% of a dose is excreted unchanged by the kidneys, while the rest undergoes hepatic metabolism to several inactive metabolites. Renal insufficiency diminishes clearance.

Although phenobarbital, phenytoin, and carbamazepine affect its elimination, topiramate generally has a favorable length of action. When given alone, it is only half eliminated in 24 hours. When given as an adjunctive therapy with enzyme inducing ASDs, twice-daily dosing is typically implemented. Topiramate has few interactions but at doses greater than 200 mg/day can increase the elimination of oral contraceptives and may result in decreased protection from pregnancy.

Topiramate was proven to be effective in decreasing the frequency of focal and secondarily generalized seizures when given in addition to other standard ASDs in patients whose seizures could not be controlled.[32] The effectiveness of topiramate appeared to be greater than that of any of the other new ASDs. However, the dose of topiramate administered was relatively higher than for gabapentin or lamotrigine in early studies and this may, in part, account for the apparent superior efficacy. Trials in generalized epilepsies with absence, myoclonic, and other seizures associated with difficult-to-control epilepsy, such as infantile spasms in infants and children, all give evidence of a broad-spectrum effectiveness.[33,34] In addition to its antiseizure properties, topiramate has demonstrated clear efficacy for prophylaxis of migraine headache, a common comorbidity of epilepsy. It can also be helpful for postural tremor.

Adverse effects were more common with the use of topiramate than with other new ASDs. Sedation and especially slowed thinking, as well as some irritability were reported in 15–20% of patients, and the number of people discontinuing the drug due to adverse effects was higher than for other new ASDs in trials. In retrospect, it seems clear that the dose selected for topiramate in these studies was much higher than necessary. The clinical benefit was evident by 400 mg/day and did not increase significantly at doses of 600, 800, and 1000 mg/day.[21] Yet, many of the patients received greater than 400 and 600 mg daily, and not surprisingly, had greater adverse effects. Greater experience with low doses being gradually increased has resulted in much improved tolerability.

Another seeming side effect of administration of topiramate is weight loss or failure to gain weight. The latter may be of some importance in children. In many adults who are overweight, this "adverse effect" may, in fact, be an advantage. Many patients will experience some tingling of the extremities, particularly when first starting the topiramate. This is a harmless effect of the drug, which will usually disappear spontaneously or with lowering of the dose.

The safety profile of topiramate appears to be very favorable. Allergic rash and associated organ toxicity have not been reported, despite fairly extensive use of the drug. Approximately 1–2% of patients given topiramate have developed renal stones, double the number expected in the general population. This has been minimized by adequate fluid intake, and it is rare that any invasive procedures have been necessary to remove the kidney stones. Acute glaucoma has rarely been encountered, manifested by some pain, blurred vision, or reddening that should warrant prompt discontinuation of the drug.

Topiramate is available in 15 and 25 mg sprinkle preparations, as well as in 25, 50, 100, and 200 mg tablets. There is no liquid formulation, but extended release formulations are available.

In summary, topiramate is a newer ASD. It has been fairly extensively used and appears to be quite effective for a wide variety of seizure types. It appears to be less well tolerated than some of the other new ASDs, although this can, at least in part, be helped by starting the medication slowly and working up the dose very gradually until it reaches an amount that provides adequate control. Its handling by the body makes it easy to use, having a favorable length of action and elimination.

21.2.19 Valproate

Valproate (Depakote/Depakene) was the last of the older drugs to be introduced, having reached the US market in 1978. Interestingly, it was actually first synthesized back in 1882, and in that regard it is probably the oldest of the ASDs. It was found by chance, as noted earlier, when its properties as a solvent were being used to study seizure effects of other drugs in France in the early 1960s.

Valproate acts via a variety of different mechanisms, including increased GABAergic transmission, reduced release and/or effects of excitatory amino acids, blockade of voltage-gated sodium channels, and modulation of dopaminergic and serotoninergic transmission.

If given as valproic acid, it is rapidly absorbed into the body through the stomach. The sodium divalproex formulation is absorbed in the small intestine, and absorption may be delayed for 2–8 h, depending on the presence of food in the stomach. It is well distributed throughout the body and brain. Its metabolic products are then excreted through the kidneys.

Particular care should be taken when valproate is taken in combination with other ASDs. The active by-products of valproate are more likely to occur if patients are concomitantly taking drugs such as carbamazepine, phenobarbital, or phenytoin. Valproate is half eliminated in approximately 12 hours when given alone, but it can be as short as half that time when given together with enzyme including drugs such as phenytoin. Valproate is not an enzyme inducer, but is an inhibitor of glucuronidation of special importance when co-administered with valproate. The metabolism of phenobarbital is also inhibited which can elevate levels and lead to adverse effects. When given alone, twice-daily dosing is sufficient.

Valproate is a broad-spectrum ASD, with some efficacy for virtually all seizure types. It is proven effective both as monotherapy and an adjunctive treatment for partial and generalized tonic–clonic seizures. In most cases, its effectiveness for partial seizures is comparable to carbamazepine and phenytoin, but in those with particularly resistant epilepsy, it seems to be slightly less effective. In addition, valproate is as effective for the treatment of absence seizures as ethosuximide; however, it was shown to cause more cognitive slowing. It is also highly effective for myoclonic seizures and tonic–clonic or clonic–tonic–clonic seizures in patients with idiopathic generalized epilepsy. It is the only one of the older drugs that is effective for all these seizure types and is also somewhat effective for more complicated atonic, tonic, and clonic seizures. In addition to formulations used for the long-term treatment of epilepsy, a liquid formulation exists that can be given intravenously very rapidly to help control acute repetitive seizures. It is effective and well tolerated.

Valproate is also useful for the prevention of migraine headaches or treatment of bipolar disorders. In patients having these conditions as well as epilepsy, valproate can be effective for both. The side effects of valproate include stomach upset upon initiation, particularly with oral formulations. This is less often experienced with the disodium valproex formulation, which is absorbed after leaving the stomach. Sedation may also occur at initiation but is usually not prominent. Overdose effects include not only some sleepiness but also, particularly, tremor of the outstretched hands. The most common side effect of valproate use is weight gain. This seems to be due primarily to an increase in appetite and food intake, but there is some evidence that valproate may change the way the body burns up fats as well. With high doses, there may also be thinning of the hair. This almost always returns with lowering of the dose and may grow back in a curly appearance and even, rarely, a different color than originally present.

In general, valproate is quite safe for administration in adults. However some rare, but serious, side effects may occur. It rarely produces rash and allergic organ problems. However, liver toxicity and failure have occurred, especially with administration in children in the first 2 years of life, particularly if taking another drug such as phenobarbital or phenytoin. The liver problems are exceedingly uncommon in adults. At times, platelet count is considerably reduced in the blood, particularly at high doses of valproate. It is rare that these changes are great enough to have any effect on blood clotting ability or consequent bleeding. Rarely, there may be some inflammation of, and even bleeding into, the pancreas. This causes nausea, vomiting, and acute pain in the pit of the stomach, often moving into the same area of the back. This is a serious medical complication, and requires prompt discontinuation of the valproate.

Particular caution should be exercised during pregnancy. There is persuasive evidence that administration of valproate early in pregnancy may result in spina bifida as well as other malformations. This occurrence is much more likely if the dose is high and perhaps may be minimized with administration of folic acid dietary supplements. However, alternative ASDs are preferable in pregnancy if they provide comparable control. A recent study evaluating the cognitive effects in children with exposure to ASDs found that children exposed to valproic acid in utero had lower mean intelligence quotients in comparison with other ASDs.[35] These teratogenicity problems indicate valproate should only be used in fertile women when measures are used to prevent pregnancy or when no other ASD can control the seizures. In the latter cases valproate should be used in the lowest doses possible to provide control.

Valproate is available as a syrup, 250 mg sprinkle capsules of valproic acid (Depakene), tablets in 125, 250, and 500 mg sodium divalproex formulation, and as a water-soluble injectable liquid. There is also an extended release formulation available.

In summary, valproate is the standard ASD for the treatment of the generalized epilepsies and associated seizures of absence, myoclonic, and tonic–clonic types. It is also effective for the treatment of focal and secondarily generalized tonic–clonic seizures. These broad-spectrum properties are unique among the older ASDs. Valproate's use is somewhat hampered by the presence of adverse effects, most of which are not serious, but important toxicity occurs occasionally.

21.2.20 Vigabatrin

Vigabatrin (Sabril) was developed by a Merrell Research laboratory in France in 1977. It was first marketed in Europe in the late 1980s. However, due to safety concerns (later detailed), its acceptance into the global market was notably delayed. It was approved in Australia in 1993 and in Canada in 1994. It was not approved in the United States until 2009.

Unlike many other seizure medicines, which were discovered serendipitously, vigabatrin was one of the first "designer medications" for epilepsy. It was specifically developed as an irreversible GABA transaminase inhibitor. Vigabatrin, gamma vinyl GABA, has a closely related chemical structure that forms an irreversible covalent bond to GABA transaminase, inactivating the enzyme, and thereby preventing the breakdown of GABA.

Vigabatrin is administered as a racemic mixture of the (R) and (S) isomers; only the (S) form is pharmacologically active. It is rapidly metabolized from the gastrointestinal tract within 1–2 hours, with about 50–60% bioavailability. Concomitant food intake has not been reported to cause any change in bioavailability. However of note, like gabapentin, the cerebrospinal fluid levels of (R, S)-vigabatrin are, on average, only 10–20% of the drug concentration in plasma.[36] It is then excreted primarily unchanged in urine.

Vigabatrin in general can be safely given with other ASDs. The only interaction of potential clinical significance that has been reported is a decrease in the plasma concentration of phenytoin. This may occur with a delay of about 5 weeks after initiation of vigabatrin and can reflect considerable interindividual variability. Vigabatrin may also slightly decrease primidone and phenobarbital levels, but this is typically of little clinical significance.

Studies have shown vigabatrin to be an effective treatment for adjunctive use in medically refractory epilepsy, focal seizures, and secondarily generalized seizures.[37] It has also been shown to be effective as monotherapy for infantile spasms in West's syndrome.

However, retrospective studies indicate that as many as 30% of patients who take vigabatrin for a year or more suffer damage to the retina, limiting the field of vision. This visual loss has been shown to be peripheral in nature and seems to be irreversible. Because of this adverse effect, the use of vigabatrin has been limited to devastating epilepsies such as infantile spasms and medically refractory epilepsy. Patients prescribed vigabatrin must undergo visual field and ophthalmological testing before treatment, frequent testing every 3 months during treatment, and then finally 3–6 months after cessation of treatment. It is recommended to discontinue the use of vigabatrin if it has not shown efficacy or substantial benefit after a 3-month trial. Vigabatrin is generally well tolerated and typically has few unwanted side effects. In a study of more than 2000 adults, the two most common side effects were drowsiness (12.5%) and fatigue (9%). The side effect most often mentioned in children taking vigabatrin is hyperactivity, which occurred in 11% of 299 children in one study.[37] These children were also taking other seizure medicines at the same time, making it possible that the hyperactivity was not due to vigabatrin alone. Finally, occasionally patients can experience an increase in their seizures after starting vigabatrin, particularly patients with myoclonic seizures.

Vigabatrin is available in 500 mg tablets and a powder formulation available for an oral solution. There is currently no intravenous formulation. Vigabatrin is often administered once or twice daily, as its duration of action exceeds its plasma half-life.

Overall, vigabatrin is an effective treatment for infantile spasms and adjunctive treatment for partial epilepsy; however, given its risk for irreversible decreased peripheral vision, its use is highly limited.

21.2.21 Zonisamide

Zonisamide (Zonegran) was first developed by Dainippon, a pharmaceutical company in Japan in 1972, during exploratory research on psychiatric drugs. However, during preclinical animal screening tests, it was incidentally found to also have anticonvulsant activity as well. Therefore, zonisamide has been commercially marketed as such in Japan since 1989, both as monotherapy and adjunctive therapy for various seizure types and syndromes in adults and children. Testing had also occurred in the United States. However, due to fears of kidney stones, studies in the United States were discontinued. It did not reemerge until

March 2000, more than a dozen years after its use in Japan, until there was reassuring evidence that the risk of kidney stones proved to be less than initially feared.

Zonisamide is a structurally novel ASD, being the only benzisoxazole derivative, chemically related to sulfa drugs. Its broad spectrum of action is attributed to its two mechanisms of action, both through its blockade of sustained firing of voltage-sensitive sodium channels and its reduction in voltage-dependent T-type calcium channel currents. A modest inhibitory effect on carbonic anhydrase has been reported, though much less than for acetazolamide. There is also some lesser effects on a number of different neurotransmitters.

Zonisamide is rapidly absorbed through the gastrointestinal tract, with nearly 100% bioavailability. It is metabolized primarily through the liver by CYP3A4 and distributed throughout the body. It is primarily eliminated directly through the kidneys. The elimination of zonisamide is quite slow when given alone; only half the drug is eliminated in 2–3 days. When administered in combination with other known inducers of CYP3A4, such as phenobarbital, carbamazepine, or phenytoin, clearance increases by about 50%; however, with such a remarkably long half-life, the slight increase of zonisamide metabolism is not expected to have any significant clinical effect. Zonisamide has no effect on other ASDs or drugs given for other medical reasons.

Zonisamide is approved in the United States and United Kingdom for adjunctive treatment of focal seizures in adults and those above the age of 12. However, it has been shown to be effective for the treatment of focal, secondarily generalized tonic–clonic seizures, and primary generalized epilepsy, with a seeming effectiveness somewhere in the middle of the other ASDs.[38] It may also be effective for other seizure types, but this is unclear.

Side effects with drug initiation include sedation, some cognitive slowing, and dizziness, which can be minimized, as with many of the other ASDs by gradual titration. Some loss of appetite has also been reported, along with symptoms typically associated with most ASDs if given at supratherapeutic doses, such as double vision, unsteady gait, tremors, and memory problems.

In general, zonisamide appears to be quite safe. Rash has been reported in approximately 3–5% of patients, somewhat less than with the older drugs, and usually is not severe. The likelihood of a rash developing is especially high in anyone having had a previous rash when using sulfa drugs. As noted above, zonisamide is associated with the development of kidney stones. This has been observed in approximately 3% of patients receiving the drug, who were carefully screened for this complication. Interestingly, subjects who were similarly screened, not taking zonisamide, had almost half as many unsuspected renal calculi discovered. This side effect can be minimized by generous intake of liquids and avoiding excessive intake of calcium.

Zonisamide is available in 100 mg capsules. The usual dose is 200–800 mg daily.

In summary, zonisamide is effective against focal and primary generalized epilepsy and has broad-spectrum value. It seems to be generally safe and well tolerated. However, few well-conducted trials are available to optimally assess this ASD (Tables 21.1—21.4).

As can be seen from the tables some ASDs have very selective effectiveness. Ethosuximide is only truly effective for absence seizures. Carbamazepine, eslicarbazepine, gabapentin, oxcarbazepine, phenobarbital, phenytoin, and tiagabine are mainly useful for focal and tonic/clonic seizures. On the other hand, clobazam, felbamate, lamotrigine, levetiracetam, topiramate, and valproate are "broad-spectrum" ASDs, and are particularly appropriate if multiple seizure types are present, as is often the case in certain epilepsies in childhood.

21.2.22 Cannabidiol

Cannabidiol (Epidiolex) is the product of the *Cannabis sativa* plant developed as a pharmaceutically active antiepileptic drug by Greenwich GC pharmaceuticals. Although extracts from the cannabis plants have been used for recreational and medical purposes for millennia, and "medical marijuana" has been approved by many states in the USA, class 1 trials have only been conducted in patients with Dravet and Lenox–Gastaut syndromes. Earlier studies suffered from unblinded nature of the trials and uncertainty of the exact contents of the medication. In 2018 the FDA approved Epidiolex for Lennox–Gastaut and Dravet syndromes.

The mechanism of action is unclear. Although endocannabinoid receptors exist in the brain, no binding has been found with cannabidiol to these sites.

The absorption after oral intake is fairly complete and is >94% protein bound. The drug is primarily cleared by biotransformation through the CYP3A4 and CSP2C19 isoenzymes. The half-life is 56–61 hours after bid dosing. Although of questionable value in Lennox–Gastaut syndrome and relatively contraindicated in Dravet syndrome, enzyme inducers such as carbamazepine and phenytoin can be expected to increase the clearance of cannabidiol. Cannabidiol is not an inducer, but inhibits CYP2C1P. This inhibition leads to clinically relevant elevated levels of desmethylclobazam if clobazam is being co-administered. It can be predicted that phenytoin clearance would also be inhibited if co-administered with cannabidiol.

Efficacy was established in three pivotal trials.[39,40,41] Drop seizures were reduced in Lennox–Gastaut syndrome at both 10 mg/kg and somewhat more at 20 mg/kg. Convulsions were significantly reduced in patients with Dravet syndrome. Controlled trials have not been published on other seizure types and epilepsy syndromes.

Adverse effects have been similar to some other ASDs. Sedation, diarrhea, and decreased appetite are most frequent. Serious life threatening toxicity has not yet been reported although elevated hepatic transaminase can be seen and is dose related. Such elevation is seen especially if patients are co-administered valproate. No definite liver failure has been associated with cannabidiol use.

Epidiolex (cannabidiol) is supplied as an oral solution containing 100 mg/ml of drug. Titration of drug is recommended at 2.5 mg/kg twice daily in weekly increments with a target of 20 mg/kg as needed and tolerated.

In summary, cannabidiol has finally been shown in to be effective in robust clinical trials in two epilepsy syndromes. Adverse effects are comparable to most other ASDs. The long-term role of this drug remains to be defined.

Table 21.1 Effectiveness of older standard antiseizure drugs

	Absence	Myoclonic	Tonic/Clonic	Focal
Carbamazepine (Tegretol)	May worsen	May worsen	Good	Very good
Ethosuximide (Zarontin)	Very good	No	No	No
Phenobarbital	No	No	Good	Good
Primidone (Mysoline)	No	Sometimes	Good	Good
Phenytoin (Dilantin)	No	No	Good	Very good
Valproate (Depakote)	Very good	Very good	Good	Moderate

Table 21.2 Effectiveness of newer antiseizure drugs

	Absence	Myoclonic	Tonic/Clonic	Partial
Clobazam (Onfi)	Good	Good	Very good	Very good
Felbamate (Felbatol)	Good	Good	Very good	Very good
Gabapentin (Neurontin)	No	No	Good	Good
Lamotrigine (Lamictal)	Good	Equivocal	Good	Good
Levetiracetam (Keppra)	Good	Good	Very good	Very good
Oxcarbazepine (Trileptal)	May worsen	May worsen	Very good	Very good
Perampanel (Fycompa)			Very good	Very good
Tiagabine (Gabatril)	May worsen	May worsen	Equivocal	Good
Topiramate (Topamax)	Equivocal	Equivocal	Very good	Very good
Zonisamide (Zonegran)	Good	Good	Very good	Very good
Pregabalin (Lyrica)	May worsen	May worsen	Very good	Very good
Vigabatrin (Sabril)	May worsen	Good	Good	Very good
Lacosamide (Vimpat)	Unclear	Unclear	Good	Good
Rufinamide (Banzel)	Unclear	Good	Good	Good

Table 21.3 Dose-related undesirable symptoms of commonly used antiseizure drugs

Drug	Average daily maintenance dose (adult)	Symptoms due to excessive dose of the antiseizure drug
Briviracetam (Briviact)	100–300 mg	Sedation, irritability
Carbamazepine (Tegretol)	600–1200 mg	Double vision, blurred vision, ataxia, dizziness
Clobazam (Onfi)	5–40 mg	Sedation drooling
Eslicarbazepine (Aptiom)		Sedation, dizziness
Ethosuximide (Zarontin)	500–2000 mg	Nausea, vomiting, gastric distress, drowsiness
Felbamate (Felbatol)	1200–3600 mg	Insomnia, loss of appetite, nausea, vomiting, headache
Gabapentin (Neurontin)	900–4800 mg	Somnolence, dizziness, weight gain
Lacosamide (Vimpat)	100–400mg	Sedation dizziness
Lamotrigine (Lamictal)	150–600 mg	Rash, dizziness, insomnia
Levetiracetam (Keppra)	1000–3000mg	Sleepiness, dizziness
Oxcarbazepine (Trileptal)	600–2400 mg	Dizziness incoordination
Phenobarbital (Luminal)	90–180 mg	Sedation thinking difficulty,
Phenytoin (Dilantin)	200–600 mg	Sedation, unsteady walking, incoordination, mental slowing

Table 21.3 (cont.)

Drug	Average daily maintenance dose (adult)	Symptoms due to excessive dose of the antiseizure drug
Perampanel (Fycompa)	8–12 mg	Dizziness, somnolence, loss of coordination, behavioral and psychiatric changes
Pregabalin (Lyrica)	150–600 mg	Drowsiness, dizziness, weight gain
Primidone (Mysoline)	500–1250 mg	Dizziness, nausea, sedation, slowed thinking
Tiagabine (Gabitril)	12–60 mg	Dizziness, sedation
Topiramate (Topamax)	200–600 mg	Sedation, slowed thinking, irritability, weight loss
Zonisamide (Zonegran)	200–600 mg	Drowsiness, loss of appetite, mental slowing, weight loss
Rufinamide (Banzel)	400–3200 mg	Drowsiness, loss of appetite
Vigabatrin (Sabril)	1000–3000 mg	Drowsiness, peripheral vision loss

Table 21.4 Pharmacokinetics of antiseizure drugs

Drug	Mechanism of action	Metabolism	Half-life
Briviracetam (Briviact)	Inhibits SV2a protein	1° hydrolysis, 2° CYP2C19; renal excretion	9 hours
Carbamazepine (Tegretol)	Na channel rapid inactivation, blocks L-type Ca channel	CYP3A4 to carbamazepine 10, 11 epoxide; excretion urine>feces.	25–65 hours initially, then 12–17 hours 3–5 weeks later (autoinduction)
Clobazam (Onfi)	GABA$_A$ receptor agonist	CYP3A4	30–40 hours
Eslicarbazepine (Aptiom)	Na channel rapid inactivation, blocks Ca HCav3.2 channel; enhances K$^+$ conductance	Eslicarbazepine acetate hydrolyzed to eslicarbazepine; renal excretion as eslicarbazepine and eslicarbazepine glucuronide (linear)	13–20 hours
Ethosuximide (Zarontin)	Low threshold slow T-Ca thalamic currents	CYP3A & CYP2E1 (saturable)	30 hours
Felbamate (Felbatol)	Enhances Na channel inactivation; blocks Ca channel, inhibits NMDA receptor, and potentiates GABA	40–50% excreted in urine unchanged; remainder converted to multiple metabolites.	22 hours

Table 21.4 (cont.)

Drug	Mechanism of action	Metabolism	Half-life
Gabapentin (Neurontin)	Binds presynaptic α2-δ of Ca channel	Renal excretion, non-linear	6 hours
Lacosamide (Vimpat)	Na channel slow inactivation	Demethylation by CYP3A4, 2C9 and 2C19; Renal excretion 95%: 40% as lacosamide and 60% as metabolites	15 hours
Lamotrigine (Lamictal)	Na channel rapid inactivation; inhibits Ca channels	Glucoronidation; renal excretion; linear	25 hours, 13 hours with EIASDs, 70 hours with valproate
Levetiracetam (Keppra)	Inhibits synaptic vesicle protein SV2A; partially inhibits N-type Ca	Enzymatic hydrolysis (non-CYP); renal excretion, 66% unchanged.	7 hours
Oxcarbazepine (Trileptal)	Enhances Na channel rapid inactivation; Blocks HCav3.2 (?M and P/Q fast) Ca channel; enhances K conductance	Hepatic reduction to MHDs: 80% S- & 20% R-liscarbazepine, then glucuronidated; Renal excretion (No autoinduction).	2 hours as oxcarbazepine, 9 hours as monohydroxy-derivative
Phenobarbital (Luminal)	Binds synaptic and extrasynaptic GABA$_A$ receptors	Hepatic parahydroxylation and glucuronidation; renal excretion: 25–50% unchanged, plus metabolites.	79 hours; newborns and children: 110 hours
Phenytoin (Dilantin)	Rapid inactivation of Na channels	CYP2C9 and 2C19; Renal excretion (zero-order kinetics)	
Perampanel (Fycompa)	Selective, noncompetitive antagonist of AMPA glutamate receptor	CYP3A4 and 3A5 to multiple metabolites	105 hours, ~24 hours with EIASDs
Pregabalin (Lyrica)	A2-δsubunit of Ca channel	Negligible metabolism; Renal excretion.	6hrs
Primidone (Mysoline)	Binds synaptic and extrasynaptic GABA A receptors	Primidone and metabolites (phenobarbital and phenylethylmalonic acid diamide) are active	12 hours
Tiagabine (Gabatril)	Selective GABA reuptake inhibitor	CYP3A4 and glucuronidation; excretion via urine and feces.	8 hours; 2–5 hours with EIASDs

Table 21.4 *(cont.)*

Drug	Mechanism of action	Metabolism	Half-life
Topiramate (Topamax)	Inhibits Na channels, kainite receptors and carbonic anhydrase; enhances GABA$_A$	Urinary excretion 70% unchanged	21 hours
Zonisamide (Zonegran)	Rapid inactivation of Na channels; dec low threshold T-type Ca current; binds GABA A ionophore; carbonic anhydrase inhibitor	Hepatic metabolism; renal excretion; linear up to 800 mg/day, then nonlinear	69 hours; 27–38 hours with EIASD, 46 hours with valproate
Rufinamide (Banzel)	Na channel rapid inactivation	PB 34%; hydrolyzed into many metabolites; renal excretion; slow nonlinear absorption due to low solubility at higher doses, better with food.	4–6 hours
Vigabatrin (Sabril)	Inhibits GABA transaminase irreversibly leading to inc GABA in CNS	Free = 100%; protein bound = 40%; extensive binding to RBCs; hepatic metabolism; renal excretion	10 hours; 5.7 hours in infants

Data from reference 42.
EIASD, enzyme inducing antiseizure drug

References

1. Fertig EJ, Mattson RH. Carbamazepine. In: Engel J, Jr., Pedley TA, eds., *Epilepsy: A Comprehensive Textbook*. Philadelphia: Wolters Kluwer; 2008:1543–1557.

2. Moseley B, Kervyn S, Nicolas J-M, Stockis A. A review of the drug-drug interactions of the new antiepileptic drug brivaracetam [abstract]. *Neurology*. 2017;88(16 Suppl):P4.109.

3. Lattanzi S, Cagnetti C, Foschi N, Provinciali L, Silvestrini M. Brivaracetam add-on for refractory focal epilepsy: a systematic review and meta-analysis. *Neurology*. 2016;86 (14):1344–1352.

4. Kasteleijn-Nolst Trenite DG, Genton P, Parain D, et al. Evaluation of brivaracetam, a novel SV2A ligand, in the photosensitivity model. *Neurology*. 2007;69 (10):1027–1034.

5. Mattson RH, Cramer JA, Collins JF, et al. Comparison of carbamazepine, phenobarbital, phenytoin, and primidone in partial and secondarily generalized tonic-clonic seizures. *N Engl J Med*. 1985;313(3):145–151.

6. Gauthier AC, Mattson RH. Clobazam: a safe, efficacious, and newly rediscovered therapeutic for epilepsy. *CNS Neurosci Ther*. 2015;21(7):543–548.

7. Wheless JW, Phelps SJ. Clobazam: a newly approved but well-established drug for the treatment of intractable epilepsy syndromes. *J Child Neurol*. 2013;28(2):219–229.

8. Geffrey AL, Pollack SF, Bruno PL, Thiele EA. Drug-drug interaction between clobazam and cannabidiol in children with

refractory epilepsy. *Epilepsia*. 2015;56 (8):1246–1251.

9. Conry JA, Ng YT, Kernitsky L, et al. Stable dosages of clobazam for Lennox-Gastaut syndrome are associated with sustained drop-seizure and total-seizure improvements over 3 years. *Epilepsia*. 2014;55(4):558–567.

10. Rickels K, Brown AS, Cohen D, et al. Clobazam and diazepam in anxiety. *Clin Pharmacol Ther*. 1981;30(1):95–100.

11. Galiana GL, Gauthier AC, Mattson RH. Eslicarbazepine acetate: a new improvement on a classic drug family for the treatment of partial-onset seizures. *Drugs R D*. 2017;17(3):329–339.

12. Hebeisen S, Pires N, Loureiro AI, et al. Eslicarbazepine and the enhancement of slow inactivation of voltage-gated sodium channels: a comparison with carbamazepine, oxcarbazepine and lacosamide. *Neuropharmacology*. 2015;89:122–135.

13. Bialer M, Soares-da-Silva P. Pharmacokinetics and drug interactions of eslicarbazepine acetate. *Epilepsia*. 2012;53 (6):935–946.

14. Nunes T, Rocha JF, Falcao A, Almeida L, Soares-da-Silva P. Steady-state plasma and cerebrospinal fluid pharmacokinetics and tolerability of eslicarbazepine acetate and oxcarbazepine in healthy volunteers. *Epilepsia*. 2013;54(1):108–116.

15. Sperling MR, French J, Jacobson MP, et al. Conversion to eslicarbazepine acetate monotherapy: a pooled analysis of 2 phase III studies. *Neurology*. 2016;86 (12):1095–1102.

16. Trinka E, Ben-Menachem E, Kowacs PA, et al. Efficacy and safety of eslicarbazepine acetate versus controlled-release carbamazepine monotherapy in newly diagnosed epilepsy: a phase III double-blind, randomized, parallel-group, multicenter study. *Epilepsia*. 2018;59 (2):479–491.

17. Gupta DK, Bhoi SK, Kalita J, Misra UK. Hyponatremia following esclicarbazepine therapy. *Seizure*. 2015;29:11–14.

18. Glauser TA, Cnaan A, Shinnar S, et al. Ethosuximide, valproic acid, and lamotrigine in childhood absence epilepsy: initial monotherapy outcomes at 12 months. *Epilepsia*. 2013;54(1):141–155.

19. Livingston S, Rodriguez H, Greene CA, Pauli LL. Systemic lupus erythematosus: occurrence in association with ethosuximide therapy. *JAMA*. 1968;204 (8):731–732.

20. Shi LL, Dong J, Ni H, Geng J, Wu T. Felbamate as an add-on therapy for refractory epilepsy. *Cochrane Database Syst Rev*. 2011(1):Cd008295.

21. Bonnet U, Richter EL, Isbruch K, Scherbaum N. On the addictive power of gabapentinoids: a mini-review. *Psychiatr Danub*. 2018;30(2):142–149.

22. Stoehr T, Freitag J, Beyreuther B, et al. (725) Lacosamide has a dual mode of action: selective enhancement of sodium channel slow inactivation [abstract]. *J Pain*. 2007;8(4 Suppl):S32.

23. Baulac M, Rosenow F, Toledo M, et al. Efficacy, safety, and tolerability of lacosamide monotherapy versus controlled-release carbamazepine in patients with newly diagnosed epilepsy: a phase 3, randomised, double-blind, non-inferiority trial. *Lancet Neurol*. 2017;16 (1):43–54.

24. Kanner AM, Ashman E, Gloss D, et al. Practice guideline update summary. Efficacy and tolerability of the new antiepileptic drugs I: treatment of new-onset epilepsy. Report of the Guideline Development, Dissemination, and Implementation Subcommittee of the American Academy of Neurology and the American Epilepsy Society. *Neurology*. 2018;91(2):74–81.

25. Nevitt SJ, Tudur Smith C, Weston J, Marson AG. Lamotrigine versus carbamazepine monotherapy for epilepsy: an individual participant data review. *Cochrane Database Syst Rev*. 2018;6: CD001031.

26. Gower AJ, Hirsch E, Boehrer A, Noyer M, Marescaux C. Effects of levetiracetam, a novel antiepileptic drug, on convulsant

activity in two genetic rat models of epilepsy. *Epilepsy Res.* 1995;22(3):207–213.

27. Brodie MJ, Perucca E, Ryvlin P, Ben-Menachem E, Meencke HJ. Comparison of levetiracetam and controlled-release carbamazepine in newly diagnosed epilepsy. *Neurology.* 2007;68 (6):402–408.

28. Smith DB, Mattson RH, Cramer JA, et al. Results of a nationwide Veterans Administration Cooperative Study comparing the efficacy and toxicity of carbamazepine, phenobarbital, phenytoin, and primidone. *Epilepsia.* 1987;28 Suppl 3 (s3):S50–58.

29. McLean MJ, Schmutz M, Pozza M, Wamil A. The influence of rufinamide on sodium currents and action potential firing in rodent neurons [abstract]. *Epilepsia.* 2005;46(Suppl 8):296.

30. Perucca E, Cloyd J, Critchley D, Fuseau E. Rufinamide: clinical pharmacokinetics and concentration-response relationships in patients with epilepsy. *Epilepsia.* 2008;49 (7):1123–1141.

31. Coppola G, Grosso S, Franzoni E, et al. Rufinamide in refractory childhood epileptic encephalopathies other than Lennox-Gastaut syndrome. *Eur J Neurol.* 2011;18(2):246–251.

32. Kanner AM, Ashman E, Gloss D, et al. Practice guideline update summary. Efficacy and tolerability of the new antiepileptic drugs II: treatment-resistant epilepsy. Report of the Guideline Development, Dissemination, and Implementation Subcommittee of the American Academy of Neurology and the American Epilepsy Society. *Neurology.* 2018;91(2):82–90.

33. Privitera MD, Brodie MJ, Mattson RH, et al. Topiramate, carbamazepine and valproate monotherapy: double-blind comparison in newly diagnosed epilepsy. *Acta Neurol Scand.* 2003;107 (3):165–175.

34. Nolan SJ, Sudell M, Tudur Smith C, Marson AG. Topiramate versus carbamazepine monotherapy for epilepsy: an individual participant data review. *Cochrane Database Syst Rev.* 2016;12: CD012065.

35. Baker GA, Bromley RL, Briggs M, et al. IQ at 6 years after in utero exposure to antiepileptic drugs: a controlled cohort study. *Neurology.* 2015;84 (4):382–390.

36. Rey E, Pons G, Olive G. Vigabatrin. Clinical pharmacokinetics. *Clin Pharmacokinet.* 1992;23(4): 267–278.

37. Xiao Y, Gan L, Wang J, Luo M, Luo H. Vigabatrin versus carbamazepine monotherapy for epilepsy. *Cochrane Database Syst Rev.* 2015(11): CD008781.

38. Baulac M, Brodie MJ, Patten A, Segieth J, Giorgi L. Efficacy and tolerability of zonisamide versus controlled-release carbamazepine for newly diagnosed partial epilepsy: a phase 3, randomised, double-blind, non-inferiority trial. *Lancet Neurol.* 2012;11(7):579–588.

39. Thiele EA, Marsh ED, French JA et al. Cannabidiol in patients with seizures associated with Lennox–Gastaut skyndrome (GWPCare4): a randomized, double-blind, placebo-controlled phase 3 trial. *Lancet,* 2018;391:1085–1096.

40. Devinsky O, Patel AD, Cross JH et al. Effect of cannabidiol on drop seizures in the Lennox-Gastaut syndrome. *N Engl J Med.* 2018;378:1888–1897.

41. Devinsky O, Cross JH, Laux L et al. Trial of cannabidiol in drug-resistant seizures in the Dravet syndrome. *N Engl J Med.* 2017; 376:2011–2020.

42. American Epilepsy Society Treatments Committee: Vossler D, Weingarten M, Gidal B. Current Review in Clinical Science: Summary of Antiepileptic Drugs Available in the United States of America. July 5, 2018.

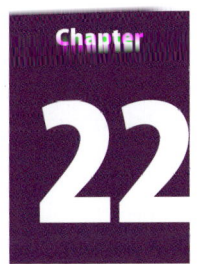

Surgical Therapies for Epilepsy

Rushna Ali and Ellen L. Air

22.1 Indications for Referral for Epilepsy Surgery

The International League Against Epilepsy (ILAE) put forth the definition for intractable epilepsy as the persistence of seizures despite "adequate trials of two tolerated, appropriately chosen and used antiseizure drug [ASD] schedules (whether as monotherapies or in combination)."[1] The definition of medically refractory epilepsy has been debated for many years,[2] and expert opinion remains divergent from common practice.[3] It has been well-documented that the chances of achieving seizure freedom are minimal with additional trials of ASDs and that increased duration of seizures before surgery is associated with decreased chance of long-term seizure freedom.[4] The American Association of Neurology 2015 Epilepsy Quality Measures recommend that each patient should have their diagnosis and treatment plan evaluated, and a referral for presurgical evaluation should be considered to a level 4 epilepsy center for those who are medically refractory about once every 2 years.[5] As part of this referral and reassessment, surgery should be considered.

Surgery for the treatment of medically refractory epilepsy remains underutilized. On average, fewer than 2000 patients undergo epilepsy surgery in the United States annually, representing less than 1% of those estimated to have refractory epilepsy.[6] Those who are referred to qualified epilepsy centers have typically experienced their initial seizure more than 20 years prior and have been medically refractory for 10 years or more.[7]

There is no set duration of epilepsy required before surgical consideration. Rather, the risks of continued seizures must be weighed against the risks and benefits of surgery. Most devastating is the risk of sudden unexpected death in epilepsy (SUDEP). A recent study by a joint subcommittee of the American Association of Neurology and American Epilepsy Society found that the risk of SUDEP is 1.2/1000 adults. This risk increases with the occurrence and increasing frequency of generalized tonic–clonic seizures.[8] Despite years of research and the identification of risk factors, SUDEP remains the primary cause of death in patients with uncontrolled epilepsy.[9] As important to the daily functioning of patients with epilepsy, continued seizures are associated with memory and cognitive impairment, depression,[10] anxiety, and impaired social function.[11] Ideally, surgical treatment for epilepsy is undertaken with the goal of achieving seizure freedom. A single, well-localized seizure focus in noneloquent territory of the brain is ideal for resection, which is potentially curative. However, seizure freedom is not an achievable or appropriate goal for many patients with medically refractory epilepsy. This may be due to multiple seizure foci, location of focus in eloquent brain, or the presence of a broad field of seizure onset. Surgical treatment can still offer significant benefit, even if palliative.

Whether a curative or palliative procedure is considered depends on the preoperative evaluation. At a minimum, patients should have undergone video electroencephalogram

(EEG), brain imaging (preferably high-quality magnetic resonance imaging (MRI)), and neuropsychologic evaluation. Long-term video-EEG confirms the presence of epileptic seizures, defines the semiology, and often identifies the region of seizure onset. MRI is invaluable in identifying structural brain abnormalities or lesions that are epileptogenic. Key amongst these are hippocampal sclerosis, tumors, and vascular malformations (e.g., cavernoma). However, attention must be paid to avoid red herrings. Lesion location should correlate with EEG findings. In addition, neuropsychologic evaluation is important, both for assessing concordance of cognitive deficits with presumed seizure onset zone (SOZ) and for documenting baseline function to characterize the potential cognitive risks of surgery. Additional studies, such as positron emission tomography, single-photon emission computed tomography, and magnetoencephalography can be performed to aid in localization as needed. Should noninvasive studies not be concordant, indicate multifocal seizure onset, or not sufficiently localize the onset zone, invasive monitoring should be considered.

The surgical options discussed in this chapter encompass ablative procedures, both curative and palliative, based on adequate preoperative assessment. Stimulation procedures will be discussed in a separate chapter.

22.2 Types of Surgical Procedures

22.2.1 Resection Procedures

As stated above, the primary goal of surgical resection is to achieve seizure freedom in patients with well-defined seizure phenomena and clear localization of the seizure onset zone (SOZ). Lesional epilepsies particularly lend themselves to surgical resection and include those caused by developmental abnormalities, tumors, vascular malformations, and trauma.[12,13] Care must be exercised not to falsely attribute seizures to an incidental lesion. Although lesional epilepsies have superior seizure-free outcomes following surgery, resection should still be considered in nonlesional epilepsies.[14] The fundamental approach of seizure characterization and localization, as has been detailed in prior chapters, should be applied to all patients in whom cortical resection is being considered, regardless of the location or etiology.

22.2.1.1 Temporal Lobe Resection

Mesial temporal lobe epilepsy (MTLE) remains the most common surgically treated cause of seizures. The classic candidate has unilateral temporal lobe seizure onset by EEG with mesial temporal sclerosis (MTS) on MRI and concordant neuropsychologic findings. The best studied surgical procedure for MTS is that of amygdalohippocampectomy. This can be accomplished via a standard anterior temporal lobectomy (ATL) or selective amygdalohippocampectomy (SAH). ATL typically involves the resection of middle and inferior temporal, fusiform, and parahippocampal gyri in addition to the amygdala and hippocampus (Figure 22.1). The extent of lateral neocortical resection is tailored depending on language dominance of the operative side; 5 cm of lateral cortex is generally considered safely resectable in the nondominant temporal lobe, while that is limited to 3.5 cm in the dominant lobe.[15]

Several approaches have been described for SAH, including subtemporal, trans-sylvian, and transcortical approaches.[16–18] The transcortical approach through the middle temporal gyrus is most widely used. In this approach, the white matter tracks of the middle temporal gyrus are followed into the temporal horn of the lateral ventricle. At this point

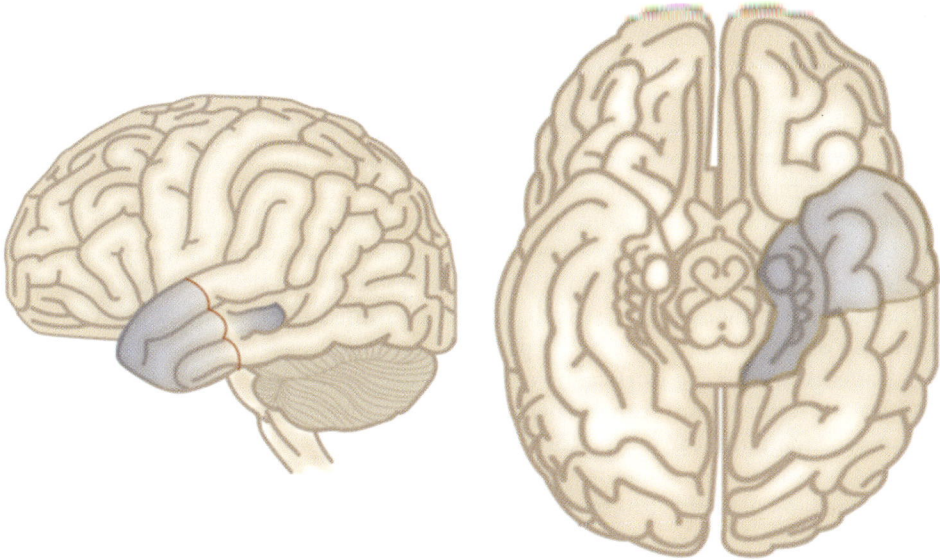

Figure 22.1 Anterior temporal lobectomy shown in (A) lateral and (B) inferior views. The shaded areas indicate the extent of the resected tissue. The dark line indicates the location of the cortical incision. Its distance from the anterior temporal tip varies depending on language dominance and neocortical seizure involvement.

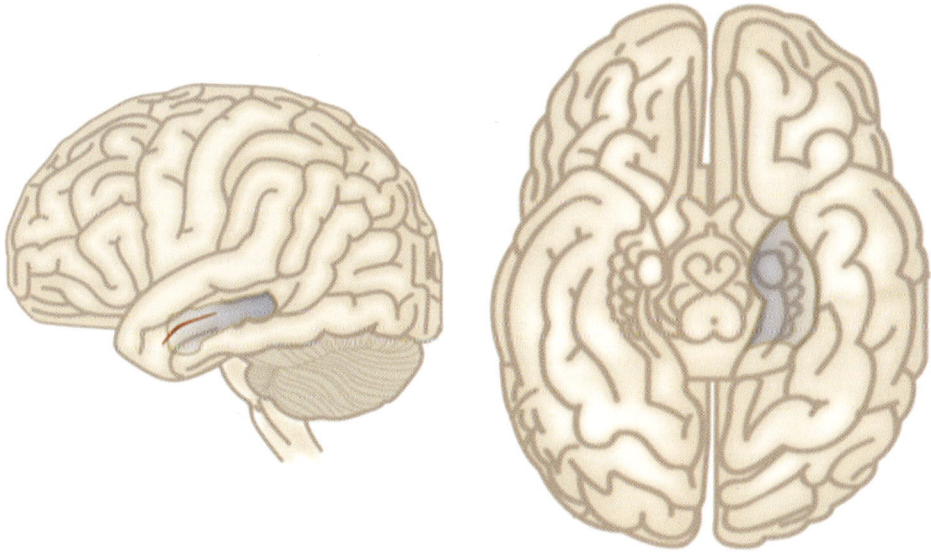

Figure 22.2 Selective amygdalohippocampectomy shown in (A) lateral and (B) inferior views. The shaded areas indicate the extent of the resected tissue. The dark line indicates the location of the cortical incision.

the hippocampus can be visualized and resected. Anterior resection is performed to remove the amygdala (Figure 22.2).[16]

There remains debate in the field as to the best approach. They have been documented to have similar rates of seizure freedom when performed by experienced surgeons, though two large meta-analyses found a higher rate of Engel Class I outcomes after ATL as compared to SAH.[19,20] In addition, the chance of seizure freedom has been directly correlated with the extent (volume) of hippocampal resection.[21,22]

SAH has been associated with improved cognitive outcomes in some, though not all, studies.[19,20] Primary consideration should be given to the risks of memory and language decline following temporal resection. Preoperative memory function is the most predictive of postoperative memory outcomes.[23]

Visual field loss, specifically contralateral superior quadranopsia, is a frequent consequence of mesial temporal resection. Meyer's loop traverses the roof of the temporal horn of the lateral ventricle; however, their anterior extent can be quite variable.[15] Patients should be advised to expect some degree of quadranopsia following surgery, though it is very well-tolerated and often not noticeable to the patient.[24]

For patients with a neocortical temporal focus, particularly those with a clearly defined lesion, lesionectomy can be performed. Electrocorticography, with or without awake speech mapping, can be performed intraoperatively to maximize the extent of resection. There remains debate as to whether mesial temporal lobe resection should be performed in patients whose lesion is adjacent to the amygdala. Sparing of the mesial structures is recommended when preoperative memory is normal on the affected side.[25]

22.2.1.2 Frontal Lobe Resection

Frontal lobectomy can be performed in patients with a broad frontal lobe SOZ. In the nondominant hemisphere, the superior, middle, and inferior frontal gyri are resected along with the anterior cingulate gyrus. Image guidance and somatosensory evoked potentials are invaluable in defining central sulcus and precentral gyrus to guide the posterior extent of resection. Generally, resection spares the gyrus immediately anterior to the precentral gyrus. In the dominant frontal lobe, the posterior aspect of the inferior frontal gyrus is spared to preserve speech. Subtotal frontal lobe resection is often performed, tailored to the SOZ. In each case, attention must be paid to the vascular anatomy. Venous infarct, particularly of the posterior frontal lobe, can lead to contralateral weakness. Resection of the supplementary motor cortex typically results in temporary contralateral hemiparesis that can last from weeks to months.[26–28]

22.2.1.3 Insular, Parietal, and Occipital Resections

Neocortical resection in these regions represent a minority of surgical procedures for epilepsy. However, surgical treatment of seizures from these regions share several challenges. Localization of the SOZ is often difficult by scalp EEG due to rapid spread to other regions. Extraoperative electrocorticography is typically necessary, in conjunction with advanced imaging techniques. Again, concordance of SOZ with lesions identified on imaging should be confirmed before lesionectomy is pursued. The associated vascular anatomy presents an additional challenge to surgery in these regions. Damage to posterior, sylvian, or interhemispheric draining veins can lead to infarction and hemorrhage. When prominent veins transverse the SOZ, subpial resection must be performed to preserve them. Finally, preoperative function, specifically speech, motor, and visual fields, should be well-defined in their relationship to the SOZ and planned resection.[29–31]

22.2.2 Disconnection Procedures

22.2.2.1 Corpus Callosotomy

The treatment of generalized seizures by sectioning the corpus callosum was first conceived in 1940, though it took several decades to become widely accepted. Its classic application is in the treatment of atonic seizures ("drop attacks"). It has also been considered for generalized tonic, myoclonic, and tonic–clonic seizures, though these seizure types do not respond as well as atonic seizures.[32,33] A focal seizure focus should be ruled out before corpus callosotomy (CC) is considered.

Partial and complete corpus callosotomies have been described. Partial CC typically involves sectioning of the anterior two-thirds of the corpus callosum: from the rostrum to the splenium, leaving the splenium and anterior commissure intact (Figure 22.3). Care is taken to stay within the midline and ensure all fibers down to the ependyma are transected. A complete CC can be performed as a single, up-front procedure or in two stages. Sectioning of the splenium, whether performed as part of a complete CC or as a separate procedure, requires great attention to preserving the interhemispheric veins. Disconnection syndrome and transient mutism have been described following CC, though they are less common after anterior CC.[34,35] Development of focal seizures with new semiology, likely the expression of seizures that can no longer generalize, is common.[36]

The decision to perform an anterior versus complete CC should be based on the underlying etiology, seizure types, and baseline cognitive function. Many have advocated for initial treatment with anterior CC due to the concern for disconnection syndrome and significant seizure reduction documented with this procedure.[33,35,37] There has also been the concern that patients with significant mental retardation fare worse with complete CC; however, studies have not supported this notion.[33] Complete CC is advocated for patients with Lennox–Gastaut whose primary seizure type is atonic due to good outcomes and lack of significant cognitive decline following surgery.[38,39]

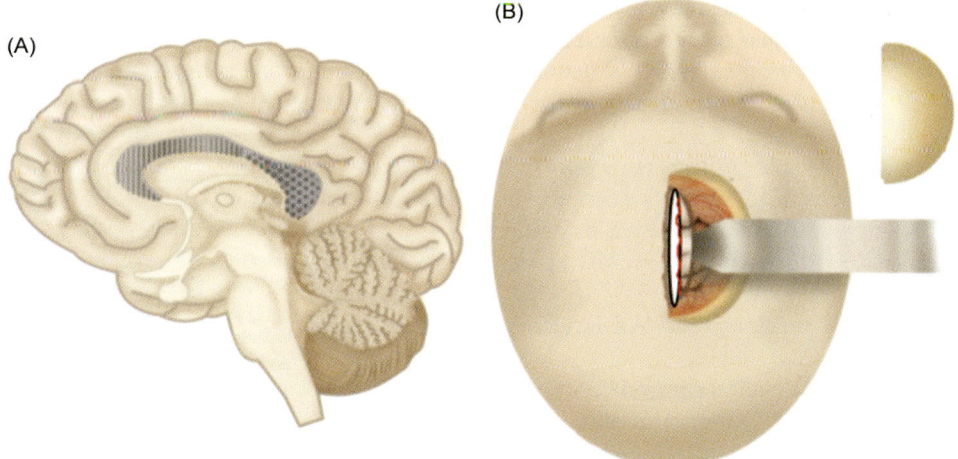

(B)

(A)

Figure 22.3 Corpus callosotomy. The sagittal view (A) depicts the extent of disconnection performed in an anterior callosotomy (striped area) and posterior or completion callosotomy (dotted area). The surgical approach (B), in which a small craniotomy is made just off midline and the corpus callosum is visualized after retraction of the cerebral hemisphere, and disconnected medial to the ipsilateral pericallosal artery.

Since the development of vagus nerve stimulation (VNS), which is surgically less invasive with relatively low morbidity, many have advocated that a patient fail VNS before CC is performed. Others have advocated that CC be considered earlier in the treatment paradigm, both because CC is potentially more effective and eligible patients have a high risk of major injury and SUDEP if untreated.[35,38,40]

22.2.2.2 Hemispherectomy

Hemispherectomy involves the removal or disconnection of one cerebral hemisphere for the treatment of hemispheric epilepsy. Hemispheric epilepsy can be caused by several congenital syndromes including Sturge–Weber syndrome, hemimegalencephaly, and infantile hemiplegic seizure syndrome. Trauma, intrauterine stroke, hemorrhage, and Rasmussen's encephalitis are acquired causes of hemispheric epilepsy.[41] Appropriate patients for hemispherectomy typically have contralateral hemiplegia and hemianopsia, though there remains debate regarding the severity of deficits required to proceed with surgery. For progressive syndromes, such as Rasmussen's encephalitis, the risk of continued seizures must be weighed against the loss of function that may occur at surgery. Generally, patients without distal motor function of the contralateral extremities can be considered candidates.[41]

Early surgical procedures were performed using an anatomic approach in which the affected hemisphere was entirely removed. This achieved excellent results in seizure control; however, many patients later deteriorated due to superficial hemosiderosis. This phenomenon, in which blood chronically seeps into the resection cavity, often results in hydrocephalus that is difficult to manage.[42] Rasmussen and others refined the approach to functionally disconnect the two hemispheres, while performing a subtotal resection. Functional hemispherectomy (also known as functional hemispherotomy) includes a large temporal lobectomy with amygdalohippocampectomy, wide resection of the peri-Rolandic cortex and complete CC with disconnection of the white matter tracts to the anterior fossa floor and tentorium.[41,43,44]

Functional hemispherectomy (Figure 22.4) is most commonly performed in young children, though it has been reported in adolescents and young adults.[45] There appears to

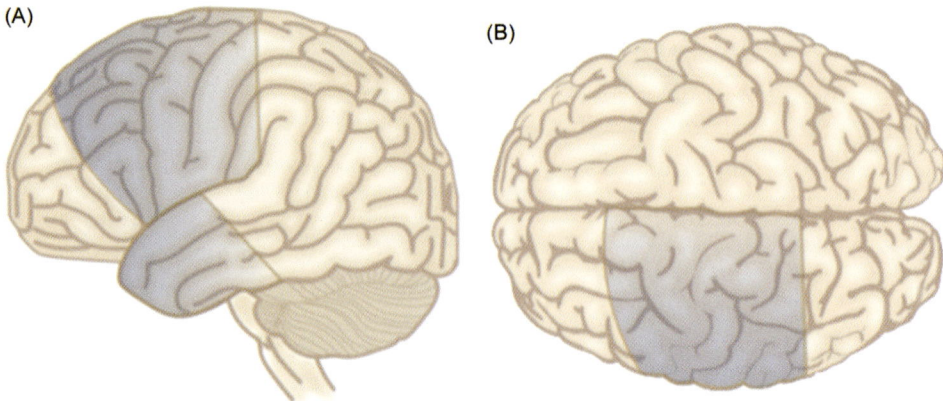

Figure 22.4 Functional hemispheriectomy shown in (A) lateral and (B) dorsal views. The shaded areas indicate the extent of resected tissue.

be a benefit to earlier surgery. Both seizure freedom and functional outcomes have been correlated with shorter preoperative duration of epilepsy. Several studies have also documented higher rates of seizure freedom among patients with acquired and progressive etiologies, as compared to those with developmental etiology.[46,47]

22.2.2.3 Multiple Subpial Transection

Multiple subpial transection (MST) is a technique aimed at disrupting the propagation of seizures by preventing the synchronization of larger populations of neurons within the cortex. It takes advantage of the organization of the cortex into vertical columns, which serve as units that convey functional output. Sectioning the cortex into such units prevents seizure spread, while preserving function of eloquent areas. It was first described by Morrell and Hanbery in 1969 for the treatment of seizures emanating from speech or motor cortex.[48] The technique involves puncturing the pia, then running an angled hook through the gray matter, beneath the pia, to transect the gray matter of individual gyri. This is repeated at 5 mm intervals creating "cortical islands," which are too small to initiate a sustained epileptic discharge.[49]

MSTs are best performed when the epileptic onset zone resides within, or includes, eloquent regions, specifically the precentral or postcentral gyri, dominant frontal operculum, the dominant posterior temporoparietal region, and primary visual cortex. Rarely have patients experienced significant loss of function as a result of this procedure, and a few have gained function due to the improved seizure control.[49] MST can be performed in isolation with significant reduction in seizures[50]; however, it is most commonly employed as an adjunct to lesionectomy. Slightly improved rates of seizure improvement have been documented in patients who have undergone MST plus lesionectomy, as compared to those who underwent MST alone.[51]

22.2.3 Minimally Invasive Ablative Procedures

The push towards less invasive procedures has dominated the evolution of surgical treatment, and the field of epilepsy surgery has been no different. In particular, laser interstitial thermal therapy (LITT) and stereotactic radiosurgery (SRS) have been applied to the ablation of epileptogenic tissue.

22.2.3.1 Stereotactic Radiosurgery

The concept of radiation treatment for epilepsy developed out of experience in the treatment of tumors and arteriovenous malformations. In many cases, patients suffered from seizures because of the underlying lesion. Radiation treatment was noted to significantly reduce, and in some cases resolve, seizures.[52,53] Subsequently, SRS has developed as a primary treatment for certain types of seizures.

Hypothalamic hamartomas, which classically cause gelastic seizures, endocrine dysfunction, and developmental delay, have long been a treatment challenge because surgical resection is associated with significant morbidity.[54] SRS has resulted in significant improvements in seizure control with minimal morbidity. Doses of at least 17 Gy to the tumor margin, while maintaining less than 8 Gy to the optic pathways, are typically given. Seizure freedom has been reported in 40% of patients and another 20% experienced only rare nondisabling seizures following treatment.[55]

SRS has also been applied to the treatment of MTLE. The anterior 2 cm of the hippocampus (head and anterior body), amygdala, and parahippocampal gyrus are targeted with a marginal dose of 20–24 Gy. Radiation dose must be limited to the adjacent brainstem and optic pathways. In both European and US studies, 60–65% of patients were seizure free at 2 years. However, seizure reduction develops over a protracted period of time, as compared to other surgical therapies. Patients generally experience an increase in auras 9–15 months after SRS, concurrent with a reduction in seizures. Significant temporal lobe edema can also occur during this time. Though typically tolerated by the patients, surgical decompression has been required in some cases.[56,57] The recently published randomized controlled ROSE trial, which compared SRS to standard ATL for MTLE, reported a seizure freedom rate of 52% with SRS versus 78% with ATL. Serious complications were reported in 16.1% of the patients in the SRS arm compared to 7% in the ATL arm.[58]

Several reports of SRS for CC have been published, though they represent a small number of patients. Reduction in seizures without significant morbidity was reported.[57,59]

22.2.3.2 Laser Interstitial Thermal Therapy

LITT involves the placement of a laser tip into the targeted area for ablation. The laser light then causes tissue heating, and ultimately, coagulation. This is monitored in real-time via MR thermometry. The indications for LITT are similar to those for SRS, however LITT offers several advantages. The extent of the final lesion can be visualized immediately and extended if needed. Seizure improvement is seen after the procedure rather than months later. In addition, LITT has been associated with low complication rates, though delayed hemorrhage has been reported, and avoids the potential long-term risk of radiation-induced, secondary malignancy.[57,60,61]

Treatment of MTLE via LITT requires stereotactic placement of the laser probe along the long axis of the hippocampus. Typically, two to three lesions are created, from anterior to posterior, to ensure adequate ablation.[62] The long-term benefits of LITT with respect to seizure control remain to be seen. Published 12-month outcomes following LITT for MTLE report 54–67% Engel I classification.[62] In one study, seizure freedom correlated with complete ablation of the mesial hippocampal head.[63] A multicenter, prospective study of LITT for MTLE is underway.

Hypothalamic hamartomas have also been treated by LITT in a small number of patients with improvement in seizures.[64] Application of LITT to the treatment of seizures due to brain tumors, cavernomas, tuberous sclerosis, as well as to perform CC, have been reported.[57,65]

22.3 Repeat Surgical Procedures

Every epilepsy program experiences their share of surgical failures, i.e., patients who continue to experience seizures after surgical resection. In evaluating such patients, two key questions are to be asked. Is the current seizure semiology the same as before surgery? Was there a significant seizure-free interval after the surgery? The answers to these questions give clues which generally fall into one of two categories: false seizure localization and inadequate surgical resection.[66,67]

Incomplete resection of the seizure focus remains the most common cause of recurrent seizures. In such cases, patients often experience a period of seizure freedom or significant seizure reduction following surgery.[68] Patients who continue to experience seizures with unchanged semiology and no postoperative seizure remittance were likely to have been incorrectly localized. Both insular seizures and contralateral temporal seizures have been falsely attributed to a resected mesial temporal lobe.[66,68]

For those patients who experience both a change in their seizure semiology and a postoperative seizure-free period, the presence of lesions or abnormalities not previously identified should be considered. This possibility should be foremost in patients whose initial surgical pathology revealed cortical dysplasia.[69–72] Progression of an underlying disease process with the development of new seizure foci should also be considered.[67]

The surgical approaches to repeat surgical treatment of epilepsy include many of the previously discussed procedures. Several have recommended that intracranial EEG be performed to better localize the seizure onset before proceeding with a second surgical procedure.[73,74] While repeat surgery can be performed safely and is reported to achieve 36–69% rate of seizure freedom, it is associated with a higher rate of complications.[69,73,74]

22.4 Complications of Surgery

Complications of intracranial surgery have been low in this modern age of neuroanesthesia and advanced surgical techniques. Pooled analysis of data from seven centers revealed an 11% complication rate with a 5% rate of infection. Of the 6% of patients who developed new neurologic deficits, only half were permanent. These were directly related to the location of resection.[75] Only one randomized controlled trial has been performed that compared surgical to medical therapy. In this study, the only reported death occurred in the medical arm.[76]

22.5 Outcomes of Surgery

Postoperative seizure outcome has long been described using the Engel classification, in which outcome is viewed with respect to seizure frequency and its impact on quality of life.[77] While quality of life, put in terms of "worthwhile improvement" in seizures, is critical to patient satisfaction after surgery, it is vague and inconsistently defined. Therefore, an ILAE commission has proposed a new classification system that defines outcome based on absolute seizure days each year.[78] The two classification systems are compared in Table 22.1.

There is similarity between the systems at the extremes of seizure outcomes. The greatest degree of variability and disagreement between these systems are highlighted in the shaded boxes. The ILAE classification is more specific at each level and can be applied for each annum following surgery.

Outcomes are best viewed relative to the location of the seizure focus (temporal versus extratemporal) and whether there was an associated lesion. Seizure freedom following epilepsy surgery remains the primary benchmark of success.

The results of temporal lobe resection have been extensively reported.[79] Two years following surgery, 60–75% of patients achieved Engel Class I outcome, which decreases to 50–60% at 10 years.[80–82] Although MTS has been associated with superior postoperative outcomes, good results have been achieved in patients with normal MRIs and should be considered for surgery.[81,83]

Extratemporal epilepsy is also divided into lesional and nonlesional types. The outcomes for both types can be highly variable in the published studies. As in temporal lobe epilepsy, surgery for pharmacoresistant epilepsy is more effective for patients with a focal epileptogenic lesion identified on MRI.[14,84–86] Lesions can consist of vascular malformations, tumors, and cortical dysplasias. Complete resection of vascular malformation, including arteriovenous malformations and cavernomas, results in 70–90% of patients becoming free

Table 22.1 Comparison of ILAE and Engel classification systems for postoperative seizure outcome

ILAE Classification	Engel Classification
Class 1: Completely seizure free, no auras	I. Free of disabling seizures A. Completely seizure free
Class 2: Only auras, no other seizures	B. Non-disabling simple partial seizures only C. Some disabling seizures after surgery, but free for >2 years D. Generalized convulsion only after ASD discontinuation
Class 3: One to three seizures days per year, ± auras	II. Rare disabling seizures A. Initially free of disabling seizures but rare seizures now B. Rare disabling seizures since surgery C. More than rare disabling seizures since surgery, but rare for last 2 years D. Nocturnal seizures only
Class 4: Four or more seizure days/year to 50% reduction of baseline seizures days/year, ± auras	III. Worthwhile improvement A. Worthwhile seizure reduction B. Prolonged seizure-free intervals amounting to > half follow-up period, but not <2 years
Class 5: Less than 50% reduction to 100% increase of baseline seizures days/year, ± auras	IV. No worthwhile improvement A. Significant seizure reduction
Class 6: More than 100% increase of baseline seizure days, ± auras	B. No appreciable change C. Seizures worse

ASD, antiseizure drug; ILAE, International League Against Epilepsy

from disabling seizures.[87] Amongst the lesional cases, cortical dysplasia has the poorest outcomes for seizure control due to the lack of a visibly clear boundary and the possibility that multiple lesions exist in close proximity to one another. The Cleveland Clinic reported a 49% Engel Class I rate in 35 patients with resections for cortical dysplasia.[88] However, a German series reported a 72% seizure-free rate in 53 patients with resections for cortical dysplasia, with completeness of the resection being a major factor contributing to successful seizure control.[89]

The reported rates of good surgical outcome for nonlesional partial epilepsy range from 37–40% for mixed mesial temporal and neocortical sites,[90] and 29–56% for extratemporal epilepsy.[85,86,91] However, outcome data in nonlesional extratemporal epilepsy is derived from a small group of highly select patients with 1-year follow-up.[85] A retrospective cohort confirmed that although seizure frequency improves in many patients with nonlesional extratemporal epilepsy, only 24% are seizure free at 1 year and 15% at 5 years.[92] The importance of early postoperative seizures, which confer a fourfold risk of later seizure recurrence, was also highlighted in this article. Factors predicting good surgical outcome in nonlesional extratemporal epilepsy include unifocal interictal epileptiform discharges, a local β-frequency ictal discharge on either a scalp or an intracranial EEG, and a localized single-photon emission computed tomography abnormality.[29,30,93]

Surgical outcomes for lesional extratemporal epilepsy are generally more favorable. When assessing for favorable outcomes based on seizure location, a recent report found long-term seizure-free rates of 27–50% for frontal, 46–80% for occipital and parietal, and 34% for grouped extratemporal resections.[90] A published study from the Cleveland Clinic shows that the seizure-free rate for frontal lobe resections drops from 56% at 1-year follow-up to 30% at 5 years.[86]

ASD withdrawal after extratemporal resection is controversial. In a retrospective study, ASDs were withdrawn in 88.7% (n = 94) of patients and 41.5% (n = 44) developed recurrent seizures. Notably, 31.8% failed to regain seizure control once the ASDs were resumed. Abnormal postoperative EEG and longer duration of epilepsy prior to resection were found to be poor prognostic factors.[94] Discussing the possibility of seizure recurrence with patients is helpful in making realistic decisions on postsurgery ASD withdrawal.

References

1. Kwan P, Arzimanoglou A, Berg AT, et al. Definition of drug resistant epilepsy: consensus proposal by the ad hoc task force of the ILAE Commission on Therapeutic Strategies. *Epilepsia*. 2010;51(6):1069–1077.

2. Tellez-Zenteno JF, Hernandez-Ronquillo L, Buckley S, Zahagun R, Rizvi S. A validation of the new definition of drug-resistant epilepsy by the International League Against Epilepsy. *Epilepsia*. 2014;55(6):829–834.

3. Wasade VS, Spanaki M, Iyengar R, Barkley GL, Schultz L. AAN Epilepsy Quality Measures in clinical practice: a survey of neurologists. *Epilepsy Behav*. 2012;24(4):468–473.

4. Yoon HH, Kwon HL, Mattson RH, Spencer DD, Spencer SS. Long-term seizure outcome in patients initially seizure-free after resective epilepsy surgery. *Neurology*. 2003;61(4):445–450.

5. Fountain NB, Van Ness PC, Bennett A, et al. Quality improvement in neurology: Epilepsy Update Quality Measurement Set. *Neurology*. 2015;84(14):1483–1487.

6. Berg AT, Vickrey BG, Testa FM, et al. How long does it take for epilepsy to become intractable?: a prospective investigation. *Ann Neurol*. 2006;60(1):73–79.

7. Kaiboriboon K, Malkhachroum AM, Zrik A, et al. Epilepsy surgery in the United States: analysis of data from the National Association of Epilepsy Centers. *Epilepsy Res*. 2015;116:105–109.

8. Harden C, Tomson T, Gloss D, et al. Practice guideline summary: sudden unexpected death in epilepsy incidence rates and risk factors. Report of the Guideline Development, Dissemination, and Implementation Subcommittee of the American Academy of Neurology and the American Epilepsy Society. *Neurology*. 2017;88(17):1674–1680.

9. Jones LA, Thomas RH. Sudden death in epilepsy: insights from the last 25 years. *Seizure*. 2017;44:232–236.

10. Rayner G, Jackson GD, Wilson SJ. Mechanisms of memory impairment in epilepsy depend on age at disease onset. *Neurology*. 2016;87(16):1642–1649.

11. Kampf C, Walter U, Rosche J. The impact of anxiety, seizure severity, executive dysfunction, subjectively perceived psychological deficits, and depression on social function in patients with epilepsy. *Epilepsy Behav*. 2016;57(Pt A):5–8.

12. Shaefi S, Harkness W. Current status of surgery in the management of epilepsy. *Epilepsia*. 2003;44 Suppl 1:43–47.

13. Willoughby JO. Mechanisms underlying partial (focal, or lesional) epilepsy. *J Clin Neurosci*. 2000;7(4):291–294.

14. Tellez-Zenteno JF, Hernandez Ronquillo L, Moien-Afshari F, Wiebe S. Surgical

outcomes in lesional and non-lesional epilepsy: a systematic review and meta-analysis. *Epilepsy Res.* 2010;89 (2–3):310–318.

15. Connolly PJ, Baltuch GH. Temporal lobectomy and amygdalohippocampectomy. In: Baltuch GH, Villemure J, eds., *Operative Techniques in Epilepsy Surgery.* New York: Thieme Medical Publishers; 2009:33–40.

16. Wheatley BM. Selective amygdalohippocampectomy: the trans-middle temporal gyrus approach. *Neurosurg Focus.* 2008;25(3):E4.

17. Adada B. Selective amygdalohippocampectomy via the transsylvian approach. *Neurosurg Focus.* 2008;25(3):E5.

18. von Rhein B, Nelles M, Urbach H, et al. Neuropsychological outcome after selective amygdalohippocampectomy: subtemporal versus transsylvian approach. *J Neurol Neurosurg Psychiatry.* 2012;83(9):887–893.

19. Josephson CB, Dykeman J, Fiest KM, et al. Systematic review and meta-analysis of standard vs selective temporal lobe epilepsy surgery. *Neurology.* 2013;80 (18):1669–1676.

20. Hu WH, Zhang C, Zhang K, et al. Selective amygdalohippocampectomy versus anterior temporal lobectomy in the management of mesial temporal lobe epilepsy: a meta-analysis of comparative studies. *J Neurosurg.* 2013;119 (5):1089–1097.

21. Joo EY, Han HJ, Lee EK, et al. Resection extent versus postoperative outcomes of seizure and memory in mesial temporal lobe epilepsy. *Seizure.* 2005;14(8):541–551.

22. Sagher O, Thawani JP, Etame AB, Gomez-Hassan DM. Seizure outcomes and mesial resection volumes following selective amygdalohippocampectomy and temporal lobectomy. *Neurosurg Focus.* 2012;32(3):E8.

23. Stroup E, Langfitt J, Berg M, et al. Predicting verbal memory decline following anterior temporal lobectomy (ATL). *Neurology.* 2003;60(8):1266–1273.

24. Georgiadis I, Kapsalaki EZ, Fountas KN. Temporal lobe resective surgery for medically intractable epilepsy: a review of complications and side effects. *Epilepsy Res Treat.* 2013;2013:752195.

25. Vives K, Lee G, Doyle W, Spencer DD. Anterior temporal rexection. In: Engel J, Jr., Pedley TA, eds., *Epilepsy: A Comprehensive Textbook.* 2nd edn. Philadelphia: Wolters Kluwer Health/ Lippincott Williams & Wilkins; 2008:1859–1867.

26. Schramm J, Kral T, Kurthen M, Blumcke I. Surgery to treat focal frontal lobe epilepsy in adults. *Neurosurgery.* 2002;51 (3):644–654; discussion 654–645.

27. Roper SN. Surgical treatment of the extratemporal epilepsies. *Epilepsia.* 2009;50 Suppl 8:69–74.

28. Olivier A. Surgery of epilepsy: methods. *Acta Neurol Scand Suppl.* 1988;117:103–113.

29. Zakaria T, Noe K, So E, et al. Scalp and intracranial EEG in medically intractable extratemporal epilepsy with normal MRI. *ISRN Neurol.* 2012;2012:942849.

30. O'Brien TJ, So EL, Mullan BP, et al. Subtraction peri-ictal SPECT is predictive of extratemporal epilepsy surgery outcome. *Neurology.* 2000;55(11):1668–1677.

31. Comair YG, Van Ness PC, Chamoun RB, Bouclaous CH. Neocortical resections. In: Engel J, Jr., Pedley TA, eds., *Epilepsy: A Comprehensive Textbook.* 2nd edn. Philadelphia: Wolters Kluwer Health/ Lippincott Williams & Wilkins; 2008:1869–1878.

32. Bower RS, Wirrell E, Nwojo M, et al. Seizure outcomes after corpus callosotomy for drop attacks. *Neurosurgery.* 2013;73 (6):993–1000.

33. Liang S, Li A, Jiang H, et al. Anterior corpus callosotomy in patients with intractable generalized epilepsy and mental retardation. *Stereotact Funct Neurosurg.* 2010;88(4):246–252.

34. Graham D, Tisdall MM, Gill D. Corpus callosotomy outcomes in pediatric patients: a systematic review. *Epilepsia.* 2016;57 (7):1053–1068.

35. Malmgren K, Rydenhag B, Hallbook T. Reappraisal of corpus callosotomy.

Curr Opin Neurol. 2015;20(2):
175–181.

36. Gates JR, Rosenfeld WE, Maxwell RE, Lyons RE. Response of multiple seizure types to corpus callosum section. *Epilepsia.* 1987;28(1):28–34.

37. Kasasbeh AS, Smyth MD, Steger-May K, et al. Outcomes after anterior or complete corpus callosotomy in children. *Neurosurgery.* 2014;74(1):17–28; discussion 28.

38. Lancman G, Virk M, Shao H, et al. Vagus nerve stimulation vs. corpus callosotomy in the treatment of Lennox-Gastaut syndrome: a meta-analysis. *Seizure.* 2013;22 (1):3–8.

39. Purves SJ, Wada JA, Woodhurst WB, et al. Results of anterior corpus callosum section in 24 patients with medically intractable seizures. *Neurology.* 1988;38(8):1194–1201.

40. Rolston JD, Englot DJ, Wang DD, Garcia PA, Chang EF. Corpus callosotomy versus vagus nerve stimulation for atonic seizures and drop attacks: a systematic review. *Epilepsy Behav.* 2015;51:13–17.

41. Peacock WJ. Hemispherectomy for the treatment of intractable seizures in childhood. *Neurosurg Clin N Am.* 1995;6 (3):549–563.

42. Oppenheimer DR, Griffith HB. Persistent intracranial bleeding as a complication of hemispherectomy. *J Neurol Neurosurg Psychiatry.* 1966;29(3):229–240.

43. Villemure J, Daniel RT. Functional hemispherectomy and periinsular hemispherotomy. In: Baltuch GH, Villemure J, eds., *Operative Techniques in Epilepsy Surgery.* New York: Thieme Medical Publishers; 2009: 138–145.

44. Danielpour M, von Koch CS, Ojemann SG, Peacock WJ. Disconnective hemispherectomy. *Pediatr Neurosurg.* 2001;35(4):169–172.

45. Schusse CM, Smith K, Drees C. Outcomes after hemispherectomy in adult patients with intractable epilepsy: institutional experience and systematic review of the literature. *J Neurosurg.* 2018;128 (3):853–861.

46. Moosa ANV, Jehi L, Marashly A, et al. Long-term functional outcomes and their predictors after hemispherectomy in 115 children. *Epilepsia.* 2013;54(10):1771–1779.

47. Jonas R, Nguyen S, Hu B, et al. Cerebral hemispherectomy: hospital course, seizure, developmental, language, and motor outcomes. *Neurology.* 2004;62 (10):1712–1721.

48. Morrell F, Hanbery JW. A new surgical technique for the treatment of focal cortical epilepsy. *Electroencephalogr Clin Neurophysiol.* 1969;26(1):120.

49. Morrell F, Whisler WW, Bleck TP. Multiple subpial transection: a new approach to the surgical treatment of focal epilepsy. *J Neurosurg.* 1989;70(2):231–239.

50. Hufnagel A, Zentner J, Fernandez G, et al. Multiple subpial transection for control of epileptic seizures: effectiveness and safety. *Epilepsia.* 1997;38(6):678–688.

51. Spencer SS, Schramm J, Wyler A, et al. Multiple subpial transection for intractable partial epilepsy: an international meta-analysis. *Epilepsia.* 2002;43(2):141–145.

52. Schauble B, Cascino GD, Pollock BE, et al. Seizure outcomes after stereotactic radiosurgery for cerebral arteriovenous malformations. *Neurology.* 2004;63 (4):683–687.

53. Schrottner O, Eder HG, Unger F, Feichtinger K, Pendl G. Radiosurgery in lesional epilepsy: brain tumors. *Stereotact Funct Neurosurg.* 1998;70 Suppl 1(1):50–56.

54. Drees C, Chapman K, Prenger E, et al. Seizure outcome and complications following hypothalamic hamartoma treatment in adults: endoscopic, open, and Gamma Knife procedures. *J Neurosurg.* 2012;117(2):255–261.

55. Regis J, Scavarda D, Tamura M, et al. Gamma knife surgery for epilepsy related to hypothalamic hamartomas. *Semin Pediatr Neurol.* 2007;14(2):73–79.

56. Bartolomei F, Hayashi M, Tamura M, et al. Long-term efficacy of gamma knife radiosurgery in mesial temporal lobe epilepsy. *Neurology.* 2008;70 (19):1658–1663.

57. Quigg M, Harden C. Minimally invasive techniques for epilepsy surgery: stereotactic radiosurgery and other technologies. *J Neurosurg.* 2014;121 Suppl:232–240.

58. Barbaro NM, Quigg M, Ward MM, et al. Radiosurgery versus open surgery for mesial temporal lobe epilepsy: the randomized, controlled ROSE trial. *Epilepsia.* 2018;59(6):1198–1207.

59. Feichtinger M, Schrottner O, Eder H, et al. Efficacy and safety of radiosurgical callosotomy: a retrospective analysis. *Epilepsia.* 2006;47(7):1184–1191.

60. Hoppe C, Witt JA, Helmstaedter C, et al. Laser interstitial thermotherapy (LiTT) in epilepsy surgery. *Seizure.* 2017;48:45–52.

61. Barber SM, Tomycz L, George T, Clarke DF, Lee M. Delayed intraparenchymal and intraventricular hemorrhage requiring surgical evacuation after MRI-guided laser interstitial thermal therapy for lesional epilepsy. *Stereotact Funct Neurosurg.* 2017;95(2):73–78.

62. Wicks RT, Jermakowicz WJ, Jagid JR, et al. Laser interstitial thermal therapy for mesial temporal lobe epilepsy. *Neurosurgery.* 2016;79 Suppl 1:S83–S91.

63. Jermakowicz WJ, Kanner AM, Sur S, et al. Laser thermal ablation for mesiotemporal epilepsy: analysis of ablation volumes and trajectories. *Epilepsia.* 2017;58(5):801–810.

64. Rolston JD, Chang EF. Stereotactic laser ablation for hypothalamic hamartoma. *Neurosurg Clin N Am.* 2016;27(1):59–67.

65. Medvid R, Ruiz A, Komotar RJ, et al. Current applications of MRI-guided laser interstitial thermal therapy in the treatment of brain neoplasms and epilepsy: a radiologic and neurosurgical overview. *Am J Neuroradiol.* 2015;36(11):1998–2006.

66. Barba C, Rheims S, Minotti L, et al. Temporal plus epilepsy is a major determinant of temporal lobe surgery failures. *Brain.* 2016;139(Pt 2):444–451.

67. Najm I, Jehi L, Palmini A, et al. Temporal patterns and mechanisms of epilepsy surgery failure. *Epilepsia.* 2013;54 (5):772–782.

68. Vale FL, Pollock G, Benbadis SR. Failed epilepsy surgery for mesial temporal lobe sclerosis: a review of the pathophysiology. *Neurosurg Focus.* 2012;32(3):E9.

69. Grote A, Witt JA, Surges R, et al. A second chance – reoperation in patients with failed surgery for intractable epilepsy: long-term outcome, neuropsychology and complications. *J Neurol Neurosurg Psychiatry.* 2016;87(4):379–385.

70. Fauser S, Essang C, Altenmuller DM, et al. Long-term seizure outcome in 211 patients with focal cortical dysplasia. *Epilepsia.* 2015;56(1):66–76.

71. Ramantani G, Strobl K, Stathi A, et al. Reoperation for refractory epilepsy in childhood: a second chance for selected patients. *Neurosurgery.* 2013;73 (4):695–704; discussion 704.

72. Palmini A, Gambardella A, Andermann F, et al. Intrinsic epileptogenicity of human dysplastic cortex as suggested by corticography and surgical results. *Ann Neurol.* 1995;37(4):476–487.

73. Bower RS, Wirrell EC, Eckel LJ, et al. Repeat resective surgery in complex pediatric refractory epilepsy: lessons learned. *J Neurosurg Pediatr.* 2015;16 (1):94–100.

74. Gonzalez-Martinez J, Bulacio J, Alexopoulos A, et al. Stereoelectroencephalography in the "difficult to localize" refractory focal epilepsy: early experience from a North American epilepsy center. *Epilepsia.* 2013;54(2):323–330.

75. Engel J, Jr., Wiebe S, French J, et al. Practice parameter: temporal lobe and localized neocortical resections for epilepsy. Report of the Quality Standards Subcommittee of the American Academy of Neurology, in association with the American Epilepsy Society and the American Association of Neurological Surgeons. *Neurology.* 2003;60(4):538–547.

76. Effectiveness, Efficiency of Surgery for Temporal Lobe Epilepsy Study Group: Wiebe S, Blume WT, Girvin JP, Eliasziw M. A randomized, controlled trial of surgery

for temporal lobe epilepsy. *N Engl J Med.*
2001;345(5):311–318.

77. Engel J, Jr., Van Ness P, Rasmussen TB,
Ojemann LM. Outcome with respect to
epileptic seizures. In: Engel J, Jr., ed.,
Surgical Treatment of the Epilepsies. 2nd
edn. New York: Raven Press; 1993:609–621.

78. Wieser HG, Blume WT, Fish D, et al. ILAE
Commission Report: proposal for a new
classification of outcome with respect to
epileptic seizures following epilepsy
surgery. *Epilepsia.* 2001;42(2):282–286.

79. West S, Nolan SJ, Cotton J, et al. Surgery
for epilepsy. *Cochrane Database Syst Rev.*
2015(7):CD010541.

80. Salanova V, Markand O, Worth R.
Longitudinal follow-up in 145 patients
with medically refractory temporal lobe
epilepsy treated surgically between
1984 and 1995. *Epilepsia.* 1999;40
(10):1417–1423.

81. Fong JS, Jehi L, Najm I, et al. Seizure
outcome and its predictors after temporal
lobe epilepsy surgery in patients with
normal MRI. *Epilepsia.* 2011;52
(8):1393–1401.

82. McIntosh AM, Kalnins RM, Mitchell LA,
et al. Temporal lobectomy: long-term
seizure outcome, late recurrence and risks
for seizure recurrence. *Brain.* 2004;127(Pt
9):2018–2030.

83. Holmes MD, Born DE, Kutsy RL, et al.
Outcome after surgery in patients with
refractory temporal lobe epilepsy
and normal MRI. *Seizure.* 2000;9
(6):407–411.

84. Bell ML, Rao S, So EL, et al. Epilepsy
surgery outcomes in temporal lobe epilepsy
with a normal MRI. *Epilepsia.* 2009;50
(9):2053–2060.

85. Bien CG, Szinay M, Wagner J, et al.
Characteristics and surgical outcomes of
patients with refractory magnetic
resonance imaging-negative epilepsies.
Arch Neurol. 2009;66(12):1491–1499.

86. Jehi LE, Najm I, Bingaman W, et al.
Surgical outcome and prognostic factors of
frontal lobe epilepsy surgery. *Brain.*
2007;130(Pt 2):574–584.

87. Piepgras DG, Sundt TM, Jr., Ragoowansi
AT, Stevens L. Seizure outcome in patients
with surgically treated cerebral
arteriovenous malformations. *J Neurosurg.*
1993;78(1):5–11.

88. Edwards JC, Wyllie E, Ruggeri PM, et al.
Seizure outcome after surgery for epilepsy
due to malformation of cortical
development. *Neurology.* 2000;55
(8):1110–1114.

89. Kral T, Clusmann H, Blumcke I, et al.
Outcome of epilepsy surgery in focal
cortical dysplasia. *J Neurol Neurosurg
Psychiatry.* 2003;74(2):183–188.

90. Blume WT, Ganapathy GR, Munoz D,
Lee DH. Indices of resective surgery
effectiveness for intractable nonlesional
focal epilepsy. *Epilepsia.* 2004;45(1):
46–53.

91. Cascino GD, Jack CR, Jr., Parisi JE, et al.
MRI in the presurgical evaluation of
patients with frontal lobe epilepsy and
children with temporal lobe epilepsy:
pathologic correlation and prognostic
importance. *Epilepsy Res.* 1992;11
(1):51–59.

92. McIntosh AM, Averill CA, Kalnins RM,
et al. Long-term seizure outcome and risk
factors for recurrence after extratemporal
epilepsy surgery. *Epilepsia.* 2012;53
(6):970–978.

93. Holmes MD, Kutsy RL, Ojemann GA,
Wilensky AJ, Ojemann LM. Interictal,
unifocal spikes in refractory extratemporal
epilepsy predict ictal origin and
postsurgical outcome. *Clin Neurophysiol.*
2000;111(10):1802–1808.

94. Menon R, Rathore C, Sarma SP,
Radhakrishnan K. Feasibility of
antiepileptic drug withdrawal following
extratemporal resective epilepsy surgery.
Neurology. 2012;79(8):770–776.

Chapter 23

Stimulation Therapies for Epilepsy

David King-Stephens and Peter Weber

23.1 Introduction

Despite the availability of more than 20 antiseizure drugs (ASDs) for the treatment of epilepsy, up to 30% of patients continue to experience disabling seizures and are classified as having medically refractory epilepsy (MRE).[1] Some patients with MRE are candidates for resective surgery or other palliative interventions, such as disconnection therapies (callosotomy or subpial transections).[2] Unfortunately, the majority of refractory patients are not candidates for these surgical options due to having multifocal epileptogenic foci, foci localized to an eloquent brain area or because the focus cannot be adequately localized.[3,4] For some of these patients, stimulation therapy (also known as neuromodulation) is an alternative palliative treatment option. This chapter will review the different neuromodulation modalities that are available as adjunctive treatment of MRE. The impact of neuromodulation on sudden unexplained death in epilepsy (SUDEP) will be explored in the final section.

The stimulation therapies used for the treatment of epilepsy can be classified according to the location where the electrodes are implanted (peripheral or central nervous system) and whether the stimulation is delivered on a set schedule (open-loop) or in response (closed-loop) to an electrophysiological signal such as the electrocorticogram (ECoG). Two such modalities are approved in the USA for treating medically refractory partial-onset seizures: vagal nerve stimulation (VNS) and brain responsive neurostimulation (RNS® System, NeuroPace, Inc.). A third modality, deep brain stimulation (DBS), has been shown to be safe and effective in a pivotal trial done in the USA but is currently not approved for use by the Food and Drug Administration (FDA). VNS therapy delivers stimulation to the peripheral nervous system in both an open and/or closed loop mode. The RNS system delivers stimulation directly to the epileptogenic focus or foci on a closed-loop mode. DBS delivers open-loop stimulation to the anterior nucleus of the thalamus. Other stimulation therapies modalities are foreseen, such as noninvasive vagus nerve stimulation, transcranial magnetic stimulation, and trigeminal nerve stimulation.[5,6]

23.2 Vagus Nerve Stimulation

Historically, the first stimulation therapy that was approved by the FDA for treatment of MRE was VNS. It is indicated for use as an adjunctive therapy in patients 4 years of age or older with focal-onset seizures that are refractory to ASDs. VNS therapy was proposed for treatment of epilepsy based on the observation that, depending on the frequency of stimulation, vagal stimulation induced EEG desynchronization and decreased interictal epileptiform discharges in animal studies.[7,8] VNS also demonstrated a significant reduction of seizure frequency in animal models that are used to predict efficacy in treatment of partial- and generalized-onset seizures, such as the pentylentetrazol and maximal electroshock models.[9,10]

The mechanism of action of VNS is not known.[11] The vagal nerve arises in the medulla and carries both afferent and efferent fibers. The afferent fibers connect in the nucleus of the solitary tract, which in turn projects connections to diverse cortical and subcortical structures, including the thalamus and medial structures of the temporal lobe.[12] Blood flow studies using positron emission tomography (PET) have demonstrated acute changes in blood flow to the various brain regions, including the thalamus, temporal cortex, and cerebellum with VNS.[13,14] Increased thalamic cerebral blood flow induced by VNS has been correlated with decreased seizure activity.[15]

Outpatient VNS implantation is done under general anesthesia. An incision is made in the left neck to expose the vagus nerve and in the left chest to create a pocket for the generator implantation. The vagus nerve is exposed for about three centimeters in its position in the carotid sheath between the carotid artery and the jugular vein. A fastening lead and two electrode leads are wrapped around the vagus nerve. Strain relief loops are created in the neck and the proximal wires are secured to the surrounding soft tissues. The distal lead is tunneled from the neck to the chest incision. The generator is connected to the distal lead wire and the construct is tested to demonstrate electrical integrity of the system. The incisions are reapproximated in layers with skin tapes or glue for the final skin closure.

The efficacy of VNS was established in two randomized, double-blind, prospective studies comparing high- versus low-intensity stimulation in patients with MRE with partial-onset seizures. The primary outcome in the USA-based study was the percentage reduction in seizure frequency compared to baseline, with a mean reduction of seizures of 24.5% for patients with high-intensity and 6.15% for patients with low-intensity stimulation.[16] Similar results were obtained in an international-based multicenter, prospective randomized double-blind study (30.9% mean seizure frequency percentage reduction with high stimulation versus 11.3% reduction with low stimulation).[17]

The most common adverse events reported in the randomized and extension phases of the trials were voice alteration (50%), increased cough (41%), paresthesia (28%), pharyngitis (27%), nausea (19%), and dyspnea (18%). In a randomized double-blind controlled study performed in the USA, the overall rate of infection was 11.6% and infection leading to explantation occurred in 1.8%.[18] Serious injuries were reported in 0.9%, including infection, respiratory injuries, including sleep apnea, dyspnea, and aspiration, cardiac events, including changes in heart rhythm, changes in blood pressure, and asystole, chest and neck pain, gastrointestinal events, including dysphagia and weight loss, and depression. Data from uncontrolled, retrospective studies report that the long-term efficacy of VNS for the 50% responder rate ($\geq$50% reduction in the seizure frequency) is as high as 70% at 5 years postimplantation.[19–21]

Based on the observation that up to 70% of focal-onset seizures demonstrate an increased heart rate prior or with the ictal onset,[22] a new iteration of the VNS device that allows both open- and closed-loop stimulation has been recently approved. This device triggers stimulation after electrocardiogram-based changes as a surrogate for seizure detection.[23,24]

Though VNS is not approved by the FDA for treatment of genetic generalized epilepsies, there is some evidence to support its use in these syndromes.[25,26] Based on data from nonrandomized studies, VNS has been reported to be effective in patients with

Lennox–Gastaut syndrome (LGS). A pooled analysis of 113 patients with LGS (including data from articles with multiple seizure types where LGS data were parsed out) yielded a 55% (95% CI 46–64%) responder rate.[27,28]

VNS therapy has been shown to be cost-effective due to the reduction in seizure frequency which translates to fewer injuries, emergency-department visits, and reduction in other healthcare costs.[29,30]

23.3 Responsive Neurostimulation System

Compared to VNS, the RNS System provides closed-loop electrical stimulation to the epileptogenic focus or foci. Stimulation is delivered in response to real-time ECoG patterns of interest. The effects of electrical stimulation on the ECoG were initially described by Penfield and Jasper.[31] Acute changes reported to occur with electrical stimulation of epileptogenic regions include local disruption of synchronous activity and modulation of short-term activity distant to the site of stimulation, affecting the epileptogenic network.[32] These acute effects of cortical stimulation might be related to changes in GABA-mediated hyperpolarization, given that high-frequency stimulation at 100 Hz appears to up-regulate glutamic acid decarboxylase and down-regulate calmodulin-dependent protein kinase II inhibition.[33] Repetitive electrical stimulation of CA3 mossy fibers has been reported to increase intracellular chloride, also consistent with a GABA-mediated mechanism. Thus, electrical stimulation seems to have an acute, local inhibitory effect.[34,35]

The acute effects of stimulation can differ depending on whether high- or low-frequency stimulation is used. Low-frequency stimulation of a white matter fiber connecting the hippocampi induces long-lasting hyperpolarization that is mediated by $GABA_B$ inhibitory postsynaptic potentials and by slow after-hyperpolarization.[36] This long-lasting hyperpolarization can inhibit seizures and the spread of epileptic activity.

High-frequency stimulation ($\geq$100 Hz) produces a local axonal block of both afferent and efferent fibers that creates a functional disconnection.[37] Sustained therapeutic effects of repeated cortical stimulation might also be related to changes in synaptic plasticity, neurogenesis, and cortical reorganization.[38]

The RNS System consists of a neurostimulator, implanted depth and cortical leads, a wireless programming wand, a physician user programmer, a patient home-use remote monitor, and a secure web-accessed database that stores ECoGs and device data sent from the programmer or remote monitor. The neurostimulator is connected to up to two flexible silicone leads that each encloses four platinum/iridium electrodes at the distal end. The electrode contacts can be programmed as either anode or cathode. The neurostimulator case can also be programmed to serve as the cathode. The physician selects from depth leads to be placed in deep structures (i.e., hippocampus, depth of a sulcus) or cortical strip leads to be placed over the neocortex, or a combination of the two. The programmer communicates with the neurostimulator using a wand with a short-range wireless radiofrequency link to program detection and stimulation parameters. The patient uses a remote monitor to communicate with the neurostimulator using a wand to collect and transmit ECoGs and device data to the web-based database.

The RNS System's neurostimulator is implanted under general anesthesia into a defect created in the skull (Figure 23.1) Depth and/or cortical electrode strip leads are located according to the seizure focus or foci. Depth leads are usually implanted using stereotactic techniques. For example, in bilateral temporal lobe epilepsy, bilateral hippocampal depth

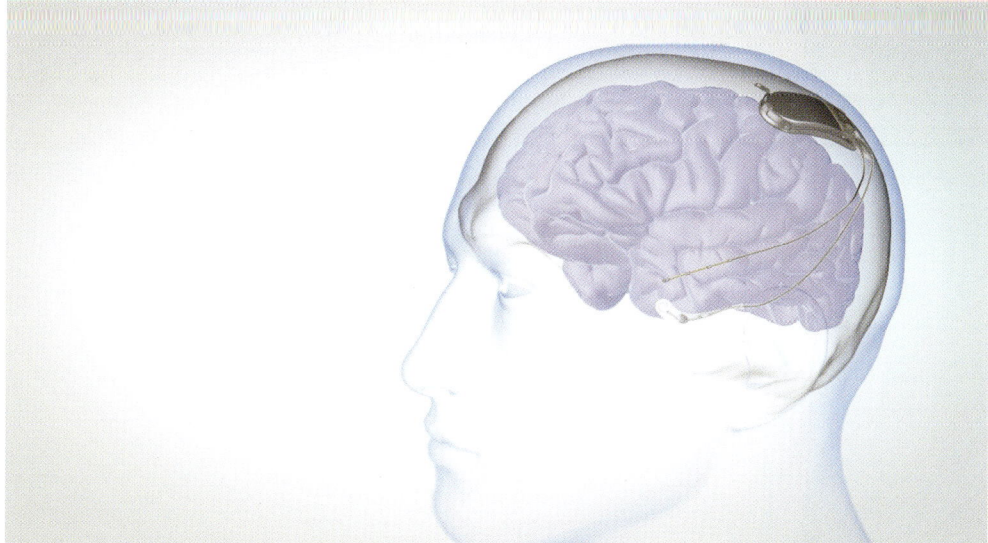

Figure 23.1 NeuroPace device and its placement in the skull. ©2017 NeuroPace, Inc. Image used with permission from NeuroPace, Inc.

Step 1: Personalized Detection

Physician determines which patterns will be detected

Figure 23.2 ECoGs capturing an ictal pattern with high-amplitude, repetitive spike activity followed by low-voltage fast activity at the LHip electrodes, with the initial detection indicated in the red square. ©2017 NeuroPace, Inc. Image used with permission from NeuroPace, Inc.

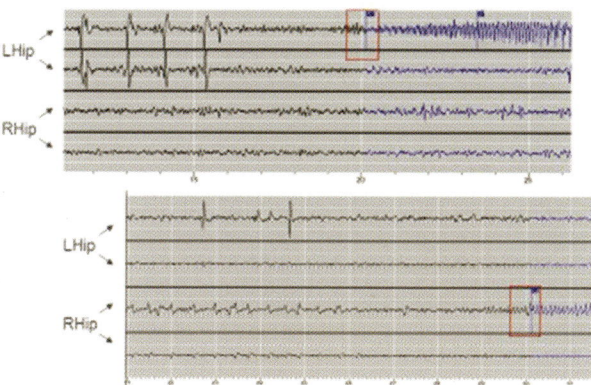

and/or strip leads are implanted. In epilepsy arising from eloquent cortex, cortical strip leads are usually placed over that region. The leads are exited from the skull and connected to the neurostimulator, which is secured into the skull defect. The skin flap is closed over the system. The patient is typically discharged on postoperative day 1.

Once implanted, the RNS System is programmed to detect patient-specific electrical patterns of interest and then continuously monitors ECoG activity through the implanted leads. Detection algorithms monitor the overall EEG signal intensity, and patient-specific electrical patterns, including dynamic changes in electrical activity and frequency, or detection of interictal discharges or activity within specific frequency bands (Figure 23.2).

Patient example: ECoGs with responsive stimulation OFF & ON

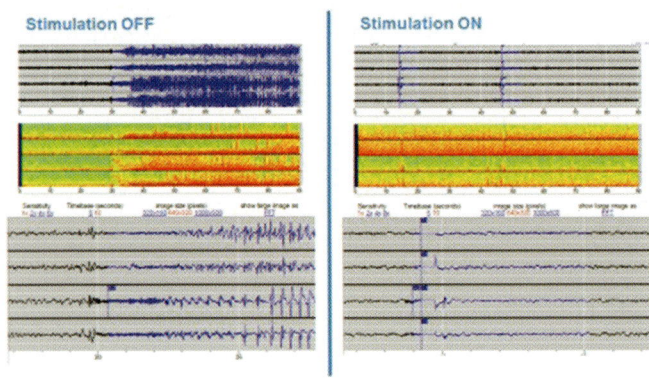

Stimulation OFF

Stimulation ON

Figure 23.3 Detection without stimulation (stimulation OFF). Stimulation is triggered by epileptiform activity with termination of the abnormal activity (stimulation ON) ©2017 NeuroPace, Inc. Image used with permission from NeuroPace, Inc.

Once the abnormal activity is detected, a current-controlled, charge-balanced biphasic electrical stimulation is delivered to the epileptogenic focus or foci (Figure 23.3).

Programmable stimulation parameters include frequency (1 Hz up to 333 Hz), current (1 mA to 12 mA), and pulse width (40 μs to 1000 μs) and duration of the stimulation. Usual parameters deliver short bursts of high-frequency stimulation of low charge density. The stimulation is subclinical and not perceived by the patient. The neurostimulator has features that ensure that charge densities remain below $<25\mu C/cm^2$, which is within the safe limits for brain tissue.[39] Stimulation can be delivered through any or all electrodes, as selected by the physician. Based on the clinical response, detection and stimulation settings are modified in an iterative manner.

A double-blind, randomized, sham-controlled, multicenter study of MRE patients established the efficacy of the RNS System in the treatment of partial-onset seizures in adults.[40] Patients with medically refractory focal-onset epilepsy were randomized to the stimulation or control group 1 month after implantation. Immediately after the implant procedure, and before randomization, there was a reduction in seizure frequency. However, the group randomized to active stimulation showed a progressive decrease in seizure frequency, whereas the group randomized to sham stimulation moved toward their pre-implant seizure frequency. Over the entire 3 months of the blinded evaluation period compared to baseline, the seizure reduction in the group treated with responsive stimula-tion (N = 97) was 37.9% compared to 17.3% in the sham stimulation group (N = 94). In the last month of the blinded evaluation period, the stimulation-treated group had a reduction in disabling seizure of 41.5% compared to a reduction of 9.4% in the sham group.

Adverse events during the first year included implant site pain (15.7%), headache (10.5%), and dysesthesias (6.3%), and were considered comparable with those seen with similar procedures, such as intracranial monitoring for seizure focus localization, and deep brain stimulation for treatment of movement disorders.[41,42]

The long-term efficacy of RNS increases over time. Long-term, prospective open-label studies found that self-reported seizures were reduced by 44% at 1 year after surgery, 53% at 2 years, and 66% at year 6.[43] The most common long-term complications reported with the RNS System over 5 years of follow-up were implant-site infection (9.0%) and

neurostimulator explantation (4.7%). The majority of infections occur shortly after the
neurostimulator initial implant or replacement; the infection risk per neurostimulator
procedure is 3.5%.[44]

Long-term studies with an average follow-up of 6.1 years report a median percentage
seizure reduction of 70% in patients with frontal or parietal seizure onsets, without
differences in the seizure reduction in patients with or without prior epilepsy surgery or
treated with VNS.[45] In addition 15% of patients experienced at least one seizure-free period
of 1 year or longer. For patients with mesial temporal lobe epilepsy, median percentage
seizure reduction was similarly 70%, with 15% of patients experiencing at least one seizure-
free period of 1 year or longer.[46]

Neuropsychological testing at 1 and 2 years of treatment has shown that the RNS system
does not have a detrimental effect on cognition. Improvements in naming, in patients with
neocortical ictal onsets, and in memory, in patients with mesial temporal lobe onsets, have
been reported.[47] These data shows significant improvements in all domains of quality of life
(QOL) and no negative effects on mood in patients with a high prevalence or pre-existing
depression.[48]

Aside from delivering responsive stimulation, the RNS System provides ECoG data in
intervals over years. Ultra-long-term ambulatory recording gives us new insights into brain
function. For example, in patients confirmed to have bilateral mesial temporal lobe seizure
onsets, the average time to record independent bilateral seizure onsets after implant was
41.6 days (median: 13 days) and over 40% required more than 3 weeks to confirm seizure
onsets in the contralateral temporal lobe. This time period cannot be easily obtained by
typical in-hospital EEG monitoring. Although the lateralization after ultra-long-term RNS
System ECoG recording confirmed the preimplant lateralization in the majority (80%) of
subjects, lateralization (unilateral versus bilateral) changed in nearly 20% of subjects.
Additionally, subjects were identified for unilateral temporal lobectomies who, prior to this
chronically recorded ECoG data, were not considered to be candidates for a surgery.[49]
Additionally, understanding the rhythmicity of interictal and ictal abnormalities might
provide insights on how to best tailor the delivery of medications and/or electrical
stimulation.[50]

23.4 Deep Brain Stimulation

DBS of the anterior nucleus of the thalamus has been shown to be effective in the treatment
of epilepsy. In a prospective, randomized, double-blind study patients with focal epilepsy
received high-frequency stimulation of the anterior nuclei of the thalamus (1 minute on,
5 minutes off) with a device similar to that used for stimulation of the subthalamic nucleus
in Parkinson's disease (Medtronic, Inc., Minneapolis, MN, USA). Patients had a 40.5%
reduction in seizure frequency compared with a 14.5% reduction in the control group.[51]

23.5 Effects of Stimulation Therapy on Reducing the Risk of Sudden Unexpected Death in Epilepsy

An important benefit of stimulation therapy is the reduction in the risk of SUDEP,
independent of whether seizure freedom is achieved. The mortality rate in patients
with epilepsy is increased three times compared to the general population.[52] One of the
most important causes of the increased mortality is SUDEP,[53] which is believed to be a

consequence of autonomic events triggered by ictal activity leading to cardiorespiratory disturbances. The incidence of SUDEP ranges from 6.3 deaths per 1000 person-years in a cohort with refractory epilepsy[54] to 9.3/1000 person-years rate in patients followed in an epilepsy surgery program.[55]

In a cohort of 1819 individuals followed 3176.3 person-years from VNS implantation, the SUDEP rate was 5.3 per 1000 over the first 2 years (CI 3.0–8.7). The rate of probable and definite SUDEP for patients treated with the RNS System is 2.0/1000 patient stimulation years (95% CI 0.7–5.2).

23.6 Conclusion

For patients with MRE who are not candidates for resective or palliative surgical therapies, stimulation therapies are viable options that have shown to be safe and effective. Peripheral stimulation with VNS and central stimulation with the RNS System or DBS are tested and accepted alternative treatment modalities for appropriately selected patients. For patients with generalized seizures in whom the foci are not localized, VNS or DBS might be the appropriate initial therapy. For patients with one or two seizure foci who are not candidates for resection or ablation, such as patients with onsets in eloquent cortex, with bilateral mesial temporal lobe onsets or with unilateral temporal onsets at risk for memory or language deficits, then the RNS System is the most appropriate initial therapy. As experience builds with the use of these modalities, it is expected that the improved ability to identify optimal candidates and outcomes will evolve with time.

References

1. Kwan P, Brodie MJ. Early identification of refractory epilepsy. *N Engl J Med.* 2000;342 (5):314–319.

2. Jobst BC, Cascino GD. Resective epilepsy surgery for drug-resistant focal epilepsy: a review. *JAMA.* 2015;313(3):285–293.

3. Engel J, Jr., Wiebe S, French J, et al. Practice parameter: temporal lobe and localized neocortical resections for epilepsy. Report of the Quality Standards Subcommittee of the American Academy of Neurology, in association with the American Epilepsy Society and the American Association of Neurological Surgeons. *Neurology.* 2003;60(4):538–547.

4. Moshe SL, Perucca E, Ryvlin P, Tomson T. Epilepsy: new advances. *Lancet.* 2015;385 (9971):884–898.

5. DeGiorgio CM, Murray D, Markovic D, Whitehurst T. Trigeminal nerve stimulation for epilepsy: long-term feasibility and efficacy. *Neurology.* 2009;72 (10):936–938.

6. Fisher RS, Velasco AL. Electrical brain stimulation for epilepsy. *Nat Rev Neurol.* 2014;10(5):261–270.

7. Chase MH, Nakamura Y, Clemente CD, Sterman MB. Afferent vagal stimulation: neurographic correlates of induced EEG synchronization and desynchronization. *Brain Res.* 1967;5(2):236–249.

8. McLachlan RS. Suppression of interictal spikes and seizures by stimulation of the vagus nerve. *Epilepsia.* 1993;34(5):918–923.

9. Woodbury DM, Woodbury JW. Effects of vagal stimulation on experimentally induced seizures in rats. *Epilepsia.* 1990;31 Suppl 2(s2):S7–19.

10. Zabara J. Inhibition of experimental seizures in canines by repetitive vagal stimulation. *Epilepsia.* 1992;33 (6):1005–1012.

11. McLachlan RS. Vagus nerve stimulation for intractable epilepsy: a review. *J Clin Neurophysiol.* 1997;14(5):358–368.

12. Rutecki P. Anatomical, physiological, and theoretical basis for the antiepileptic effect

of vagus nerve stimulation. *Epilepsia.* 1990;31 Suppl 2(s2):S1–6.

13. Ko D, Heck C, Grafton S, et al. Vagus nerve stimulation activates central nervous system structures in epileptic patients during PET H2^{15}O blood flow imaging. *Neurosurgery.* 1996;39(2):426–431.

14. Henry TR, Bakay RA, Votaw JR, et al. Brain blood flow alterations induced by therapeutic vagus nerve stimulation in partial epilepsy: I. Acute effects at high and low levels of stimulation. *Epilepsia.* 1998;39 (9):983–990.

15. Henry TR, Votaw JR, Pennell PB, et al. Acute blood flow changes and efficacy of vagus nerve stimulation in partial epilepsy. *Neurology.* 1999;52(6):1166–1173.

16. Vagus Nerve Stimulation Study Group. A randomized controlled trial of chronic vagus nerve stimulation for treatment of medically intractable seizures. *Neurology.* 1995;45(2):224–230.

17. Ben-Menachem E, Mañon-Espaillat R, Ristanovic R, et al. Vagus nerve stimulation for treatment of partial seizures: 1. A controlled study of effect on seizures. First International Vagus Nerve Stimulation Study Group. *Epilepsia.* 1994;35(3):616–626.

18. Handforth A, DeGiorgio CM, Schachter SC, et al. Vagus nerve stimulation therapy for partial-onset seizures: a randomized active-control trial. *Neurology.* 1998;51 (1):48–55.

19. Elliott RE, Morsi A, Tanweer O, et al. Efficacy of vagus nerve stimulation over time: review of 65 consecutive patients with treatment-resistant epilepsy treated with VNS > 10 years. *Epilepsy Behav.* 2011;20 (3):478–483.

20. DeGiorgio CM, Schachter SC, Handforth A, et al. Prospective long-term study of vagus nerve stimulation for the treatment of refractory seizures. *Epilepsia.* 2000;41 (9):1195–1200.

21. Kuba R, Brazdil M, Kalina M, et al. Vagus nerve stimulation: longitudinal follow-up of patients treated for 5 years. *Seizure.* 2009;18(4):269–274.

22. Eggleston KS, Olin BD, Fisher RS. Ictal tachycardia: the head-heart connection. *Seizure.* 2014;23(7):496–505.

23. Fisher RS, Afra P, Macken M, et al. Automatic vagus nerve stimulation triggered by ictal tachycardia: clinical outcomes and device performance – the U.S. E-37 Trial. *Neuromodulation.* 2016;19(2):188–195.

24. Kostov H, Larsson PG, Roste GK. Is vagus nerve stimulation a treatment option for patients with drug-resistant idiopathic generalized epilepsy? *Acta Neurol Scand Suppl.* 2007;187(s187):55–58.

25. Morris GL, 3rd, Gloss D, Buchhalter J, et al. Evidence-based guideline update: vagus nerve stimulation for the treatment of epilepsy. Report of the Guideline Development Subcommittee of the American Academy of Neurology. *Neurology.* 2013;81(16):1453–1459.

26. Shahwan A, Bailey C, Maxiner W, Harvey AS. Vagus nerve stimulation for refractory epilepsy in children: more to VNS than seizure frequency reduction. *Epilepsia.* 2009;50(5):1220–1228.

27. Zamponi N, Passamonti C, Cesaroni E, Trignani R, Rychlicki F. Effectiveness of vagal nerve stimulation (VNS) in patients with drop-attacks and different epileptic syndromes. *Seizure.* 2011;20(6):468–474.

28. Boon P, D'Have M, Van Walleghem P, et al. Direct medical costs of refractory epilepsy incurred by three different treatment modalities: a prospective assessment. *Epilepsia.* 2002;43(1):96–102.

29. Helmers SL, Duh MS, Guerin A, et al. Clinical outcomes, quality of life, and costs associated with implantation of vagus nerve stimulation therapy in pediatric patients with drug-resistant epilepsy. *Eur J Paediatr Neurol.* 2012;16(5):449–458.

30. Penfield W, Jasper H. *Epilepsy and the Functional Anatomy of the Human Brain.* Boston, MA: Little, Brown; 1954.

31. D'Arcangelo G, Panuccio G, Tancredi V, Avoli M. Repetitive low-frequency stimulation reduces epileptiform synchronization in limbic neuronal

networks. *Neurobiol Dis.* 2005;19 (1–2):119–128.

32. Liang F, Isackson PJ, Jones EG. Stimulus-dependent, reciprocal up- and downregulation of glutamic acid decarboxylase and Ca2+/calmodulin-dependent protein kinase II gene expression in rat cerebral cortex. *Exp Brain Res.* 1996;110(2):163–174.

33. Thompson SM, Gahwiler BH. Activity-dependent disinhibition. I. Repetitive stimulation reduces IPSP driving force and conductance in the hippocampus in vitro. *J Neurophysiol.* 1989;61(3):501–511.

34. Thompson SM, Gahwiler BH. Activity-dependent disinhibition. III. Desensitization and GABAB receptor-mediated presynaptic inhibition in the hippocampus in vitro. *J Neurophysiol.* 1989;61(3):524–533.

35. Toprani S, Durand DM. Long-lasting hyperpolarization underlies seizure reduction by low frequency deep brain electrical stimulation. *J Physiol.* 2013;591 (22):5765–5790.

36. Feng Z, Zheng X, Yu Y, Durand DM. Functional disconnection of axonal fibers generated by high frequency stimulation in the hippocampal CA1 region in-vivo. *Brain Res.* 2013;1509:32–42.

37. Stone SS, Teixeira CM, Devito LM, et al. Stimulation of entorhinal cortex promotes adult neurogenesis and facilitates spatial memory. *J Neurosci.* 2011;31 (38):13469–13484.

38. McCreery DB, Agnew WF, Yuen TGH, Bullara L. Charge density and charge per phase as cofactors in neural injury induced by electrical stimulation. *IEEE Trans Biomed Eng.* 1990;37(10):996–1001.

39. RNS System in Epilepsy Study Group: Morrell MJ. Responsive cortical stimulation for the treatment of medically intractable partial epilepsy. *Neurology.* 2011;77(13):1295–1304.

40. Wong CH, Birkett J, Byth K, et al. Risk factors for complications during intracranial electrode recording in presurgical evaluation of drug resistant partial epilepsy. *Acta Neurochir (Wien).* 2009;151(1):37–50.

41. Weaver FM, Follett K, Stern M, et al. Bilateral deep brain stimulation vs best medical therapy for patients with advanced Parkinson disease: a randomized controlled trial. *JAMA.* 2009;301(1):63–73.

42. Heck CN, King-Stephens D, Massey AD, et al. Two-year seizure reduction in adults with medically intractable partial onset epilepsy treated with responsive neurostimulation: final results of the RNS System Pivotal trial. *Epilepsia.* 2014;55 (3):432–441.

43. Bergey GK, Morrell MJ, Mizrahi EM, et al. Long-term treatment with responsive brain stimulation in adults with refractory partial seizures. *Neurology.* 2015;84(8):810–817.

44. Jobst BC, Kapur R, Barkley GL, et al. Brain-responsive neurostimulation in patients with medically intractable seizures arising from eloquent and other neocortical areas. *Epilepsia.* 2017;58(6):1005–1014.

45. Geller EB, Skarpaas TL, Gross RE, et al. Brain-responsive neurostimulation in patients with medically intractable mesial temporal lobe epilepsy. *Epilepsia.* 2017;58 (6):994–1004.

46. Loring DW, Kapur R, Meador KJ, Morrell MJ. Differential neuropsychological outcomes following targeted responsive neurostimulation for partial-onset epilepsy. *Epilepsia.* 2015;56(11):1836–1844.

47. RNS® System Pivotal Trial Investigators: Meador KJ, Kapur R, Loring DW, Kanner AM, Morrell MJ. Quality of life and mood in patients with medically intractable epilepsy treated with targeted responsive neurostimulation. *Epilepsy Behav.* 2015;45:242–247.

48. King-Stephens D, Mirro E, Weber PB, et al. Lateralization of mesial temporal lobe epilepsy with chronic ambulatory electrocorticography. *Epilepsia.* 2015;56 (6):959–967.

49. Spencer DC, Sun FT, Brown SN, et al. Circadian and ultradian patterns of epileptiform discharges differ by seizure-onset location during long-term

ambulatory intracranial monitoring.
Epilepsia. 2016;57(9):1495–1502.

50. Fisher R, Salanova V, Witt T, et al.
Electrical stimulation of the anterior
nucleus of thalamus for treatment of
refractory epilepsy. *Epilepsia.* 2010;51
(5):899–908.

51. Lhatoo SD, Sander JW. Cause-specific
mortality in epilepsy. *Epilepsia.* 2005;46
Suppl 11(s11):36–39.

52. Tomson T, Walczak T, Sillanpaa M, Sander
JW. Sudden unexpected death in epilepsy: a
review of incidence and risk factors.
Epilepsia. 2005;46 Suppl 11(s11):54–61.

53. Nilsson L, Ahlbom A, Farahmand M M,
Tomson T. Mortality in a population-based
cohort of epilepsy surgery patients.
Epilepsia. 2003;44(4):575–581.

54. Dasheiff RM. Sudden unexpected death in
epilepsy: a series from an epilepsy surgery
program and speculation on the
relationship to sudden cardiac death. *J Clin
Neurophysiol.* 1991;8(2):216–222.

55. Annegers JF, Coan SP, Hauser WA, et al.
Epilepsy, vagal nerve stimulation by the
NCP system, mortality, and sudden,
unexpected, unexplained death. *Epilepsia.*
1998;39(2):206–212.

Practical and Psychosocial Considerations in Epilepsy Management

Russell A. Derry

24.1 Introduction

The American Academy of Neurology has developed epilepsy quality measures[1] that should serve as a minimum standard for epilepsy care and can also serve as a template for clinical interactions with patients. This chapter will discuss how using these quality measures can enhance patient and family education, and how clinicians can influence patient outcomes beyond just seizure control.

24.2 Patient and Family Education

24.2.1 Determination of Seizure Frequency

In discussing seizure frequency, probing questions may be needed to compensate for the inherent inaccuracy of self-reporting. In a study by Hoppe et al.,[2] patients in an epilepsy monitoring unit (EMU) failed to document 32% of daytime seizures, 73% of focal seizures with impaired awareness, and over 85% of nocturnal seizures. Failure to report focal seizures with impaired awareness or nocturnal seizures is most likely a result of seizure-induced seizure unawareness. In such cases, through a combination of memory disruption and postictal confusion, patients simply do not realize that they've had a seizure, unless there was a witness or an obvious consequence (e.g., tongue lacerations, incontinence, etc.). This reason for under-reporting is particularly likely in patients who live alone or spend significant periods of time alone. Living with someone, however, does not guarantee that accuracy of seizure reporting will be substantially better. In a study by Akman et al., parents who were asked to report every seizure they witnessed while their child was in the EMU, correctly identified only 38% of recorded seizures.[3] Unless specifically asked, patients may neglect to mention seizures that they consider "mild" or "minor," such as absence, myoclonic, or focal aware seizures. Asking the patient to keep a seizure diary or use a seizure tracking app on a mobile device, may help improve the accuracy of reporting on seizure type and frequency. Until seizure detection technology becomes more affordable and accurate, clinicians will have to rely on reports from patients and caregivers. The accuracy of these reports will depend on the skill of the clinician in eliciting relevant details from the patient.

24.2.2 Offering Interventions to Reduce Seizure Frequency

In offering interventions to patients who are not seizure-free, it's important to discuss seizure patterns and triggers before simply increasing medication dosage, adding a new antiseizure drug (ASD), or discussing other treatment options. A seizure diary can help with the identification of seizure triggers and patterns. If seizures occur at a certain time of day, adjusting the dosing schedule may help. If seizures are more common at certain points in the menstrual cycle (i.e., catamenial epilepsy), a different set of interventions may be offered. In addition, identification of seizure triggers can open the door to a number of behavioral and medical interventions. For example, querying about sleep quality, quantity, and habits may reveal the possibility of a sleep disorder, unidentified nocturnal seizures, sleep-related medication side effects, or poor sleep hygiene, all of which can be addressed behaviorally or medically. Similarly, if stress is identified as a common trigger, clinicians can provide basic information on relaxation techniques or, if an anxiety disorder is suspected, make a referral to a mental health professional.

Perhaps the most common seizure trigger is missed medication. Patients may under-report problems with medication adherence in an effort to please their doctor, out of embarrassment, or simply because they don't recall missing doses. As a result, clinicians may incorrectly assume ineffectiveness of the current treatment regimen and therefore increase the dose or add another medication. Informing patients of this potential consequence can help to promote honest and accurate reporting of medication adherence. Other factors that may affect adherence include depression, memory difficulties, side effects, medication costs, and lack of belief in the value of the medication. Because these factors vary from patient to patient, there are no foolproof strategies to assess and improve adherence. Interventions should be tailored to each patient's unique pattern of nonadherence, and multiple strategies may need to be employed.[4]

24.2.3 Specifying Seizure Type and Epilepsy Syndrome or Etiology

Many patients with epilepsy cannot accurately identify their seizure types, and have limited understanding of the nature of their epilepsy (i.e., cause, localization, epilepsy syndrome, etc.). Clinicians should share the diagnosis and discuss ways to provide further diagnostic clarity. In addition, clinicians should avoid using vague or outdated terms while explaining the diagnosis.

24.2.4 Asking About Antiseizure Drug Side Effects

Perhaps one of the greatest challenges in discussing medication side effects in patients with epilepsy is that many potential side effects can also be symptoms of epilepsy itself or common comorbid conditions. Depression, cognitive dysfunction, and drowsiness are a few examples of this. In the case of drowsiness, it is certainly reasonable to consider medication side effects as a likely cause; however, nocturnal seizure activity or a comorbid sleep disorder could disrupt the sleep cycle and also result in daytime drowsiness. Therefore, in determining whether a symptom is a medication side effect, it's important to consider whether the onset of the symptom truly correlates with the initiation of the medication, or if a patient is simply noticing a pre-existing symptom as a result of being hypervigilant for possible side effects. When initiating a new medication, it may be helpful to ask about the patient's expectations about medications in general. Doing so may reveal a bias against medication that could result in a nocebo effect – a negative effect resulting from negative expectations. The goal of treatment should always be "no seizures and no side effects," but different patients may have different preferences on their way to that goal.

In addition to ongoing side effects, clinicians should address potential long-term effects of ASDs, as this is a common concern among patients and family members. Although evidence is limited, ASDs (particularly older ones) may have an impact on bone health, cardiovascular risk factors, and endocrine function.[5] Such risks and steps to reduce them should be discussed with patients, especially those who have been or are expected to be on ASDs for a long time.

24.2.5 Personalized Discussion of Epilepsy-Specific Safety Issues

Safety-related discussions in patients with epilepsy should be individualized and should take into account the risk tolerance and the goals of the patient. Too often, people with epilepsy live their lives in isolation and fear, in part due to overprotection from family members and excessive restrictions placed on them by clinicians. The purpose of such discussions is to reduce the risk of injury and mortality, both for the patient and for the public, while supporting the patient's independence and quality of life. Clinicians should familiarize themselves with their state's driving regulations, including how long a patient must be seizure-free (for operator's, chauffeur's, and commercial licenses), physician reporting requirements, and exceptions. Decisions about driving must take into account medication adherence, potential inaccuracy in the patient's seizure reporting, and the possible impact of cognitive impairments and medication side effects on driving ability. Clinicians should discuss sudden unexpected death in epilepsy (SUDEP) with every epilepsy patient, even those who are considered to be at low risk. Household safety discussion should include bathroom safety (e.g., taking showers instead of baths, using a shower chair if appropriate, checking drain function, reducing water temperature, etc.), kitchen safety (e.g., using a microwave or the back burners on an electric stove, using a food processor or buying prechopped ingredients instead of using a knife, etc.), and fall protection (e.g., avoiding or covering sharp corners, adding carpeting, avoiding glass tables, wearing a helmet if seizure-related falls are common, etc.). Workplace safety discussions should focus on accommodations rather than restrictions. Both the American Epilepsy Society and the Job Accommodation Network have resources available to help clinicians draft employment letters that do just this.

24.2.6 Screening for Psychiatric or Behavioral Health Disorders

Psychiatric disorders, including depression, anxiety disorders, and psychotic disorders, are more common in patients with epilepsy than in the general population. Depression, the most common psychiatric comorbidity in people with epilepsy, is estimated to occur in 20–50% of patients.[6] Depression, anxiety, and psychosis can be experienced ictally, interictally, or peri-ictally. Several factors contribute to the increased prevalence of these conditions, including neurobiological factors, the challenges of living with a stigmatizing chronic health condition, social isolation and activity restriction, and treatment side effects. If not identified and adequately treated, these disorders can have a major impact on medication adherence, seizure control, and quality of life. While there is no consensus regarding which conditions to screen for, what tools to use, how often to screen, or how to respond when someone screens positively, clinicians should develop and consistently follow some sort of screening protocol. Free and publicly available tools that have been validated in people with epilepsy and can be quickly administered include the PHQ-9 and the Neurological Disorders Depression Inventory for Epilepsy (NDDI-E) for depression, and the Generalized Anxiety Disorder 7-Item Scale (GAD-7) for generalized anxiety disorder.

Cognitive dysfunction (including problems with memory, attention, executive function, language, and processing speed) is common in patients with epilepsy, can be subtle, and have a significant impact on quality of life. In many cases, this impact can be greater than the impact of seizures themselves. Because self reporting of cognitive function is highly susceptible to distortion and the influence of mood and anxiety disorders, it is advisable to screen for it and solicit input from close relatives as well.[7] When clinicians identify significant cognitive dysfunction, referral to a neuropsychologist for further evaluation and intervention is recommended.

24.2.7 Counseling on Contraception and Pregnancy for Women of Childbearing Potential

The Quality Indicators for Epilepsy Treatment in adults (QUIET) study showed that only 34% of women with epilepsy received counseling on aspects of epilepsy and its treatment that are specific to women.[8] In addition to reviewing the impact of enzyme-inducing ASDs on oral contraceptives and pregnancy risks associated with epilepsy and its treatment, clinicians should broaden the discussion to include the potential impact of reproductive hormones on seizure frequency throughout the lifespan (i.e., puberty, catamenial epilepsy, pregnancy, and menopause), increased incidence of reproductive endocrine disorders such as polycystic ovarian syndrome, and increased risk for sexual dysfunction. Both Epilepsy Foundation and the American Epilepsy Society offer discussion guides that can assist clinicians in such counseling.

24.2.8 Referral of Patients with Intractable Epilepsy to a Comprehensive Epilepsy Center

Delays in obtaining appropriate epilepsy specialty care are common, but avoidable. Patients with intractable epilepsy, patients whose diagnosis is in question, women with epilepsy considering pregnancy, and patients experiencing intolerable side effects should all be referred to an epileptologist, preferably at a comprehensive epilepsy center. A survey of neurologists showed that 47% who did refer patients to a comprehensive epilepsy center reported that they did not receive sufficient clinical feedback from the center.[9] Prompt and respectful communication can go a long way toward promoting trust and appropriate referral practices.

24.3 School and Employment

The spectrum of symptoms in epilepsy is reflected in the diversity of experiences patients encounter in school, the workplace, and the community. It is often with some degree of difficulty that a majority of patients are able to thrive in school and the workplace. The laws created to protect the rights of individuals with disabilities in the school and the workplace (the Individuals with Disabilities Education Act, Section 504 of the Rehabilitation Act of 1973, and the Americans with Disabilities Act) are necessary and often effective; however, stigma, discrimination, and misconceptions often persist in spite of these laws, and a considerable amount of advocacy is still needed to succeed. Epilepsy Foundation affiliates, vocational rehabilitation agencies, county-level school districts, and a variety of advocacy organizations can provide a great resource for support.

Impaired cognitive function is one of the most common barriers to employment and school success. Assessments of cognitive function used by school psychologists and vocational rehab counselors are often fairly generic in nature, and rarely take into account the unique presentation and causation of cognitive difficulties in epilepsy. A high-quality neuropsychological evaluation with recommendations can make a world of difference in both settings.

Assisting patients and families with the development of a seizure response plan is another important role of clinicians, particularly for school-aged patients. While there are many available templates that can be used to draft a seizure response plan, the key objectives of such a plan should be to maximize safety and minimize the impact of seizures on the student's learning. Plans should be thorough and unambiguous so as to limit the need for guesswork among school staff, but they should also be concise so as to be helpful in stressful and urgent situations. Plans should also account for the possibility that a school may not have a school nurse in the building at all times. In such cases, the local Epilepsy Foundation affiliate may be able to provide hands-on rescue medication training to designated non-medical school personnel. In all cases, seizure plans should clearly delineate between when to call 911 and when to allow the student to rest and then return to school activities.

When patients suspect they are unable to work because of their epilepsy, they may decide to apply for Social Security disability benefits. Both Social Security Disability Insurance (SSDI) and Supplemental Security Income (SSI) require that an individual meet the Social Security Administration's disability criteria. The simplest way to meet the SSA's disability criteria is to meet the *Listing of Impairments*. For people with epilepsy this includes those who have at least one generalized tonic–clonic seizure per month, or at least one complex partial seizure per week, for three consecutive months, despite adherence to prescribed treatment. With less frequent seizures, individuals may still meet the *Listing of Impairments* if they also have physical, cognitive, social, or self-care challenges. Clinicians can help by making sure that seizure type and frequency, medication adherence, and, if necessary, other limitations are accurately and consistently documented in the patient's medical records. In cases where patients do not meet the *Listing of Impairments*, they may still qualify, but doing so may require a more individualized description of how the patient's disability interferes with the ability to maintain employment. Encouraging the use of an advocate or lawyer who specializes in Social Security disability benefits is generally a good idea, particularly in cases where the patient doesn't clearly meet the *Listing of Impairments* or lacks the initiative and attention to detail needed to submit an accurate and thorough application. Even when patients qualify for benefits, clinicians should consider engaging the patient and caregivers in a discussion about employment, particularly if the patient is highly motivated to work and has significant potential for improved seizure control in the near future.

24.4 Quality of Life

Numerous factors influence quality of life to varying degrees in patients with epilepsy. With this in mind, clinicians should consider more than simply seizure frequency and medication side effects when assessing the effectiveness of the care they provide. A variety of emotional, interpersonal, and environmental forces combine with neurobiology and treatment to shape each individual's experience of living with epilepsy. Emotional factors can influence quality of life both directly and indirectly. Fear can be pervasive, even among those with well-controlled seizures. When will that next seizure happen? What will other people think? Will I lose my license and my job? What if I don't wake up? These fears exert a heavy emotional burden and often limit one's activities and willingness to try new things. Effective risk communication by clinicians can help patients take appropriate precautions without allowing their lives to be dictated by fear. Closely related to fear is stress, which can affect seizure control, physical health, and emotional wellbeing. Stress is part of a vicious cycle. Seizures cause stress, which, in turn, causes further seizures. Encouraging patients to regularly practice relaxation techniques and referring to mental health professionals when necessary can help break this cycle. The unpredictability of seizures not only creates fear and stress, but it can also lead to an external locus of control followed by overdependence on others, helplessness, and apathy. Acknowledging the emotional impact of epilepsy, encouraging patience, and consistently providing options for improved seizure control (even minor improvements) can prevent these feelings from spiraling into depression.

For those patients who have been socially isolated due to the severity of their epilepsy and with comorbid conditions that affect social skills (e.g. autism, traumatic brain injury), social situations beyond the family can also be challenging. In such cases, clinicians can encourage participation in safe, facilitated social activities such as those offered by local Epilepsy Foundation affiliates, or, if necessary, refer to professionals who can provide social skills training.

Even those with less severe forms of epilepsy may struggle with trust and developing new relationships because the possibily of seizures still persists. This may be particularly true in dating. Fear of having a seizure during sexual activity can be a strong deterrent to intimacy. Anxiety regarding sex can be exacerbated by the fact that sexual dysfunction is more common in people with epilepsy, due to medication side effects, or in part due to the pathophysiology of epilepsy itself. The first step clinicians can take to alleviate these fears and address dysfunction is to simply screen about the topic. Once patients are comfortable reporting sexual concerns, clinicians can intervene by offering behavioral, psychological, and medication-related strategies to improve sexual function.

Among the many environmental factors that influence quality of life for people with epilepsy, those that impact one's ability to be self-sufficient are most notable. This includes fragmented and insufficient public transportation, a health insurance system that often leads to financial difficulties and suboptimal treatment, employment discrimination laws that are underenforced and contain too many loopholes for employers, and a lack of appropriate, supported residential options for people with epilepsy (with most being tailored to seniors or people with intellectual disabilities). People with poorly controlled seizures and comorbid disorders often fall through the holes in the public safety net and continue to struggle with independence and community integration. Social workers and similar professionals, both within and outside of the health system, are essential to providing the long-term follow-up and advocacy that's often required to piece together resources from a system that is ill-equipped to support people with epilepsy.

24.5 Prognosis and Counseling

Prognosis is a fluid concept that evolves as the many factors that influence it change. Therefore, prognosis should be part of an ongoing conversation with patients over the course of their epilepsy. Clinicians must strike a balance between painting a realistic picture of potential challenges on the horizon and promoting hope and optimism.

Perhaps the most common questions patients and families want answered upon receiving a diagnosis of epilepsy involve the extent to which seizures and epilepsy will persist. At initial diagnosis, clinicians can, at a minimum, share general statistics on seizure control in patients with epilepsy. More tailored information on the likelihood of seizure freedom and resolution of epilepsy may be provided if a specific epilepsy syndrome has been identified. For example, 83% of patients with juvenile myoclonic epilepsy will need lifelong treatment,[10] but over 90% will achieve seizure freedom with that treatment.[11] For many severe forms of epilepsy, like Dravet syndrome and Lennox–Gastaut syndrome, both seizure freedom and resolution are unlikely. In contrast, almost all children who have benign epilepsy with centro-temporal spikes achieve resolution, with seizures ending by age 15, regardless of treatment. For other syndromes and unclassified epilepsies, there may be considerable variation from patient to patient in terms of prognosis, and clinicians need to rely on other factors to predict future outcomes. In addition, the often-cited study by Kwan and Brodie[12] serves as an important guide for both prognosis and treatment. The study showed that 47% of patients achieved seizure control with the first drug tried, 13% achieved seizure control through monotherapy with the second drug tried, and only 4% achieved seizure control through monotherapy with a third drug or through subsequent polytherapy. Reviewing this study with patients at initial diagnosis can help to prepare them for the possibility that surgery, neurostimulation, or a ketogenic diet may be needed if two medications have failed to control seizures.

Prognosis should provide additional information beyond simply the likelihood of seizure freedom and resolution of epilepsy. In cases where epilepsy is likely to be progressive in nature or shorten the lifespan, the patient and family should be informed of the suspected mechanisms behind this, the projected timeline, and what can be done to slow or halt this progression.

There is an art to relaying discouraging news at an appropriate time, in a sensitive manner, and with a realistic amount of hope. Difficult conversations are made easier when both the patient and the clinician are prepared. Preparation prevents patients and families from being blindsided by information that is in stark contrast with their expectations. Clinicians also need to provide sufficient time to digest the information and ask questions. After asking if the patient and family are ready, closing the conversation with a discussion of next steps may help to eventually guide them to a more positive and productive place; however, it's important to acknowledge that receiving a diagnosis of epilepsy and a disappointing prognosis often involves a grieving process. It is normal for patients who develop epilepsy as teens or adults to mourn the actual, perceived, or anticipated loss of independence, control, security, activities, and abilities. Parents may mourn the loss of the dreams that they may have had for their child. Clinicians should allow time for this grieving process, but they should also be sure to provide evidence to refute distorted or exaggerated beliefs. They can also reframe perceived permanent losses as temporary challenges that they will work with the patient to overcome.

References

1. Fountain NB, Van Ness PC, Bennett A, et al. Quality improvement in neurology: Epilepsy Update Quality Measurement Set. *Neurology.* 2015;84(14):1483–1487.

2. Hoppe C, Poepel A, Elger CE. Epilepsy: accuracy of patient seizure counts. *Arch Neurol.* 2007;64(11):1595–1599.

3. Akman CI, Montenegro MA, Jacob S, et al. Seizure frequency in children with epilepsy: factors influencing accuracy and parental awareness. *Seizure.* 2009;18 (7):524–529.

4. Brodtkorb E, Samsonsen C, Sund JK, et al. Treatment non-adherence in pseudo-refractory epilepsy. *Epilepsy Res.* 2016;122:1–6.

5. Novy, J. Long term somatic adverse events of antiepileptic drugs. *Epileptologie.* 2015;32:65–69.

6. Kanner AM, Palac S. Depression in epilepsy: a common but often unrecognized comorbid malady. *Epilepsy Behav.* 2000;1(1):37–51.

7. Karkoska A, Hallmeyer-Elgner S, Berth H, Reichmann H, Schmitz-Peiffer H. Improving the assessment of everyday cognitive functioning in patients with epilepsy by means of proxy reports. *Epilepsy Behav.* 2015;44:55–58.

8. Pugh MJ, Berlowitz DR, Rao JK, et al. The quality of care for adults with epilepsy: an initial glimpse using the QUIET measure. *BMC Health Serv Res.* 2011;11:1.

9. Hakimi AS, Spanaki MV, Schuh LA, Smith BJ, Schultz L. A survey of neurologists' views on epilepsy surgery and medically retractory epilepsy. *Epilepsy Behav.* 2008;13(1):96–101.

10. Baykan B, Martínez-Juárez IE, Altindag EA, Camfield CS, Camfield PR. Lifetime prognosis of juvenile myoclonic epilepsy. *Epilepsy Behav.* 2013;28(Suppl 1):S18–24.

11. Chowdhury A, Brodie MJ. Pharmacological outcomes in juvenile myoclonic epilepsy: support for sodium valproate. *Epilepsy Res.* 2016;119:62–66.

12. Kwan P, Brodie MJ. Early identification of refractory epilepsy. *N Engl J Med.* 2000;342(5):314–319.

Comorbidities with Epilepsy

Ramon Edmundo D. Bautista, Shannon M. LaBoy,
Imran Farooqui, and Samuel S. Giles

25.1 Introduction

In this chapter, we present some of the common comorbidities frequently encountered in persons with epilepsy (PWE). We begin by examining the cognitive and behavioral issues, then focus on sleep disorders, headaches, and bone health, and end by discussing the topic of sudden unexpected death in epilepsy (SUDEP). We hope that this chapter will assist physicians in providing better care to PWE.

25.2 Cognitive and Behavioral Issues

25.2.1 Cognitive Issues

There are multiple factors determining the cognitive abilities of PWE. These include the type of epilepsy, level of seizure control, presence and location of a structural lesion, and the presence of interictal epileptiform discharges (IEDs).[1–11] Individuals, particularly those with symptomatic (structural-metabolic) generalized epilepsies, such with as Lennox–Gastaut syndrome, often have severe cognitive dysfunction, frequently referred to as epileptic encephalopathy. The type of epilepsy often affects the individual's baseline levels of cognition, such as IQ, as well as knowledge accumulation over time.[1,3] During a study evaluating the effect of the various facets of epilepsy on cognition, individuals with focal epilepsies performed worse on educational achievement tests in arithmetic and reading when compared to those with generalized epilepsies. Reading skills were profoundly delayed in focal epilepsy patients and only mildly affected in those with idiopathic generalized epilepsy.[1] When full-scale IQ was examined in children, the control group had a mean IQ of 112.3. The IQ of those with idiopathic generalized epilepsy was lower at 101.9, but children with temporal lobe epilepsy had an even lower IQ at 96.5.[8] These changes to cognition occur even before the onset of epilepsy, as enrollment in special education is high in a significant percentage of children even prior to their first seizure.[4] While the age of epilepsy onset by itself has not been found to significantly impact cognition levels per se, when paired with pharmacoresistance, younger age of seizure onset correlates with worse cognitive performance.[2] Poor seizure control appears to be particularly harmful to the developing brain, as shown in a study by Bjornaes and colleagues who compared serial IQ testing in children and adults with refractory epilepsy that showed children with refractory epilepsy with progressive declines in IQ on serial testing, whereas adults with refractory epilepsy showed no such decline.[5]

Mesial temporal lobe sclerosis, a causative lesion in mesial temporal lobe epilepsy, is associated with remote memory impairment. Furthermore, among temporal lobe epilepsy patients, those with high seizure frequency have poorer anterograde memory testing compared to low seizure frequency patients.[11] In addition to seizures affecting mentation, IEDs have been shown to affect cognition. Patients with frequent IEDs have impaired attention and speed of information processing.[1] Highly frequent IEDs, when comprising at least 10% of an awake electroencephalogram (EEG), is associated with slowing of central information processing speed, impaired short-term verbal memory, and impaired visual motor integration.[6] During a follow-up study, central information processing speed improved with control of IEDs and worsened during increased frequency of discharges.[7] IEDs in the nondominant hemisphere is associated with impaired visuospatial function and recall.[6] In patients with genetic generalized epilepsies, increased IEDs during sleep was associated with poor IQ performance, while long-term memory dysfunction was seen more often in patients whose IEDs occurred in wakefulness.[9]

Cognitive difficulties can be particularly severe in some childhood epilepsy syndromes. In a Canadian study examining childhood-onset symptomatic generalized epilepsy, 88% of those affected showed some degree of psychomotor retardation.[12] A population-based study in South Carolina showed significantly higher rates of autism spectrum disorder among PWE less than 18 years old (4.3%) compared to less than 0.1% of controls. Attention deficit hyperactivity disorder was found in 12.8% in PWE who were less than 18 years old.[13] A study from the Netherlands showed that PWE have a lower IQ when compared to age-matched controls, and this defect was especially encountered among patients with symptomatic localization-related epilepsy.[1] A community-based prospective incident cohort study evaluated the IQ levels among PWE and found that only 73.6% were within normal limits.[3]

Beyond snapshot evaluations of cognitive capability, studies have demonstrated progressive cognitive decline over time that correlates with the degree of seizure control and seizure type. Severe intractable epilepsy patients consistently have progressively worsening performance on serial neuropsychological testing. Patients with increasing frequency of seizures also demonstrate progressive cognitive decline. Patients with generalized tonic–clonic seizures show deficits in verbal IQ, performance IQ, verbal learning, delayed verbal recall, naming, and semantic fluency. Those with focal seizures with impaired awareness showed problems with memory but no difference in intellect. A history of status epilepticus is also associated with declines in both verbal learning and recall. Fortunately, achieving a state of seizure remission, despite years of intractability in some situations, results in an improvement in cognition.[10]

25.2.2 Psychiatric Issues

Even as epilepsy affects cognition, there are also profound effects on the mind as it relates to psychiatric comorbidities. PWE have increased rates of depression, anxiety, psychosis, substance abuse, and attention deficits. A population study in Sweden examined the occurrence of psychiatric comorbidities among epilepsy patients. Psychiatric diagnoses were encountered more frequently among PWE (40.7%) compared to individuals without epilepsy (10.3%), and substance use was seen in 11.5% in epilepsy patients compared to 2.9% of those without epilepsy. About 18% of PWE already had pre-existing psychiatric disorders, while 6.8% displayed substance abuse behavior even before their first seizure. In contrast, among individuals without epilepsy, 3.5% had a diagnosed psychiatric condition and 1% had a substance abuse disorder.[14] The impact of epilepsy on mood disorders varies based on the type of epilepsy. Rates of depression were higher in children and adolescents with temporal lobe epilepsy compared to frontal lobe epilepsy.[15]

Because depression and anxiety are common in various chronic illnesses, a population-based study in South Carolina by Sellasie and colleagues compared the psychiatric comorbidities of epilepsy patients, chronic migraine patients, and otherwise healthy controls who were treated for a lower extremity fracture. The study revealed a significantly higher rate of psychiatric comorbidities among PWE. The rates of depression was highest among PWE (32.3%) compared to both the control group (15.3%) and migraine patients (28.5%). Anxiety disorders were also more frequently encountered among PWE at 20.1%, compared to 13.3% of healthy controls. Schizophrenia was significantly more prevalent at 5.6% among PWE, compared to 1.2% of individuals with migraine and 1.3% of healthy controls. Substance abuse was elevated in a similar trend.[13]

Suicidal ideation as well as suicidal attempts are more common in chronic epilepsy patients compared to the general population, and increases further in PWE with comorbid depression. In a multicenter study, the current rate of suicidal ideation among PWE was 12.2%, and the lifetime prevalence of suicide attempts was 20.8%. In contrast, the suicide rate in the general population was around 1.2%.[16] In a population study from Sweden, the estimated odds for suicide among PWE who had comorbid depression was 23 times higher when compared to nondepressed population controls.[14] The increased risk for suicide attempt is already present prior to developing epilepsy and occurs despite the absence of a formal psychiatric diagnosis.[17]

It is important for providers to address symptoms of depression and anxiety in epilepsy patients and to treat it appropriately. Due to the historical FDA warning against the use of many psychopharmacological agents in patients with epilepsy, a study was performed evaluating clinical trial data to determine the actual risk to seizure threshold in medications indicated for depression, psychosis, and obsessive-compulsive disorder. Depression itself seems to lower the seizure threshold. Medications such as bupropion should be avoided in PWE as there is a significantly increased risk of seizures. However, other antidepressants (citalopram, fluoxetine, venlafaxine, paroxetine, nefazodone, mirtazapine, escitalopram, duloxetine, and sertraline) are generally well-tolerated by PWE and should be considered for depression treatment in patients with epilepsy. When treating psychosis, practitioners should avoid clozapine, olanzapine, and quetiapine as they have shown an increase in seizure incidence. Ziprasidone, aripiprazole, and risperidone did not affect seizure frequency and should be considered when necessary for treatment in epilepsy patients. When treating PWE who have obsessive-compulsive disorder, practitioners should avoid clomipramine, as it has shown an increase in seizure frequency when compared to placebo.[18]

Patients with epilepsy should be frequently screened for comorbid psychiatric conditions and treated appropriately with medications, education, and alternative therapies, in order to improve their quality of life, well-being, and degree of seizure control.

25.3 Sleep and Epilepsy

For over a century, the association between sleep and epilepsy has been well established. In 1885, William Gowers, studying 850 institutionalized patients, observed that 42%

had seizures occurring only from wakefulness, 21% solely from sleep, while the rest had seizures during both wakefulness and sleep.[19] In 1929, John Langdon Down and William Russell Brain showed that in patients with convulsions, seizures tend to occur in two waves, the first occurring approximately 2 hours following sleep onset and the second taking place between 4 and 5 o'clock in the morning. They also noted that the majority of daytime seizures occurred within the first hour upon awakening.[20] The advent of the EEG in 1929 allowed researchers to further analyze this relationship. Gibbs identified patterns of IEDs during both wake and asleep states.[21] Other investigators have shown that IEDs occur more frequently during stages 1–2 of non-rapid eye movement (NREM) sleep and less frequently during rapid eye movement (REM) sleep.[22,23]

Various theories have been postulated to explain the relation between seizures and sleep. According to Terzano and colleagues, each stage of NREM sleep can be divided into periods of transient fluctuations of arousal referred to as cyclic alternating patterns (CAP). CAP consists of two phases. The first (CAP-A) contains paroxysmal phasic activity and represents a state of increased arousal. The second phase (CAP-B) represents a return to background EEG activity and decreased arousal. These phases alternate during CAP, which then alternates with non-CAP sleep. By calculating the percentage of CAP from the total sleep time, a CAP rate can be established that provides a measure of elevated arousal during sleep.[24] Gigli and colleagues later showed that, when compared to individuals without epilepsy, patients with both primary generalized and focal epilepsy had an increased amount of CAP.[25] In a later study, Terzano and colleagues identified a significant relation between CAP-A phase NREM sleep and the presence of IEDs. Their study showed that during sleep, focal motor seizures arose solely during CAP-A stages.[26]

In both human and animal models, there is an inverse relation between the presence of seizures and sleep quality. In 1962, Janz showed that patients with awakening epilepsy often had difficulty falling asleep, increased NREM stages 1 and 2, and a decrease in stage 3–4. He also noted that patients with nocturnal seizures had increased stages 3–4 NREM sleep.[27] Cohen and Dement electrically induced generalized seizures in cats causing a suppression of REM sleep.[28] Raol and Meti showed that after stimulating amygdala-kindled rats, resulting in seizures, the animals had a decrease in REM duration during sleep, an effect which persisted for 28 days (despite no additional seizures).[29] Other authors have shown that among amygdala- and hippocampal-kindled cats, even a single seizure results in a decrease in the amount of REM sleep.[30,31]

Obtaining sleep recording has now become a routine part of EEG analysis and provides additional findings in patients who have otherwise normal awake-only studies. In 1947, Gibbs showed that 19% of patients had IEDs when an awake EEG was obtained, but this number increased to 63% in patients who fell asleep.[21] Across various studies, the ability of sleep EEGs to detect IEDs ranges from 26.7–63.8%.[32–34] The use of sleep deprivation (3–4 hours sleep maximum) or sleep induction via chloral hydrate to induce NREM activity increases the occurrence of IEDs.

As the relationship between sleep and epilepsy has become well established, it is no surprise then that good sleep hygiene plays a vital role in helping PWE maintain good seizure control. Many epilepsy specialists advise their patients to limit the use of alcohol and caffeine and to avoid sleep deprivation as these can decrease the amount of REM sleep.[35,36]

Effective management of obstructive sleep apnea (OSA) has been shown to significantly improve seizure control. Several authors have showed that PWE with OSA treated with continuous positive airway pressure, protriptyline, and tracheostomy had an improvement in both seizure control and daytime alertness.[37,38] Wyler and Weymuller showed that PWE who received surgical intervention for coexisting OSA had a decrease in the amount of seizure activity.[39]

Ehrenberg studied PWE with periodic leg movements/restless leg syndrome treated with gabapentin and showed that 50% of patients who had decreased leg movements also had an improvement in seizure control, while only 1 of 17 patients who did not have an improvement in leg movement had improved seizure control.[40]

In addition to their therapeutic effects on seizures, antiseizure drugs (ASDs) have also been shown to play a positive role in improving sleep quality.[41,42] ASDs appear to improve the sleep quality of PWE with daytime seizures and decrease the deeper stages of NREM among patients with nocturnal seizures.[43] However, only limited data exists on this topic and further research is needed to better elucidate these findings.

25.4 Headaches

Headache is a well-established comorbidity in epilepsy. The incidence of migraines in the general population is around 12%.[44] However, the incidence of migraines is two to three times higher among PWE compared to the general population.[45] Likewise, seizures are approximately three times more commonly seen in pediatric patients with migraines compared to the general pediatric population.[46] A study by Ottman and Lipton indicates that nearly a quarter of PWE report having migraines. In fact, more than 80% of PWE report having headaches.[47] Children with benign epilepsy with centro-temporal spikes and those with juvenile myoclonic epilepsy more frequently complain of headaches.[48] Cai and colleagues found that over 40% of PWE patients reported having peri-ictal headaches.[49] It is well established that both migraine patients and PWE share common triggers including sleep deprivation, hormone fluctuations (particularly in females), visual stimulation/light fluctuations, and alcohol use.[35,36]

The proposed underlying pathophysiology is thought to be due to a complex relationship between ion channel dysfunction, glutamate activity, and mitochondrial dysfunction. In migraines, positive symptoms (cortical hyperexcitability) can be followed by negative ones (cortical spreading depression). These occur independently of synaptic transmission and are linked to N-methyl-D-aspartate (NMDA) glutamate receptor activity. On the other hand, the occurrence of seizures is dependent on the rate of synaptic transmission via glutamate activity on alpha-amino-3-hydroxyl-5-methyl-4-isoxazole-propionate (AMPA) receptors.[50] While these processes appear to occur independently of one another, the presence of channel dysfunction involving Na/K ATPase has been proposed as a common link and may explain in part the usefulness of ASDs for both conditions.[51] Another proposed hypothesis relates to mitochondrial dysfunction. Though not well understood, the occurrence of both migraines and epilepsy in patients with mitochondrial disease suggests a common pathophysiologic process.[52]

Often the ability to successfully control both migraines and seizures in a single individual depends on the ability to manage both conditions. Therefore, it is important to screen PWE for accompanying headaches. Fortunately, certain ASDs, such as topiramate or valproate can be utilized in both conditions, thus reducing the risk of complications associated with polypharmacy.

25.5 Bone Health

Over the past decades, it has become apparent that there is an increased incidence of bone fractures among PWE.[53] A study by Vestergaard showed that PWE had twice the risk of fractures compared to the general population. Though initially thought to be due to primary bone diseases unrelated to epilepsy, such as rickets, osteomalacia, or age-related osteoporosis, or to falls associated with seizures, it has become apparent that these situations do not entirely explain the increased risk of fractures among PWE.[54]

The proposed mechanism for bony fractures among PWE is increased bone fragility, primarily linked to vitamin D metabolism and its role in calcium homeostasis. ASDs that are cytochrome p450 inducers increase vitamin D metabolism. However, ASDs that are not strong cytochrome p450 inducers have also been shown to decrease levels of available vitamin D, although the reasons for this are less understood.[55]

Bone deterioration can be seen in both children and adults.[56–58] Genetic and developmental risk factors for bone deterioration include age, impairment of bone accrual in children, duration of ASD therapy, postmenopausal hormone depletion, and polypharmacy. In addition, immobility, thyroid and liver disease, alcohol dependence, and tobacco also increase the risks of bony fractures.[59–62]

Women, especially those who are menopausal, are especially vulnerable. A study by Ensrud and colleagues showed that despite the use of replacement estrogen in postmenopausal women, ASD usage resulted in lower bone mineral density and increased risk of fracture.[56]

The use of ASDs in the pediatric population is especially problematic given that peak bone mass and growth development occur during this time. Studies have shown that the long-term use of valproate and lamotrigine in children is associated with shorter stature.[63,64] A study by Chou and colleagues examined the effect of carbamazepine on bone development of children age 5-18 years and showed significantly reduced bone density.[65] In a recent study by Albaghadadi and colleagues, 50 young PWE who were taking valproate were compared to healthy age- and sex-matched individuals and assessed for bone health using a variety of parameters (dual-energy X-ray absorptiometry (DEXA) scanning, serum 25-hydroxyvitamin D, parathyroid hormone, calcium, phosphate, and alkaline phosphatase). Their study showed that patients taking valproate had significantly lower bone mineral densities.[66]

Due to the increased risk of bony fracture among PWE, bone health assessment should be a standard part of epilepsy care. In adults, screening should begin immediately following the onset of ASD use by obtaining a bone densitometry T-score (goals between –1.0 and –2.5). In order to reduce radiation exposure in the pediatric population, the use of the Fracture Risk Assessment Tool (FRAX) may serve as a screening tool.[67] When assessing for 25-hydroxyvitamin D deficiency, it is essential to first rule out liver and renal disease, calcium metabolism disorders, thyroid disease, cancer, or exogenous hormones (parathyroid hormone, estradiol, testosterone). Adults with serum 25-hydroxyvitamin D levels of less than 80 nmol/l should receive vitamin D supplementation of 2000 IU/day. In addition, these patients will need a calcium intake of 600–1000 mg/day.[67,68]

25.6 Sudden Unexpected Death in Epilepsy

It has long been recognized that PWE have a shorter life expectancy compared to the general population.[69] At times, death among PWE can occur without an obvious inciting event. The term SUDEP was coined to define those circumstances by which death at times occurs in epilepsy without any obvious cause.[70] SUDEP is one of the leading neurological causes of death in the United States, second only to stroke.[71] In 1997, Nashef later formally defined SUDEP as "the sudden, unexpected, witnessed or unwitnessed, non-traumatic and non-drowning death in patients with epilepsy, with or without evidence of a seizure, and excluding documented status epilepticus, in which post-mortem examination does not reveal a toxicological or anatomic cause for death."[72]

More recently, the term SUDEP has evolved into a classification scheme. Definite SUDEP plus is defined as "death satisfying the criteria for SUDEP, if a concomitant condition other than epilepsy is identified before or after death, if the death might have been due to the combined effect of both conditions, and if autopsy or direct observations or recording of the terminal event did not prove the concomitant condition to be the cause of death." Probable SUDEP is also characterized by the previous definition but without autopsy findings. Possible SUDEP occurs when "a competing cause of death is present." Near SUDEP occurs when "a patient with epilepsy survives resuscitation for more than an hour after cardiorespiratory arrest and no structural cause is identified after investigation." Not SUDEP occurs when a clear alternative of death is identified.[73]

SUDEP is encountered more frequently among males and occurs more often at night. There is a decreased prevalence among children and the condition occurs more frequently in young adults aged 20–45 years. In fact, SUDEP is 27 times more likely to occur in this age group compared to a control population.[74] There are other associated risk factors for the development of SUDEP. These include having poorly controlled primary or secondary generalized tonic–clinic seizures, seizure onset before 16 years of age, disease duration of greater than 15 years, and an increased frequency of seizures.[75,76] Additional risk factors include sleeping in a prone position and noncompliance with treatment, as well as developmental delay.[77,78]

The pathophysiology of SUDEP remains poorly understood and research is ongoing to identify an etiology. There are several theories to explain its underlying mechanism. These are broadly classified as genetic, cardiac, respiratory, and central. Genetic causes have been postulated to result in treatment-resistant epilepsies for which afflicted individuals have an increased risk of SUDEP. Potential genes that have been identified include *SCN1a*, *SCN2a*, *SCN8a*, *TSC1*, *TSC2*, and *CSTB*.[79] Other genetic disorders thought to be implicated include Dup15q syndrome and 5q14.3 deletion.[80] Defects in sodium channel subunit (SCN) genes are associated with Dravet syndrome, a syndrome of febrile seizures occurring within first year of life in otherwise normal infants who develop subsequent developmental delay, coordination issues, and refractory epilepsy.[79,81] Cathpsin B is a protein that encodes stefin (type 1 cystatin) that inhibits intracellular thiol protease. This is associated with Unverricht–Lungborg syndrome, a genetic epilepsy characterized by progressive myoclonic seizures that can progress into tonic–clonic seizures and lower life expectancy.[82] Tuberous sclerosis complex is divided into Type 1 (hamartin) and 2 (tuberin). TSC2 is thought to down-regulate the mTORC1 pathway, leading to diffuse sclerosis of brain parenchyma with resultant increased seizure frequency. All these genes have been shown to be expressed in the brain, heart, and lungs.[83] Dup15q11 is an epileptic encephalopathy associated with extra copies of *UBE3A* and *GABRB3* that causes increased seizure frequency and neurological impairment. The 5q14.3 deletion results in various severities of epilepsy with neurological disability and is associated with a dysfunction of *myocyte-specific enhancer factor 2C (MEF2C)* and *ephrin-A5 precursor (EFNA5)* genes. Both of these genetic disorders are also expressed in the brain, heart, and lungs.[79,80]

An underlying cardiac etiology for SUDEP has also been proposed. A study by Chyou and colleagues compared electrocardiogram findings among cases of SUDEP and epilepsy control patients over a span of 10 years and found abnormal ventricular conduction patterns in the SUDEP subset.[84] Arrhythmias have been shown to occur during seizures that range from benign sinus tachycardia and bradycardia, to more fatal arrhythmias such as asystole, bundle branch block, ST depression or elevation, T wave inversion, and prolongation or shortening of the QT interval.[85,86] It is postulated that these arrhythmias may be due to defects of cardiac genes such as *KCNQ1*, *KCNH2*, *SCN5A*, *NOS1AP*, *RYR2*, and *HCN4*. Most of these genes have been found in cases of SUDEP, except for *KCNQ1* and *KCNH2*. Overall, it has been difficult to prove that these genes are the exclusive causes of SUDEP due to their concomitant expression in the brain and lungs.[83,87]

Respiratory causes have also been postulated as a potential etiology for SUDEP. Using animal studies, Hajek and Buchanan identified changes in measures of respiration during certain sleep states and postulated that this dysfunction could be used as a biomarker for SUDEP.[88] They applied maximal electroshock-induced seizures to mice with underlying respiratory dysfunction. Mice who had seizures during REM sleep had 100% mortality. Buchanan and colleagues showed that animals who died after seizures during sleep demonstrated respiratory rate variability during sleep.[89] Data from the Mortality in Epilepsy Monitoring Unit Study (MORTEMUS) indicated that SUDEP occurred after a sequence of events that began with a generalized tonic–clonic seizure and postictal generalized EEG suppression resulting in decreased cardiopulmonary function, apnea and hypoventilation, and ultimately asystole.[90] It remains unclear if the underlying respiratory dysfunction is the sole cause of SUDEP as cardiac and respiratory processes typically work in tandem with one other.

SUDEP has also been thought to have an underlying central nervous system etiology. It has been postulated that the underlying mechanism of SUDEP may be related to depressed brainstem function during the ictal and postictal periods. Lower brainstem systems driven by serotonin are thought to play a role in cardiorespiratory changes during and after seizures. In contrast, upper brainstem systems are involved with regulation of arousal. In established rat seizure models, multiunit and single-unit recordings from the medullary raphe nuclei and midbrain dorsal raphe nuclei demonstrated decreased firing rates during ictal and postictal periods.[91] Zhan and colleagues have demonstrated that seizures may be associated with decreased serotonin firing in the lower brainstem, resulting in depressed breathing, and this feature has been shown to correlate with SUDEP. Other brainstem neurotransmitters have also been implicated in SUDEP. Along with serotonin, norepinephrine, acetylcholine, and glutamate are also involved in the ascending and descending projections of brainstem function that regulate arousal, modulate respiratory output, and carbon dioxide chemoreception.[92] Adenosine's role has also been of interest due to its down-regulatory effect on centrally controlled cardiorespiratory drive. Adenosine antagonists such as caffeine have been thought to inhibit this down-regulation, and are targets of interest, but currently do not yet have clinical relevance and require further research.[93]

Other researches have focused on the pathological changes associated with SUDEP. Cardiac and pulmonary abnormalities are commonly seen in cases of SUDEP on postmortem exam. P-Codrea Tigaran and colleagues performed histopathologic examination on 52 cases of SUDEP: 11 cases (21%) showed mild to moderate myocyte hypertrophy while 22 (42%) showed varying extent of focal myocardial fibrosis. All of these cases displayed moderate to severe pulmonary congestion and edema.[94]

Mild brain swelling has also been shown to occur in about 28% of SUDEP cases. In 55% of cases of SUDEP, acute hypoxic eosinophilic changes involving the CA1 region have been demonstrated, but similar changes have been shown to occur diffusely in the cortical and subcortical regions as well. These neuronal changes were more frequently seen when seizures occurred within 24 hours of death, when the body was in a prone position, the external airway was obstructed, or if brain swelling was present. However, at this time, no specific lesion types or locations have been associated with an increased risk of SUDEP.[95]

To date, there is no specific treatment for SUDEP. While the optimization of ASD therapy and ensuring patient's treatment adherence is of utmost importance, it does not necessarily prevent the occurrence of SUDEP.[75] However, it has been shown that patients with refractory seizures who optimize their medical therapy decrease their overall risk of SUDEP.[90] Safety checklists to help prevent SUDEP have been developed for smart-phone applications and are increasing in popularity.[69] In hospital settings, the MORTEMUS study demonstrated that prompt resuscitation prevents the occurrence of SUDEP.[90,96] Therefore at this time, the mainstay of SUDEP prevention is focused on optimizing treatment, as well as patient and family counseling and education. It is also important that healthcare providers are adequately educated on the topic. Among the apprehensions healthcare providers have in discussing SUDEP are the fear of causing anxiety among patients and the perceived inability to improve overall outcomes.[97,98] Despite this hesitation, it has been shown that more than 90% of patients want to be educated about the topic. Indeed, the role of patient and family education, with an emphasis on treatment adherence and lifestyle modification may go a long way in decreasing the occurrence of SUDEP.[79]

25.7 Conclusion

In this chapter we have discussed some of the common comorbidities seen among PWE. In addition to being well-versed with seizure management, physicians treating PWE should be comfortable in dealing with the multiple comorbidities that accompany this condition. Only by doing so are they able to optimize the care they provide PWE, improve seizure control, and improve their patient's quality of life.

References

1. Aldenkamp A, Arends J. The relative influence of epileptic EEG discharges, short nonconvulsive seizures, and type of epilepsy on cognitive function. *Epilepsia.* 2004;45(1):54–63.

2. Berg AT, Zelko FA, Levy SR, Testa FM. Age at onset of epilepsy, pharmacoresistance, and cognitive outcomes: a prospective cohort study. *Neurology.* 2012;79 (13):1384–1391.

3. Berg AT, Langfitt JT, Testa FM, et al. Global cognitive function in children with epilepsy: a community-based study. *Epilepsia.* 2008;49(4):608–614.

4. Berg AT, Smith SN, Frobish D, et al. Special education needs of children with newly diagnosed epilepsy. *Dev Med Child Neurol.* 2005;47(11):749–753.

5. Bjornaes H, Stabell K, Henriksen O, Loyning Y. The effects of refractory epilepsy on intellectual functioning in children and adults: a longitudinal study. *Seizure.* 2001;10(4):250–259.

6. Ebus S, Arends J, Hendriksen J, et al. Cognitive effects of interictal epileptiform discharges in children. *Eur J Paediatr Neurol.* 2012;16(6):697–706.

7. Ebus SC, DM IJ, den Boer JT, et al. Changes in the frequency of benign focal spikes accompany changes in central information processing speed: a prospective 2-year follow-up study. *Epilepsy Behav.* 2015;43:8–15.

8. Gascoigne MB, Smith ML, Barton B, et al. Attention deficits in children with epilepsy: preliminary findings. *Epilepsy Behav.* 2017;67:7–12.

9. Loughman A, Seneviratne U, Bowden SC, D'Souza WJ. Epilepsy beyond seizures: predicting enduring cognitive dysfunction in genetic generalized epilepsies. *Epilepsy Behav.* 2016;62:297–303.

10. Thompson PJ, Duncan JS. Cognitive decline in severe intractable epilepsy. *Epilepsia.* 2005;46(11):1780–1787.

11. Voltzenlogel V, Vignal JP, Hirsch E, Manning L. The influence of seizure frequency on anterograde and remote memory in mesial temporal lobe epilepsy. *Seizure.* 2014;23(9):792–798.

12. Camfield CS, Camfield PR. The adult seizure and social outcomes of children with partial complex seizures. *Brain.* 2013;136(Pt 2):593–600.

13. Selassie AW, Wilson DA, Martz GU, et al. Epilepsy beyond seizure: a population-based study of comorbidities. *Epilepsy Res.* 2014;108(2):305–315.

14. Fazel S, Wolf A, Langstrom N, Newton CR, Lichtenstein P. Premature mortality in epilepsy and the role of psychiatric comorbidity: a total population study. *Lancet.* 2013;382(9905):1646–1654.

15. Schraegle WA, Titus JB. The relationship of seizure focus with depression, anxiety, and health-related quality of life in children and adolescents with epilepsy. *Epilepsy Behav.* 2017;68:115–122.

16. Jones JE, Hermann BP, Barry JJ, et al. Rates and risk factors for suicide, suicidal ideation, and suicide attempts in chronic epilepsy. *Epilepsy Behav.* 2003;4(Suppl 3): S31–38.

17. Hesdorffer DC, Ishihara L, Webb DJ, et al. Occurrence and recurrence of attempted suicide among people with epilepsy. *JAMA Psychiatry.* 2016;73(1):80–86.

18. Alper K, Schwartz KA, Kolts RL, Khan A. Seizure incidence in psychopharmacological clinical trials: an analysis of Food and Drug Administration (FDA) summary basis of approval reports. *Biol Psychiatry.* 2007;62(4):345–354.

19. Foldvary N. Sleep and epilepsy. *Curr Treat Options Neurol.* 2002;4(2):129–135.

20. Malow BA. Sleep and epilepsy. *Neurol Clin.* 2005;23(4):1127–1147.

21. Gibbs FA. Electroencephalography. *Am J Psychiatry.* 1947;103(4):519–522.

22. Touchon J, Baldy-Moulinier M, Billiard M, Besset A, Cadilhac J. Sleep organization and epilepsy. *Epilepsy Res Suppl.* 1991;2:73–81.

23. Crespel A, Baldy-Moulinier M, Coubes P. The relationship between sleep and epilepsy in frontal and temporal lobe epilepsies: practical and physiopathologic considerations. *Epilepsia.* 1998;39(2):150–157.

24. Terzano MG, Mancia D, Salati MR, et al. The cyclic alternating pattern as a physiologic component of normal NREM sleep. *Sleep.* 1985;8(2):137–145.

25. Gigli GL, Placidi F, Diomedi M, et al. Nocturnal sleep and daytime somnolence in untreated patients with temporal lobe epilepsy: changes after treatment with controlled-release carbamazepine. *Epilepsia.* 1997;38(6):696–701.

26. Terzano MG, Parrino L, Spaggiari MC, Barusi R, Simeoni S. Discriminatory effect of cyclic alternating pattern in focal lesional and benign rolandic interictal spikes during sleep. *Epilepsia.* 1991;32(5):616–628.

27. Janz D. The grand mal epilepsies and the sleeping-waking cycle. *Epilepsia.* 1962;3:69–109.

28. Cohen HB, Dement WC. Sleep: suppression of rapid eye movement phase in the cat after electroconvulsive shock. *Science.* 1966;154(3747):396–398.

29. Raol YH, Meti BL. Sleep-wakefulness alterations in amygdala-kindled rats. *Epilepsia.* 1998;39(11):1133–1137.

30. Rondouin G, Baldy-Moulinier M, Passouant P. The influence of hippocampal kindling on sleep organization in cats. Effects of alpha-methylparatyrosine. *Brain Res.* 1980;181(2):413–424.

31. Tanaka T, Naquet R. Kindling effect and sleep organization in cats. *Electroencephalogr Clin Neurophysiol.* 1975;39(5):449–454.

32. White P, Dyken M, Grant P, Jackson L. Electroencephalographic abnormalities during sleep as related to the temporal distribution of seizures. *Epilepsia*. 1962;3:167–174.

33. Mattson RH, Pratt KL, Calverley JR. Electroencephalograms of epileptics following sleep deprivation. *Arch Neurol*. 1965;13(3):310–315.

34. Niedermeyer E, Rocca U. The diagnostic significance of sleep electroencephalograms in temporal lobe epilepsy: a comparison of scalp and depth tracings. *Eur Neurol*. 1972;7(1):119–129.

35. Chabriat H, Danchot J, Michel P, Joire JE, Henry P. Precipitating factors of headache: a prospective study in a national control-matched survey in migraineurs and nonmigraineurs. *Headache*. 1999;39 (5):335–338.

36. Tan JH, Wilder-Smith E, Lim EC, Ong BK. Frequency of provocative factors in epileptic patients admitted for seizures: a prospective study in Singapore. *Seizure*. 2005;14(7):464–469.

37. Ezpeleta D, Garcia-Pena A, Peraita-Adrados R. [Epilepsy and sleep apnea syndrome]. *Rev Neurol*. 1998;26 (151):389–392.

38. Devinsky O, Ehrenberg B, Barthlen GM, Abramson HS, Luciano D. Epilepsy and sleep apnea syndrome. *Neurology*. 1994;44 (11):2060–2064.

39. Wyler AR, Weymuller EA, Jr. Epilepsy complicated by sleep apnea. *Ann Neurol*. 1981;9(4):403–404.

40. Ehrenberg B. Importance of sleep restoration in co-morbid disease: effect of anticonvulsants. *Neurology*. 2000;54(5 Suppl 1):S33–37.

41. Declerck AC, Martens WL, Wauquier A. Evaluation of the effects of antiepileptic drugs on sleep-wakefulness patterns following 1 night total sleep deprivation in epileptic patients. *Neuropsychobiology*. 1985;13(4):201–205.

42. Shouse MN, da Silva AM, Sammaritano M. Circadian rhythm, sleep, and epilepsy. *J Clin Neurophysiol*. 1996;13(1):32–50.

43. Janz D. Epilepsy with grand mal on awakening and sleep-waking cycle. *Clin Neurophysiol*. 2000;111(Suppl 2):S103–110.

44. Oakley CB, Kossoff EH. Migraine and epilepsy in the pediatric population. *Curr Pain Headache Rep*. 2014;18(3):402.

45. Forderreuther S, Henkel A, Noachtar S, Straube A. Headache associated with epileptic seizures: epidemiology and clinical characteristics. *Headache*. 2002;42 (7):649–655.

46. Ludvigsson P, Hesdorffer D, Olafsson E, Kjartansson O, Hauser WA. Migraine with aura is a risk factor for unprovoked seizures in children. *Ann Neurol*. 2006;59 (1):210–213.

47. Ottman R, Lipton RB. Comorbidity of migraine and epilepsy. *Neurology*. 1994;44 (11):2105–2110.

48. Kelley SA, Hartman AL, Kossoff EH. Comorbidity of migraine in children presenting with epilepsy to a tertiary care center. *Neurology*. 2012;79(5):468–473.

49. Cai S, Hamiwka LD, Wirrell EC. Peri-ictal headache in children: prevalence and character. *Pediatr Neurol*. 2008;39(2):91–96.

50. Rogawski MA. Common pathophysiologic mechanisms in migraine and epilepsy. *Arch Neurol*. 2008;65(6):709–714.

51. Ryan DP, Ptacek LJ. Episodic neurological channelopathies. *Neuron*. 2010;68 (2):282–292.

52. Yorns WR, Jr., Hardison HH. Mitochondrial dysfunction in migraine. *Semin Pediatr Neurol*. 2013;20(3):188–193.

53. Valmadrid C, Voorhees C, Litt B, Schneyer CR. Practice patterns of neurologists regarding bone and mineral effects of antiepileptic drug therapy. *Arch Neurol*. 2001;58(9):1369–1374.

54. Vestergaard P. Epilepsy, osteoporosis and fracture risk – a meta-analysis. *Acta Neurol Scand*. 2005;112(5):277–286.

55. Tekgul H, Serdaroglu G, Huseyinov A, Gokben S. Bone mineral status in pediatric outpatients on antiepileptic drug monotherapy. *J Child Neurol*. 2006;21 (5):411–414.

56. Ensrud KE, Walczak TS, Blackwell TL, et al. Antiepileptic drug use and rates of hip bone loss in older men: a prospective study. *Neurology*. 2008;71(10):723–730.

57. Ensrud KE, Walczak TS, Blackwell T, et al. Antiepileptic drug use increases rates of bone loss in older women: a prospective study. *Neurology*. 2004;62(11):2051–2057.

58. Sheth RD, Binkley N, Hermann BP. Progressive bone deficit in epilepsy. *Neurology*. 2008;70(3):170–176.

59. Sheth RD, Binkley N, Hermann BP. Gender differences in bone mineral density in epilepsy. *Epilepsia*. 2008;49(1):125–131.

60. El-Hajj Fuleihan G, Dib L, Yamout B, Sawaya R, Mikati MA. Predictors of bone density in ambulatory patients on antiepileptic drugs. *Bone*. 2008;43(1):149–155.

61. Vestergaard P. Changes in bone turnover, bone mineral and fracture risk induced by drugs used to treat epilepsy. *Curr Drug Saf*. 2008;3(3):168–172.

62. Pack AM, Walczak TS. Bone health in women with epilepsy: clinical features and potential mechanisms. *Int Rev Neurobiol*. 2008;83:305–328.

63. Timperlake RW, Cook SD, Thomas KA, et al. Effects of anticonvulsant drug therapy on bone mineral density in a pediatric population. *J Pediatr Orthop*. 1988;8(4):467–470.

64. Farhat G, Yamout B, Mikati MA, et al. Effect of antiepileptic drugs on bone density in ambulatory patients. *Neurology*. 2002;58(9):1348–1353.

65. Chou IJ, Lin KL, Wang HS, Wang CJ. Evaluation of bone mineral density in children receiving carbamazepine or valproate monotherapy. *Acta Paediatr Taiwan*. 2007;48(6):317–322.

66. Albaghdadi O, Alhalabi MS, Alourfi Z, Youssef LA. Bone health and vitamin D status in young epilepsy patients on valproate monotherapy. *Clin Neurol Neurosurg*. 2016;146:52–56.

67. Heaney RP. Vitamin D: criteria for safety and efficacy. *Nutr Rev*. 2008;66(10 Suppl 2):S178–181.

68. Drezner MK. Treatment of anticonvulsant drug-induced bone disease. *Epilepsy Behav*. 2004;5(Suppl 2):S41–47.

69. Shankar R, Cox D, Jalihal V, et al. Sudden unexpected death in epilepsy (SUDEP): development of a safety checklist. *Seizure*. 2013;22(10):812–817.

70. Nashef L, Sander JW. Sudden unexpected deaths in epilepsy – where are we now? *Seizure*. 1996;5(3):235–238.

71. Thurman DJ, Hesdorffer DC, French JA. Sudden unexpected death in epilepsy: assessing the public health burden. *Epilepsia*. 2014;55(10):1479–1485.

72. Nashef L. Sudden unexpected death in epilepsy: terminology and definitions. *Epilepsia*. 1997;38(11 Suppl):S6–8.

73. Nashef L, So EL, Ryvlin P, Tomson T. Unifying the definitions of sudden unexpected death in epilepsy. *Epilepsia*. 2012;53(2):227–233.

74. Holst AG, Winkel BG, Risgaard B, et al. Epilepsy and risk of death and sudden unexpected death in the young: a nationwide study. *Epilepsia*. 2013;54(9):1613–1620.

75. Langan Y, Nashef L, Sander JW. Case-control study of SUDEP. *Neurology*. 2005;64(7):1131–1133.

76. Hesdorffer DC, Tomson T, Benn E, et al. Do antiepileptic drugs or generalized tonic-clonic seizure frequency increase SUDEP risk?: a combined analysis. *Epilepsia*. 2012;53(2):249–252.

77. Nilsson L, Farahmand BY, Persson PG, Thiblin I, Tomson T. Risk factors for sudden unexpected death in epilepsy: a case-control study. *Lancet*. 1999;353(9156):888–893.

78. Berg AT, Nickels K, Wirrell EC, et al. Mortality risks in new-onset childhood epilepsy. *Pediatrics*. 2013;132(1):124–131.

79. Devinsky O. Sudden, unexpected death in epilepsy. *N Engl J Med*. 2011;365(19):1801–1811.

80. Yang YJ, Yao X, Guo J, et al. Interstitial deletion 5q14.3q21.3 associated with lethal epilepsy. *Am J Med Genet A*. 2015;167A(4):866–871.

81. Veeramah KR, O'Brien JE, Meisler MH, et al. De novo pathogenic SCN8A mutation identified by whole-genome sequencing of a family quartet affected by infantile epileptic encephalopathy and SUDEP. *Am J Hum Genet*. 2012;90(3):502–510.

82. Shannon P, Pennacchio LA, Houseweart MK, Minassian BA, Myers RM. Neuropathological changes in a mouse model of progressive myoclonus epilepsy: cystatin B deficiency and Unverricht-Lundborg disease. *J Neuropathol Exp Neurol*. 2002;61(12):1085–1091.

83. Glasscock E. Genomic biomarkers of SUDEP in brain and heart. *Epilepsy Behav*. 2014;38:172–179.

84. Chyou JY, Friedman D, Cerrone M, et al. Electrocardiographic features of sudden unexpected death in epilepsy. *Epilepsia*. 2016;57(7):e135–139.

85. Surges R, Adjei P, Kallis C, et al. Pathologic cardiac repolarization in pharmacoresistant epilepsy and its potential role in sudden unexpected death in epilepsy: a case-control study. *Epilepsia*. 2010;51 (2):233–242.

86. Brotherstone R, Blackhall B, McLellan A. Lengthening of corrected QT during epileptic seizures. *Epilepsia*. 2010;51 (2):221–232.

87. Bagnall RD, Crompton DE, Petrovski S, et al. Exome-based analysis of cardiac arrhythmia, respiratory control, and epilepsy genes in sudden unexpected death in epilepsy. *Ann Neurol*. 2016;79 (4):522–534.

88. Hajek MA, Buchanan GF. Influence of vigilance state on physiological consequences of seizures and seizure-induced death in mice. *J Neurophysiol*. 2016;115(5):2286–2293.

89. Buchanan GF, Murray NM, Hajek MA, Richerson GB. Serotonin neurones have anti-convulsant effects and reduce seizure-induced mortality. *J Physiol*. 2014;592 (19):4395–4410.

90. Ryvlin P, Nashef L, Lhatoo SD, et al. Incidence and mechanisms of cardiorespiratory arrests in epilepsy monitoring units (MORTEMUS): a retrospective study. *Lancet Neurol*. 2013;12 (10):966–977.

91. Tsai CY, Chan JY, Hsu KS, Chang AY, Chan SH. Brain-derived neurotrophic factor ameliorates brain stem cardiovascular dysregulation during experimental temporal lobe status epilepticus. *PLoS One*. 2012;7(3):e33527.

92. Zhan Q, Buchanan GF, Motelow JE, et al. Impaired serotonergic brainstem function during and after seizures. *J Neurosci*. 2016;36(9):2711–2722.

93. Shen HY, Li T, Boison D. A novel mouse model for sudden unexpected death in epilepsy (SUDEP): role of impaired adenosine clearance. *Epilepsia*. 2010;51 (3):465–468.

94. P-Codrea Tigaran S, Dalager-Pedersen S, Baandrup U, Dam M, Vesterby-Charles A. Sudden unexpected death in epilepsy: is death by seizures a cardiac disease? *Am J Forensic Med Pathol*. 2005;26 (2):99–105.

95. Thom M, Michalak Z, Wright G, et al. Audit of practice in sudden unexpected death in epilepsy (SUDEP) post mortems and neuropathological findings. *Neuropathol Appl Neurobiol*. 2016;42 (5):463–476.

96. Rugg-Gunn F, Duncan J, Hjalgrim H, Seyal M, Bateman L. From unwitnessed fatality to witnessed rescue: Nonpharmacologic interventions in sudden unexpected death in epilepsy. *Epilepsia*. 2016;57 (Suppl 1):26–34.

97. Friedman D, Donner EJ, Stephens D, Wright C, Devinsky O. Sudden unexpected death in epilepsy: knowledge and experience among U.S. and Canadian neurologists. *Epilepsy Behav*. 2014;35:13–18.

98. Miller WR, Young N, Friedman D, Buelow JM, Devinsky O. Discussing sudden unexpected death in epilepsy (SUDEP) with patients: practices of health-care providers. *Epilepsy Behav*. 2014;32:38–41.

System-Based Issues in Epilepsy

Yeeck Sim and David M. Labiner

26.1 Introduction

Individuals with epilepsy, and their family and friends, are impacted by system-based barriers arising from public policies, affecting their quality of lives. Policies on driving, education, employment, ethics, and research are widespread, and often lead to unwarranted complications.

26.2 Driving

Driving has always been a difficult topic for individuals with epilepsy, as at least one study has shown that they may have an increased risk for fatal crashes if no limitations are imposed.[1] In the United States, each state has different laws regarding mandatory reporting of individuals with epilepsy, as well as duration of seizure freedom required prior to resuming driving following a seizure.

Only six states still require mandatory physician reporting (California, Delaware, Nevada, New Jersey, Oregon, and Pennsylvania) at the time of this writing, while the remaining states support "good faith" immunity for reporting where the patient is responsible for notifying the motor vehicle division.[2] States require anywhere from 3 to 12 months of seizure freedom before an individual may resume driving. The physician's role is typically to provide medical data to the State to support the resumption of driving whereas the ultimate decision lies with the State. This is an improvement from the total prohibition for individuals with epilepsy from driving that existed prior to the 1940s. Model legislation that balances public safety with the need for transport has been proposed by the American Academy of Neurology, American Epilepsy Society, and the Epilepsy Foundation.[3]

Driving regulations for individuals with epilepsy continue to improve as more research supports driving for individuals with controlled epilepsy. Fatal accidents due to seizures are far less likely than those due to alcohol (0.2% versus 30%).[4] In fact, the vast majority of accidents involving individuals with epilepsy are not seizure-related.[4] An Arizona study compared car accidents before and after a decrease in mandatory seizure-free duration from 12 months to 3 months and found no significant increase in crashes.[5] Conversely, delaying the resumption of driving for the individual has been found to be detrimental to quality of life, with negative effects on socialization.[6]

Even among states that go by "good faith" immunity, physicians may be liable should adverse events occur associated with a patient with epilepsy driving. Hence, the physician should discuss, and document the discussion, with patients the details of the laws of the local jurisdiction regarding seizures and driving. The discussion should include informing the patients that they may be liable if they drive against medical advice and suffer from a seizure that causes an adverse event.

26.3 Education

Although most children with epilepsy are able to function normally throughout their school years, children with uncontrolled epilepsy may encounter difficulties within the education system and are more likely not to graduate high school.[7] It is important for physicians and teachers to identify these barriers, as mandated by the United States Department of Education through the Individuals with Disabilities Education Act (IDEA). The Act protects individuals with disabilities by ensuring that free public education is provided without restrictions in access. The physician's role is to provide such information to the family, as well to assist in designing an individual education program (IEP) tailor-made for the child and the school.[8] It is important that the IEP is designed to have the child's best educational interests in mind. Parents always have the right to contest the school's educational program in a court of law.

Students and parents of children with epilepsy should seek support online as there are available resources to utilize. The Epilepsy Foundation provides free courses for school personnel that trains staff to recognize seizures, how to apply first aid during seizures, and how to assist with academic support for students with seizures and epilepsy. Social support is encouraged and helps staff to recognize bullying and identify social stigmas that are often experienced by students with seizures.[9]

26.4 Employment

It is well understood that people with epilepsy have numerous difficulties with employment. Individuals with complicated epilepsy are disadvantaged in the job market before the interviewing process even begins, as they are less likely to have graduated high school, with even fewer having a college or higher degree.[7] They also may endure hardships with transportation to and from the workplace, as fewer individuals with epilepsy have active driver licenses, feel uncomfortable with driving, or are not allowed to drive.[10] Once actually employed, psychosocial issues such as self-perceived stigma, family overprotection, and coping with work stressors can hinder the individual's work performance. Additionally, the types of seizure the individual has may also play a role, with generalized seizures having more of a significant impact.[11]

Individuals with well-controlled epilepsy have more work opportunities compared to those with uncontrolled epilepsy.[10] Less stigma, depression, restrictions on driving, and improved workplace quality of life are also positive outcomes of well-controlled epilepsy.[10] For individuals with epilepsy who suffer from discrimination in the workplace, school, or community life, the Epilepsy Foundation has a legal defense fund to assist with fighting discriminatory practices.[12]

The clinician plays a critical role in educating individuals with uncontrolled epilepsy with regards to workplace safety. The American Epilepsy Society provides a comprehensive guide on worksite safety.[13] There the clinician may find safety considerations for the patient, medical documentation often sought by employees including sample responses, and common questions from both the employer and employee. Individuals with epilepsy unable to overcome these workplace barriers are not without assistance, however, as the Americans with Disability Act (ADA) provides them protections (Section 26.5).

26.5 The Americans with Disability Act

The ADA was modeled after the Rehabilitation Act of 1973, which was enacted to prohibit discrimination on the basis of disability in programs conducted by federal agencies, in programs receiving federal financial assistance, in federal employment, and in the employment practices of federal contractors.[14] The ADA was enacted in 1990 to expand the scope of provisions to not only protect government-employed individuals, but to assist all persons with disability regarding employment, state and local government activities (including education), public accommodations, commercial facilities, transportation, and telecommunications. It is important to note, however, that not all persons with epilepsy qualify as disabled under the ADA.

Disability as defined by the ADA describes an individual with a physical or mental impairment that substantially limits one or more major life activities, who has a history or record of such impairment, or a person who is perceived by others as having such impairment. Although the ADA does not specifically name all of the impairments covered, epilepsy was a covered entity in the Rehabilitation Act of 1973. Major life activities include, but are not limited to, caring for oneself, performing manual tasks, seeing, hearing, eating, sleeping, walking, learning, communicating, and working. Major bodily functions are also regarded as life activities, including functions of brain and neurological systems. The ADA further provides that an impairment that is episodic or in remission (much like epilepsy) is a disability if it would substantially limit a major life activity when active. The impairment itself, however, must exceed an expected duration of 6 months. The determination of whether an impairment limits a major life activity should be made without regard to ameliorative effects, such as antiepileptic medications, surgery, diet, or other adaptive neurological modifications such as neuromodulatory treatments.[14]

After the ADA was enacted, numerous issues arose, such as inconsistencies regarding the definition of handicapped individuals between the ADA and Rehabilitation Act of 1973, as well as court rulings that substantially limited the scope of protection originally sought by the ADA. Thus, the ADA was amended in 2008 to fulfill the original intent of the legislation by providing a clear and comprehensive mandate addressing discrimination and by reinstating a broad scope of protection.

The ADA provides three major accommodations for qualified individuals with disability: employment, public transportation and government activities, and public accommodations. The first title, within the law, regarding employment has the greatest impact on individuals with epilepsy. It requires employers with 15 or more employees to provide the same employment opportunities to individuals with disabilities as to those without. These opportunities include prohibiting discrimination in recruitment, hiring, promotions, training, pay, and social activities. For example, during the hiring process, employers are not allowed to ask questions regarding an applicant's disability, prior to making a job offer. This allows the individual with disability the freedom to not disclose their disability prior to accepting the job offer. If certain tests are required for recruitment such as drug screening, it must be applied to all applicants.

Once employed, individuals with disabilities are expected to function at their job at the same level of those without disability. Reasonable accommodations should be provided to assist the individual with the disability to perform the essential functions of the job, as long as it does not create undue hardships for the employer. A federally funded resource regarding appropriate accommodations is available by calling 1-800-ADA-WORK (1-800-232-9675).

Providers should encourage these reasonable accommodations for patients with epilepsy, such as minimizing sleep disturbances within the schedule (i.e., graveyard shifts), removing flashing lights from the workplace, minimizing possibly dangerous situations such as climbing, operating dangerous equipment, and training coworkers about seizure precautions and first aid administration.

26.6 Research Funding

Although seizures are the fourth most common neurological disorder, epilepsy research is persistently underfunded by the National Institutes of Health (NIH) compared to other prevalent neurologic disorders.[15] The scarcity in research funds and allocation of resources is seen both locally and globally. Although the global prevalence increases as epilepsy becomes acknowledged as a medical issue and is now better diagnosed in Third World countries, disparity in research funding continues.[16] Additionally pharmaceutical companies whose studies are often not considered academic, only address issues directly related to therapy.[17] The Center for Disease Control and Prevention also supports epilepsy research and focuses on epidemiologic studies, but with a much smaller budget than the NIH. Other organizations target varying research topics such as the American Epilepsy Society, which focuses on basic and clinical studies, CURE (Citizens United for Research in Epilepsy), which focuses on treatment and public awareness, NINDS (National Institute of Neurological Disorders and Stroke), which focuses on biomedical studies, and the Epilepsy Foundation, which focuses on new frontiers in epilepsy research. There are ongoing measures to bring awareness of epilepsy and its disease burden to the public. We believe that it is the physician's responsibility, as well as others in the epilepsy community, to continue advocating for research support to continue advancing the field.

26.7 Medical Ethics and Epilepsy

While the routine treatment of epilepsy does not typically raise ethical dilemmas, treatment of refractory status epilepticus is one example that does, specifically regarding whether or not to withdraw care. Most institutions have a protocol for treating status epilepticus. However, there is no consensus on the treatment of status epilepticus that does not respond to the prescribed protocol. Different neurologists have varying approaches to this problem. Inasmuch as this is often medically futile, a protocol should be in place to determine when it is appropriate to withdraw care, following institutional guidelines and typically in consultation with a bioethics committee.

26.8 Conclusion

There are multiple systemic barriers to optimizing care for individuals with epilepsy. However, there are many tools, legal and advocacy-based, that allow physicians to help enhance the quality of life for their patients. It is important for the physician to not only know the rules in their state that may affect their patients (regarding driving, employment, education, etc.) but to also have a basic understanding of what tools are available to allow patients to best function within the system. They should also be aware of support and educational services provided by patient advocacy groups, such as the Epilepsy Foundation. By utilizing the resources available, healthcare providers can assist their patients with epilepsy in achieving the best quality of life possible.

References

1. Sheth SG, Krauss G, Krumholz A, Li G. Mortality in epilepsy: driving fatalities vs other causes of death in patients with epilepsy. *Neurology*. 2004;63(6):1002–1007.

2. Epilepsy Foundation. State driving laws database. http://www.epilepsy.com/driving-laws. Accessed April 3, 2019.

3. American Academy of Neurology, American Epilepsy Society, Epilepsy Foundation of America. Consensus statements, sample statutory provisions, and model regulations regarding driver licensing and epilepsy. *Epilepsia*. 1994;35 (3):696–705.

4. Krumholz A. Driving issues in epilepsy: past, present, and future. *Epilepsy Curr*. 2009;9(2):31–35.

5. Drazkowski JF, Fisher RS, Sirven JI, et al. Seizure-related motor vehicle crashes in Arizona before and after reducing the driving restriction from 12 to 3 months. *Mayo Clin Proc*. 2003;78(7):819–825.

6. Myers L, Lancman M, Laban-Grant O, Lancman M, Jones J. Socialization characteristics in persons with epilepsy. *Epilepsy Behav*. 2017;72:99–107.

7. Baca CB, Barry F, Vickrey BG, Caplan R, Berg AT. Social outcomes of young adults with childhood-onset epilepsy: a case-sibling-control study. *Epilepsia*. 2017;58 (5):781–791.

8. Office of Special Education Programs, Office of Special Education and Rehabilitative Services, US Department of Education. Individuals with Disability Education Act. https://sites.ed.gov/idea/. Accessed April 3, 2019.

9. Epilepsy Foundation. Seizure training for school personnel. https://www.epilepsy.com/living-epilepsy/our-training-and-education/seizure-training-school-personnel. Accessed April 3, 2019.

10. Josephson CB, Patten SB, Bulloch A, et al. The impact of seizures on epilepsy outcomes: a national, community-based survey. *Epilepsia*. 2017;58(5):764–771.

11. Wo MC, Lim KS, Choo WY, Tan CT. Factors affecting the employability in people with epilepsy. *Epilepsy Res*. 2016;128:6–11.

12. Epilepsy Foundation. Legal help. https://www.epilepsy.com/living-epilepsy/legal-help. Accessed April 3, 2019.

13. Garcia PA. Physician's guide to worksite safety. https://www.aesnet.org/clinical_resources/practice_tools/employment_resources/physicians_guide_to_work_site_safety. Accessed April 3, 2019.

14. Disability Rights Section, Civil Rights Division, US Department of Justice. A guide to disability rights laws. https://www.ada.gov/cguide.htm. Accessed April 3, 2019.

15. Meador KJ, French J, Loring DW, Pennell PB. Disparities in NIH funding for epilepsy research. *Neurology*. 2011;77 (13):1305–1307.

16. Chin JH. The global fund for epilepsy: a proposal. *Neurology*. 2013;80(8): 754–755.

17. Privitera M. Large clinical trials in epilepsy: funding by the NIH versus pharmaceutical industry. *Epilepsy Res*. 2006;68(1):52–56.

Index